53. 00

A Glossary of
Anesthesia and
Related Terminology

Second E

D1380744

Sanford L. Klein

A Glossary of Anesthesia and Related Terminology

Second Edition

With 228 Illustrations

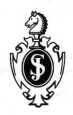

Springer-Verlag

New York   Berlin   Heidelberg   London   Paris
Tokyo   Hong Kong   Barcelona   Budapest

Sanford L. Klein, DDS, MD
Professor and Chairman
Department of Anesthesia
University of Medicine and Dentistry of New Jersey
Robert Wood Johnson Medical School
New Brunswick, NJ 08903-0019 USA

The first edition was published by Medical Examination Publishing Co., Inc.

Library of Congress Cataloging-in-Publication Data

Klein, Sanford L.
    A glossary of anesthesia and related terminology / Sanford L. Klein—2nd ed.
      p.   cm.
    Includes bibliographical references.
    ISBN 0-387-97831-3.—ISBN 3-540-97831-3
    1. Anesthesia—Dictionaries. 2. Anesthesia—Terminology. I. Title.
    [DNLM: 1. Anesthesia—terminology. WO 213 K64q]
    RD78.5.K54   1992
    617.9'6'03—dc20
    DNLM/DLC
    for Library of Congress   92-2223

Printed on acid-free paper.

Production managed by Christin R. Ciresi; manufacturing supervised by Jacqui Ashri.
Typeset by Princeton Editorial Associates, Princeton, NJ.
Printed and bound by Edwards Brothers Inc., Ann Arbor, MI.
Printed in the United States of America.

9 8 7 6 5 4 3 2 1

ISBN 0-387-97831-3 Springer-Verlag New York Berlin Heidelberg
ISBN 3-540-97831-3 Springer-Verlag Berlin Heidelberg New York

This book is dedicated in all humility to Dr. William F. Harrigan, my first chief, who not only rescued me from polishing Pontiacs in Passaic, but who also set an example for achievement that I continue to admire. This book is also dedicated to Dr. Harry Wollman, without whose many kindnesses and, in some instances, deliberate lapses of attention, I could not be where I am today.

Preface to the Second Edition

The second edition of this text catches the specialty of anesthesia at what will probably prove to be the apex of its influence and recognition amongst the specialties of medicine. The scientific basis of the specialty is becoming increasingly well delineated. Anesthesiologists have established themselves in local, regional, and national forums as spokespersons not only for the specialty, but also for medicine in general. And the specialty at last may be emerging from the stereotype of a faceless, inarticulate, shy and retiring figure, whose outstanding characteristic was the cloying odor of diethel ether!

Technology has moved into the specialty on seven league boots. Just as an example, the basic design of the anesthesia machine was stable between the early 1950s and certainly the late 1970s. Suddenly, in the blink of an eye, our anesthesia machines are becoming intelligent, are utilizing heads-up displays, and are becoming more and more capable of writing the anesthesia record. Monitoring standards for anesthesia have burgeoned to the point that almost every aspect of the specialty is impinged upon by some rule and some "thou will or thou will not." The importation and creation of terminology is exploding. In fact, one of the problems in updating this book was deciding when to stop.

The author hopes that the goal of creating a snapshot in time through definitions of commonly used words and phrases has been achieved. Furthermore, I hope this book will be very helpful to new and old practitioners of the specialty by meeting its primary goal of providing a common language and a common understanding of language in the specialty without which clear discourse is impossible.

In conclusion, I would like to thank Ms. Lenore Stewart, who was of immense help with her perseverance, her artistry, and her editing and assembling skills in making this new edition a real living and breathing entity, and the other members of my department, from the residents to the senior staff, who contributed their time and efforts in reviewing and critiquing the various elements of this text.

A

AAA:

See Anesthesia Administrative Assembly.

AANA:

See American Association of Nurse Anesthetists.

AAPD:

See Association of Anesthesiology Program Directors.

ABA:

See American Board of Anesthesiology.

Abandonment:

Refusal, in a medicolegal context, on the part of a physician or dentist to continue caring for a patient without the patient's consent.

Abdominal Electrocardiography:

Obstetric technique for determining the fetal electrocardiogram by the application of electrodes to the mother's abdominal wall. Difficulty is encountered owing to electrical interference from the maternal electrocardiogram and abdominal wall musculature and gross interference from fetal movement.

Abdominal Nerve Syndrome:

See Abdominal wall pain.

Abdominal Wall Pain, Abdominal Nerve Syndrome:

Little understood cause of chronic abdominal pain, this syndrome is due to entrapment of the intercostal nerves as they emerge through the rectus sheath. The pain is characterized as sharp or burning and can persist for a long time.

Abducens:

Sixth cranial nerve and the most likely to be affected by a drop in cerebrospinal fluid pressure after a spinal anesthetic. Paralysis of the abducens causes diplopia. *See* Cranial nerves.

Ablation:

Process of removing material from the surface of an object, usually by vaporization or decomposition. Ablation may also mean complete mechanical destruction; cryosurgery is used for total ablation of a tumor. Ablation-type heat shielding is used on the nose cones of rockets returning to earth.

Abort:

Abrupt termination of an ongoing event.

ABS Plastic:

Class of plastics that is identified as belonging to the acrylonitrile-butadiene-styrene group. They are usually of good rigidity, high impact strength, and fair hardness over a wide temperature range. ABS is a typical plastic used in helmets, luggage, and machine parts, where abrasion resistance is not a prerequisite.

Absolute Zero:

Temperature that, according to theory, is the lowest physically possible. This temperature has been closely approached but never reached in practice. In units it is zero Kelvin (°K), minus 273.15 degrees Celsius (°C), and minus 459.67 degrees Fahrenheit (°F).

Absorbent Channeling:

Phenomenon occurring in poorly packed absorbent canisters that can severely affect the proper absorption of CO_2. The cross-sectional area of absorbent to which the gas stream is exposed is reduced dramatically by small passageways, or channels that course through the absorbent from one end to the other, bypassing the bulk of active absorbent. It can lead to a relatively rapid yet insidious buildup of CO_2 in the gas mixture the patient breathes.

Absorber:

See Carbon dioxide absorption.

Absorber Bypass:

Fitting that allows exhaled gases to be routed around the CO_2 absorber material in the circle system. Dangerous if not understood (allows for CO_2 rebreathing). *See* Circle system.

Absorption:

Process by which a substance becomes available to the circulating fluids of the body. The rate of absorption depends on the physical characteristics of the substances being absorbed and the nature of the barriers and membranes between the site of initial deposit and the circulation.

Absorption Atelectasis:

Phenomenon that occurs when the air passageway to the alveolus is blocked. If the patient has been breathing air, it can be assumed that at the instant of blockage the PAO_2 is approximately 100 mm Hg, $PACO_2$ is approximately 40 mm Hg, alveolar pressure of nitrogen is 573 mm Hg, and partial pressure of water vapor is 47 mm Hg. In capillary blood flowing past the alveolus, the partial pressure of nitrogen and water vapor are the same; however, PO_2 is about 40 mm Hg and PCO_2 is about 45 mm Hg. On balance, this gives a net positive pressure to the alveolus, which loses gas to the pulmonary blood and gradually collapses. This gradual collapse is splinted by nitrogen which shifts slowly to the alveolus from the blood flowing past it, tending to keep the alveolus open. In any situation where alveolar O_2 has been augmented to take the place of alveolar nitrogen, absorption atelectasis occurs more quickly because the partial pressure difference between alveolar O_2 and capillary O_2 is much greater. In fact, when a healthy individual breathes 100% O_2, the PAO_2 approaches 668 mm Hg, $PACO_2$ is 45 mm Hg, and water vapor is 47 mm Hg. *See* Atelectasis.

Absorption Indicator:

Any of a number of chemicals added to CO_2 absorption granules to demonstrate progressive diminution of absorptive capacity. A commonly used indicator is the chemical ethyl violet. As absorption capacity decreases, this indicator changes from white to purple. The deeper the purple, the less absorption capacity is available. Ethyl violet has a critical pH (the pH at which the color changes) of 10.3. Absorption indicators are only qualitatively accurate; a purple granule may turn white again when exposed to air owing to the limited regeneration capacity of some absorbents. Any absorption chamber that is color-tinged should be refilled. *See* Carbon dioxide absorption.

Abusive Legal Process (Barratry):

Use of the courts to harass an individual. Along with defamation, it is grounds for a countersuit in patient-initiated malpractice action.

Accelerations:

See Fetal monitor.

Accumulation:

Phenomenon resulting from repeated drug administrations that are spaced so closely together that neither metabolism nor excretion is fast enough to prevent the drug from increasing in concentration in the body. For example, succinylcholine is a drug that undergoes rapid metabolism in the plasma. However, a fast-running intravenous infusion of succinylcholine can actually cause the plasma concentration of succinylcholine to rise continuously until the infusion is stopped or a plateau is reached (based on an equilibrium between administration and metabolism).

Accumulator:

Mildly obsolescent alternative to 'reservoir tank,' 'reservoir,' or 'storage container.'

Accuracy:

Measurement or, when applied to laboratory equipment, specification of the freedom from error of a device. Most often it is expressed as a percentage over a particular range. For example, a 2% error on a scale of 100, in whole numbers, means that '98' may be registered on the machine as 96, 97, 98, 99, or 100, and the machine is still operating within design limits. *See* Precision.

ACD:

See Acid citrate dextrose, Blood storage, Blood types, CPD blood preservation.

Acebutolol:

Cardio-selective beta-blocker that has intrinsic sympathomimetic effect and membrane stabilizing effect. *See* Intrinsic sympathomimetic activity; Membrane stabilizing activity.

Acetaminophen (Tylenol):

Effective alternate drug to the salicylates when analgesic and antipyretic actions are needed. Acetaminophen is a breakdown product of phenacetin. It is well tolerated by the gastrointestinal tract, but overdosage may cause severe hepatic or renal damage or death.

Acetazolamide (Diamox):

Drug that inhibits the enzyme carbonic anhydrase. By inhibiting this enzyme, acetazolamide prevents the combination of H_2O and CO_2 from forming carbonic acid, which then dissociates into hydrogen ion and bicarbonate. It functions as a diuretic and mild antihypertensive agent. The drug at times has found controversial use as a preanesthetic agent for open eye injuries, as it is known to decrease intraocular pressure. Acetazolamide interferes with the CO_2 transport mechanism and may, at least transiently, give rise to increased CO_2 tension in the peripheral tissues and decreased CO_2 tension in the pulmonary alveoli.

Acetylation:

Form of drug metabolism in which an acetyl group, $COCH_3$, is added to a drug or other pharmacologically active compound to change its reactivity.

Acetylcholine (ACh):

Neurotransmitter substance released at autonomic nerve endings by cholinergic neurons. Synthesis of ACh is controlled by the enzyme choline acetyltransferase, which mediates transfer of an acetyl group from acetyl coenzyme A to choline. Following release at cholinergic nerve endings, ACh is rapidly hydrolyzed and inactivated by the enzyme acetylcholinesterase. Acetylcholine produces peripheral vasodilation (flushing of the face, increased skin temperature); stimulates secretion from exocrine glands (sweating, salivation, tearing); causes bronchoconstriction, decreased heart rate, and pupillary constriction; and stimulates gastrointestinal smooth muscle (peristalsis), defecation, and urination. *See* Neuromuscular blocking agent, Succinylcholine.

$$(CH_3)_3N^+-CH_2-CH_2-O-\overset{\overset{\textstyle O}{\|}}{C}-CH_3$$

Acetylcholine (ACh).

Acetylcholine Receptor Antibody:

See Anti AChR antibodies.

Acetylcholinesterase:

Cholinesterase enzyme found in red blood cells and nerve terminals that is responsible for the hydrolysis of acetylcholine to choline and acetic acid. Nerve terminal acetylcholinesterase is usually referred to as true cholinesterase. It is also found in the placenta, where its function is unknown. *See* Pseudocholinesterase.

Acetylene (C_2H_2):

Colorless gas with a distinct odor, that can explode spontaneously when compressed at room temperature. Its primary use is for welding and cutting metals with flame. It is 92.3% carbon and can therefore be considered nearly gaseous carbon; mixed with O_2 it can reach a torch tip temperature of 3500°F. Employed as a general anesthetic earlier in the twentieth century, acetylene was discontinued because of its combustibility and because better anesthetics were developed.

Acetylsalicylic Acid (Aspirin):

One of a series of salicylates that is usually taken orally as an analgesic, an antipyretic, or an antiinflammatory agent. In small doses, it also causes inhibition of platelet aggregation and prolongation of bleeding time; it is therefore a significant preoperative drug.

ACh:

See Acetylcholine.

Acid:

Substance that, according to the Bronsted-Lowry definition, tends to dissociate and release hydrogen ions (H^+) when in solution. The substance itself may be either positively or negatively charged or neutral.

Acid-Base Balance:

General term for the way in which the body maintains its hydrogen ion concentration (pH) despite the constant production of cationic end products by metabolic processes. The acid-base status is ensured in three major ways: (1) maintenance of a large buffering capacity, (2) manipulation of the volatile acid (carbonic acid), and (3) elimination of excess

Acid-Base Balance: Acid-base normal values.

	Average	Range
Hemoglobin		12.5 - 16.0 gm%
pH arterial	7.4	7.35 - 7.45
PCO_2	40 mm Hg	34 - 45 mm Hg
Total CO_2 (plasma)	28 mmol	23 - 33 mmol
Bicarbonate (plasma)	24 mEq	22.8 - 27.5 mEq/L
Buffer base (whole blood)		43 - 47 mEq/L

acid or base (over a period of a few days) by the kidneys. *See* Table. *See* Acidemia; Alkalemia; Buffer; Buffer base; Carbon dioxide transport in blood; Henderson-Hasselbalch equation; Metabolic acidosis; Metabolic alkalosis.

Acid-Base Compensation:

Adaptive response made by the body to adjust to a primary disturbance in acid-base equilibrium. A primary disturbance is a change from normal caused by a nonphysiologic or pathologic process that precedes any body adaptation to the disturbance. The initial rapid response is due to changes in ventilation that alter $PaCO_2$ (the secondary disturbance) so as to return the hydrogen ion concentration to normal. For example, in the patient with metabolic acidosis, ventilation increases allowing CO_2 to be exhaled and arterial pH to return to normal. The slower response, completed in a number of days, occurs when the kidney either excretes more acid or conserves more bicarbonate to oppose the primary disorder. *See* Acid-base balance; Henderson-Hasselbalch equation; Metabolic acidosis; Metabolic alkalosis.

Acid-Citrate-Dextrose (ACD):

See Blood storage; Blood types; CPD blood preservation.

Acid-Citrate-Dextrose Anticoagulant:

See Blood storage; Blood types; CPD blood preservation.

Acidemia:

Condition existing when the arterial blood pH is less than 7.35 or hydrogen ion concentration is above the normal range of 35–45 nEq/L.

Acidosis:

Physiologic condition that would cause acidemia (pH < 7.35) if not compensated by respiratory or metabolic changes. *See* Acid-base balance; Metabolic acidosis; Respiratory acidosis.

Acquired Immunodeficiency Syndrome:

See AIDS.

Acrylic Cement:

See Methyl methacrylate.

ACT:

See Activated clotting time.

Action Potential (Spike Potential):

Change in the electric state of a nerve membrane (the critical part of nerve impulse transmission). During the action potential, the polarity of the inside of the nerve membrane (relative to the outside) changes from approximately minus 60 mV to approximately +40 mV because of an influx of sodium ions. The electrical change of the membrane from

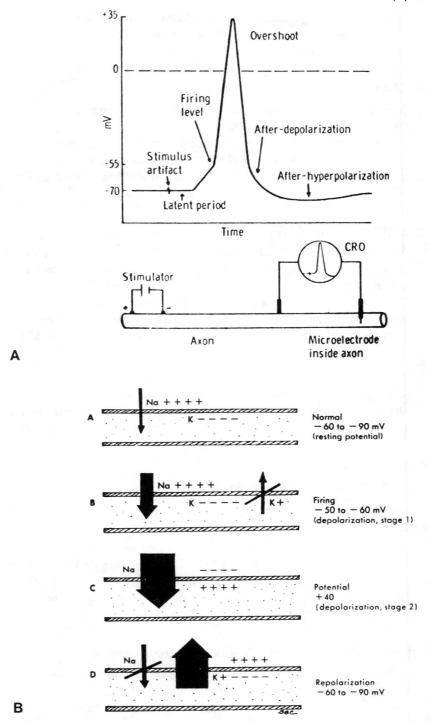

Action Potential: (A) Recorded with one electrode inside and one electrode outside the cell membrane. (B) Ionic shifts across the cell membrane which causes changes in electric potential.

negative to positive is referred to as depolarization. Repolarization occurs when the sodium is transferred back to the outside of the membrane. Large nerve fibers can depolarize and repolarize at a rate of 1000 times/second. *See* Figure.

Activated Charcoal:

Material that is nearly pure amorphous carbon. Its unique properties are due to its incredible internal surface area. Depending on its method of manufacture and the source from which it comes (which can range from petroleum and coal to peach pits and coconut shells), it can be designed to trap molecules of a particular size. Canisters of activated charcoal are commonly used to remove halogenated hydrocarbons from operating room air. The binding of material to activated charcoal can, to a certain extent, be reversed by heating.

Activated clotting time (ACT):

Blood test to determine the adequacy of heparinization for cardiopulmonary bypass patients. A blood sample is drawn into a special test tube that contains a magnet. The tube is then placed in an incubator timer device, such as Hemachron (International Technidyne Corporation), where it is warmed. The time is noted from the start of the drawing of the blood sample until the machine detects changes in the position of the magnet as it is moved by fibrin strand formation. With proper heparinization, the ACT should approach infinity.

Actomyosin:

Combination of actin and myosin, two proteins found in muscle cells. It is the longitudinal shortening of these two proteins as they interdigitate with each other that is responsible for muscle contraction. *See* Figure.

Actual Bicarbonate:

See Carbon dioxide total in blood.

Acupuncture:

Ancient Chinese system of medical therapy based on stimulation of the skin at previously designated points, usually by needles, to treat disease. It has generated considerable enthusiasm as a means of anesthesia. Widely conflicting claims for efficacy and effectiveness have been voiced. Some evidence exists that the effects of acupuncture are caused by central nervous system release of endorphins. *See* Figure.

Acute Idiopathic Polyneuritis (Guillain-Barré Disease):

Disease process characterized by a sudden onset of weakness or paralysis, typically manifesting in the legs. It then spreads, over a number of days, and ultimately may involve the muscles of the arms, trunk, and head. Respiration can be severely compromised. The paralysis is flaccid owing to lower motor neuron involvement. Autonomic nervous system dysfunction is a prominent finding in these patients. Current treatment is primarily supportive as the disease process is not understood.

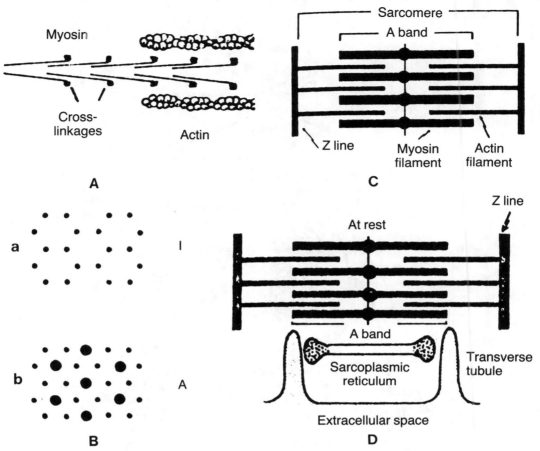

Actomyosin: (A) Arrangement of actin and myosin filaments in skeletal muscle. (B) Cross-section through the I band. Cross-section through the lateral portion of the A band. (C) Detailed structure of myosin and actin. (D) Muscle contraction Ca^{2+} ions (black dots) are normally stored in the cisterns of the sarcoplasmic reticulum. The action potential spreads via the transverse tubules and releases Ca^{2+}. The actin filaments slide on the myosin filaments and the Z lines move closer together. Ca^{2+} is then pumped into the sarcoplasmic reticulum and the muscle relaxes.

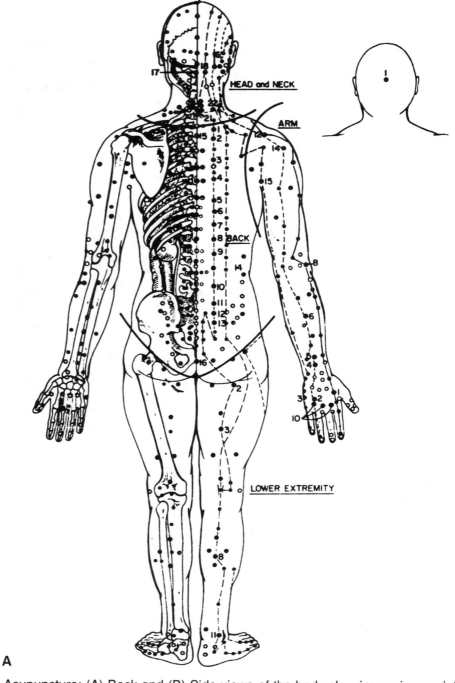

A

Acupuncture: (A) Back and (B) Side views of the body showing various points for the application of acupuncture. (C) Index of selected points.

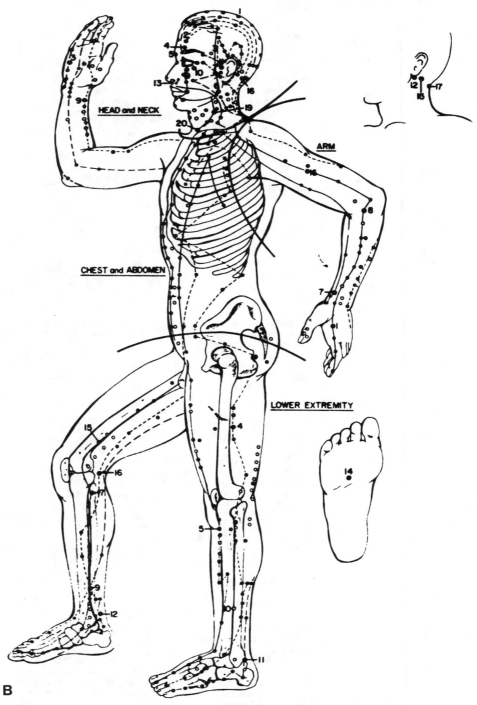

B

Acupuncture *(continued)*

Acute Idiopathic Polyneuritis (Guillain-Barré Disease)

Head and Neck

1.	Vertex	hyakue, pai hui (GV20)
2.	Supraorbital	yohaku, yang-pei (GB14)
3.	Temporal	taiyo, tai-yang
4.	Mid-eyebrow	bichiyu, chien
5.	Glabella	Indo, yin-tang
6.	Inferior Masseter	kyoshiya, chia-che (S3)
7.	Infratemporal	Gekan, hsia-kuan (S2)
8.	Median canthus	seimei, chang-ming (B1)
9.	Midinfraorbital	shiyokyu, cheng-chi (S4)
10.	Lateral infraorbital	kyugo, chiu-hon
11.	Superior tragus	jimon, erh-men (T21)
12.	Posterior earlobe	eifu, I-feng (T17)
13.	Infranasal	jinchiyu, jen-chung (L1)
14.	Lateral oral angle	chiso, ti-ts'ang (S7)
15.	Inframastoid	Imei I-mong
16.	High lateral trapezius	Fuchi, fengs-chi (GB31)
17.	C1-C2	Amon, ya-men (GV15)
18.	Para C1-C2	Tenchyu, tien-chu (B10)
19.	Lateral thyroid	jingei jen-ying (S9)
20.	Supra Sternal	tentotsu, t'ien-t'u (CV22)
21.	C7-T1	Daizui, ta-ch'ui (GV14)
22.	Para C7-T1	Chizen

Chest and Abdomen

1.	Midsternum	danchyu, shan-chung (CV17)
2.	Subxyphoid	κyubi chiu-wei (CV15)
3.	Sub Breast	nyukon, Ju-keng (S18)
4.	Midepigastrium	chyukan, chung-wuan (CV12)
5.	Lateral umbilicus	tensu, t'ien-shu (S25)
6.	Upper hypogastrium	kikai, chi-hai (CV)
7.	Low hypogastrium	kangen, kuan-yuan (CV4)
8.	Lower hypogastrium	chyu kyoku, chung-chi (CV3)
9.	Suprapubic	kyoku kotsu chu-ku (CV2)
10.	Lateral inguinal	Iho

Back

1.	para T2-T3	fumon, feng-men (B12)
2.	para T3-T4 (lung)	haiyu, fei-yu (B13)
3.	para T5-T6 (heart)	shinyu, hsin-yu (B16)
4.	para T7-T8 (diaphragm)	kakuyu, ke-yu (B17)
5.	para T9-T10 (liver)	kanyu, kenye (B18)
6.	para T10-T11 (gallbladder)	tanyu, tanyu (B19)
7.	para T11-T12 (spleen)	hiyu, p'i-yu (B20)
8.	para T12-L1 (stomach)	Iyu, wei-yu (B21)
9.	para L2-L3 (kidney)	jinyu, shen-yu (B23)
10.	para L4-L5 (colon)	daichyoyu, ta-chang-yu (B25)
11.	para L5-S1	Kangenyu kuan-yuan-yu (B26)
12.	para S1-S2 (small bowel)	shyochyoyu, hsiao-ch'ang-yu (B27)
13.	para S2-S3 (bladder)	bokoyu, p'ang-k'uang-yu (B28)
14.	Lateral L2-L3	shishitsu chih-shih (B47)
15.	T3-T4	mumei
16.	Posterior anal	chyokyo, ch'ang-ch'iang (GV1)

Upper Extremities

1.	First dorsal web	gokoku, ho-ku (L14)
2.	Fourth dorsal web	chyushyo, chung-chu (T3)
3.	Fifth lateral metacarpal	kokei, hou-chi (SI3)
4.	Dorsal distal forearm	gaikan, waikuan (T5)
5.	Dorsal low forearm	shiko, chih-kou (T6)
6.	Dorsal upper forearm	shitoku szu-tu (T9)
7.	Radial styloid process	letsuketsu, lieh-ch'uen (L7)
8.	Lateral cubital crease	kyokuchi, chu-ch'ih (LI11)
9.	Volar distal forearm	naikan, neikuan (P6)
10.	Inter M.P. joint	hachija, pa-hsieh
11.	Finger tip	jissen, shih-hsuan

C

Acupuncture *(continued)*

Acute Intermittent Porphyria:

See Porphyria.

Acute Laboratory:

Laboratory (operating room, blood gas, intensive care) usually staffed around-the-clock to deliver accurate quantitative evaluations of patient samples within a time period that is only slightly longer than the analysis apparatus cycle time and the administrative bookkeeping time combined. Reasonable objectives of an acute laboratory are the determinations of blood gases, serum electrolytes, ionized calcium, serum glucose, fluid osmotic pressures, hemoglobin, and hematocrit. As an example, semiautomated analyzers for blood gas measurement usually cycle within 2 to 3 minutes. Therefore an acute laboratory can reasonably be expected to report on every blood gas specimen received in less than 5 minutes.

Acute Plasmapheresis:

See Plasmapheresis.

Acute Toxic Encephalopathy:

See Reye syndrome.

Adaptation:

See Nociceptor.

Adaptor:

Specialized form of connector joining two or more components that are otherwise physically incompatible.

Addiction:

Pattern of behavior characterized by compulsive and undeniable use of a drug by self-administration for pharmacologically, physically, or socially unacceptable reasons.

Addison Anemia:

See Anemia.

Adenohypophysis:

See Hormone.

Adenosine Triphosphate (ATP):

Ubiquitous, labile compound that is present in all cells of the body. It provides energy for many of the body's biochemical reactions. ATP can function as an energy transfer molecule because the two phosphate molecules of ATP are joined to adenosine monophosphate by "high-energy bonds" (i.e., making or breaking this molecular bonding requires a large amount of energy, in this case 8000 calories). *See* Figure.

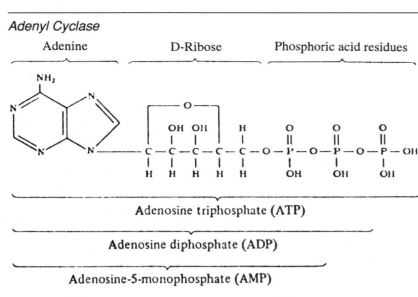

Adenyl Cyclase

Adenine   D-Ribose   Phosphoric acid residues

Adenosine triphosphate (ATP)

Adenosine diphosphate (ADP)

Adenosine-5-monophosphate (AMP)

$$R - \overset{\overset{\displaystyle OH}{|}}{\underset{\underset{\displaystyle O}{||}}{P}} - OH + H_2O \longrightarrow R - H + HO - \overset{\overset{\displaystyle OH}{|}}{\underset{\underset{\displaystyle O}{||}}{P}} - OH + Energy$$

Hydrolysis of energy-rich phosphate bonds

Adenosine Triphosphate: Adenosine triphosphate, its subunits and the basic chemical reaction for energy release.

Adenyl Cyclase:

Enzyme activated in many combinations of hormone and receptor sites, which in turn causes the conversion of cytoplasmic adenosine triphosphate (ATP) to cyclic adenosine 3',5' monophosphate (cAMP). *See* Receptor/receptor site.

ADH:

See Antidiuretic hormone.

Adiabatic

Occurring without loss or gain of heat. Anesthetically, adiabatic processes occur during the expansion and compression of a gas. During adiabatic compression of a gas, no heat is added from the surroundings during compression. However, the temperature of the gas rises according to the following ratio: final temperature/initial pressure × final volume/initial volume. This relation which is seen in Regulator accidents, occurs when high-pressure O_2 is admitted to a Regulator that has been inadvertently oiled. The gas already in the regulator is compressed rapidly in an adiabatic process. As it is compressed, its temperature rises, surpassing the ignition temperature of the oil, causing a fire which is then O_2-fed.

Adrenal Cortex:

See Corticosteroid.

Adrenalin:

Term used by the British Pharmacopeia for epinephrine. *See* Epinephrine.

14

Adrenergic Blocking Agent:

See Autonomic nervous system; Receptor/receptor site.

Adrenergic drug:

See Autonomic nervous system.

Adrenergic Nervous System:

See Autonomic nervous system.

Adrenocortical Steroids:

Collective term for the steroid hormones synthesized and secreted by the adrenal cortex. (They are all derivatives of cholesterol.) The two classes of steroids are the corticosteroids (with 21 carbons, C_{21}) and the adrenal androgens (with 19 carbons, C_{19}). The corticosteroids are subclassified into mineralocorticoids and glucocorticoids. *See* Corticosteroid.

Adult Respiratory Distress Syndrome (ARDS):

Symptom complex with many etiologies that is typified by severe hypoxia, increasing hypercapnia, interstitial infiltrates and edema, microemboli, alveolitis, and, as the disease progresses, frank filling of the alveoli with fluid and the appearance of alveolar hyaline membranes. Pathophysiologically, the most striking phenomenon observed is the severe reduction of lung compliance, or "stiff lung," which is due to the interstitial infiltrates, filled alveoli, and an increase in absolute lung water. Stiff lung increases the work of breathing. The functional residual capacity progressively decreases, ventilation/perfusion mismatch increases, and alveolar deadspace increases. Treatment is aimed toward immediate relief of the hypoxic condition, it usually requires mechanical ventilation and often accompanied by positive end-expiratory pressure, while acid-base derangements caused by hypoxia and hypercapnia are brought under control. *See* Infant respiratory distress syndrome; Surfactant.

Adverse Reaction:

Reaction that is not desired following administration of a drug.

AEP:

See Auditory evoked potential.

Aerobic:

Requiring the presence of O_2 to exist or grow.

Aerobic Metabolism:

Degradation of food molecules and subsequent energy production carried out in the presence of abundant O_2. From aerobic metabolism of glucose the body gains 38 ATP molecules per glucose molecule metabolized. The net efficiency of this reaction is 44%, with 56% of the total energy available released as heat. The end-products are CO_2 and H_2O. When O_2 is not available, many body tissues can continue some energy production via anaerobic metabolism. *See* Anaerobic metabolism.

Aerosol:

Suspension of discrete particles in air.

Afferent:

Going toward or moving toward the center. For example, afferent sensory nerves from the skin return information to the central nervous system. Afferent and efferent (going or moving away from the center) depend on the point of reference.

A Fiber:

See Nerve fiber, anatomy and physiology of.

Afibrinogenemia:

Marked deficiency in the blood fibrinogen levels, encountered most dramatically in disseminated intravascular coagulation. *See* Disseminated intravascular coagulation.

After Cooler:

Device to separate compressed air from condensed moisture, usually found installed downstream of air compressors used to provide compressed air.

Afterload:

One determinant of cardiac output. It is the resistance to left ventricular ejection and can be approximated by aortic diastolic pressure. Afterload is directly related to myocardial O_2 consumption.

After-Pain:

Term covering the uncomfortable, long, dull sensation (which may be described as burning) that persists after an initial noxious stimulus. It is probably transmitted to the central nervous system by less discrete afferent pathways.

Agent-Specific Filling Device:

Apparatus designed to prevent accidental filling of vaporizers with anesthetic agents that they are not meant to contain. The major part of the device is an adaptor tube that fits between a specifically collared bottle and the custom designed fill port of the vaporizer. The adaptor tube and the bottle and vaporizer are usually color coded. *See* Figures.

Ageusia:

See Dysgeusia.

Agent-Specific Filling Device: (A) Filling the vaporizer; (B) draining the vaporizer; (C) adaptor tube. The bottle cap is at left and the filler block at right. Note the groove (slot) in the side and the two holes on the flat surface of the filler block. Keyed filling device with two front screws.

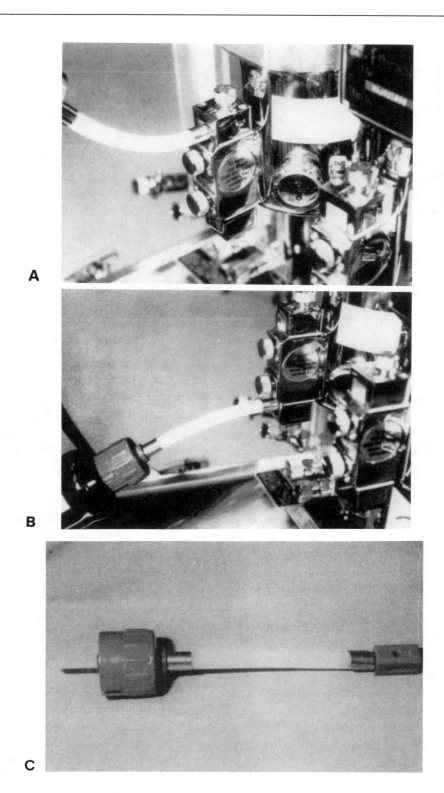

Agglutinin:

See Blood types.

Agglutinogen:

See Blood types.

Agonist:

Pharmacologic agent or physiologic product that causes a clearly defined biologic response. Its biologic effect is proportional to the number of receptor sites it occupies on the cells for which it is targeted. *See* Antagonist; Receptor; Receptor site.

AHA:

See Anesthesia History Association.

AICD:

See Automatic implantable cardioverter—defibrillator.

AIDS (Acquired Immunodeficiency Syndrome):

Disease characterized by severe depression of the immune system. AIDS is caused by the human immunodeficiency virus (HIV), a retrovirus. Of low but real infectious potential by contaminated needle stick or contact with contaminated blody fluids, AIDS is primarily transmitted by sexual contact and from infected mother to offspring. It also has been transmitted by contaminated blood products. The fear of AIDS has single-handedly forced operating room personnel to adopt "universal precautions" when dealing with patients. *See* Universal precautions.

Air:

Mixture of gases that make up the atmosphere in which life on Earth exists. For the purposes of anesthesia, three components of air are important: N_2 (which makes up 78.08% of air), O_2 (20.94%), and CO_2 (0.03%). The remainder of the gases that make up air are primarily argon, neon, helium, krypton, xenon, and radon in total amounts of less than 1%.

Airco Medical & Specialty Gases:

Large company with a home base in Huntington Valley, Pennsylvania. They are responsible for many medical products including medical gases, as well as welding supplies.

Air Embolus:

Presence of air in the circulation. It is not a natural occurrence and is almost invariably seen, albeit rarely, in trauma cases and as a potential problem in certain surgical cases. It can occur in any procedure in which a negative intrathoracic pressure is communicated to the periphery by means of a large vein. The most common example occurs when the cervical veins are exposed during a sitting cervical laminectomy, and the negative pressure can draw air in from the atmosphere surrounding the surgical wound. The air passes centrally quickly to the right side of the heart. If the air volume is high enough, and it occupies the right atrium or the right ventricle and right outflow tract, it can completely block the right side of the heart, precipitating failure. In other circumstances, it may pass out of the right side of the heart, go far into the periphery of the lungs, and cause a block by preventing blood flow to large segments of the lungs. In this situation, a severe ventilation/perfusion abnormality would result with possible disastrous consequences to the patient. Air can also traverse a patent foramen ovale embolizing the systemic arteries. *See* Ventilation/perfusion abnormality.

Air Encephalography:

Neuroradiologic technique by which the ventricles of the brain are outlined via withdrawal of cerebrospinal fluid and the injection of air below the dura, usually by lumbar puncture. It is significant to anesthesiologists because, as the air can rarely be drawn out effectively, the residual volume of remaining air grows appreciably if the patient is subjected to an anesthetic with N_2O. *See* Nitrous oxide.

Air Equivalent:

Measurement of the efficiency of a material to absorb radiation expressed as the thickness of the layer of air that causes the same amount of absorption.

Air Monitoring:

Type of air sampling for waste anesthetic gases in an operating room to determine leaks in the high-pressure gas supply side of the anesthesia machine. It is done when the room is empty and a long enough time has elapsed for N_2O to equilibrate in the room air. When functioning flowmeters on the low-pressure side of the machine are turned off, any N_2O that is detected is from the high-pressure side. This type of monitoring is most conveniently done in the morning just before surgery begins. *See* Air sampling.

Air Products & Chemicals, Inc.:

Worldwide manufacturing supplier of industrial gases and chemicals based in Allentown, Pennsylvania.

Air Sampling:

Intermittent or continuous monitoring of waste anesthetic vapors in the operating room. Considerations of air sampling include not only the type of instrument used to obtain the sample but the timing of the sample, the location to be sampled, and the gas to be detected. The conventional procedure monitors the air within the breathing zone of the anesthetist sampling before, during, and after anesthetics are administered. An average inhaled concentration is obtained by continuous sample collection during this period, and storage in a gas-tight bag. Determination of the concentration of anesthetic vapor gives a "time-weighted average."

Air Test:

Technique for determining unintentional intravenous placement of epidural catheters. It uses the injection of 1 ml of air through the epidural catheter, while heart tones are continually monitored by Doppler ultranography. Detection of air in the heart by this Doppler indicates intravenous placement of the catheter.

Airway; Airway Management:

Maintenance of the functional integrity of the air passageways from their anatomic beginning in the nose and mouth through the multiple divisions of the pulmonary tree to the alveolus. In common usage, airway refers to only the upper airway, which ends at the trachea. "Lost" airway refers to the blockage of all or part of the anatomic air passageways. Maintenance of an open airway is one of the most basic reflex responses. This reflex response is severely attenuated by general anesthesia. *See* Cardiopulmonary resuscitation.

Airway Heat and Moisture Exchanger (Artificial Nose):

Mechanical device for trapping exhaled moisture normally lost owing to bypass of the nasal passages by an endotracheal tube. This moisture is then available to be added to the next inspiratory breath.

Airway Obstruction:

Pathologic condition occuring when foreign bodies or trauma close down an air passageway; used preferentially for the upper airway. The example of this occurrence seen in everyday life is the "cafe coronary," in which food is aspirated and blocks the larynx at an otherwise social occasion. The Heimlich maneuver, or subdiaphragmatic abdominal thrusts is the recommended procedure to open the airway of a conscious or unconscious adult victim where equipment is limited. *See* Figures. *See* Cardiopulmonary resuscitation; Heimlich manuever.

Airway Pressure Release Ventilation (APRV):

Technique of ventilation that differs from conventional mechanical ventilation. It intermittently decreases lung volume while maintaining oxygenation. This type of ventilation may be particularly appropriate for lung-damaged neonates susceptible to barotrauma.

Airway Resistance:

See Resistance, airway.

Airway Score:

Technique for forecasting ease of intubation as determined by patient examination. Class I-IV is determined by number of posterior-structures seen through the open mouth.

Akathisia:

Unfortunate side effect of a number of centrally acting depressants. Akathisia is a sense of uncomfortable physical restlessness. It most often manifests as an inability to sit still. (Schpilcus in Yiddish.)

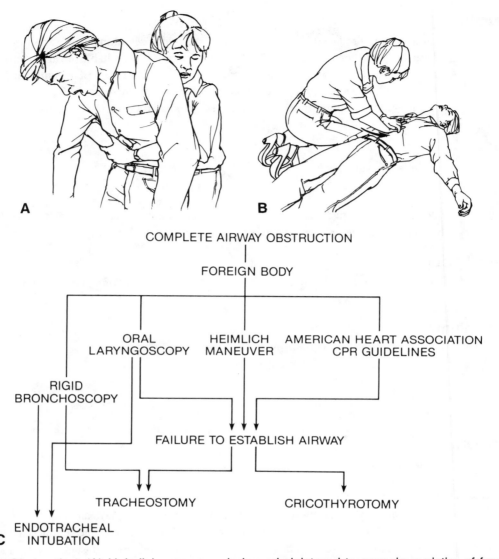

COMPLETE AIRWAY OBSTRUCTION

FOREIGN BODY

ORAL LARYNGOSCOPY   HEIMLICH MANEUVER   AMERICAN HEART ASSOCIATION CPR GUIDELINES

RIGID BRONCHOSCOPY

FAILURE TO ESTABLISH AIRWAY

TRACHEOSTOMY   CRICOTHYROTOMY

ENDOTRACHEAL INTUBATION

C

Airway Obstruction: (A) Heimlich maneuver being administered to conscious victim of foreign-body airway obstruction. (B) Heimlich maneuver being administered to unconscious victim of foreign-body airway obstruction. (C) Management of complete airway obstruction.

Akinetic Seizure:

Type of seizure characterized by a sudden short loss of consciousness and an absence of postural muscle tone.

Al:

See Aluminum.

Albumin:

Serum protein produced by the liver; one of the major determinants of serum osmolarity. Normally blood contains about 3.5–5.5 gm per 100 ml. It is available in various proprietary preparations, such as plasma protein precipitate, Plasmanate, or 25% albumin, and is used as a volume expander following blood loss. It is a human serum protein and therefore expensive. When appropriately heat-treated it does not transmit the hepatitis virus.

Albuterol:

See Beta blocker.

Alcohol:

Oldest known sedative drug. Medical use includes intravenous administration to stop labor. It markedly potentiates all central nervous system depressants, especially the benzodiazepines.

Alcohol Neuritis:

Intense burning pain that occurs after incomplete destruction of a nerve by an injection of alcohol for neurolysis.

Alcuronium:

Nondepolarizing, competitive muscle relaxant related to curare. *See* Neuromuscular blockade, assessment of; Neuromuscular blocking agent.

Aldactone:

See Spironolactone.

Aldomet:

See Methyldopa.

Aldosterone:

Potent, naturally occurring steroid. It acts on the kidney and plays an important role in the regulation of sodium and potassium balance in the body. Aldosterone, a mineralocorticoid, is excreted by the adrenal cortex and acts to conserve sodium. Aldosterone antagonists are often used for the control of hypertension. *See* Figure.

Aldosterone.

Aldrete Score:

Means of determining postanesthetic recovery, it assigns a quantitative value between 0 and 2 for respiration, circulation, consciousness, color, and patient activity. *See* Figure. *See* Postanesthesic recovery room.

ROBERT WOOD JOHNSON UNIVERSITY HOSPITAL
NEW BRUNSWICK, N.J. 08901

POST ANESTHESIA CRITICAL CARE RECORD
PA 49 r 8/84

DATE:	TIME IN:
ADMITTING NURSE	
ANESTHESIOLOGIST	
SURGEON	
ANESTHESIA	
SURGERY	
VENTILATOR ☐ ETT ☐ NTT ☐ TRACH ☐	
O₂ _____ TIME EXTUBATED _____	
O₂ NASAL _____ MASK _____ TIME ON _____	
AIRWAY ☐ NASAL ☐ ORAL ☐ TIME OUT _____	
LOC	SIDERAILS:
PRE-OP BP _____	P _____

POST ANESTHESIA RECOVERY SCORE (ALDRETE SCORE)

		A	D
ABLE TO MOVE 4 EXTREMITIES VOLUNTARILY OR ON COMMAND — 2			
ABLE TO MOVE 2 EXTREMITIES VOLUNTARILY OR ON COMMAND — 1	ACTIVITY		
ABLE TO MOVE 0 EXTREMITIES VOLUNTARILY OR ON COMMAND — 0			
ABLE TO DEEP BREATHE AND COUGH FREELY — 2			
DYSPNEA OR LIMITED BREATHING — 1	RESPIRATION		
APNEIC — 0			
BP ± 20% OF PREANESTHETIC LEVEL — 2			
BP ± 20-50% OF PREANESTHETIC LEVEL — 1	CIRCULATION		
BP ± 50% OF PREANESTHETIC LEVEL — 0			
FULLY AWAKE — 2			
AROUSABLE ON CALLING — 1	CONCIOUSNESS		
NOT RESPONDING — 0			
PINK — 2			
PALE, DUSKY, BLOTCHY, JAUNDICED, OTHER — 1	COLOR		
CYANOTIC — 0			
	TOTALS		

NEURO-VASC ✓									
TIME									
INIT									
PULSES TYPE									
MOBILITY									
SENSATION									
CAP REFILL									
COLOR									
TEMP									

Aldrete Score: Post anesthesia recovery score (Aldrete Score).

Alfentanil:

Derivative of the synthetic narcotic fentanyl, which is approximately one-third as potent. It has a much smaller volume of distribution and a significantly shortly elimination half-time.

These factors prevent significant accumulation of alfentanil during a typical continuous infusion. *See* Fentanyl.

Algesimeter:

Device used to measure a subject's sensitivity to pain produced by precise pricking with a sharp point.

Algogenic Substance:

Substance released upon noxious stimulation of the skin or viscera; it either excites or sensitizes nociceptors. Known algogenic substances include serotonin, bradykinin, and prostaglandin E.

Algorithm:

Set of directions, rules, and procedures for solving a particular problem or accomplishing a particular process. For example, both the series of internal directions that would allow a blood gas machine to calculate base deficit from blood sample values and the series of steps used to deliver contaminated material to the central sterilizing department are algorithms.

Alkalemia:

Condition of the blood in which the pH is higher than 7.44 or the hydrogen ion concentration is below the normal range of 36–44 nEq/L.

Alkali Reserve:

Derived value for the buffering capacity of the blood that corresponds to actual bicarbonate. An archaic means of reporting acid-base status. *See* Carbon dioxide total in blood. *See* Acid-base balance.

Alkalosis:

Pathophysiologic condition that would cause alkalemia (pH >7.44) if not compensated by respiratory or metabolic changes. *See* Acid-base balance; Metabolic alkalosis; Respiratory alkalosis.

Allander Air Curtain:

Sophisticated high-technology operating room air filtration system. The Allander air curtain provides large flows of slowly moving air originating from vents in the ceiling over the operating table. The intent is to sweep contaminated particle-laden air down and away from the operative site. The return ducts for the air curtain are located low in the operating room walls. All recirculated air goes through a HEPA filter. Air is recirculated at a rate of 100–400 changes per filter. *See* HEPA filter.

Allen Test:

Clinical test performed at the wrist to determine the patency of the radial and ulnar arterial blood supply to the hand. The patient is asked to make a tight fist, thereby expressing the blood from the hand. The examiner compresses the ulnar and radial arteries at the wrist, and the patient then opens the hand. Compression is maintained on one vessel while the other is released. The procedure is repeated to test the second artery. If flow to the hand is shared by the radial and ulnar arteries, color should return to the palm and fingers in roughly equal time when supplied by one vessel only. If, however, one vessel dominates supply, the color returns only when this vessel is released, with the hand remaining white when the non-contributory vessel is released. This test is used to determine if artery catheterization at the wrist is likely to result in ischemia of the hand. As an example, if the Allen test shows that the ulnar artery does not significantly contribute to the blood supply of the hand, catheter-ization of the dominant radial artery at the wrist would have an increased risk of ischemic damage to the hand.

Allergen:

Agent that induces an allergic response.

Allergic Response:

Inappropriate, apparently self-destructive response to an innocuous stimulus to an organ-ism. It can range from respiratory discomfort by contact with various pollens to respiratory and cardiovascular collapse in severe reactions to, for example, penicillin. Allergic re-sponses are mediated in part through the immune system. *See* Allergen; Bradykinin; Histamine.

Allodynia:

Perception of pain when a nonnoxious stimulus is applied to normal skin.

Allogenic Transplant:

See Transplantation.

All-Or-None Law:

Principle relating to the functioning of nervous tissue that states there is no partial response to a stimulus. If the stimulus is strong enough, the nervous system responds with a maximum action potential, or it does not respond at all. The similarity to binary systems (in which the signal state is either 1 or 0, positive or negative) is apparent.

Allosteric Inhibition:

Distortion of the three-dimensional configuration of the active sites of enzymes that causes them to function less than optimally. By nonspecifically binding close to the active sites on enzymes, anesthetic molecules may cause allosteric inhibition which may, in turn, be part of the mechanism of action of anesthetics.

Alloy:

Material that is not a pure element but that exhibits metallic properties. At least one major component of the alloy must be a metal. For example, amalgams are alloys which have the metal mercury as one component; steels are alloys of iron and carbon.

Almitrine Bismesylate:

Agent that functions as a peripheral chemoreceptor agonist. It is said to improve arterial oxygen tension and reduce arterial carbon dioxide tension in those patients with chronic respiratory failure caused by obstructive pulmonary disease. It may function by enhancement of hypoxic pulmonary vasoconstriction. *See* Hypoxic pulmonary vasoconstriction.

Alpha$_1$-Acid Glycoprotein:

See Binding proteins.

Alpha$_2$-Agonists:

New to anesthesia; a class of drugs that have sedative, anxiolytic, and analgesic properties. They originally were used for their hypotensive effects. Some of the newer agents have great promise.

Alpha Blocker:

See Autonomic nervous system, Receptor/receptor site.

Alphadolone:

See Althesin.

Alpha-Endorphin:

See Endorphins.

Alpha Particle:

Nucleus of a helium atom containing two protons and two neutrons. A stream of alpha particles is called an alpha ray(s) and is the result of the breakdown processes of certain radioactive nuclei. Alpha particles are relatively large, can travel only a few centimeters in air, and can be stopped by such materials as paper or skin. They remain dangerous, however, because the stoppage of an alpha particle requires transfer of a large amount of energy to the material stopping the particle. Alpha particles can pose a significant health hazard.

Alphaprodine (Nisentil):

Meperidine-like narcotic formally used frequently in obstetrics for pain relief and as a substitute for meperidine or morphine in balanced anesthesia technique. It was formerly used in combination with a narcotic antagonist as a general anesthetic, with or without N_2O. *See* Narcotic.

Alpha Receptor:

See Receptor/receptor site.

Alpha$_1$-Acid Glycoprotein (AAG):

See Binding proteins.

Alpha Stat Management:

Treatment strategy during cardiopulmonary bypass hypothermia. It maintains $PaCO_2$ and pH at 40 mm Hg, and 7.40, respectively, when they are measured in the blood gas analyzer at 37 degrees centigrade. *See* Table. *See* pH stat management (strategy).

Alphaxalone:

See Althesin.

Alpha-Stat Management: pH Stat Management.

	*p*H-Stat	*α*-Stat
Pa$_{CO_2}$ (at 28.5° C body temperature)	40 mmHg	27 mmHg
Pa$_{CO_2}$ (at 37° C, blood gas analyzer)	60 mmHg	40 mmHg

Alprazolam:

One of the benzodiazepine series of antianxiety agents; trade name Xanax. *See* Benzodiazepine.

ALS:

See Amyotrophic lateral sclerosis.

Alternating Pulse:

See Pulsus alternans.

Althesin:

Combination of two steroids, alphadolone and alphaxalone, administered as a short-acting intravenous anesthetic. It is a clear, colorless, isotonic solution of neutral pH. The drug is used clinically in England but is available only for research purposes in the United States. It can cause anaphylactoid-type reactions. Cremophor El is the solvent for althesin, which may in part be responsible for the severe allergic reactions.

Aluminum (Al):

Element with an atomic weight of 26.97, a specific gravity of 2.70, and a melting point in excess of 658 degrees Celsius. It is resistant to corrosion and a number of chemicals. It can be attacked by alkalis and hydrochloric acid. After O_2 and silicon, it is the most abundant element. By various alloying processes it can be made into a material with good conductivity (about two-thirds that of copper), high tensile strength (on the order of 20,000 lb/in^2), and a good strength/weight ratio.

Alveolar Air, Alveolar Gas:

Percent contribution of the gases that make up the air filling the ideal alveolus at sea level. Of a total of 760 mm Hg, the partial pressure of N_2 is 563 mm Hg, the partial pressure of water vapor at 100% humidity is 47 mm Hg, and the PCO_2 (which can be assumed to be equal to normal arterial CO_2 tension) is 40 mm Hg. Subtracting these three values from a total of 760 mm Hg leaves 110 mm Hg as the alveolar O_2 tension. Alveolar O_2 tension, however, is exquisitely sensitive to ventilation/perfusion (V/Q) ratios. In one extreme situation, the V/Q abnormality known as shunt occurs when no gas exchange between

27

alveolar gas and the blood takes place. Alveolar O_2 tension rises toward its inspired tension of 159 mm Hg partial pressure (21% of 760). In the V/Q abnormality known as deadspace (the other extreme), no ventilation of the affected alveoli takes place, and the gas in the alveoli ultimately comes into equilibrium with the blood flowing past it such that the PO_2 approaches 40 mm Hg and the PCO_2 approaches 45 mm Hg. *See* Absorption atelectasis; Alveolar air equation; Ventilation/perfusion abnormality.

Alveolar Air Diagram (Oxygen-Carbon Dioxide Diagram; Rahn and Fenn Diagram):

Complex graphic representation of the interrelation of O_2 saturation and CO_2 content that combines all of the O_2 and CO_2 dissociation curves. The former varies with the changing PCO_2 (Bohr effect), and the latter varies with the O_2 saturation (Haldane effect).

Alveolar Air Equation; Alveolar Gas Equation; Alveolar Partial Pressure of Oxygen Equation

Mathematic method for determinating the mean alveolar partial pressure of oxygen (PAO_2). The formula depends on knowing the partial pressure of oxygen inspired (PIO_2). It assumes that (1) the partial pressure of inspired carbon dioxide ($PICO_2$ is zero, (2) arterial partial pressure of carbon dioxide ($PaCO_2$) is a good representation of alveolar carbon dioxide partial pressure ($PACO_2$), (3) nitrogen partial pressure is not changed by ventilation as nitrogen is not metabolized and therefore is at a steady state, (4) the respiratory quotient (R) is either measured or can be assumed to be 0.8, (5) the partial pressure of water vapor at 37 degrees Celsius is 47 mm Hg, and (6) barometric pressure is 760 mm Hg minus 47 (water vapor) = 713 mm Hg. Under these conditions,

$$PAO_2 = FIO_2(713) - PaCO_2 \left[FIO_2 + \frac{1 - FIO_2}{R} \right]$$

The expression in brackets is a correction for R, as the volume of O_2 consumed per minute is greater than the volume of CO_2 produced.

Alveolar-Arterial Carbon Dioxide Difference:

Difference in CO_2 tension found in the alveolus versus arterial blood. This difference is rarely greater than 1 mm Hg, as CO_2 is rarely affected by V/Q abnormalities or diffusion block in the lung. *See* Alveolar end-capillary difference.

Alveolar-Arterial Oxygen Difference (PAO_2-PaO_2):

Measurement in millimeters of mercury that describes the inequality between PAO_2 and PaO_2 in normal young individuals breathing room air. The PaO_2 is approximately 97 mm Hg. At the same time, the normal average PAO_2 is about 101 mm Hg. The difference between the two, approximately 4 mm Hg, is known as the alveolar-arterial O_2 difference. The difference becomes larger as age increases, reaching 20 to 25 mm Hg in the elderly. The alveolar-arterial O_2 difference also increases with larger percentages of inspired O_2. The difference is explained by the fact that not all arterial blood has been exposed to the alveoli. *See* Alveolar air, alveolar gas; Alveolar air equation; Alveolar end-capillary difference; Shunt; Ventilation/perfusion abnormality.

Alveolar Cell Types:

Five distinct cell types are identified in normal alveoli. Type 1 pneumocytes are flattened, pavement-like cells. Type 2 pneumocytes are rounded cells that contain granules. They synthesize pulmonary surfactant, which is vital for decreasing the fluid tension at the fluid-air interface of the alveoli, thereby facilitating full expansion of the alveoli. The remaining types are brush cells, alveolar macrophages (foreign particle scavengers), and mast cells, which secrete heparin, histamine, and serotonin. Alveoli are lined by one cell layer of epithelium (septal cells) attached to a basement membrane that separates the alveoli from the underlying endothelial cells of the capillaries.

Alveolar Concentration Curve:

Graphic display of the relation between the fractional alveolar (F_A) and inspired (F_I) anesthetic concentration as a function of time. The approach of F_A to F_I varies inversely with blood solubility of the agent: the greater the solubility, the slower the rise in the alveolar concentration. *See* Alveolar concentration of anesthetics.

Alveolar Concentration of Anesthetics:

Percentage of alveolar gas that is anesthetic vapor. The concentration of anesthetic vapor or gas in the alveolus depends on the following variables: concentration at which it is delivered, rate and depth of ventilation of the alveolus, and rate at which it diffuses across the alveolar membrane and enters the arterial blood. Because there is rarely a diffusion barrier preventing the passage of anesthetics into the blood, the last variable is based on the solubility of the agent in the blood. The more soluble the anesthetic agent, the greater the amount that enters the blood during a fixed period of time without raising its partial pressure appreciably. The greater the amount entering the blood, the less there is left in the alveolus. The less left in the alveolus, the lower is the alveolar tension, or concentration, of the agent. Paradoxically, then, highly soluble agents take much longer to induce anesthesia than poorly soluble agents (low alveolar partial pressure → low arterial partial pressure → low brain partial pressure → little anesthetic effect).

Alveolar Deadspace:

Volume of air within unperfused alveoli that does not take part in inspiratory exchange. It is of little significance in the healthy individual. *See* Anatomic deadspace; Ventilation/perfusion abnormality.

Alveolar Diffusion Measurement:

See Diffusion.

Alveolar End-Capillary Difference:

Potential difference between the partial pressures of gases in the alveolus and in the capillary exiting the alveolar capillary interspace. Under normal circumstances, the difference between the PO_2 of the alveolus and the PO_2 of the capillary is so small as to be undetectable. However, when diffusion is disrupted and the transfer of O_2 across the alveolar membrane is slowed, the PO_2 of the capillary blood may not reach the PO_2 of the alveolar gas in the time available for O_2 transfer. In this case, a diffusion block is said to exist. With CO_2 which is 20 times as diffusible as O_2, little diffusion block occurs, even under extreme circumstances. *See* Figure.

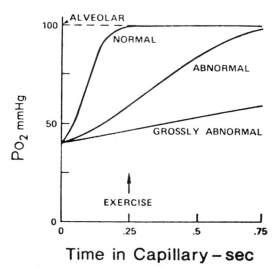

Time in Capillary – sec

Alveolar End-Capillary Difference: Graph showing the effect of a barrier to O_2 transport across the alveolar membrane. The X axis is blood transit time in the capillary; the Y axis is capillary PO_2. Exercise lowers transit time to about 0.25 sec. If diffusion is normal then there is still enough time for capillary PO_2 to equilibrate with alveolar PO_2.

Alveolar Gas Equation:

See Alveolar air equation.

Alveolar Macrophage:

See Alveolar cell types.

Alveolar Partial Pressure of Oxygen Equation (Mean Alveolar PAO₂):

See Alveolar air equation; Respiratory exchange ratio.

Alveolar Plateau:

(1) Period occurring during end expiratory N_2 analysis when N_2 content is nearly uniform. The gas measured at this time is considered pure alveolar gas. (2) The portion of a capnograph trace which is positive and nearly horizontal, indicates a steady exhalation of CO_2 from the alveoli. *See* Single-breath test.

Alveolar Ventilation:

Portion of tidal volume that reaches the alveoli and is involved in gas exchange in the lung. If alveolar ventilation is halved, the P_ACO_2 usually is doubled. *See* Alveolar deadspace.

Alveolar Vessels:

Network of capillaries traversing lung septa that plays an integral role in diffusion of gases.

Alveolus:

Terminal air sac of the lung in which gas exchange occurs between alveolar air and pulmonary capillary blood. There are approximately 300 million alveoli in the healthy human lung. Approximately 0.3 mm in diameter, the alveoli have a combined surface area of 50–100 m^2. In any disease process which tends to destroy the septa between alveoli, the surface area becomes tremendously diminished. The alveolar wall separating blood from gas is less than 1 m thick. *See* Figure. *See* Diffusion.

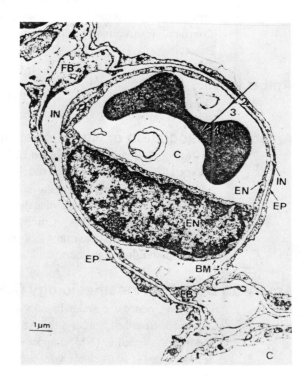

Alveolus: Electron micrograph showing the alveolus, pulmonary capillary interface (C), erythrocyte (EC), alveolar epithelium (EP), interstitium (IN), capillary endothelium (EN), fibroblasts (FB), basement membrane (BM), and plasma. The long arrow shows the diffusion path for O_2.

AMA:

See American Medical Association.

Amaurosis:

Blindness without an organic eye defect. Amaurosis fugax: unilateral centrally caused transient blindness.

Amblyopia:

Defective vision without an organic eye defect.

Amblyopia Ex Anopsia:

Loss of vision due to suppression of one image of the two presented to the cortex because of the misalignment of the visual axes due to strabismus. Usually seen in children under age 6; if it is not corrected before this age, the loss of vision usually becomes permanent. *See* Strabismus (squint).

Ambu Bag:

See Ambu resuscitator.

Ambu Resuscitator (Ambu Bag):

One brand of self-inflating bag for resuscitation purposes that has almost become a generic term. The bag is usually sold in combination with a nonrebreathing valve. In one modification, an O_2 reservoir is added to the tail of the bag to increase inspired O_2 concentration. *See* Breathing bag.

Ambu Valve:

See Nonrebreathing valve.

American Association of Nurse Anesthetists (AANA):

Professional organization founded in 1931, with a membership of over 19,000 registered nurses (RNs) who have received between 1 and 2 years of post-RN training in the administration of anesthesia and who have passed a nationally administered qualifying examination. RNs who have met these qualifications are designated Certified Registered Nurse Anesthetists (CRNA). Currently nurse anesthetist training programs are at least 18 months long and may last up to 27 months. Some schools grant a bachelor's or master's degree in addition to the certificate in anesthesia.

American Board of Anesthesiology (ABA):

Certifying board for specialists in anesthesiology. Originally (1937) an affiliate of the American Board of Surgery, the Advisory Board for medical specialties of the American Medical Association (AMA) approved the establishment of the ABA as a separate major board in 1941. Individuals who are certified by the ABA are designated diplomates in anesthesiology. Certification is established by passing the board examination to become a diplomate, but the requirements also include 12 months of post-MD/DO clinical training in an area other than anesthesiology and 36 months of training in clinical anesthesia. Eligible candidates must pass a written examination that qualifies them to take an oral examination. Currently, the ABA has certified over 20,000 diplomates. The office of the Board is located in Hartford, Connecticut.

American Dental Society of Anesthesiology:

Founded in 1953, this organization is made up of dentists who have a special interest in anesthesiology. The organization starts the 1990s with a current membership of more than 3200. The society has numerous goals, among which are to develop high standards of education in dental schools for teaching acute and chronic pain control and elevating the standards of anesthesiology in dental practice. The current location of the organization is Chicago, Illinois.

American Medical Association (AMA):

National organization founded in Philadelphia in 1847, that represents the American medical profession. The AMA acknowledges Dr. Nathan Smith Davis as its founder because of his early work in organizing the association. The AMA started the decade of the 1990s with approximately 240,000 members from a total of approximately 550,000 physicians in the United States.

American National Standards Institute (ANSI):

Organization that evolved from the merger in 1918 of five leading engineering societies with segments of the Departments of War, Navy, and Commerce. It provides a voluntary unit for coordinating the development of engineering and related standards. (ANSI has developed extensive standards for anesthesia equipment.) Based in New York City, it comprises the nation's trade, technical, professional, consumer, and labor groups. It is a private, nonprofit organization that operates in the public interest and in close cooperation with the federal government.

American Osteopathic College of Anesthesiologists:

Organization started in 1952 that is made up of osteopathic physicians who have had formal training in anesthesiology. It started the decade of the 1990s with more than 550 members. The objective of the organization is to advance the standards of practice in the specialty of anesthesiology and promote the osteopathic concept of disease states related to anesthesia. Its current address is in Independence, Missouri.

American Society of Anesthesiologists (ASA):

Organized in 1905 by nine physicians from Long Island, New York, the ASA was the first professional anesthesia society. Its named evolved from the New York Society of Anesthetists to the American Society of Anesthetists in 1936. Then, in 1945, it became the American Society of Anesthesiologists. The organization began the 1990s with more than 28,000 members. ASA's National headquarters is in Park Ridge, Illinois.

American Society of Critical Care Anesthesiologists:

Organization open to all physicians who are members of the American Society of Anesthesia who have an interest in critical care medicine. The organization began the decade of the 1990s with more than 600 members.

American Standard Compressed Gas Cylinder Valve Outlet Connections:

Safety system that applies to large gas cylinders, i.e., sizes F, M, G, H, and K. Because tanks of these sizes do not use yokes and connections are made by direct piping to their valves, the gas cylinder valve outlet connections are made in 12 combinations of diameter and number of threads per inch. The threads can vary, being right-handed or left-handed and internal or external. This safety system is used between the valves of the cylinder and the regulator; the Diameter Index Safety System (DISS) is used on the low-pressure side of the regulator. Although these systems all rely, in part, on differences in threading, they cannot be interchanged.

Amethocaine:

Alternate name for the local anesthetic tetracaine. *See* Tetracaine hydrochloride.

Amicar:

See H-Aminocaproic acid.

Amidone:

See Methadone.

Amigen:

Brand name for preparations of protein hydrolysates (a sterile solution of amino acids and short-chain polypeptides) used for parenteral feeding (hyperalimentation), and administered through a large central vein. Amigen is commonly used during the postoperative period when patient nutrition is hampered owing to inability to feed orally. It is physically incompatible with many other drugs and solutions. Other brand names are Aminosyn and Travasol.

Amikacin (Amikin):

Semisynthetic aminoglycosidic antibiotic related to streptomycin. It is used for serious gram-negative infections. It may be implicated in enhancing neuromuscular blockade.

Amino Acid Solutions:

See Amigen.

H-Aminocaproic Acid (Amicar):

A drug used to inhibit plasminogen activators and plasmin. It is helpful for treating bleeding disorders in which hemorrhage occurs owing to premature lysis of clots. *See* Disseminated intravascular coagulation; Hemorrhage; Primary fibrinolysis.

Aminoglycoside:

Class of antimicrobial antibiotic agents primarily used to treat gram-negative infections. In addition to the class leader streptomycin, neomycin, gentamicin, kanamycin, tobramycin, amikacin, and paromomycin are useful aminoglycosidic agents. Adverse side effects include significant ototoxicity and nephrotoxicity. *See* Table. *See* Antibiotics; Streptomycin.

Aminophylline:

Soluble salt of the xanthine compound theophylline. Its major effect is the relaxation of bronchial smooth muscle and stimulation of the myocardium. It is used during anesthesia primarily to treat bronchial constriction.

Aminoglycosides.

Generic Name (Trade Name)	Spectrum of Activity	Comments
Streptomycin SO$_4$ IM	Fairly broad spectrum of activity. It is used in the treatment of tuberculosis and infections caused by G$^-$ microbes, including tularemia and bubonic plague.	Streptomycin, like all the aminoglycosides, is generally bactericidal in action, especially in larger doses. It is most notably effective against G$^-$ rods. Side effects include ototoxicity, a generally reversible nephrotoxicity, and rarely, neuromuscular blockade which can lead to respiratory paralysis. This blockade is most likely to occur if an aminoglycoside is given soon after the administration of general anesthesia or of neuromuscular blocking agents. Streptomycin can also cause allergic reactions, eosinophilia and optic nerve dysfunction. Rapid bacterial resistance occurs.
Kanamycin (Kantrex) IM IV PO	Fairly broad spectrum. It is used in the treatment of infections caused by G$^-$ microbes. Pseudomonas is not sensitive to kanamycin.	Kanamycin is related to streptomycin but resistance is slower to develop. It is ototoxic, nephrotoxic and can cause eosinophilia, as well as neuromuscular blockade.
Gentamicin (Garamycin) IM Topical	Broad spectrum. It is the drug of choice for many serious G$^-$ bacillus infections. Effective against many Pseudomonas species.	Gentamicin is ototoxic, though this is mostly vestibular as opposed to auditory. It can also produce neuromuscular blockade, GI upset, headache, proteinuria, acute renal insufficiency and tubular necrosis.
Tobramycin (Nebein) IM IV	Closely related to gentamicin and effective against Pseudomonas.	Side effects similar to gentamicin.
Amikacin (Amikin) IM IV	Similar to gentamicin.	Side effects similar to gentamicin.
Neomycin (Neosporin) IM Topical	Broad spectrum.	The toxic effects of neomycin include nerve deafness, renal damage and possible neuromuscular blockade.

4-Aminopyridine:

Agent that acts presynaptically markedly enhances acetylcholine release. However, it is not often used owing to its ability to cross the blood-brain barrier and cause untoward CNS effects.

35

Amitriptyline:

>*See* Tricyclic antidepressant.

Ammonium Sulfate:

>Neurolytic drug effective in relieving pain associated with unmyelinated nerve fibers. It is used most frequently for treatment of intercostal neuralgia.

Amniotic Fluid Embolism:

>Catastrophic event in which amniotic fluid enters the maternal circulation. It involves rupture of the amniotic membranes or a tear at the placental margin. The syndrome produced by this condition is a combination of mechanical blocking of the pulmonary vessels by the particulate matter in the amniotic fluid and an anaphylactic reaction to the foreign substances in the fluid. There is a sudden decrease in blood return to the heart, a sharp rise in pulmonary vascular resistance, and marked (to extreme) ventilation abnormalities. Part of the syndrome may be caused by the high concentration of various prostaglandins in the amniotic fluid. Aside from the immediate cardiovascular problems, amniotic fluid embolism can lead to disseminated intravascular coagulation. Amniotic fluid embolism is fatal in approximately 50% of cases. *See* Disseminated intravascular coagulation.

Amniotic Fluid Foam Test:

>Test performed by agitating a solution of amniotic fluid and alcohol. If the fetal lung has produced a normal amount of lecithin, the foam produced is stable compared to a standard.

Amobarbital:

>*See* Barbiturate.

Ampere (AMP, A):

>Unit of electric current in the standard international (SI) system. It defines 1 amp as that current maintained in two parallel conductors, 1 m apart in a vacuum and of negligible cross-section, that produces between the conductors a force equal to 2×10^{-7} newton/m of length. An older and approximately equivalent definition of ampere is a current of 6.25×10^{18} electrons/second past a single point in a circuit or 1 ampere = 1 coulomb/second.

Amphetamine:

>Class of powerful central nervous system drugs that also stimulate alpha and beta receptors peripherally. They have been used orally as antidepressants and fatigue suppressants. Parenterally, they have been used acutely for hypotensive crisis. Because of their severe abuse potential the amphetamines have fallen into disfavor. Preoperatively, chronic abusers of amphetamines and amphetamine-like compounds may exhibit disordered thinking, inappropriate behavior, and extreme wasting due to an appetite suppression effect. Abusers are prone to possible cardiovascular collapse under anesthesia.

Amplifier:

Device that takes an input signal such as light, sound, or current flow and produces an output higher in magnitude. This is usually accomplished by using the variations in the input signal to control the variations in the output signal. In physical terms, the input signal can be viewed as the control function on a floodgate or a stream. A strong input raises the gate, and the stream output rises. The reverse also occurs. Changes in the stream flow exactly mirror changes in the gate position. This term is most often used in relation to electrical or electronic systems. *See* Operational amplifier.

Amrinone:

Prototype of the phosphodiesterase inhibitor class of drugs which combines strong inotropic activities with vasodilatation.

AMV:

See Assisted mechanical ventilation.

Amygdala:

Bilateral ovoid mass of gray matter located in the anterior part of the temporal lobes of the brain. In humans it appears to be associated with violent emotion.

Amyotrophic Lateral Sclerosis (ALS):

Motor neuron disease characterized by progressive muscle weakness and wasting due to the degeneration of corticospinal tract neurons and brainstem and spinal cord anterior horn motor cells. ALS affects twice as many men as women, with the peak incidence between 50 and 60 years of age. ALS patients may exhibit an exaggerated response to nondepolarizing muscle relaxants, and they may become hyperkalemic when depolarizing muscle relaxants are administered. Variants of ALS are progressive spinal muscular atrophy, a less severe disease with much longer survival, and progressive bulbar palsy, a more severe disease that affects the muscles innervated by the cranial nerves and corticobulbar tracts. Death usually occurs within 3 years and is frequently due to respiratory problems.

Amytal:

See Barbiturate.

Anacrotic Notch:

Notch in the ascending limb of the pulse-pressure tracing usually seen only if the sample site is close to the aortic valve. It is believed to represent the interaction of the pulse-pressure wave with the slower but larger fluid movement wave. *See* Pulse-pressure tracing.

Anaerobic:

Having the capacity to exist or grow with little or no O_2.

Anaerobic Metabolism:

Degradation of and energy production from food molecules without the presence of O_2. This type of metabolism is low in recoverable (non-heat-producing) energy because it forms only two molecules of ATP per molecule of glucose. The end-products of anaerobic glucose metabolism are pyruvic acid and hydrogen ions. These two products combine to form lactic acid, which can be reconverted to glucose or directly used for energy when O_2 is again available. The brain has a limited ability to function anaerobically. The heart has essentially no anaerobic capacity, but it can directly use lactic acid for energy efficiently. This mechanism provides a margin of safety for the heart during heavy exercise. *See* Aerobic metabolism.

Analeptic:

Drug or agent that acts to increase central nervous system activity. *See* Pentylenetetrazol.

Analog:

Physical variable representing either a physiologic parameter or a numeric value. A thermometer filled with mercury is an analog device in that temperature is represented by the expansion of the volume of mercury along a scale.

Analog Computer:

Fundamental computer class that operates on the principle that both input and output are continuously changing quantities. It is distinct from the digital computer, which represents each input as a binary number and then manipulates the number by the rules of mathematics. In the analog computer, input variables are translated into equivalent electrical or mechanical circuits as analogs for the physical phenomena under investigation.

Analog-to-Digital Converter (Analog-to-Digital Conversion):

Device designed to take a continuous quantity or value and convert it into a discrete quantity or value. It is most frequently used in medicine to convert physiologic data (e.g., heart rate, blood pressure) into discrete binary numbers for use on a digital computer. *See* Binary code.

Analysis of Variance (ANOVA):

Statistical technique that consists of rules for creating test statistics to describe the means of more than two groups of experimental data.

Anasarca:

See Edema.

Anatomic Deadspace (VD):

Portions of the respiratory tract (from the nose and mouth to the terminal bronchioles) that do not participate in gas exchange and in which two-way flow exists. In healthy individuals, anatomic deadspace usually is calculated as 2 ml/kg. A 70-kg man has a deadspace of

140 ml/tidal volume under normal conditions. *See* Alveolar dead space; Physiologic deadspace; Ventilation/perfusion abnormality.

Anatomic Shunt:

See Shunt.

Ancrod:

Anticoagulant collected from the venom of the Malayan pit viper. It selectively depletes the plasma of fibrinogen. It may be clinically useful as an alternative to heparin anticoagulation. It may also have some use in the treatment of peripheral vascular disease or deep venous thrombosis.

Androgen:

Chemical substance that promptes masculinization. *See* Adrenocortical steroids.

Anectine:

See Succinylcholine.

Anemia:

Condition in which there is a reduction, below normal, in the number of circulating erythrocytes or in the quantity of hemoglobin. Anemias may be classified on the basis of etiology: (1) excessive blood loss; (2) deficient red blood cell (RBC) production (erythropoiesis or bone marrow inhibition); (3) excessive RBC destruction; and (4) decreased production together with increased destruction of RBCs. Anemias can be acquired or congenital. Thalassemia (Cooley, Mediterranean) is a congenital type in which there is a decreased rate of production of one polypeptide chain of hemoglobin. With pernicious anemia (Addison anemia), a type of anemia with a strong familial component, there is a lack of secretion of intrinsic factor, a constituent of normal gastric juice. This condition does not allow for normal absorption of vitamin B_{12}, which is vital for normal RBC formation. An example of acquired anemia is hemolytic anemia, a progressive, often rapid destruction of RBCs which can be a catastrophic consequence of mismatched blood transfusion or a result of various poisons or toxins.

Anemometer, Hot Wire (Hot-Wire Respirometer):

Device for measuring the volume of moving gas. It works by the following principle. A wire is placed in an airstream. A constant voltage is applied across the ends of the wire. With no movement of the airstream, a known current flows through the wire (depending on its resistance) and heats the wire to a known temperature. The continuous heating of the wire is balanced by heat transfer from the wire to the nonmoving air around it. As the air around the wire begins to move, its ability to cool the wire rises in proportion to its velocity past the wire. Within reasonable limits, the drop in temperature of the wire can be read as air velocity. Alternately, the change in electrical resistance of the wire, which occurs as it cools, can also be interpreted the same way.

Aneroid:

Functioning without a fluid. An aneroid gauge for measuring blood pressure does not contain mercury.

Anesthesia Administrative Assembly (AAA):

Special interest group within the Medical Group Management Association (MGMA) that provides information resources plus networking opportunities between MGMA members in anesthesia group practices. AAA was created in 1983 and began the decade of the 1990s with nearly 400 members. *See* Medical Group Management Association (MGMA).

Anesthesia, Awareness During (Recall):

Phenomenon of a patient who has undergone a general anesthetic recalling single or multiple events that occurred during anesthesia. Several reports have indicated that the problem of recall is increased in N_2O/O_2/narcotic relaxant techniques. Although careful evaluation can usually show some incidence of recall irrespective of the general anesthetic technique, most studies show recall to be on the order of 1–2%. Dreams, hallucinations, and unpleasant sensations connected with the anesthetic period have been reported to occur 2–20% of the time, depending on the situation and the anesthetic technique employed. Anecdotal reports exist of patients who were assumed anesthetized but were actually paralyzed and awake during a prolonged surgical procedure. They suffered for hours from the pain of the operation but were totally incapable of doing anything about it and subsequently became mentally disturbed. These reports are difficult to verify.

Anesthesia Chart:

Record of anesthesia that is ongoing, on-line, and in "real time." Harvey Cushing, the famed neurosurgeon, and Ernest Amory Codman, a surgeon, are credited with introducing the first record of the vital signs, pulse, and respiratory rate during anesthesia while they were still sophomore medical students at Harvard during the early 1890s. The modern anesthesia chart records not only vital signs but contains a description of induction procedures, gas flows as necessary, and all other monitored modalities. A number of attempts have been made through the years to automate this charting procedure. It is interesting to note that anesthesia is one of the few areas of personal service in which the practitioner is expected to write up his or her work and perform it simultaneously. *See* Figure.

Anesthesia Circuit Filter:

Passive device that filters any particulate matter (e.g., bacteria, dust) circulating within the breathing circuit.

Anesthesia Dolorosa:

Pain sensation reported in an area of the body known to be anesthetized.

ROBERT WOOD JOHNSON UNIVERSITY HOSPITAL
New Brunswick, NJ 08901

ANESTHESIA RECORD

| DATE | PAGE OF | AGE | SEX | WT. | HT. | NPO SINCE |

| PRE-MEDICATION | TIME | EFFECTS: ☐ SATIS. ☐ LIGHT ☐ HEAVY |

DRUG ALLERGIES ☐ NKA | PERTINENT HISTORY

AIRWAY ASSESSMENT | CURRENT MEDICATIONS

| BP | PULSE | HGB/HCT | DIAGNOSIS (pre-op and intra-op) | ASA CLASS: *(CIRCLE ONE)* I II III IV V VI E | TECHNIQUE: ☐ GENERAL ☐ REGIONAL ☐ MAC |

SPECIAL PROCEDURES
☐ ART LINE
☐ CVP
☐ SWAN GANZ
☐ ENDOBRONCHIAL
☐ HYPOTENSIVE
☐ CARDIOPUL. BYPASS
☐ ABG
☐ FLUID WARMER
☐ WARMING BLANKET
☐ CELL SAVER
☐ OTHER

EKG
FiO_2
$ETCO_2$
SaO_2
Temp
TVRR/ PIP
PA

☐ Patient identified, chart reviewed
☐ Anesthesia machine #
☐ Machine & equipment checked
☐ IV site ___ size ___
☐ Monitors applied
☐ Uterine displacement

INDUCTION
☐ Pre O_2
☐ IV ☐ Inhalation
☐ Rapid sequence ☐ Cricoid pressure
☐ Satisfactory ☐ Other (see remarks)

INTUBATION
☐ Easy
☐ Other (see remarks)
☐ Breath sounds equal bilaterally
☐ ET size ___ depth ___
☐ Cuffed ☐ Nasal
☐ Uncuffed ☐ Direct
☐ Oral ☐ Blind

REGIONAL ANESTHESIA
☐ Type ___ ☐ Site ___
☐ Position ___ ☐ Sterile prep
☐ Agent ___
☐ Needle ___ ☐ LOR technique
☐ Test drug/dose ___
☐ Easy ☐ Other (see remarks)
☐ Level
☐ Lot # of kit ___

AGENTS | TIME
O_2
N_2O / AIR
Hal / Enf / Iso

REMARKS:

MONITORS/EQUIPMENT
☐ ECG lead ___
☐ Steth precord
☐ Steth esoph
☐ Cuff BP
☐ Art. BP
☐ CVP
☐ PA
☐ Temp. (sites ___)
☐ FiO₂
☐ ETCO₂
☐ MS Spec
☐ SaO₂
☐ NMB
☐ EEG
☐ Precordial doppler
☐ Airway pressure
☐ Apnea monitor
☐ Ventilation volume monitor
☐ Mechanical ventilator
☐ Semiclosed circle
☐ Non rebreathing
☐ Fetal monitor
☐ Other ___

240 220 200 180 160 140 120 100 80 60 40 20 10 0

OPEN HEART
CPB Time ___ Xclamp time ___
OB
Uterine ___ Delivery ___
ins ___ Apgars ___

REMARKS

FLUID TOTALS

FLUIDS

BLOOD LOSS
URINE OUTPUT

| POST-OP PLAN: ☐ PACU ☐ ICU ☐ Pain SVC | ARRIVAL IN PACU: | TIME | BP | P. | R. | CONDITION |

| SURGICAL PROCEDURE | | ANESTH. TIME | START: am pm | END: am pm | DURATION: hrs min |

| SURGICAL TEAM | ANESTHESIA TEAM | SURG. TIME | START: am pm | END: am pm | DURATION: hrs min |

A

Anesthesia Chart: (A) Front View: Anesthesia Record used at the Robert Wood Johnson University Hospital, New Brunswick, NJ. The Anesthesia Record contains standard grid of time versus ongoing events; as well as other information such as: review of preoperative status, monitors and equipment used intraoperatively, cumulative and final totals of intake and output for all fluids, and completion of the procedure with arrival in the post-anesthesia care unit.

PRE-ANESTHESIA EVALUATION
ROBERT WOOD JOHNSON UNIVERSITY HOSPITAL

DATE ___ TIME ___ □ AM □ PM

PRE-OPERATIVE DIAGNOSIS

PROCEDURE PLANNED

HISTORY OF PRESENT ILLNESS / REVIEW OF SYSTEMS / PAST MEDICAL HISTORY

SURGICAL / ANESTHETIC HISTORY

FAMILY ANESTHETIC HISTORY

OBSTETRIC / PRENATAL / PERINATAL HISTORY (IF APPLICABLE)

MEDICATIONS

ALLERGIES / ADVERSE DRUG REACTIONS

TOBACCO / ALCOHOL / DRUG ABUSE

NPO SINCE

PERTINENT POSITIVE FINDINGS:
□ Head / Face
□ EENT
□ Dental
□ Neck
□ Airway
□ Neurologic CNS/PNS/Psychiatric
□ Cardiac
□ Vascular
□ Pulmonary
□ Tobacco Use
□ Gastrointestinal
□ 'Full Stomach'
□ Hepatic
□ Alcohol Use
□ Renal
□ Genitourinary
□ Gynecologic
□ Pregnant
□ Obstetric
Gravida ___ Para ___
Cervix ___ / ___ / ___
□ Pediatric / Perinatal / Neonatal
□ Endocrine
□ Diabetes Mellitus
□ Hematologic
□ Immunologic
□ Orthopedic / Musculoskeletal

VITAL SIGNS / DATA T | P | R | B/P | HEIGHT | WEIGHT | BSA

PHYSICAL EXAMINATION (INCLUDING AIRWAY ASSESSMENT)

LABS / STUDIES

ASSESSMENT: ASA I II III IV V VI E
PLAN

□ PRE-MEDICATION:

□ The choice of anesthesia, alternatives, risks and benefits were discussed with the patient and/or family. All questions were answered. The goals of the Anesthesia Team are understood and agreed upon. Anesthesia care will be provided by an attending anesthesiologist who may be assisted by a resident anesthesiologist and Certified Registered Nurse Anesthetist.

PATIENT REPRESENTATIVE (SPECIFY) IF PATIENT UNABLE TO SIGN   PATIENT SIGNATURE
□ POST-ANESTHESIA PLANNING:

ICU ___ Ventilator ___ Pain Service ___   ANESTHESIOLOGIST

POST-ANESTHESIA EVALUATION

DATE	TIME	□AM □PM	□ NO ANES. COMPL. KNOWN.	DATE	TIME	□AM □PM	□ ADDITIONAL EVAL.

SIGNATURE: SIGNATURE:

B

Anesthesia Chart *(continued):* Back View: This side contains the pre-anesthesia evaluation, a concise but comprehensive review of pertinent medical history, physical findings and technologic data needed to formulate an assessment of risk and an anesthesia plan. The evaluation form also contains an informed consent statement and space for the post-anesthesia follow-up.

Anesthesia Foundation:

Organization dedicated to the advancement of anesthesiology. Established under the sponsorship of the American Society of Anesthesiologists in 1956, it is a nonprofit foundation that uses its available funds to provide financial assistance to needy anesthesiology residents. It promotes programs to encourage medical students and young physicians to consider a career as an anesthesiologist. It also supports educational programs and research related to anesthesiology, and it preserves and recognizes the American heritage of anesthesiology.

Anesthesia, General (Components of):

See General anesthesia.

Anesthesia History Association (AHA):

Objective of this organization, which held its first official meeting in 1983, is to bring together those interested to promoting research on anesthesia historical issues. The organization started the decade of the 1990s with approximately 500 members. AHA is based in Bainbridge Island, Washington.

Anesthesia Machine, Continuous Flow:

See Continuous flow anesthesia machine.

Anesthesia Patient Safety Foundation (APSF):

Incorporated in 1985, the APSF is headquartered in Park Ridge, Illinois and membership has grown now to include all members of the American Society of Anesthesiologists (ASA). The goal of the organization is to emphasize and improve patient safety during anesthesia. *See* American Society of Anesthesiologists (ASA).

Anesthesia, Pressure Reversal of:

An unusual phenomenon, discovered in the laboratory, that may give insight into the mechanism of action of anesthetics. As a generality, very high hydrostatic pressures have been observed to increase the amount of anesthetic needed to maintain the anesthetic state. This phenomenon has been demonstrated on tadpoles immobilized by ethyl alcohol. When the pressure is raised high enough-on the order of tens to hundreds of atmospheres-the tadpoles revive and begin to swim about. The same phenomenon has been shown in newts when anesthetized by halothane or pentobarbital and subjected to high pressures. A striking demonstration of the pressure reversal of anesthesia is seen when high pressures reverse anesthetic depression of chemiluminescence. The relation between hydrostatic pressure and anesthesia appears to be biphasic, at least with N_2O. When administered at a 70% concentration at atmospheric pressure, N_2O is not an anesthetic; while keeping the concentration of N_2O constant and raising pressure to approximately 2 atmospheres, N_2O becomes a complete general anesthetic. As seen experimentally in mice, if the pressure is raised further, particularly by the addition of helium, the relative partial pressure of N_2O must be increased in order to maintain the same level of anesthesia. The complex interrelation between the anesthetic effect and increased pressure is being used as a research tool to investigate the mechanism by which anesthetics exert their effects. One theory proposes that anesthetics act by expanding critical areas of the cell membrane to produce the anesthetic effect. Elevated pressures reverse this action on the cell membrane and therefore reduce the anesthetic effect.

Anesthesia Simulator-Recorder:

Teaching and evaluation tool that runs as a computer program on an IBM-compatible machine. It trains and evaluates anesthetist management of critical anesthesia incidents.

Anesthesia System, Closed:

System, in strict definition, in which the patient rebreathes all expired gases with the exception of CO_2, which is absorbed. Oxygen taken up by the patient is restored by a continuous low O_2 inflow to the breathing system. Closed systems are the most economical for conserving fresh gas supplies. Clinical practice usually requires the inflow of more than the estimated 250 ml of O_2 that the average adult human requires per minute plus replacement of any O_2 or anesthetic agent that might escape from the patient through the skin or through open body cavities. Slightly excess O_2 provides a margin of safety. Closed-system techniques also eliminate much of the load on the scavenger systems used to dispose of waste anesthetic gases. *See* Anesthesia system, open; Low-flow anesthesia.

Anesthesia Subspecialties:

Since the mid-1970s, the specialty of anesthesia has been forced to divide itself into subspecialty areas because of expanding knowledge to the point where it appears no longer possible for a generalist to be up to date on all the information available to the specialty. Recognized subspecialties of anesthesia include Pediatric, Neurosurgical, Obstetric, Pain Management, and Intensivist, among others. Each subspecialty deals with a growing body of knowledge that differentiates it from the other subspecialties. *See* Table.

Anesthesia System, Open:

System, by strict definition, in which the patient rebreathes no expired gas. *See* Table.

Anesthetic Administration, Subjective Effects of:

Catchall phrase that applies to the complaints of anesthetists concerning increased fatigue, difficulty concentrating, headache, nausea, and feeling of disequilibrium connected with the administration of anesthesia. The fact that these effects are reported is one of the arguments for scavenging waste gases in the operating room.

Anesthetic Gas:

See Gaseous anesthetic agent.

Anesthetist:

Generic term commonly applied to any individual who administers anesthesia.

Anexate:

See Flumazenil

44

Anesthesia Subspecialties: Cardiorespiratory Data In Neonate and Adult.

	Neonate	Adult
Cardiovascular		
Stroke volume (ml)	4–5	70–80
Heart rate/min	120–140	70
Cardiac output (ml/min)	500–600	4000–6000
Metabolic rate (cal/kg/hr)	2	1
Respiratory*		
FRC (ml/kg)	30	34
FRC/TLC (ml/kg)	0.48	0.40
Tidal volume (ml/kg)	6	7
Dead space (ml/kg)	2.2	2.2
Respiratory rate	40	20
Alveolar ventilation (ml/kg/min)	100–150	60
Arterial Blood Gas		
pH	7.38	7.38
$Paco_2$ (mm Hg)	32–35	38–40
Pao_2 (mm Hg)	60–80	80–100
$AaDO_2$ (mm Hg)	25 (105–80)	10 (105–95)

*From Nelson NM. Pediatr Clin North Am 1966; 13:769.

Abbreviations: FRC = functional reserve capacity; TLC = total lung capacity; $AaDO_2$ = alveolar-arterial oxygen difference.

Angel Dust:

See Phencyclidine.

Angina Pectoris:

Pain, arising from a relatively hypoxic myocardium, that results from a relative mismatch of myocardial oxygen demand and oxygen supply. It is usually described as "crushing" or "constricting." Worsened by exercise, it is usually treated with nitroglycerin, which appears to work by both dilating the coronary arteries and decreasing afterload. Nitroglycerin can be administered either sublingually or by dermal paste or patch. An anesthetically significant angina variant is unstable angina, which occurs at rest and is not necessarily relieved by nitroglycerin. It often exacerbates to an infarction.

Angiography:

Radiographic visualization of blood vessels following injection of a radiopaque dye. The technique is useful as a diagnostic aid in cerebrovascular attacks, coronary artery disease, and myocardial infarctions.

Angioplasty:

Radiographically controlled process of opening constricted blood vessels by externally manipulated catheter.

Angiotensin:

Potent vasoconstrictor hormone that exists in the circulation as a precursor molecule known as angiotensinogen. This molecule is acted on by renin, a proteolytic enzyme secreted by

Anesthesia System, Open: Comparison of the various anesthesia gas delivery system nomenclatures.

	Insufflation	Nonrebreathing Valves	T-piece	Magill and Mapleson B, C, & D Systems	Open Drop	Circle System	To and Fro
Dripps	Insufflation	Open	Semi-open	Semi-open	Semi-open	Semi-closed Closed	Semi-closed Closed
Collins	Open	Semi-closed nonrebreathing	Open (no exp. arm) Semi-open (with exp. arm)	Semi-closed partial rebreathing nonrebreathing	Open Semi-open if towels added	Semi-closed partial rebreathing Closed	Semi-closed partial rebreathing Closed
Adriani	Insufflation	Semi-closed nonrebreathing	Semi-closed (if no air dilution)	Semi-closed	Open	Semi-closed Closed	Semi-closed Closed
Conway	Open	Semi-closed nonrebreathing	Semi-closed rebreathing Semi-open (low gas flow and short exp. limb)	Semi-closed rebreathing nonrebreathing	Semi-open with occlusive packing	Semi-closed absorption Closed	Semi-closed absorption Closed
Moyers	Open	Semi-open	Open (no exp. limb) Semi-open (with exp. limb and high fresh gas flow)	Semi-open (high fresh gas flow) Semi-closed (low fresh gas flow)	Open Semi-closed with towels or thick mask	Semi-closed Closed	Semi-closed Closed

Wright	Open	Semi-closed (with exp. limb and low fresh gas flow)	Semi-closed without absorption Semi-open (if exp. limb occluded during inspiration)	Semi-closed without absorption	Open Semi-open with occlusive packing	Semi-closed with absorption Closed	Semi-closed with absorption Closed
McMahon	Open	Open	Open Semi-closed	Open Semi-closed	Open Semi-closed	Semi-closed Closed	Semi-closed Closed

the juxtaglomerular cells of the kidneys. The results of the action of renin on angiotensinogen is formation of a decapeptide, angiotensin I. This molecule is physiologically inert. It is converted, however, to angiotensin II, an octapeptide, by the action of converting enzyme. The half-life of the latter molecule is less than 1 minute because of the action of multiple degradation enzymes located in most tissues of the body. *See* Renin.

Angstrom:

A unit of measurement of wavelength equal to one ten-billionth meter (10^{-10} m).

Anileridine (Leritine):

Meperidine-like narcotic drug used as a morphine substitute. *See* Narcotic.

Animal Research Review Committee:

See Human Subjects Review Committee.

Anion:

Negatively charged ion. The principal anions in the body are Cl^-, HCO_3^-, PO_4^-, and SO_4^-.

Anion Gap (Unmeasured Anions):

Difference between the quantity of measured anions and measured cations in the blood. Serum is electrically neutral with an equal number of anions (–) and cations (+). The major cations measured in the laboratory are sodium and potassium; the major anions are chloride and CO_2 (as HCO_3^-). The sum of sodium plus potassium is always greater than the sum of bicarbonate and chloride. The missing unmeasured anions (anion gap) are nonvolatile organic and inorganic acids, such as sulfates and phosphates (HPO_4^-). The anion gap is usually 12 + 2 mEq/L. A low anion gap (<10 mEq/L) is rare and, occurs in situations in which abnormal unmeasured proteins replace sodium as serum cations (e.g., IgG myeloma). An increased anion gap is found in bromism (elevated serum Br^2 seen with overdose of proprietary over-the-counter medications). Other significant increases in anion gap occur when metabolic acidosis is caused by ketone bodies, excessive lactate, or salicylate overdose.

Ankle Block:

Blocking the saphenous nerve, superficial peroneal nerve, deep peroneal nerve, posterior tibial nerve and sural nerve in appropriate combination or singly, to facilitate surgery on the foot.

Anociassociation:

Loosely defined theory that surgery and other noxious stimuli cause more than direct damage to the surgical sites involved but also disturb the central nervous system which is bombarded by noxious stimuli that are poorly defined. The consequence of this theory is that regional anesthesia is "better" for the patient than general anesthesia because regional blocks pain sensations from reaching the CNS, whereas general anesthesia merely suppresses the response of the central nervous system to these stimuli.

Anode Tube, Spiral Embedded Tube:

See Armored endotracheal tube.

Anopsia:

Failure to use one eye, even though it is anatomically usable. Occurs with such diseases as strabismus in which the brain suppresses the image from one eye, which cannot be brought into line with the primary eye. *See* Amblyopia Ex Anopsia.

Anova:

See Analysis of variance.

Anoxia:

Condition in which there is not enough oxygen to meet metabolic needs. It is also called O_2 deficiency and is used interchangeably with hypoxia.

ANSI:

See American National Standards Institute.

Antacid:

Compound that is given orally to neutralize stomach acid. Aluminum hydroxide and magnesium trisilicate are two often used ingredients of antacids. Unfortunately, because of the unpredictability of gastric mixing, antacids cannot be relied on 100% to neutralize all available stomach acid.

Antagonism:

Pharmacologic effect seen when two or more drugs administered concurrently produce an effect that is less than the sum of their individual actions. Often the drugs compete for the same receptor site, thereby interfering with drug activity. *See* Potentiation; Summation; Synergism.

Antagonist:

Pharmacologic opposite of agonist. A molecule which blocks the action of an agonist at a receptor. *See* Agonist; Receptor/receptor site.

Anterograde Amnesia:

Interference with the ability to learn new information for a variable period of time. The benzodiazepine family of drugs are particularly noted for this action as a side effect. *See* Retrograde amnesia.

Anti AChR Antibodies:

Antibodies considered specific for myasthenia gravis. They are also called acetylcholine receptor antibody. Of significance to anesthesia is the fact that the greater the anti-acetylcholine receptor antibody titer is, the more sensitive is a patient to muscle relaxants.

49

Antianalgesic:

Drug or preparation that appears to lower the pain threshold, i.e., it seems to make a standard stimulus more painful. This phenomenon is most often seen with sedatives, hypnotics, barbiturates, and phenothiazines and appears in doses below those that produce unconsciousness.

Antianxiety:

See Table. *See* Anxiety.

Antiarrhythmic Drugs:

Agents that oppose electrical (rhythm) disturbances of the heart. Whereas many drugs have some antiarrhythmic action, the three major classes are local anesthetics, beta-blockers, and calcium channel blockers.

Antibiotics:

Compound used to fight infectious diseases. Multiple subclasses and molecules exist. Almost without exception, the first of any series of antibiotic was discovered in nature; and then, through chemical manipulation, multiple congeners were created. The physical and chemical incompatibilities of antibiotics must be kept in mind when they are injected intravenously. A number of antibiotics, prepared as sodium or potassium salts, may also affect the body's electrolyte balance. *See* Table. *See* Cephalosporins.

Anticoagulant:

Drug that interferes with the clotting process and causes prolonged bleeding. Two major types of anticoagulant exist. The first type, of which parenteral heparin is the only clinically available drug, works directly at multiple levels of the clotting mechanism but most directly in preventing the conversion of prothrombin to thrombin. The second type, the coumarin derivatives (usually given orally), depresses synthesis in the liver of various coagulation factors, particularly factors II, VII, IX, and X. Coumarins antagonize vitamin K, which is needed for the synthesis of these factors. Heparin is used for rapid anticoagulation. For surgery it is most often used in cases of extracorporeal circulation in which prevention of coagulation is essential. It is also used for microvascular surgery, where anticoagulants are assumed to prevent clotting in the microvascular circulation. Heparin can be directly antagonized by the drug protamine (a fish protein). Coumarin derivatives can be reversed in two ways: (1) by vitamin K, which requires 6 hours to increase liver production, and (2) by fresh frozen plasma.

Antidepressant:

See Tricyclic antidepressant.

Antianxiety Agents.

Generic Name (Trade Name)	Structure	Comments
A. Benzodiazepines		The benzodiazepines are widely used antianxiety drugs having anticonvulsant properties. They are also used as skeletal muscle relaxants (particularly diazepam). They do not produce significant extrapyramidal or autonomic side effects. They are pharmacologically similar to the barbiturates but are not as likely to produce physical dependence and tolerance, and are less lethal when taken in very large dosages. Side effects include fatigue, ataxia, paradoxical excitement, nausea, rash, and altered libido. The differences between the benzodiazepines include half-life, pain on injection, tendency to accumulate, and the route of degradation and elimination.
Chlordiazepoxide (Librium)		
Diazepam (Valium)		
Oxazepam (Serax)		
Clorazepate (Tranxene)		
Lorazepam (Ativan)		

Antianxiety Agents *(continued)*

Generic Name (Trade Name)	Structure	Comments
Prazepam (Verstran)		
Nitrazepam (Mogadon)		
Flurazepam HCl (Dalmane)		Flurazepam HCl is considered a sedative hypnotic. It has some advantages over barbiturates in that it does not immediately suppress REM sleep and causes very little rebound REM upon its discontinuation. It does not induce hepatic microsomal enzymes and has a very high therapeutic index and low addiction potential.
Midazolam		A new water-soluble, short half-life benzodiazepine which may assume significance as an induction agent.

Triazolam (Halcion)

A new short-acting benzodiazepine used as a hypnotic.

B. Butyrophenones

Droperidol (Inapsine)

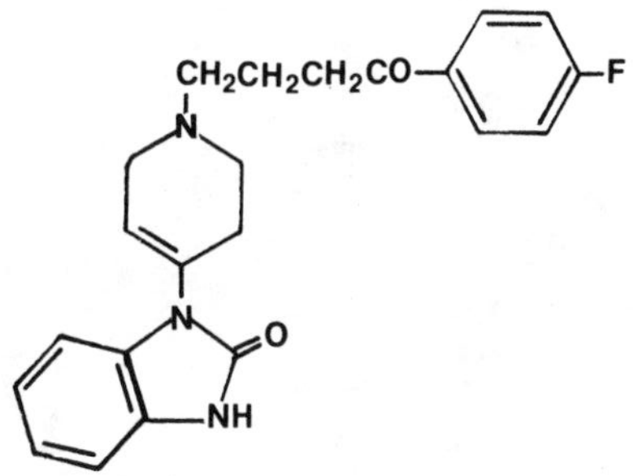

Used at times as a preoperative anti-anxiety drug, droperidol is most commonly used in conjunction with fentanyl (Sublimaze), a narcotic analgesic. This combination (Innovar) is used to produce neuroleptanesthesia. The droperidol produces calmness and drowsiness. It also reduces the incidence of postoperative nausea and vomiting.

Antidepressant

Antibiotics.

Drug	Available (parenteral)		Usually Thought of First for These Infective Agents
	Children	Adults	
Acyclovir	Y	Y	Herpes simplex
Amdinocillin	N	Y	
Amikacin	Y	Y	
Amoxicillin with clavulanic acid	N	N	
Amoxicillin	N	N	Haemophilus influenzae Salmonella typhi
Amphotericin	Y	Y	
Ampicillin	Y	Y	Enterobacter Enterococcus Listeria monocytogenes Proteus mirabilis
Ampicillin with sulfactam	Y	Y	
Azlocillin	Y	Y	
Aztreonam	Y	Y	Proteus vulgaris Providencia Pseudomonas aeruginosa (other systemic)
Bacampicillin	N	N	
Carbenicillin	Y	Y	
Cefaclor	N	N	
Cefadroxil	N	N	
Cefamandole	Y	Y	
Cefazolin	Y	Y	
Cefoperazone	Y	Y	Pseudomonas aeruginosa (other systemic)
Ceforanide	Y	Y	
Cefotaxime	Y	Y	
Cefotetan	N	Y	
Cefoxitin	Y	Y	
Ceftazidime	Y	Y	Pseudomonas aeruginosa (other systemic) Pseudomonas aeruginosa (other systemic)
Cefuroxime	Y	Y	
Cephalexin	N	N	
Cephalothin	Y	Y	
Cephapirin	Y	Y	
Cephradine	Y	Y	
Chloramphenicol	Y	Y	
Ciprofloxacin	N	N	
Clindamycin	Y	Y	Bacteroides other than B. Fragilis
Cloxacillin	N	N	
Cyclacillin	N	N	
Dicloxacillin	N	N	
Doxycycline	N	Y	

Antibiotics *(continued)*

Drug	Available (parenteral) Children	Available (parenteral) Adults	Usually Thought of First for These Infective Agents
Erythromycin	Y	Y	Bordetella
			Corynebacterium diphtheriae
			Legionella
			Mycoplasma pneumoniae
Ethambutol	N	N	
Flucytosine	N	N	
Gentamicin	Y	Y	
Imipenem plus cilastatin	Y	Y	Citrobacter freundii
Isoniazid	Y	Y	
Kanamycin	Y	Y	
Ketoconazole	N	N	
Methicillin	Y	Y	
Metronidazole	Y	Y	Bacteroides fragilis
			Gardnerella vaginalis
Mezlocillin	Y	Y	
Miconazole	Y	Y	
Minocycline	N	Y	
Moxalactam	Y	Y	
Nafcillin	Y	Y	
Nalidixic acid	N	N	
Netilmicin	Y	Y	
Nitrofurantoin	N	N	
Norfloxacin	N	N	
Oxacillin	Y	Y	
Penicillin G	Y	Y	Actinomyces
			Correlia burgdorferi
			Clostridium perfringens
			Eubacterium
			Fusobacterium
			Neisseria meningitidis (illness)
			Pasteurella multocida
			Peptococcus
			Peptostreptococcus
			Spirillum
			Streptobacillus
			Streptococcus agalactiae (Group B)
			Streptococcus bovis (Group D)
			Streptococcus pneumoniae
			Streptococcus pyogenes (Group A)
			Streptococcus viridans
			Treponema pallidum
Penicillin V	N	N	
Piperacillin	Y	Y	

(continued)

Drug	Available (parenteral)		Usually Thought of First for These Infective Agents
	Children	Adults	
Rifampin	Y	N	Mycobacterium marinum Mycobacterium tuberculosis Neisseria meningitidis (carrier)
Spectinomycin	N	N	
Streptomycin	Y	Y	Francisella tularensis Yersinia pestis
Sulfonamides	Y	Y	Nocardia
Tetracycline	N	Y	Borrelia burgdorferi Borrelia recurrentis Chlamydia Francisella tularensis Propionibacterium acnes Rickettsia Ureaplasma Vibrio vulnificus Vibrio cholerae
Ticarcillin	Y	Y	
Ticarcillin w/clavulanic acid	Y	Y	
Tobramycin	Y	Y	
Trimethoprim	N	N	
Trimethoprim-Sulfamethoxazole	Y	Y	
Vancomycin	Y	Y	Clostridium difficile Corynebacterium species JK Staphylococcus aureus Methicillin resistant Staphylococcus epidermidis

Antidiuretic Hormone (ADH, Vasopressin):

Hormone of the posterior pituitary that regulates free water clearance by acting on the distal nephrons of the glomeruli. As secretion of the hormone increases, urinary volume decreases and electrolyte concentration of the urine rises. In higher concentrations (greater than that required for antidiuresis), vasopressin causes contraction of smooth muscles in the vasculature, particularly in capillaries and venules. *See* Diabetes insipidus; Inappropriate antidiuretic hormone (ADH) secretion syndrome.

Antiemetic:

Pharmacologic agent used to prevent nausea or vomiting (emesis). The most commonly used agents for this purpose are antihistamines or phenothiazine derivatives. Two characteristics of antiemetics are noteworthy: (1) The antiemetic effect is not usually the primary effect of the drug. (2) Because antiemesis is not an absolute, what appears to be an adequate dose of an antiemetic may not prevent vomiting.

Antihistamine:

Pharmacologic substance that is a competitive antagonist of endogenous histamine. The classic antihistamines, e.g., diphenhydramine, antagonize the effects of histamine at H_1 receptors which are located in the smooth muscle of the intestines, blood vessels, and bronchi. H_2 receptors, significant primarily in the gastric parietal cells, are blocked only by the newer antihistamines, e.g., cimetidine. H_1 blockers are not completely effective at routine clinical dosages. Central sedation is often an unwanted side effect. *See* Table. *See* Histamine.

Antihypertension Drugs:

Any and all pharmaceutic agents used to treat hypertension. *See* Table. *See* Hypertension.

Antilirium:

See Physostigmine.

Antioxidant:

Material added to a compound to retard oxidation and deterioration. It is found primarily in rubber and other organic products.

Antipollution Assembly:

See Scavenger system.

Antipsychotic Agents:

Pharmacologic products, also known as major tranquilizers, that are used to treat severe psychotic illness, such as schizophrenia. The major classes of antipsychotic agents are phenothiazines, thioxanthenes, and butyrophenones. *See* Table. *See* Droperidol; Phenothiazine.

Antisialagogue:

Agent that prevents salivation. Classically used as a premedicant particularly when diethyl ether, a potent sialagogue (promoting salivation), was to be administered. With the newer, more modern general anesthetics, the practice of prescribing antisialagogues prior to anesthesia has been questioned. The most commonly used antisialagogues are atropine, scopolamine, and glycopyrrolate.

Antihistamines: H_2-antagonist.

Prototype Generic Name (Trade Name)	Structure	Comments
Cimetidine (Tagamet)		Available in oral and parenteral forms, it can decrease gastric secretion by 50% and can cause CNS dysfunction, constipation, and diarrhea. It is becoming more popular as a preoperative premedicant.

Antihistamines: H$_1$-antagonists.

CH$_2$CH$_2$NH$_2$ (histamine structure)

Prototype Generic Name (Trade Name)	Structure	Comments
A. Alkylamines Chlorpheniramine (Chlor-Trimeton)		The alkylamines are among the most potent of the H$_1$ antagonists while they also show a low incidence of drowsiness. They show strong anticholinergic effects.
B. Ethanolamines Diphenhydramine (Benadryl)		The ethanolamines are potent antihistamines which possess anticholinergic, antiemetic, and sedative properties. Diphenhydramine is used as an antiparkinsonism agent as well as being widely used parenterally for moderate to severe allergic reactions.
C. Ethylenediamines Pyrilamine (Neo-Antergan)		The ethylenediamines show some incidence of drowsiness as well as occasional dizziness. GI upset is common.

Antisialagogue

D. Phenothiazines

Promethazine (Phenergan)

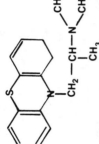

The phenothiazines can have many side effects, including extrapyramidal effects, orthostatic hypotension, and endocrine changes. Promethazine has been advocated for the treatment of motion sickness, for relief of nausea and vomiting, and for sedation.

E. Piperazines

Cyclizine (Marezine)

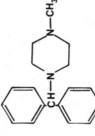

The piperazines are used in the treatment of motion sickness and for relief of postoperative nausea and vomiting. They show a relatively low incidence of drowsiness.

F. Miscellaneous

Cyproheptadine (Periactin)

Cyproheptadine has antiserotonin, anticholinergic, and sedative properties. It can cause some degree of epigastric distress.

59

Antihypertension Drugs: Drugs used in treatment of hypertension.

Drug	Site of Action	Contraindications	Significant Side Effects
Amiloride	Renal tubule	Renal Failure	Hyperkalemia, nausea, vomiting, leg cramps, nephrolithiasis, hyperkalemia, GI disturbances
Atenolol	Beta receptors	Congestive heart failure, asthma, diabetes mellitus (on hypoglycemic therapy), MAO inhibitor administration	Dizziness, depression, bronchospasm, nausea, vomiting, diarrhea, constipation, heart failure
Captopril	Vascular smooth muscle	Renal failure (reduction of dose)	Leukopenia, pancytopenia, proteinuria, nephrotic syndrome, membranous glomerulopathy, urticarial rash, fever, loss of taste, acute renal failure in bilateral renal artery stenosis
Clonidine	Central nervous system		Postural hypotension, drowsiness, dry mouth, rebound hypertension after abrupt withdrawal; insomnia, lupuslike syndrome
Diazoxide	Vascular smooth muscle	Diabetes mellitus, hyperuricemia, congestive heart failure	Hyperglycemia, hyperuricemia, sodium retention
Enalapril	Vascular smooth muscle		Same as Captopril, but no evidence for leukopenia, nephrotic syndrome, or taste loss
Furosemide	Renal tubule	Hyperuricemia, primary aldosteronism	Potassium depletion, hyperuricemia, nausea, vomiting, diarrhea
Guanabenz	Central nervous system		Postural hypotension, drowsiness, dry mouth, rebound hypertension after abrupt withdrawal, insomnia, lupuslike syndrome
Guanadrel Guanethidine	Nerve endings	Pheochromocytoma, severe coronary artery disease, cerebrovascular insufficiency, MAO inhibitor administration	Postural hypotension, bradycardia, dry mouth, diarrhea, impaired ejaculation, fluid retention, asthma
Hydralazine	Vascular smooth muscle	Lupus erythematous, severe coronary artery disease	Headache, tachycardia, angina pectoris, anorexia, nausea, vomiting, diarrhea, lupuslike syndrome
Labetalol	Beta receptors	Congestive heart failure, asthma diabetes mellitus (on hypoglycemic therapy), MAO inhibitor administration.	Less resting bradycardia than other beta blockers
Methyldopa	Centra nervous system/sympathetic nerves	Pheochromocytoma, active hepatic disease, MAO inhibitor administration	Postural hypotension, sedation, fatigue, diarrhea, impaired ejaculation, fever, gynecomastia, lactation, positive Coombs tests (occasionally associated with hemolysis), chronic hepatitis, acute ulcerative colitis

Drug	Site of action	Contraindications	Side effects
Metoprolol	Beta receptors	Congestive heart failure, asthma, diabetes mellitus (on hypoglycemic therapy), MAO inhibitor administration	Dizziness, depression, bronchospasm, nausea, vomiting, diarrhea, constipation, heart failure
Minoxidil	Vascular smooth muscle	Severe coronary artery disease	Tachycardia, aggravates angina, marked fluid retention, hair growth on face and body, coarsening of facial features, possible pericardial effusions
Nadolol	Beta receptors	Congestive heart failure, asthma, diabetes mellitus (on hypoglycemic therapy), MAO inhibitor administration	Dizziness, depression, bronchospasm, nausea, vomiting, diarrhea, constipation, heart failure
Nitroprusside	Vascular smooth muscle		Apprehension, weakness, diaphoresis, nausea, vomiting, muscle twitching
Phenoxybenzamine	Alpha receptors		Postural hypotension, tachycardia, miosis, nasal congestion, dry mouth
Pindolol	Beta receptors	Congestive heart failure, asthma, diabetes mellitus (on hypoglycemic therapy), MAO inhibitor administration	Dizziness, depression, bronchospasm, nausea, vomiting, diarrhea, constipation, heart failure
Prazosin	Alpha receptors		Sudden syncope, headache, sedation dizziness, tachycardia anticholinergic effect
Propranolol	Beta receptors	Congestive heart failure, asthma, diabetes mellitus (on hypoglycemic therapy), MAO inhibitor administration	Dizziness, depression, bronchospasm, nausea, vomiting, diarrhea, constipation, heart failure
Reserpine	Nerve endings	Pheochromocytoma, peptic ulcer, depression, MAO inhibitor administration	Depression, nightmares, nasal congestion, dyspepsia, diarrhea, impotence
Spironolactone	Renal tubule	Renal failure	Hyperkalemia, diarrhea, gynecomastia, menstrual irregularities
Thiazides	Renal tubule	Diabetes mellitus, hyperuricemia, primary aldosteronism	Potassium depletion, hyperglycemia, hyperuricemia, dermatitis, purpura
Timolol	Beta receptors	Congestive heart failure, asthma, diabetes mellitus (on hypoglycemic therapy), MAO inhibitor administration	Dizziness, depression, bronchospasm, nausea, vomiting, diarrhea, constipation, heart failure
Triamterene	Renal tubule	Renal failure	Hyperkalemia, nausea, vomiting, leg cramps, nephrolithiasis, hyperkalemia, GI disturbances
Trimethaphan	Autonomic ganglia	Severe coronary artery disease, cerebrovascular insufficiency, diabetes mellitus (on hypoglycemic therapy), glaucoma, prostatism	Postural hypotension, visual symptoms, dry mouth, constipation, urinary retention, importence

Antipsychotic Agents.

Prototype Generic Name (Trade Name)	Structure Substitutions	Comments
A. Phenothiazines		All phenothiazines can produce atropine-like effects (though pupil dilatation and tachycardia are uncommon), postural hypotension, lowering of body temperature, and various endocrine effects. They are not physically addicting.
General Structure		
Aliphatic Derivatives Chlorpromazine (Thorazine)	$R_1 = CH_2-CH_2-CH_2-N(CH_3)_2$ $R_2 = -Cl$	The class leader of the phenothiazines, chlorpromazine can produce moderate extrapyradimal effects and severe sedative effects. It has antiemetic properties.
Piperazine Derivatives Fluphenazine (Permitil)	$R_1 = -CH_2-CH_2-CH_2-N\underset{}{\boxed{}}N-CH_2-CH_2OH$ $R_2 = -CF_3$	Fluphenazine can produce severe extrapyramidal effects, mild hypotension, and mild sedative effects.
Prochlorperazine (Compazine)	$R_1 = -CH_2-CH_2-CH_2-N\underset{}{\boxed{}}N-CH_3$ $R_2 = -Cl$	Prochlorperazine can produce severe extrapyramidal effects, mild hypotension, and moderate sedative effects. It also has antiemetic properties.
Piperidine Derivatives Thioridazine (Mellaril)	$R_1 = -CH_2-CH_2-$ [piperidine ring with $N-CH_3$] $R_2 = -SCH_3$	Thioridazine produces mild extrapyramidal effects, moderate hypotension, and severe sedative effects.

B. Thioxanthenes

Chlorprothixene
(Taractan)

Thiothixene
(Navane)

The thioxanthenes are less potent than the phenothiazines though their efficacy is the same.

Chlorprothixene has moderate extrapyramidal effects, moderate to severe hypotensive and sedative effects, and has antiemetic properties.

Thiothixene can cause severe extrapyramidal effects, mild hypotension, and mild sedation. It has antiemetic effects.

C. Butyrophenones

Haloperidol
(Haldol)

Haloperidol can produce severe extrapyramidal effects, mild hypotension, and mild sedation.

D. Dibenzoxazepines

Loxapine
(Loxitane)

Loxapine can produce severe extrapyramidal effects, mild hypotension, and mild sedation.

E. Dihydroindolones

Molindone
(Moban)

Molindone can produce moderate extrapyramidal effects, mild hypotension, and moderate sedation. It also has antiemetic properties.

Antistatic Material:

Substance that cannot accumulate electrons (static charge) because of its inherent molecular makeup. Most surfaces can be made antistatic by proper coatings. *See* Capacitor.

Anuria (Anuresis):

Condition in which there is absence of urine excretion. Clinically, however, anuria is said to exist when less than 100 ml of urine is excreted daily by the average adult.

Anxiety:

Subjective feeling of uncertainty or apprehension that appears detached from, or out of proportion to, an apparent cause. Anxiety produces physiologic changes, such as hypertension, tachycardia, muscle tremors, sweating, and gastrointestinal disturbances. A patient is frequently premedicated prior to surgery in an effort to lessen anxiety. *See* Antianxiety.

Aortic Balloon:

See Cardiac Assist device.

Aortic Insufficiency:

Condition in which the aortic valve is variably incompetent and a regurgitant stream from the aorta is added to the normal ventricular filling from the left atrium. When attempting to adapt to aortic insufficiency, the left ventricle increases in wall thickness and chamber size.

Aortic Stenosis:

Narrowing of the cross-sectional area of the aortic valve. It is primarily an obstruction to ventricular emptying, causing a tremendous increase in the pressure/work the left ventricle must produce to maintain cardiac output. The area of the normal adult aortic valve is approximately 3 cm^2; the symptoms of stenosis may begin when this area falls below 1 cm^2. The left ventricular wall thickens, but the heart chamber remains the same size. This thick wall is highly vulnerable to ischemic insult.

Aortocaval Syndrome:

Group of circulatory deficiencies seen in the pregnant patient near term and possibly also in the grossly obese, patients with ascites, and patients with abdominal masses. The enlarged abdominal mass in the supine patient can partially occlude (1) the aorta (aortic compression), decreasing flow to the uterus and lower body; or (2) the inferior vena cava (inferior vena cava syndrome), decreasing blood return to the heart, thereby diminishing cardiac output (supine hypotensive syndrome). Tilting the patient to the left minimizes the compression. A mechanical uterine displacer (Kennedy displacer) may also be used.

Aperiodic Analysis of the Electroencephalogram (EEG):

Analysis technique for compression and presentation of EEG information usually associated with the name Demetrescu. EEG frequency and amplitude information is presented as a pseudo-three-dimentional plot, and color is used as one of the information parameters.

Apex Accelerometry:

Technique that determines the rate of change in velocity of heart muscle during ventricular contractility. This measurement of acceleration is correlated with aortic blood acceleration, which in turn is a reflection of cardiac contractility.

Apexcardiography:

Technique for mechanically transducing the movement of the heart through the intact chest with one simple technique, a transducer (using the skin as a diaphragm) is placed over the apex of the heart. Two modifications of apexcardiography are kinetocardiography, which attaches the sensing transducer to a fixed point in space, and cardiokymography, which uses a capacitance transducer that is held slightly separated from the skin.

Apgar Score:

Scoring system for evaluating the condition of a newborn infant. The five factors that determine the Apgar score are heart rate, respiratory effect, muscle tone, reflex irritability, and color. All five factors are rated on a scale of 0–2, with the best possible score 10, and the worst 0. Usually, active efforts at resuscitation are required in infants with an Apgar score below 5. Taken at 1 and 5 minutes after delivery, the score appears to correlate well with long-term outcome. The mnemonic for APGAR is: appearance, pulse, grimace (reflex irritability), activity, respiration. *See* Table.

Apgar score.

Sign	0	1	2
Heart rate	Absent	Slow (<100)	>100
Respiratory effort	Absent	Weak Cry; Hypoventilation	Good; Strong Cry
Muscle tone	Limp	Some Flexion of Extremities	Well Flexed
Reflex irritability	No Response	Some Motion	Cry
Color	Blue; Pale	Body Pink; Extremities Blue	Completely Pink

Apnea:

Absence of respiration.

Apneic Oxygenation (Diffusion Respiration; Apneic Diffusion Oxygenation):

Physiologic finding pertaining to respiration. A healthy patient denitrogenated by 100% O_2 can maintain arterial O_2 saturation while paralyzed and apneic if left connected to the O_2 source. Experimentally, periods of apnea of 30–55 minutes have been tolerated in humans. The maintenance of hemoglobin saturation has been ascribed to the mass movement of O_2 down the trachea following the pressure gradient from the reservoir bag (760 mm Hg PO_2) to the cells (40–60 mm Hg PO_2). CO_2 builds up because its pressure gradient in the reverse direction is much less. This buildup limits the technique because pH falls to low levels. The

65

concept of apneic oxygenation is the basis for ventilating respirator patients with 100% O_2 before suctioning.

Apneustic Breathing:

Breathing pattern characterized by a prolonged inspiratory plateau. Inspiration may be maintained for as long as 30 seconds. Pontine infarction is a common cause. *See* Biot breathing.

Apneustic Center:

See Respiratory Centers.

Apomorphine:

Chemical derivative of morphine used primarily to induce vomiting. After subcutaneous administration, nausea, salivation, and vomiting occur within a few minutes. Because, like morphine, it can produce central nervous system depression, it must be used with care in the already unconscious patient. (Precautions must be taken for securing the airway to prevent aspiration.)

APP:

See Plasmapheresis.

Apparent Death:

State of complete interruption of all bodily processes from which the patient can be restored or resuscitated to independent function.

Aprotinin:

Naturally occurring enzyme inhibitor. It is usually derived commercially from bovine lungs. It acts on plasmin, trypsin, and tissue kallikrein. It is used to slow down blood loss and reduce homologous blood requirements, as it reduces thrombotic and fibrinolytic activity.

APRV:

See Airway pressure release ventilation.

APSF:

See Anesthesia Patient Safety Foundation.

Arachnoiditis:

Inflammation of the arachnoid, which is the membrane located between the dura mater and the pia mater, covering the brain and spinal cord. It is separated from the pia mater by the subarachnoid space. Arachnoiditis is one of the most feared complications of spinal anesthesia, as the inflammation can become adhesive and strangle nerve trunks or the spinal cord itself. *See* Arachnoiditis, chronic adhesive; Cauda equina syndrome.

Arachnoiditis, Chronic Adhesive:

Pathologic condition in which congestion and thickening of the dura mater occur along with adhesions to the spinal cord and nerves. With advanced forms the cord, nerve, and blood vessels are strangulated. This condition can occur as a result of nonspecific, relatively minor spinal cord injuries and may be caused anesthetically by the inadvertent injection of toxic or contaminated materials during a spinal block. *See* Arachnoiditis.

Aramine:

See Metaraminol.

Archimedes Principle:

Principle stating that a body floating in a fluid displaces a weight of fluid equal to its own weight.

ARDS:

See Adult respiratory distress syndrome.

Arduan:

See Pipecuronium.

Area Under the Curve (AUC):

Area bounded by the x-axis and y axis and the plotted curve of information points. A numeric value can be given to this area by cutting and weighing the AUC or by the mathematic techniques of trapezoidal rule or integration. The AUC is useful for comparing the metabolism of two drugs if plasma levels (x) and time of sampling (y) are known.

Arfonad:

See Trimethaphan.

Argon:

Inert gaseous element found in the atmosphere. It is obtained commercially by the differential fractionalization of liquid air. The gas has been used experimentally in studies of anesthetic potency.

Armored Endotracheal Tube:

Endotracheal tube usually composed of latex or, more recently, Silastic. It has a stainless steel or nylon spring incorporated into the wall to prevent kinking. These tubes follow the shape of the airway in even the most unusual positions and almost invariably require a stylet for placement because of their flexible nature. *See* Endotracheal tube.

Arnold-Chiari Deformity:

Congenital anomaly in which the tonsils of the cerebellum and the medulla oblongata protrude through the foramen magnum into the spinal canal. This malformation blocks cerebrospinal fluid outflow from the fourth ventricle and causes hydrocephalus. *See* Figure.

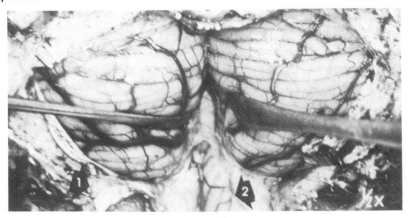

Arnold-Chiari Deformity: Gross specimen of the Arnold-Chiari malformation. Note thickened meninges (1) and the abnormally low cerebellar tonsils (2) projecting into the cervical canal.

Arousal Response:

See Habituation.

Arousal Values:

See Habituation.

Arrhythmia:

Irregularity of the heartbeat or the pulse rate. The normal rhythm can become irregular owing to heart disease, anoxia, or catecholamine stimulation. *See* Figure. *See* Atrial fibrillation; Atrial flutter; Electrocardiogram; Ventricular fibrillation.

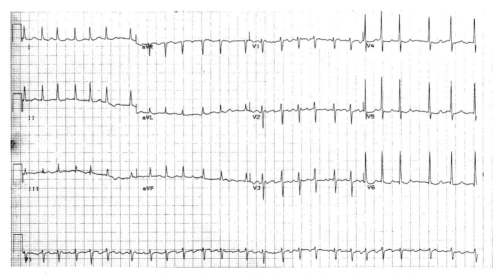

Arrhythmia: A 12-lead ECG showing atrial fibrillation with rapid ventricular response.

Arterial Blood Pressure:

Pressure of the blood on the walls of the arteries. This pressure is contingent on the force of contraction of the heart, the elasticity of the arterial walls, and the volume and viscosity of the blood. Sampling site, sampling technique, and equipment used also cause variation in the absolute value of the arterial pressure obtained. This pressure is measured in terms of millimeters of mercury above atmospheric pressure. As a measurement, it is considered one of the "vital signs." In the supine patient, arterial pressure measured in the leg is 10 to 20 mm Hg higher than arterial pressure measured in the arm. This difference is due, in part, to a complex resonance phenomenon in the aorta in which each new pressure wave is reinforced by echoes in the fluid column caused by the preceding waves. The numeric value of "normal" resting blood pressure in adults is controversial. It is generally accepted, however, that diastolic pressures above 90 mm Hg and systolic pressures above 160 mm Hg are abnormal and require investigation. *See* Table. *See* Central venous pressure; Diastolic pressure; Hypertension, Hypotension; Mean arterial pressure; Systolic pressure.

Arterial Pressure Determination by Palpation:

System based on palpating an artery proximal to which a blood pressure cuff is inflated and slowly deflated, with the pressure of the cuff being monitored by a gauge or mercury column. The systolic pressure is read when the first pulse is felt. Systolic measurements are usually slightly lower than those determined by listening for Korotkoff sounds. The cuff adds a resistance drop, which lowers the pressure distal to it. Diastolic pressures are not obtainable by this method. *See* Arterial blood pressure.

Arterialization for Blood Sampling:

Procedure done when direct puncture of an artery for a blood sample is contraindicated or impossible, particularly in infants. It entails heating a skin site to maximize its capillary blood flow, followed by a skin stick. The rapidly flowing blood, not having time to equilibrate with the tissue as to PO_2, PCO_2, and pH, approximates arterial blood in these parameters. The pH is the most accurate determination obtained from this type of sampling.

Arterialization of Blood:

Process by which venous blood receives O_2 from the alveolar gas and in turn gives up CO_2 in the lungs. *See* Figure.

Arteriole:

Final branches of the arterial system just proximal to a capillary. The walls of arterioles contain smooth muscle capable of contracting sufficiently to cut off flow completely. They can also dilate to several times their normal size. They are the major source of vascular resistance and account for 60–70% of total peripheral resistance. Well supplied with alpha receptors, they are a primary site of action for norepinephrine and its antagonists. *See* Figure.

Arteriovenous Capillary:

See Microcirculation.

Arterial Blood Pressure: Methods of determining blood pressure.

Method	Equipment Needed	Technique	Advantages and Disadvantages

Auscultation	1. Inflatable bladder with attached pressure gauge (blood pressure cuff and sphygmomanometer).	1. Cuff is wrapped snugly around upper arm and inflated by air pressure to a pressure high enough to collapse artery through entire cardiac cycle. Stethoscope head is placed over distal artery segment and pressure is slowly released. A distinctive rushing sound is heard over the artery as the cuff pressure drops below systolic pressure. These sounds continue changing in quality until the pressure is so low that the artery is open during all the cardiac cycle. These sounds then disappear. The sounds are called Korotkoff sounds (frequency range approximately 4 to 50 hz).	1. Cuff width should be 20% greater than the diameter of the arm (1/3 circumference).
			  a) A cuff too wide gives false low readings.
			  b) A cuff too narrow gives false high readings.
			2. Technique is more accurate for systolic than diastolic measurement.
			3. Confusion can occur because Korotkoff sounds are often "lost" for three or four heart beats after they are first heard and with cuff pressure still dropping. This poorly understood phenomenon is called the "auscultatory gap".
			4. Sounds may be too low to be heard during periods of low pressure.

Oscillation (Oscillotonometrics)	1. Inflatable bladder with attached pressure gauge (blood pressure cuff and sphygmomanometer).	1. As above, except movement of pressure gauge needle is observed. For oscillations with artery completely occluded, these movements are small. As blood first spurts past the deflating cuff, oscillations increase. This point is regarded as systolic pressure. The point at which oscillations are maximal is considered mean pressure. Diastolic pressure is poorly perceived by this method.	1. Most accurately done with a double cuff apparatus (Riva-Rocci). 2. Not easily done consistently by different examiners. 3. The concept is easily automated by electrically transducing the cuff pressure oscillations (Dinamap™).

Method	Description	Comments
Palpation	1. As above	1. The most straightforward method. 2. Diastolic endpoint not ascertainable.
	1. As above, except a palpating finger is placed over a distal artery and the first pulse felt is considered the systolic pressure.	
Photoelectric	1. As above	1. Detects change in light transmitted from skin surface by color change of each pulse beat.
	1. A light source and photocell replaces the palpating finger (usually placed on wrist or finger).	
Doppler Ultrasound	1. Blood pressure cuff and pressure gauge and Doppler Ultrasound crystal receiver.	1. The Doppler device is technically sophisticated and relatively expensive. 2. Ascertaining diastolic pressure requires even more sophisticated electric equipment and repeatability is open to question.
	1. As above, except that Doppler technique is used to detect distal arterial wall movement instead of a palpating finger.	
Arterial Puncture	1. Percutaneous catheter directly cannulating an artery interfaced to a transducer via a fluid path.	1. An invasive technique with known morbidity. 2. Inherently very accurate but open to many technical problems such as clotting, kinking.
	1. The arterial pressure is interfaced to a fluid path which affects the output of a pressure transducer proportionally.	
Very Low Frequency Sound (Infrasound)	1. Cuff and electronic stethoscope.	1. Most accurate at low pressures (pediatrics).
	1. Automated apparatus which detects Korotkoff sounds too low in frequency to be heard.	

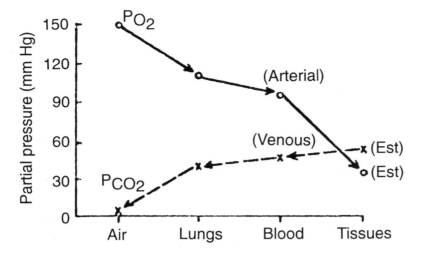

| Gas | ml/dl of Blood Containing 15 g of Hemoglobin | | | |
| | Arterial Blood (P_{O_2} 95 mm Hg; P_{CO_2} 40 mm Hg; Hb 97% Saturated) | | Venous Blood (P_{O_2} 40 mm Hg; P_{CO_2} 46 mm Hg; Hb 75% Saturated) | |
	Dissolved	Combined	Dissolved	Combined
O_2	0.29	19.5	0.12	15.1
CO_2	2.62	46.4	2.98	49.7
N_2	0.98	0	0.98	0

Arterialization of Blood: Gas content of blood.

Artificial Hibernation:

Drug-induced state of dormancy characterized by reduced metabolism, muscle relaxation, and a twilight sleep resembling narcosis. High doses of phenothiazines and narcotics are used. This state theoretically renders the patient insensitive to pain without gross alteration of the vital signs. However, in practice, achieving this state (without overshoot to cardiovascular or respiratory collapse) is extremely difficult. *See* Lytic cocktail.

Artificial Neural-Networks:

Technique of computer hardware and software that mimics the simpler architecture of the brain in electronic terms. These networks can be "trained" to detect and identify various patterns of transduced signals.

Artificial Nose:

See Airway heat and moisture exchanger.

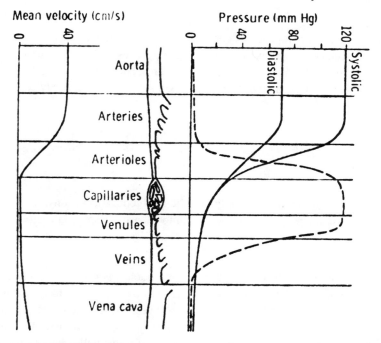

Arteriole: Diagrammatic representation of changes in velocity and pressure as blood flows through the systemic circulation. The dashed line indicates the total cross-sectional area of the vessels; 4.5 cm^2 in the aorta to 4500 cm^2 in the capillaries.

Artificial Pneumothorax:

Deliberate introduction of air (under sterile conditions) into the pleural cavity to collapse the lung. An obsolete treatment for tuberculosis to "rest the lung."

Aryepiglottic Folds:

See Laryngospasm.

Arytenoid Cartilage:

Paired cartilages that occupy the upper surface of the lamina of the cricoid cartilage to which the posterior ends of the vocal cords are attached. Important for speech, they can be damaged relatively easily by intubation. *See* Cricoid cartilage; Larynx.

ASA:

See American Society of Anesthesiologists.

ASA Physical Status Classifications:

See Physical status classifications, ASA.

Asbestos:

Fibrous mineral composed of combinations of silicon, magnesium, and O_2. Because of its heat resistance and acoustic dampening properties, it has been used extensively for the manufacture of fabrics, paper, insulating boards, and wall covering. Known as a potent lung carcinogen when inhaled over prlonged periods, its use is severely curtailed.

ASD:

See Atrial septal defect.

Asphyxia:

State that denies a normal supply of O_2 to the blood. It is synonymous with suffocation. In the practice of anesthesia, the most common cause of asphyxia is airway obstruction.

Aspiration:

Introduction of any foreign matter into the trachea and upper airways. The aspiration of stomach contents remains one of the most serious complications of anesthesia. It is usually brought about by the reflux of material up the esophagus and the obtundation of the airway reflexes that normally seal the upper airways against reflux. Aspiration pneumonitis (Mendelson syndrome) results when the material actually reaches the bronchioles. The severity of injury depends primarily on the pH of the gastric contents. Other factors are volume, particulate matter, and bacterial count. Above pH 2.5, little injury occurs beyond that caused by airway closure by solid or liquid blockage. Below pH 2.5, however, there is direct toxic injury to the lining of the air passageways, causing an immediate exudation of fluid, bronchospasm, and severe ventilation/perfusion abnormalities.

Aspiration Pneumonitis:

See Aspiration.

Aspirin:

See Acetylsalicylic acid.

Assault:

Seemingly violent attempt or willful offer (with violence or force) to do harm to another person, without actually doing the harm threatened. Assault is one of the grounds for malpractice suits. *See* Battery.

Assist/Control Ventilation:

Mechanical ventilating technique that combines assisted mechanical ventilation (AMV) and controlled mechanical ventilation (CMV). The ventilator is triggered by whichever comes first: a spontaneous inspiratory effort or by a timing device, timing out. In this configuration, controlled mechanical ventilation acts as a backup if the patient becomes apneic. *See* Assisted mechanical ventilation, Ventilator.

Assisted Breathing:

See Ventilation, assisted.

Assisted Mechanical Ventilation (AMV):

More properly referred to as patient-triggered mechanical positive-pressure ventilation. It refers to the type of mechanical ventilation for which the patient (by creating a negative airway pressure) must initiate an inspiratory flow from the ventilator. It may be used as a weaning technique from mechanical ventilation. It can be dangerous, as nondetection of spontaneous breathing or lack of spontaneous breathing can lead to hypoxia. *See* Ventilator.

Association of Anesthesiology Program Directors (AAPD):

Membership in this association is open to chairmen of departments of anesthesiology that have an anesthesiology residency program accredited by the Accreditation Council for Graduate Medical Education (ACGME). The association had 159 members at the beginning of the decade of the 1990s. This association's main objective is to provide a forum for discussion and development of education, finance, and administrative policies concerning graduate medical education in anesthesiology. AAPD is headquartered in Park Ridge, Illinois. *See* Society of Academic Anesthesia Chairmen (SAAC).

Association of University Anesthesiologists:

Organization formed to promote research in teaching in the specialty of anesthesia. Founded in Philadelphia in 1953, the organization started out the decade of the 1990s with nearly 600 members. Membership is open to anesthesia faculty of affiliated teaching hospitals in the United States and Canada and is headquartered in Seattle, Washington.

Asthma:

Disease characterized by various degrees of bronchial constriction, thickened secretions, increased work of ventilation, wheezing, and impaired gas exchange. The duration of an asthmatic attack may be from a few minutes to many hours, in which case it is referred to as *status asthmaticus*. The latter may be severe enough to threaten life. Attacks appear to be triggered by airway irritation, which can be environmental (airborne pollen) or iatrogenic (anesthetic vapors). An asthmatic attack is a feared complication during the induction of anesthesia.

Asystole:

Lack of cardiac contraction; standstill of the heart.

Atelectasis:

Collapse of the lung caused by bronchial obstruction or external compression. This collapse may affect only a lobe (lobar atelectasis) or a specific segment (segmental atelectasis) of the lung. The blockage may be due to bronchial exudate, foreign bodies, tumor, lymph nodes, or aneurysms compressing the bronchi, or to bronchial distortions. Atelectasis may also be brought about by loss of surfactant such that the fluid lining of the alveoli develops a significant surface tension and literally pulls the alveoli in on themselves. *Patchy atelectasis* is a term used to describe small, diffuse, radiopaque areas seen on a chest roentgenogram that represent collapsed alveoli. Primary atelectasis describes a lung that has not expanded at birth. *See* Figure.

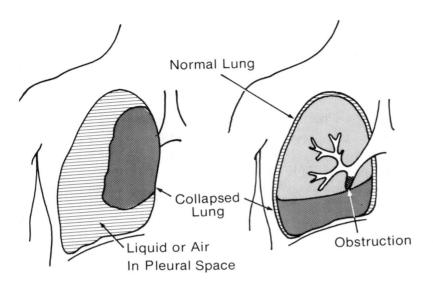

Atelectasis: Atelectasis produced by external compression (left) and bronchial obstruction (right).

Atelectasis, Absorption:

See Absorption atelectasis.

Atelectatic Shunt:

See Shunt.

Ativan:

See Benzodiazepine.

Atmosphere:

Gaseous medium that envelops the earth. At sea level, it exerts a uniform pressure equal to 760 mm Hg.

Atomic Number:

See Nucleus, atomic.

ATP:

See Adenosine triphosphate

Atracurium:

Nondepolarizing muscle relaxant of intermediate duration of action. It is a distant derivative of d-tubocurarine.

Atrial Fibrillation:

Cardiac arrhythmia in which the atria randomly contract at a high rate. *See* Figure.

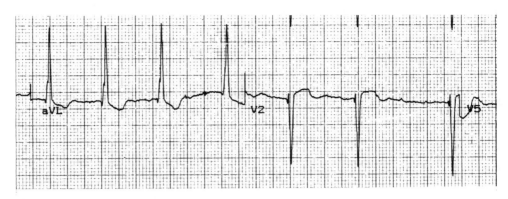

Atrial Fibrillation: Rhythm strip.

Atrial Flutter:

Cardiac arrhythmia in which the atria contract at a rapid but regular rate, ranging from 200 to 300 times/minute. *See* Figure.

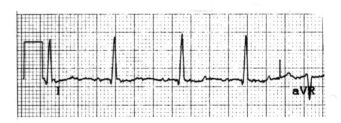

Atrial Flutter: Rhythm strip.

Atrial Septal Defect (ASD):

Congenital heart anomaly characterized by a patent atrial septum. ASDs are described according to their position in the septum and their embryologic origin. Secundum defects are in the area of the fossa ovalis and result from failure of the septum secundum to develop. Ostium primum defects occur in the lower portion of the septum. Other less common ASDs occur as well. Frequently infants and children have minimal or no symptoms; however, surgical correction is recommended during childhood. *See* Endocardial cushion defect, Ventricular septal defect.

Atrioventricular Bundle:

See Heart, conduction system of.

Atrioventricular Node:

See Heart, conduction system of.

Atropine:

Naturally occurring alkaloid originally prepared from the belladonna plant (deadly nightshade). As an anticholinergic, atropine (in large doses): (1) blocks the parasympathetic-mediated vagal effect on the adult heart causing tachycardia in the range of 115–120 (increased sympathetic nervous system activity can further increase heart rate); (2) inhibits salivary secretion, causing mouth dryness and difficulty swallowing; and (3) decreases gastric secretion and gastrointestinal motility. In small doses it may incite central vagal stimulation, causing bradycardia. In large, nonpharmacologic doses, it can cause central nervous system excitation and frank seizure activity. At any dosage, its effects are of short duration. *See* Figure.

$$H_2C\text{---}CH\text{---}CH_2 \quad CH_2OH$$
$$\text{NCH}_3 \quad CH\text{-}O\text{-}\overset{\overset{O}{\|}}{C}\text{-}CH$$
$$H_2C\text{---}CH\text{---}CH_2 \quad C_6H_5$$

Atropine.

Atenolol:

Drug that is a beta-blocker, similar to metoprolol. It is relatively cardio-selective and has no intrinsic sympathomimetic effect or membrane stabilizing effect.

AUC:

See Area under the curve.

Auditory Evoked Potential (AEP):

Evoked potential caused by stimulating the auditory nerve. The early part of the AEP tracing is called the brainstem auditory evoked potential (BAEP). *See* Evoked potential.

Autocoids:

See Prostaglandin.

Autologous:

Coming from one's self. For example, an autologous blood transfusion is one in which patient gave his or her own blood and it was stored up to 1 month earlier. Autologous blood is used therapeutically in cases of spinal headache. *See* Autologous blood; Epidural patch; Spinal headache. *See* Transplantation.

Autologous Blood:

Blood storage technique in which a potential surgical patient donates his or her own blood preoperatively for possible transfusion during the perioperative period. Most reasonably healthy patients can donate up to three units at 7- to 10-day intervals. *See* Autologous; Blood storage; Blood types; Type and crossmatch; Type and screen.

Automated Analysis Instrument
(Sequential Multiple Analyzer: SMA 1260; SMA 660):

Device that determines on a single serum sample levels of electrolytes, enzymes, cholesterol, or inorganic ions. Usually the tests are based on reaching a particular color intensity after appropriate chemical reactions with a small portion of the sample. The exceptions are those tests that require ion-specific electrodes. The SMA 1260 can run 12 tests/sample, 60 samples/hour.

Automated Anesthesia Record:

Technique for maintaining an anesthetic record by means of an automatic writer that routinely enters on a preprinted form values from various patient monitors. Several forms of this device have been available for a number of years. They have not so far seen widespread use because of concerns about their ability to reject artifact without continuous oversight. *See* Figure.

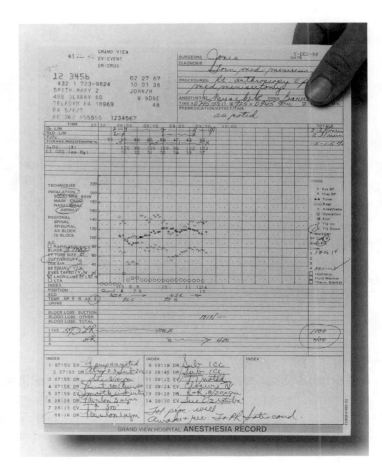

Automated Anesthesia Record: Illustration of a prototypical Automated Record.

Automated Cell Counter:

Device that determines a precise count of a desired cellular element in a sample of blood. Usually the sample is pretreated to destroy rather than count all unwanted cellular elements. Two types of automated cell counter exist. The electro-optical counter (e.g., Technicon Autocounter) utilizes a photomultiplier tube to detect light bounced from cells. The voltage pulse machine (e.g., Coulter counter) counts cells as they change electrolyte conductivity by moving between two electrodes immersed in that electrolyte.

Automatic Baseline Centering:

Electronic modality (available on oscilloscopic displays of the electrocardiogram) in which the machine centers the trace on its screen without intervention of the operator.

Automatic Blood Pressure Device (Dinamap^{TM}):

Automatic device that uses the oscillometric method to determine blood pressure. *See* Figure.

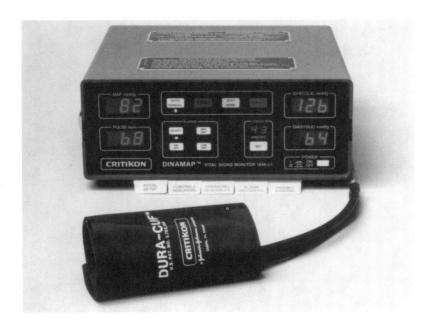

Automatic Blood Pressure Device (Dinamap^{TM}): Blood pressure monitor, Model 1846SX.

Automatic Implantable Cardioverter—Defibrillator (AICD):

An implantable device for the treatment of patients with malignant ventricular tachydysrhythmias that are otherwise refractory to more conventional forms of therapy. The device functions to detect and cardiovert these dysrhythmias automatically. *See* Pacemaker.

Autonomic Hyper-Reflexia:

See Mass reflex.

Autonomic Nervous System:

Part of the central nervous system that controls the involuntary functions of the body, including regulation of the heart, blood vessels, smooth muscles, and many glands. The autonomic nervous system consists of two parts that balance and antagonize each other, the sympathetic and parasympathetic systems. Because sympathetic nervous system activity is mediated by the release and uptake of epinephrine, norepinephrine, and related adrenergic hormones, it is sometimes called the adrenergic nervous system. (Two apparent exceptions, the sweat glands and the adrenal medulla, although activated by the sympathetic nervous system, are controlled by acetylcholine release.) Because parasympathetic nervous system activity is mediated by the release of acetylcholine, it is also known as the cholinergic nervous system. *See* Figure and Table. *See* Central nervous system; Cranial nerves; Receptor/receptor site.

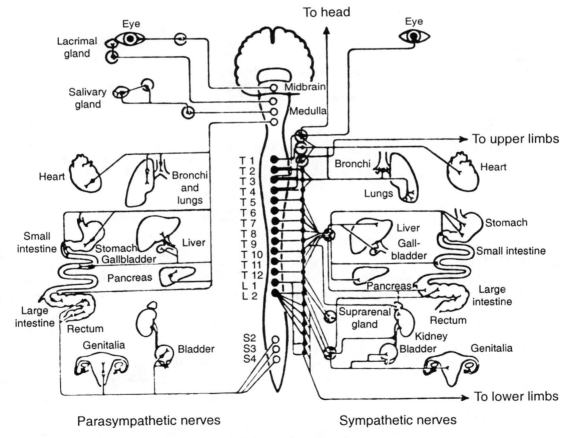

Autonomic Nervous System: Autonomic innervation of various organs.

Autonomic Nervous System: Selected actions of the autonomic nervous system.

Site of Effector Cells	Activation of Sympathetic Division (Thoracolumbar) Tends to:	Activation of Para-sympathetic Division (Craniosacral) Tends to:
Heart	Increase rate and output	Decrease rate and output
Coronary arteries	Dilate	Dilate
Blood vessels in nose, salivary glands, and pharynx	Constrict	Dilate
Cutaneous vessels	Constrict	
Bronchi	Dilate	Constrict
Gastrointestinal motility and secretion	Decrease peristalsis and muscle tone; constrict sphincters	Increase; relax sphincters
Glycogenolysis by the liver	Increase	
Glands	Decrease secretion	Increase secretion
Sweat glands	Increase (some authorities classify this as parasym-pathetic function)	
Pupil of eye	Dilate	Constrict
Ciliary muscles	Lessen tone, eyes accommodate to see at a distance	Contract ciliary muscle, eyes accommodate to see near objects
Mental activity	Increase	

Auto-PEEP:

Phenomenon seen during mechanical ventilation when positive pressure is present at end-expiration *without* being deliberately caused. It usually is due to a too short expiratory time.

Autoregulation:

Ability of tissue, in relation to circulation, to maintain constant blood flow despite variations in mean arterial blood pressures. Normal cerebral circulation offers the most striking example of autoregulation in that the cerebral blood flow will remain unchanged between mean arterial pressures of 60 mm Hg to at least 160 mm Hg. The kidney also autoregulates at a range of 10–15 mm Hg higher than the brain. In hypertensive individuals the range of autoregulation rises. All halogenated hydrocarbon anesthetics increase cerebral blood flow

(CBF) and abolish cerebral autoregulation. Hypercapnia increases CBF and overrides autoregulation, whereas hypocapnia decreases CBF but also overrides autoregulation. *See* Cerebral blood flow, Intracranial pressure measurement.

Average:

Value that is typical of or represents a set of values. In common usage, it is identified with the arithmetic mean or the sum of all the values in a set divided by the number of values within that set.

Avertin:

See Rectal anesthesia.

Avogadro Number:

Number of molecules contained in 1 mole of substance. It is expressed as 6.02×10^{23}.

Awareness:

Taking note of one's surroundings, it includes being watchful, informed, and vigilant. Awareness is relative to the idea of the awake state of a patient who is totally paralyzed and given a general anesthetic. One of the more controversial concepts in anesthesia, it has been demonstrated that a patient can be "aware" during general anesthesia but has little or no memory of surgery or being in the operating room. On the other hand, it is a potential tragedy if a patient does not appear awake or aware in the operating room and yet has memory of surgical procedures and pain. *See* Isolated forearm technique.

Axillary Nerve Block:

Name of a particular approach to anesthetizing the brachial plexus, it is the most popular approach because of the ease of technique and its reliability for hand and forearm anesthesia. It is also a safe approach, as the incidence of pneumothorax is low. It is not suitable for surgical procedures on the upper arm or shoulder. The technique involves injecting of a local anesthetic solution in the sheath surrounding the axillary artery high up in the axilla. Several methods,including localization by paresthesias,have been suggested. *See* Supraclavicular block.

Axon:

Part of a neuron that transmits impulses away from a cell body. *See* Action potential; Depolarization.

Axoplasm:

Cytoplasm of a nerve axon.

Ayre T-Piece: (A)Modifications to the T-piece.

Name	Shape*	Patient Limb Diameter	Expiratory Limb Diameter	Dealers	Comment
Ayre T-piece		10 mm or 12.5 mm	10 mm or 12.5 mm	Dupaco Foregger	
Bissonnette		15 mm	Small 3/8" Large 1/2"	Dupaco Foregger	To facilitate attachment to endotracheal tube.
T-piece mask		25 mm OD	10 mm	Dupaco	Can accommodate mask or endotracheal tube.
Summers T-tube		15 mm ID	15 mm OD	Dupaco	Fresh gas flow directed toward patient by shape of inlet tube.
Norman mask elbow (Norman elbow)		22 mm OD 15 mm ID	15 mm OD	Dupaco	Gas inlet ends 9/16" above mask fitting, reducing dead space. Fresh gas feed blows jet of gas into the mask. Dead space with a 3 L/min flow is 0.2 ml.
Fletcher T-tube		15 mm ID	15 mm ID	Dupaco	Fresh gas inflow tube is bent 90° after leaving tube.
Washington T-tube		15 mm ID	15 mm OD	Dupaco	Used with male-female sequence of fittings.

	Dimensions		Manufacturer	Notes
Rabbit ears	15 mm ID	3/4 or 7/16" OD	Anesthesia Associates	
Magill connection	4 mm OD and 2.5 mm ID or 5 mm OD and 3 mm ID		Anesthesia Associates	
Keets modification of Hanks-Rackow elbow (Keets type Hanks-Rackow elbow)	22 mm OD 15 mm ID	15 mm OD	Anesthesia Associates	Fits endotracheal tube. Patient end 90° to Y.
Hanks-Rackow elbow with side inlet	22 mm OD 15 mm ID	15 mm OD	Anesthesia Associates	Modified to blow a jet of gas into the mask. Fresh gas inlet at side or top.
Neoprene modified Ayre T-tube	22 mm OD 15 mm ID	15 mm OD	Anesthesia Associates	Gas inflow tube does not extend into lumen at side or top.

Ayre T-Piece: (A) (continued)

Name	Shape	Patient Limb Diameter	Expiratory Limb Diameter	Dealers	Comment
NRPR elbow (Non-rebreathing pressure relieving elbow) (Hustead Elbow)		15 mm ID 22 mm OD	15 mm ID 22 mm OD	Puritan-Bennett Corporation	Modified to blow a jet of fresh gas into the mask. Bag can be connected directly to elbow. Pressure relief outlet on top of elbow. Dead space with a 3 L/min flow is 0.2 ml.

*P, patient limb; E, expiratory limb: and I, fresh gas inlet limb.

Ayre T-Piece: (B) Modifications to the expiratory limb of the T-piece system.

Equipment	Functional Analysis	Reference
Double-ended bag is fitted to the expiratory limb. The open end of the bag is fitted with an adjustable tap. Corrugated tubing is often used between the T-piece and bag.	Bag allows breathing to be assisted or controlled and spontaneous breathing to be monitored. The tap is adjusted so that intermittent pressure applied to the bag expels the amount of gas required to maintain the equilibrium of the system.	Jackson-Rees G: Anaesthesia in the newborn. Br. Med. J. 2:1419–1422, 1950.
Two T-pieces are used: one at the patient end and one between the reservoir tube and the bag.	If fresh gas flow is delivered to the proximal T-piece, the system functions similar to the Jackson-Rees modification. To control respiration, the anesthesiologist's thumb is put over the sidearm of the distal T-piece. This system may also be used as a Magill system if fresh gas flow is delivered to the distal T-piece.	Baraka A, Brandstater B, Muallem, M, et al.: Rebreathing in a double T-piece system. Br. J. Anaesth. 41:47–53, 1969.
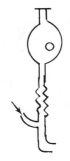 The bag contains two exits–flap valve on bag and an adjustable tap.	For assisted or controlled ventilation, the adjustable tap is closed and the flap valve is covered by the anesthesiologist's thumb during inspiration.	Davenport HT. Pereze E: Infant anesthesia set. Anesthesiology 21:776, 1960.

87

Ayre T-Piece:(B) (continued)

Equipment	Functional Analysis	Reference
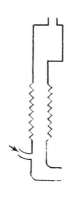 Georgia valve is attached proximal to the breathing bag. Bag is closed ended.	During spontaneous respiration, the valve remains open. When the breathing bag is compressed, the sudden increase in pressure closes the valve.	Freifeld S: Modification of the Ayre T-piece system. Anesth. Analg. 42:575–577, 1963.
Nonexpansile hose leading to ventilator is attached to expiratory limb of the T-piece.	Ventilator supplies positive pressure during inspiration.	Kuwabara S, McCaughey TJ: Artificial ventilation in infants and young children using a new ventilator with the T-piece. Can. Anaesth. Soc. J. 13:576–584, 1966.
		Munson ES, Eger EI: Controlled ventilation in the newborn. Anesthesiology 24:871–872, 1963.
		Smith C: Controlled ventilation employing a modified Ayre's technic. Anesth. Analg. 44:842–845. 1965.

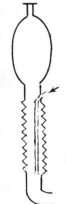

The fresh gas inflow tubing is incorporated inside the exhalation limb.

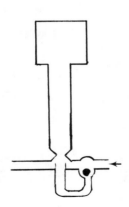

Fresh gas flow is divided into portions: one going directly to the patient, the other into the Venturi-shaped outlet. Position of stopcock determines relative flow to each.

Manual compression of the bag may be used, or a respirator can be attached for controlled or assisted ventilation.

The flow through Venturi outlet provides a negative pressure during expiration. Position of stopcock regulates amount of negative pressure. Ventilator may be attached to provide positive pressure during inspiration.

Bain JA, Spoerel WE: A streamlined anaesthetic system. Can. Anaesth. Soc. J. 19:426-435. 1972.

Keuskamp DHG: Automatic ventilation in paediatric anaesthesia using a modified Ayre's T-piece with negative pressure during expiratory phase. Anaesthesia 18:46-56, 1963.

Ayre T-Piece:

Apparatus used to modify standard anesthesia equipment in pediatric cases. The prime purpose of the Ayre device is to prevent the pediatric patient from expending excessive energy, which would be the case if the valved adult circuit were used. Many modifications of the Ayre T-piece system have been made. At the same time, by supplying high flows, nonrebreathing of expired gas may be accomplished. *See* Tables.

Azeotrope:

Physical mixture of two or more liquids that cannot be separated by distillation. Halothane and diethyl ether form an azeotrope that was used as a general anesthetic. It is no longer utilized as only slight differences in clinical effect were observed when it was compared with either agent alone, and it was a flammable mixture.

B

BAB:

See n-Butyl p-aminobenzoate.

Background Noise:

Any nonspecific unwanted random sound or electric activity.

Background Radiation:

Radiation due to radioisotopes in soil, bombardment of cosmic rays, and trace radioactive gases in the atmosphere. It must be taken into account when quantitating total radiation dose. *See* Electromagnetic spectrum.

BAEP:

See Auditory evoked potential.

Bain Circuit:

Popular modification of the Mapleson D system that uses a coaxial fresh gas inflow hose internal to a corrugated expiratory hose. Used for both controlled and spontaneous ventilation, this circuit is flexible, lightweight and convenient. Possible problems occur with disconnection or kinking of the inner tube. *See* Ayre T-piece.

Bainbridge Reflex:

Phenomenon demonstrated best in laboratory animals and seen inconstantly in humans. It occurs when a rapid infusion of intravenous fluids increases a low resting heart rate.

Balanced Anesthesia (Combined Anesthesia):

Term introduced in 1926 that refers to the induction of anesthesia using a combination of agents, each for its specific effect, rather than using a single agent with multiple effects. Diethyl ether inhaled with room air is the prototypic single-agent anesthetic. A combination of muscle relaxants, intravenous barbiturates, narcotics, and N_2O/O_2 is an example of balanced anesthesia, which is characterized by relaxation and unconsciousness, but not necessarily areflexia. Balanced anesthesia has been disparagingly referred to as "garbage anesthesia" because of the ease with which the drug combinations may change depending on which drugs are readily available in a particular operating room on a particular day.

Ballast:

See Fluorescent lamp.

Ballistocardiograph:

Device used to record the movement of the entire body caused by the movement of the heart during contraction. Laboratory techniques exist to convert these body movements into a direct readout of cardiac output.

Balloon Pumping:

See Intraaortic balloon pump.

Bandwidth:

The range within a band of wavelengths, frequencies, or energies. *See* Frequency.

Bar:

A unit of pressure equal to 10^6 dynes/cm^2. It is roughly the air pressure measured at mean sea level, which is actually 1.013250×10^6 dyne/cm^2.

Baralyme:

Trade name for barium hydroxide lime. *See* Carbon dioxide absorption; Carbon dioxide absorption canister; Soda lime.

Barbital:

See Barbiturate.

Barbitone:

British term for barbital. *See* Barbiturate.

Barbiturate:

Class of drugs, derived from barbituric acid, that act as generalized depressants of cellular function. The first barbiturate, barbital, was introduced into clinical practice in 1903, and since then many other derivatives have been prepared by substitutions of the side chains on the basic molecule. Clinically, the onset, duration of action, and, to a lesser extent, speed of degradation are the determining factors for use of a particular barbiturate. All barbiturates have been classified as ultrashort acting, short to intermediate acting, and long acting. However, a large dose of an ultrashort acting barbiturate has an effect indistinguishable from a moderate dose of a long-acting barbiturate. *See* Table.

Barbituric Acid:

See Barbiturate.

Barbotage:

Repeated withdrawal and injection of cerebrospinal fluid mixed with a local anesthetic to ensure maximal distribution of the anesthetic.

Barbiturate: Structure of barbituric acid and classification of common barbiturates.

```
              H   O
              N———C
            1 |     | 6  H
      O=C 2  |     5 C
            3 |     | 4  H
              N———C
              H   O
```

Generic Name (Trade Name)	Substituents in Position 5	Duration of Action
Thiopental* (Pentothal)	Ethyl, 1-methylbutyl	Ultrashort
Thiamylal* (Surital)	Allyl, 1-methylbutyl	(intravenous
Hexobarbital** (Evipal)	Methyl, cyclohexenyl	anesthetics)
Secobarbital (Seconal)	Allyl, 1-methylbutyl	Short
Pentobarbital (Nembutal)	Ethyl, 1-methylbutyl	
Butabarbital (Butisol)	Ethyl, sec-butyl	Intermediate
Amobarbital (Amytal)	Ethyl, isoamyl	
Vinbarbital (Delvinal)	Ethyl, 1-methyl-1-butenyl	
Phenobarbital (Luminal)	Ethyl, phenyl	Long
Mephobarbital** (Mebaral)	Ethyl, phenyl	
Barbital (Veronal)	Ethyl, ethyl	

* Thiobarbiturate.
** A CH_3 group is attached to the nitrogen atom.

Barium Hydroxide Lime (Baralyme):

See Carbon dioxide absorption; Carbon dioxide absorption canister; Soda lime.

Barium Sulfate (BaSO₄):

Bulky, fine powder that is odorless and tasteless and is used (dissolved in water) as a contrast medium for radiology of the digestive tract. A contrast medium, by filling a hollow space, outlines and differentiates specific areas. Other barium salts, including bromide, carbonate, and chloride, were previously used in medicine for the treatment of various diseases. These practices have been discarded.

Barlow Syndrome:

See Mitral valve prolapse.

Barometer:

Instrument used to measure atmospheric pressure.

Baroreceptor (Pressure Receptor):

Stretch receptor in the walls of the heart and all large arteries. These receptors are stimulated by distention of the structures in which they are located; they discharge at an increased rate as

93

the pressure rises in these structures. Their afferent nerve fibers pass via the glossopharyngeal and vagus nerves to the vasomotor center and the cardioinhibitory center. Baroreceptor impulses inhibit vasoconstrictor nerves and excite the cardioinhibitory center, eliciting vasodilatation, a decrease in blood pressure, bradycardia, and a decreased cardiac output.

Basal Anesthesia:

Technique of giving preoperative medication beyond the point where consciousness is lost. An early technique of anesthesia that has fallen into disuse because of its dangerous consequences. It was originally advocated for children, who were likely to be frightened by the surgical suite.

Base Deficit:

See Base excess.

Base Excess (BE):

Base concentration of whole blood. It is measured in milliequivalents per liter by titrating of blood to pH 7.4 with a strong acid at PCO_2 40 mm Hg at 37°C. Negative BE values (blood deficient in base) must be titrated with a strong base. The base excess or deficit can also be derived by calculation (rather than by titration) or by using a nomogram if the pH, PCO_2, and hemoglobin concentration are known. The base excess or deficit is used clinically to determine appropriate corrections for metabolic acid-base derangements. In the case of base deficit (by far the most common), the total correction is calculated as BE × calculated extracellular fluid compartment volume (usually 25–33% of total body weight) to arrive at the milliequivalents of bicarbonate needed. Usually one-third to one-half of this amount is administered, and then acid-base status is redetermined after the body has had time to equilibrate. Complete restoration of a normal (zero) base deficit should not be attempted with a single large dose of bicarbonate because of the danger of overshoot. *See* Bernard rules.

Base:

Substance that binds hydrogen ions (H^+) when in solution. Strong bases bind H^+ much more readily than weak bases. It may be positively charged, negatively charged, or neutral. *See* Acid; Acid-base balance.

Base Units:

See Relative value guide.

Basic:

Easy-to-learn computer language that is an acronym for beginner's all-purpose symbolic instruction code.

Basic Life Support:

See Cardiopulmonary resuscitation.

Battery:

Unlawful beating of, or use of force against, another person without his or her consent. It may be grounds for a malpractice suit. *See* Assault.

Battery, Electric:

Device that in its simplest form consists of two dissimilar plates placed in an electrolyte bath. Electricity (current flow) is produced by the chemical reaction of the electrolyte on the plates. Current strength and duration depend on plate composition and size. A primary battery is one in which the electric current is produced without prior electric charging. A secondary battery must be charged by sending a current through it in the reverse direction of its discharge, which reverses the chemical reaction of the electrolyte on the metal plates. Consequently, a primary cell can deliver current immediately but cannot revert to its original state after complete discharge; the secondary cell is reversible and can be re-charged and discharged repeatedly. An example of a primary cell is the standard carbon-zinc flashlight battery; an example of a secondary cell is the rechargeable nickel-cadmium battery.

Baud:

Unit of signaling data or transmission speed; in the binary system 1 baud is equal to 1 bit/second. *See* Binary code; binary number system; Bit.

BBB:

See Blood-brain barrier.

BE:

See Base excess.

Beckman Analyzer:

See Oxygen analyzer.

Beclomethasone (Vanceril Inhaler):

Potent steroid, related to prednisolone, usually given to asthmatics in a dose-metering aerosol unit. It can be given to patients who are unsuitable for treatment with systemic steroids because of potential adverse reactions.

Bel:

Logarithmic unit of measurement comparing the ratio of two amounts of power. The most commonly used unit is the decibel (one-tenth of a bel), which measures sound intensity. A 3-decibel change upward doubles and a 3-decibel change downward halves signal strength.

Belladonna (Belladonna Alkaloids):

See Atropine.

Bends:

> *See* Caisson disease.

Benzedrine:

> *See* Amphetamine.

Benzocaine:

> Ester-type local anesthetic. It is often combined with other agents, such as tetracaine, and is useful as a topical preparation in a gel, liquid, or ointment form. *See* Local anesthetic.

Benzodiazepine:

> Class of sedative, hypnotic, antianxiety drugs. The derivative diazepam (Valium) is one of the most frequently prescribed drugs. Other examples of benzodiazepines are oxazepam (Serax), chlordiazepoxide hydrochloride (Librium), flurazepam hydrochloride (Dalmane), nitrazepam (Mogadon), and lorazepam (Ativan). The popularity of this drug class appears to stem from the fact that central nervous system depression and antianxiety action occur at dosages much lower than those causing total body cellular depression. *See* Anxiety; Midazolam.

Benzoic Acid:

> Naturally occurring acid used as a food preservative and antifungal agent.

Benzoquinonium (Mytolon):

> Neuromuscular blocking agent that combines some features of the nondepolarizing and depolarizing types. It currently has little clinical use.

Benzquinamide:

> Antiemetic drug used with limited success to control postanesthetic vomiting.

Benztropine Mesylate (Cogentin):

> Antiparkinsonian agent with atropine-like effects. It is also used for treatment of the Parkinson-like syndrome induced by the phenothiazines.

Benzyl Alcohol:

> Compound formed by combining benzene and methyl alcohol. It has some local anesthetic effects and may be useful in patients who have demonstrated sensitivity to the more common local anesthetics.

Bernard Rules:

> Three principles that govern the estimate of the appropriate change in serum bicarbonate levels when $PaCO_2$ changes. When the estimated appropriate bicarbonate level differs from the measured level, the contribution of metabolism to acid-base status can be determined. Rule 1 states that the increase in serum bicarbonate that accompanies an acute elevation in $PaCO_2$ is approximately 1 mEq/L for each 10 mm Hg rise in $PaCO_2$ over 40 mm Hg. Rule 2

states that the decrease in serum bicarbonate that accompanies an acute decline in $PaCO_2$ is approximately 2 mEq/L for each 10 mm Hg fall in $PaCO_2$ below 40 mm Hg. Rule 3 states that the increase in serum bicarbonate that accompanies a chronic increase in $PaCO_2$ is approximately 4 mEq/L for each 10 mm Hg increase in $PaCO_2$ above 40 mm Hg.

Bernoulli Law:

Relationship of velocity of fluid flow to cross-sectional diameter in a horizontal pipe. Stated simply, a fluid gains speed as it passes from a wide to a narrow portion of the pipe. Conversely, the pressure is lowest where the velocity is highest and vice versa. If a horizontal pipe contains a constriction and then opens out to its original diameter slowly, the fluid slows but regains its original pressure. This situation describes a Venturi tube. The Venturi tube generates a negative pressure at the constriction. The relation between the negative pressure at the constriction and the positive pressure upstream can be related to flow. This pressure difference is used to measure gas flow in the water depression flow-meter.

Beta₁, Beta₂ Adrenergic Agent:

See Receptor/receptor site.

Beta-Blocker:

Class of pharmaceutical agents that act by competitively antagonizing the action of beta stimulating drugs. *See* Isoproterenol; Receptor/receptor site.

Beta-Endorphin:

See Endorphins.

Beta Particle:

Rapidly moving, energetic electron or positron emitted by some radioisotopes during decay. Each element capable of beta decay emits beta particles over a characteristic range of energies. *See* Alpha particle, Gamma ray.

Betamethasone:

Potent glucocorticoid, often encountered as a topical preparation.

Bethanechol:

See Methylcholine.

Bethanechol Chloride (Urecholine):

Parasympathomimetic drug (not destroyed by cholinesterase) that has a specific effect on the smooth muscles of the gastrointestinal tract and urinary bladder. It is used to treat postoperative abdominal distention (due to loss of muscle tone and impairment of peristalsis) and urinary retention (due to loss of muscle tone).

B Fiber:

See Nerve fiber, anatomy and physiology of.

Bicuculline:

Convulsant that acts as an antagonist for the inhibitory neurotransmitter gamma-aminobutyric acid (GABA). It binds directly to GABA receptors, preventing GABA action and leading to seizure activity.

Bier Block:

Technique for anesthesia of an extremity. It entails venous cannulation, draining of blood from the extremity, and replacing the blood with a dilute solution of local anesthetic; the limb remains isolated by a tourniquet. *See* Nerve fiber; anatomy and physiology of.

Bilirubin:

Complex molecule produced in the reticuloendothelial system as a breakdown product of hemoglobin. Free bilirubin is bound to albumin to be transported in plasma to the liver. In the liver it is conjugated with glucuronic acid, which makes it water-soluble. The ratio of conjugated to unconjugated bilirubin is used as an indicator of liver function. The absolute amount of bilirubin is an indicator of red blood cell breakdown.

Binary Code; Binary Number System:

Mathematical notation using a numbering system made up of two digits, 0 and 1, called bits. The position of the bit determines the value of the bit string. (The binary code is the universal method for moving data in digital computers.) *See* Figure.

Binding Proteins:

Plasma-borne proteins primarily responsible for drug binding in the circulating blood. The two main ones are albumin and $alpha_1$-acid glycoprotein (AAG). To a much lesser extent, drugs also bind to globulins, plasma lipoproteins and erythrocytes. Albumin is the mort important drug binding-protein. *See* Albumin.

Bioavailability:

Measure of the degree to which an administered substance becomes available to the target tissue.

Biologic Death:

Cessation of life; the irreversible termination of cerebral function, spontaneous respiration, and spontaneous function of the circulatory system (the totally metabolically challenged).

Bionics:

Science concerned with relating living systems to artificial devices and machinery. The goal of bionics is to simulate, duplicate, and enhance biologic functions.

Binary	Decimal
0	0
+ 1	+ 1
1	1
+ 1	+ 1
10	2
+ 1	+ 1
11	3
+ 1	+ 1
100	4
+ 1	+ 1
101	5
+ 1	+ 1
110	6
+ 1	+ 1
111	7
+ 1	+ 1
1000	8
+ 1	+ 1
1001	9
+ 1	+ 1
1010	10

10,000,000	1,000,000	100,000	10,000	1,000	100	10	1

Value of each position in the decimal system

Binary Code; Binary Number System: The example adds one ten times in succession in both binary and decimal. Note that the binary method has more carries than the decimal method. In binary, 1 and 1 are 0 with a carry of 1.

128	64	32	16	8	4	2	1

Value of each position in the binary system

Biot Breathing (Respiratory Ataxia):

Completely random pattern of ventilation; shallow and deep breaths occur in any sequence, pauses are variable. Apnea is a frequent complication. An indicator of severe brain injury. *See* Apneustic breathing.

Biotransformation:

Alteration of an administered pharmacologic agent due to metabolic processes. *See* Elimination, drug.

Bird Medical Technicians, Inc. (BMTI):

This organization based in Palm Springs, California, was founded in 1954 by Dr. Forrest M. Bird under the name of Bird Corporation. It started manufacturing and selling respiratory care products such as the MARK 7 through the MARK 10 series. Later derivatives are the BABYbird, the IMVbird, and the MINbird. This successful company was sold and became public in August 1990 and is now traded on the NASDAQ as Bird Medical Technicians Incorporated.

Bit:

Abbreviation of "binary digit" used in computer technology to signify either digit, (1 or 0). *See* Binary code, binary number system.

Bizzarri-Guiffrida Laryngoscope Blades:

Modification of the basic Macintosh blade in which much of the flange has been removed to limit damage to the upper teeth.

Black Box:

Electronic device that performs its function so automatically it appears magical to its user. It may also denote the unobtainable, ideal solution to a difficult problem (i.e., "Let's black box the solution").

Blalock-Hanlon Procedure:

Palliative surgical procedure for treating a congenital cardiac anomaly in which there is transposition of the great arteries. It consists of resecting the right lateral portion of the interarterial septum. Segments of the right and left atria and septum are clamped prior to the excision so there is no interruption of blood flow. This procedure is performed only on patients who are not good candidates for intracardiac repair. *See* Figure.

Blalock-Taussig Shunt:

End-to-side anastomosis of the subclavian artery with the pulmonary artery. It is a palliative procedure used in pediatric patients with defects that reduce pulmonary blood flow, such as tetralogy of Fallot, pulmonary atresia with a ventricular septal defect, or transposition of the great vessels coupled with pulmonary stenosis. This shunt allows a controlled increase of pulmonary blood flow. *See* Figure.

Bleeding Disorder:

Condition in which the normal clotting function of the blood is compromised partially or completely. It can be either primary or secondary, congenital or acquired. Under certain circumstances (e.g., open heart surgery), it can be the result of pharmacologic management of the patient. *See* Anticoagulant, Blood coagulation, Blood storage, Disseminated intra-vascular coagulation, Hemophilia, Von Willebrand disease.

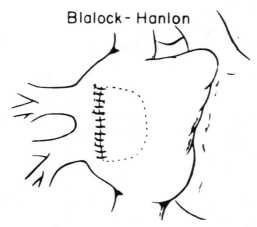

Blalock - Hanlon

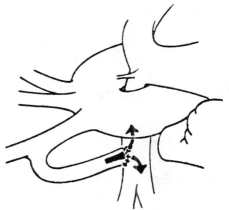

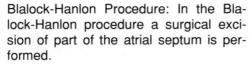

Blalock-Hanlon Procedure: In the Blalock-Hanlon procedure a surgical excision of part of the atrial septum is performed.

Blalock-Taussig Shunt: In the Blalock-Taussig, there are three common types of procedures to increase pulmonary blood flow in congenital cardiac defects.

Bleeding Time:

Screening test to determine coagulability. Typically, a puncture is made on the earlobe (Duke method), and the wound is blotted at 30-second intervals until the bleeding is stopped. The total time elapsed from onset to cessation of bleeding is considered the bleeding time. The "normal values" are difficult to standardize because of probable variations in puncture technique by different individuals. The Ivy method of measuring bleeding time requires an incision to be made distal to an inflated blood pressure cuff on the forearm. The blood drops are absorbed at 30-second intervals. The normal time for the cessation of bleeding is under 8 minutes.

Blend Current:

Setting on electrosurgical machines that combines the damped, sinusoidal wave pattern of the coagulation setting with the continuous undamped output of the cutting setting. This combination allows for some cutting and some coagulating simultaneously. *See* Coagulation current.

Bleomycin:

Antineoplastic agent that appears to cause chronic lung damage. The damage manifests when a patient who has been treated with the drug receives inspired oxygen concentrations higher than 30%.

Blind Nasal Intubation:

Technique of introducing an endotracheal tube through the nose without visualizing the trachea.

Block:

Deposition of a local anesthetic near a nerve trunk to prevent nerve conduction. *See* Brachial plexus block; Caudal anesthesia; Digital block; Epidural anesthesia; Field block; Spinal anesthesia.

Blockade Monitor:

Device that delivers various configurations of electric current across skin electrodes to evaluate neuromuscular blockade. These devices have open-circuit voltages of approximately 250 volts. *See* Peripheral nerve stimulator.

Blood-Brain Barrier (BBB):

Functional impediment to molecular diffusion that separates the brain and the cerebrospinal fluid from the blood. In the brain, endothelial cells of the capillaries are joined by tight junctions. Only lipid-soluble molecules easily penetrate into the brain and rapidly equilibrate between the blood and the brain. Lipid-insoluble molecules and proteins penetrate brain tissue extremely slowly. When the brain is damaged (irradiation, infection, tumor, or surgical retraction), this selective permeability of the blood-brain barrier breaks down. *See* Figure.

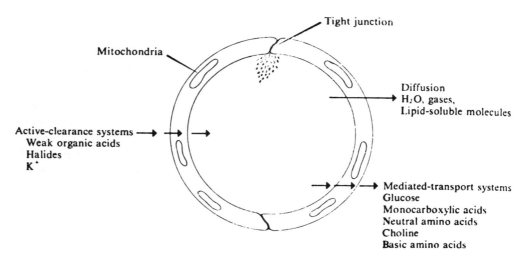

Blood-Brain Barrier: Transport processes across capillary endothelial cells in brain parenchyma. The tight junctions between endothelial cells preclude movement of large molecules.

Blood Coagulation:

Process by which blood forms a fibrin clot. One of the most elegant and complex physiologic functions, coagulation depends on the interaction of multiple proteins. These proteins, either circulating in the blood or contained in platelets, are induced to form a multiple chemical cascade upon encountering an environment other than the interior of blood vessels. *See* Figure and Table. *See* Blood storage.

Blood Coagulation: Clotting factors and some of their common names.

FACTOR	SYNONYM	CLINICAL SYNDROME CAUSED BY DEFICIENCY
I	Fibrinogen	Yes
II	Prothrombin, prethrombin	Yes
III	Tissue factor, tissue thromboplastin	No
IV	Calcium	No
V	Labile factor, proaccelerin, plasma accelerator globulin (ac-G)	Yes
VI	NO FACTOR ASSIGNED TO THIS NUMERAL	
VII	Stable factor, proconvertin, autoprothrombin I, serum prothrombin conversion acceleration (SPCA)	Yes
VIII	Antihemophilia globulin (AHG) Antihemophilic factor (AFG) Thromboplastinogen, platelet cofactor I, antihemophilia Factor A	Yes
IX	Plasma thromboplastin component (PTC), Christmas Factor, autothrombin II, antihemophilic Factor B, platelet cofactor II	Yes
X	Stuart-Prower factor, autoprothrombin C (or III)	Yes
XI	Plasma thromboplastin antecedent (PTA), Rosenthal syndrome, antihemophilic Factor C	Mild
XII	Hageman factor, glass factor	No
XIII	Fibrin stabilizing factor (FSF) Laki-Lorand factor, fibrinase serum factor, urea-insolubility factor	Yes

Blood Flow; Blood Flow Velocity:

Movement of blood by cardiac contraction determined by the change in pressure (delta P) along a given vessel length divided by the resistance to flow (R). The velocity of blood flow in each segment of the arterial circulation is inversely proportional to its area in cross-section. *See* Blood flow, methods for measuring.

Blood Flow, Methods for Measuring:

Various techniques used to measure blood flow. (1) The rotameter (experimental use only) is a device inserted into a cut vessel enabling the previously anticoagulated blood to flow through. The rotameter float reading is directly calibrated to blood flow. (2) The electromagnetic flowmeter (clinically useful) operates on the principle that an electric conductor, such as blood, moving in a magnetic field generates a weak electric current within itself. This current can be measured between two electrodes placed on the vessel wall and is proportional to the blood flow velocity. (3) The ultrasonic flowmeter is a crystal transmitter/receiver combination that is placed around a vessel. The transmitter alternates sending sound waves up and down the vessel length. The sound waves are altered in frequency by the Doppler shift in an amount proportional to the blood velocity. (4) The plethysmograph is used for estimating volume change of a limb, organ, or part. When used to estimate blood flow, a limb (e.g., forearm) is inserted into an airtight chamber and a blood pressure cuff is placed on the arm and inflated to less than 40 mm Hg; this prevents pressure venous return but not arterial inflow. The rate of forearm swelling is proportional to the rate of blood flow into the forearm.

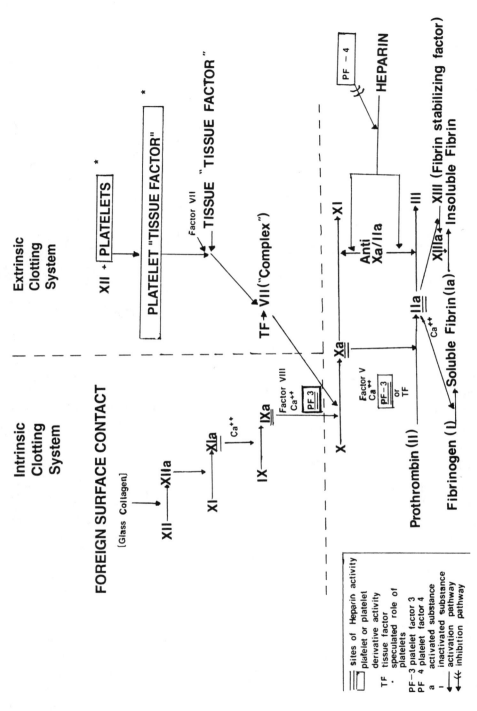

Blood Coagulation: Generally accepted scheme of the coagulation cascade modified to emphasize the sites of platelet and heparin activity. Substances enclosed in boxes represent platelet or platelet derivative activity. Underlined factors identify sites of heparin activity. The right portion of the final common pathway illustrates the theoretic interaction of heparin with PF-4. Heparin in combination with circulating antiXa/IIa inactivates Xa and IIa. PF-4 antagonizes this heparin activity.

Blood Gas Factor:

Percentage of error exhibited by an O_2 electrode calibrated by a known gas mixture which then measures PO_2 in a known blood sample. It is expressed as PO_2 gas minus PO_2 equilibrated blood/PO_2 gas $\times$ 100. (This error can be as large as 10–20%.)

Blood Gas Machine:

Device for determining PO_2, PCO_2, and pH of a blood sample using specific electrodes. *See* Figure.

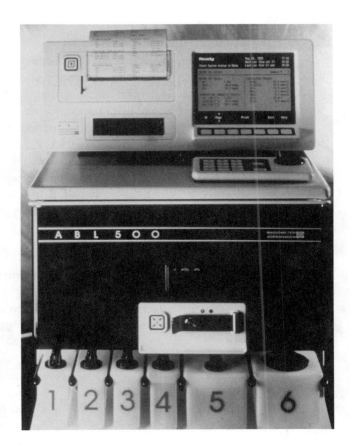

Blood Gas Machine: ABL™ 500 Acid Base Laboratory.

Blood Groups:

See Blood types.

Blood Loss, Estimate of:

Attempt to determine as accurately as possible the amount of blood lost from the patient during surgery. The most accurate and practical technique involves weighing all the sponges and pads as they are used during the procedure and keeping a running total (1 ml blood weighs about 1 mg). Blood removed (suctioned) from the incision site is placed in a calibrated chamber and its volume is determined (subtracting the volume of wash and irrigation solutions used). More elaborate situations involve operating tables that continually weigh the patient with various corrections for drapes and instruments, and washing machines that wash all the drapes, pads, and so on after the procedure, with the hemoglobin content of the rinse water being determined.

Blood Patch:

See Epidural patch.

Blood Pressure:

See Arterial blood pressure; Arterial pressure determination by palpation; Central venous pressure; Mean arterial pressure; Photoelectric determination of blood pressure.

Blood Pressure Cuff Size Selection:

Choice of cuff size as it relates to accurate blood pressure measurement. Sizing of the blood pressure cuff is a common source of error in auscultatory methods of blood pressure determination. If the cuff is too narrow in relation to the arm, it must be blown up to a falsely high pressure in order to produce the proper tissue pressure on the artery. An inappropriately wide cuff, in contradistinction, gives relatively low readings. Loose wrapping of the cuff gives the same effect as a narrow cuff. The air bladder should occupy at least one-half of the arm circumference. In general, the minimum width of the cuff should be approximately 20% greater than the diameter of the arm, which usually works out to be anywhere from one-half to two-thirds the length of the upper arm. A cuff size that is incorrectly selected similarly affects all indirect methods for determining blood pressure.

Blood Storage:

Saving of whole blood or its various components for use in transfusions. Whole blood is stored on a unit basis. One unit contains approximately 450 ml of whole blood to which 50 ml of an anticoagulant, acid-citrate-dextrose (ACD) or citrate-phosphate-dextrose (CPD), are added. Anticoagulants are not added when storing components of blood. Until recently, ACD was added most frequently. When compared with whole blood, ACD-stored blood has a much lower pH, a much higher PCO_2, a very low 2,3-diphosphoglycerate (2,3-DPG) level, a decrease of factors V and VIII, and a serum potassium in excess of 15 mEq/L. Stored at 4°C, it has a shelf life of approximately 21 days. CPD-stored blood, at 4°C, has at least a 7-day longer shelf life. It is less acidic, it has lower potassium levels, and its 2,3-DPG levels are not as depressed as in acid-stored blood. Neither ACD- nor CPD-stored blood contains viable platelets. With component therapy, only the specific blood fraction needed is administered; e.g., concentrated factor VIII is given to patients with classic hemophilia. Other commonly used fractions include fresh frozen plasma (FFP), which is used to restore clotting factors. Platelet concentrates (stored at room temperature), are useful for treating thrombocytopenia. Albumin, the major blood protein, is used to expand volume; red blood cell concentrates (stored at 4°C) replace lost hemoglobin and thereby increase O_2-carrying capacity. Red blood cells may also be suspended in glycerin and deep-frozen for an indefinite period. Once thawed, they must be used within 24 hours. *See* Blood coagulation.

Blood Substitutes:

Any agent that works to replace blood, particularly its capacity to carry oxygen. These agents currently include perfluorochemicals (PFCs). One of them, an emulsion, is Fluosol-

DA which has received limited FDA approval. Modified or encapsulated hemoglobins are also being tested as blood substitutes.

Blood Types (Blood Groups):

Characterization of the blood by type of antigen on the red blood cell (RBC) surface and type of antibody found in the serum. These antigen-antibody combinations are genetically determined. A major blood type system is the ABO grouping, which depends on the presence or absence of the two antigenic factors A and B. (O signifies that neither A nor B is present.) Agglutinogens are the antigens located on the membranes of human RBCs; antibodies against these agglutinogens are called agglutinins. Individuals with type A blood have agglutinogen A on their RBCs and anti-B agglutinins in their serum. Therefore if their plasma is mixed with type B cells, clumping and destruction of the blood occur. The reverse is true for people with type B blood. Individuals with type O blood have circulating anti-A and anti-B agglutinins whereas those with type AB blood have no circulating agglutinins. Another major blood-typing system is concerned with the Rh factor. This system is composed of many antigens, the most important being D. (Alternate terminology for the Rh factor is blood group D.) The Rh+ (positive) person has agglutinogen D on the RBCs and the Rh– (negative) person has no D antigen. Transfusion reactions occur when a patient is given incompatible blood resulting in hemolysis. This result leads to hemolytic anemia. Clinically, in the awake patient, signs and symptoms may include hives, chills, chest pain, shortness of breath, headache, and skin flushing. (Reactions vary in severity depending on such factors as the degree of incompatibility and the amount of blood transfused.) During general anesthesia many of the symptoms may be masked. In both the awake and anesthetized patient, coagulation disorders, cardiovascular collapse, and hemoglobinuria may be seen when incompatible blood is given. Researchers have identified a plethora of tissue and blood antigen-antibody systems, but 90% of all transfusion reactions occur as a result of incompatibility within the ABO and Rh systems. In most hospitals, three levels of preparation for transfusion are maintained preoperatively. (1) "Type and hold," in which a patient's blood type only is characterized, is the lowest level of preparedness. (2) With "type and screen" the blood is characterized and checked for ABO and Rh incompatibilities against a panel of standard antigens. (3) With "type and crossmatch," all possible antigen-antibody reactions are determined between the recipient and all possible donors. Compatible units are then stored and used only for that particular patient. *See* Table.

Blood Volume Measurement:

Estimate of circulating blood volume. This measurement can be made by either of two radioactive tracer techniques: the radioiodine-tagged albumin technique or the chromium-tagged red blood cell technique. Both methods measure dilution of radioactive material by the blood pool of nontagged albumin in one test and of red blood cells in the other. Both are subject to errors because of an unequal dilution of the radioactive material. Clinically, relative blood volume is determined by measuring the filling pressure of the right and left ventricles, the cardiac output, and the total peripheral resistance. In addition, when a baseline series of these pressures and outputs is known, blood volume trends can be monitored.

107

Blood Types: (A) The relationship between major ABO red cell antigens and reciprocal serum antibodies. (B) Frequency of occurrence of ABO blood types.

A

Blood Group	Antigen(s) on RBC	Antibodies in Serum
A	A	Anti-B
B	B	Anti-A
AB	A and B	Neither anti-A nor anti-B
O	Neither A nor B	Both anti-A and anti-B

B

	Approximate Frequency (%)	
Phenotype	Whites	Blacks
O	44	49
A	45	27
B	8	20
AB	3	4

Bloomquist Pediatric Circle System:

First described in 1957; the Bloomquist circuit is a miniature version of an adult system employing smaller components.

BMI:

See Body mass index.

BMTI:

See Bird Medical Technicians, Inc.

Body Fluid Compartment:

Model for body fluid distribution that assumes water is present in two compartments: intracellular (within cells) and extracellular (outside cells). The extracellular compartment is further subdivided into interstitial (between cells) and intravascular (within the blood vessels). Fluid transfer between compartments is determined by electrolyte gradients, which in turn are controlled by cellular membranes, at times with energy expenditure. *See* Figures.

Body Mass Index (BMI):

Measurement of obesity. It is the weight in kilograms divided by the height in meters. In most U.S. adults 20–30 years old the BMI averages around 27.

Body Plethysmograph:

Apparatus for ascertaining changes in body volume. It is useful for measuring the functional residual capacity of the lung, i.e., the volume of gas in the lung after a normal expiration. The patient sits in a large airtight chamber and is asked to force ventilation at the end of expiration against a closed mouthpiece. The gas in the lungs is compressed and lung volume decreases. The gas volume in the box increases as the box pressure decreases.

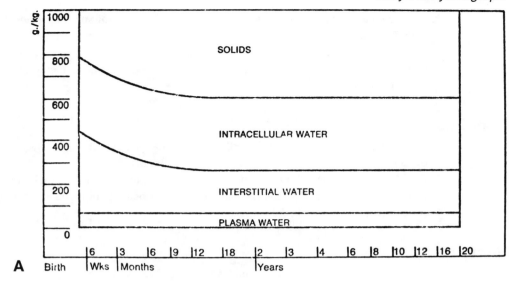

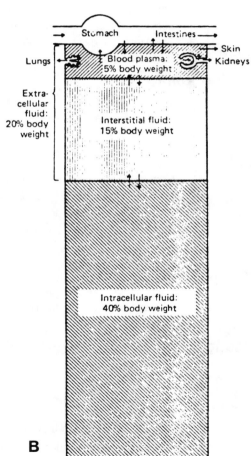

Body Fluid Compartment: (A) Body content and distribution of water at various ages. (B) Adult body fluid compartments. The arrows show fluid movement. Transcellular fluids, a very small part of total body fluid, are not shown.

According to Boyle law, at a given temperature, pressure × volume is constant. Therefore if the initial pressure in the airway and in the box, the initial volume, and the new pressure in the box are known, the functional residual capacity of the lungs can be calculated. The body plethysmograph measures the total volume of gas in the lungs, including gas trapped behind closed airways.

Bohr Effect:

Phenomenon exhibiting the increased affinity of O_2 for hemoglobin at low concentrations of CO_2 and the decreased affinity of O_2 for combining with hemoglobin at high levels of CO_2. The Bohr effect aids O_2 transport by favoring O_2 loading onto hemoglobin in the lungs (decreased PCO_2) and by favoring unloading from hemoglobin in the peripheral tissues (increased PCO_2). *See* Haldane effect.

Bohr Equation:

Method for determining physiologic deadspace. The equation states that the deadspace volume divided by the tidal volume equals the $PaCO_2$ minus the expiratory gas $PECO_2$. In normal subjects the physiologic deadspace approximates that of the anatomic deadspace. *See* Anatomic dead space; Physiologic deadspace.

Boiling Point:

Temperature at which a vaporizing liquid has a vapor pressure equal to atmospheric pressure. As a consequence bubbles of gas form throughout the volume of liquid.

Bolus:

Concept that an action is taken, and in particular, that a drug is given "all at once." For example, it might be appropriate during patient-controlled analgesia to give a drug intermittently or, at least at the beginning of pain management, give it as a bolus to gain an initial drug level rapidly. *See* Patient-controlled analgesia.

Bond Energy:

Energy required to break a chemical bond between two atoms in a molecule. The amount of energy depends on the type of atom and the nature of the molecule.

Bouncing Ball:

See Oscilloscope.

Boundary Layer:

Fluid layer most proximal to the solid boundaries restraining that fluid, e.g., the layer of blood immediately adjacent to the inner wall of a blood vessel. Its thickness is determined by the viscosity of the blood, the friction between the blood and the vessel wall, and the speed at which the blood is moving. *See* Reynolds number.

Bourdon Tube Pressure Gauge:

Device measuring cylinder gas pressure. It incorporates a curved tube, and elevation of the internal tube pressure tends to straighten the tube. This straightening in turn may be mechanically linked to move a pointer across a dial. *See* Figure.

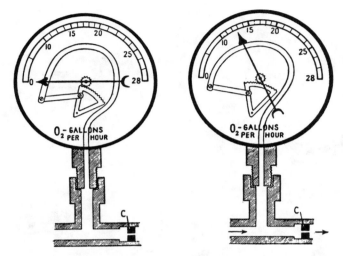

Bourdon Tube Pressure Gauge: Cross section of a Bourdon gauge type of flowmeter. A gas flowing from its source passes through the orifice (C) to a delivery tube. A pressure builds up proximal to (C) and is transmitted to the hollow spring tube which straightens. This movement operates a clockwork mechanism and the gas flow is indicated on a calibrated scale by a dial needle.

Bovie, Bovie Machine:

Generic misnomer for an electrosurgical unit (ESU). *See* ESU.

Boyle Bottle:

Early vaporizer that can be classified as a variable-bypass, flow-over, or bubble-through vaporizer. The amount of gas allowed into the vaporizer is controlled by the position of the on-off lever. The path of the gas through the vaporizing chamber depends on the height of the plunger, which redirects flow across or under the surface of the liquid in the vaporizer. The Boyle bottle has no temperature compensation and may be used with multiple anesthetic agents. Anesthetic concentration is basically regulated by monitoring the clinical signs. This vaporizer produces unpredictable results owing to the many variables involved in its usage. *See* Figure.

Boyle Law:

Principle stating that if a given mass of gas is compressed at a constant temperature (T) but the pressure (P) is increased or decreased, the volume (V) of gas varies inversely to pressure. (At constant T: $PV = P'V'$.) Although the law is only an approximation for real gases, it is accurate enough for most clinical circumstances.

111

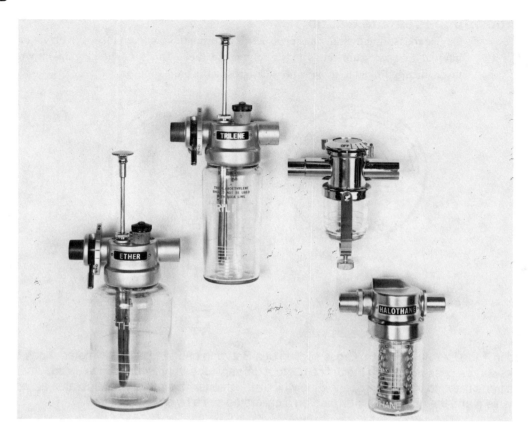

Boyle Bottle: Courtesy of the Medishield Corporation Limited, Essex, England.

BPD:

See Fetal biparietal diameter.

Brachial Plexus Block:

A regional nerve block used for surgical procedures of the hand, forearm, and upper arm in which a local anesthetic is injected unilaterally near the brachial plexus. There are essentially three approaches to brachial plexus block: supraclavicular, interscalene (a variation of the supraclavicular), and axillary. Phrenic nerve paralysis, Horner syndrome, and hematoma are potential complications of the supraclavicular and interscalene approaches. Pneumothorax occurs in 1–3% of cases with the supraclavicular approach. Intravascular injection and nerve injury are potential complications of the axillary approach. *See* Figures.

Bradycardia:

Low pulse rate; usually below 60 beats per minute. Sinus bradycardia is seen when the slow electrical pattern is initiated in the sinoatrial node. In athletes, sinus bradycardia can be perfectly normal and reflects a well functioning cardiovascular system.

Bradykinin:

Polypeptide found in precursor form in plasma; also known as plasma kinin. It is bound to the α_2-globulin fraction of the plasma, but the action of the proteolytic enzyme kallikrein enables the bradykinin to be released. Bradykinin causes profound relaxation of vascular smooth muscle and an increase in capillary permeability. It is assumed to play a role in inflammatory processes and anaphylactic shock syndromes. *See* Allergic response.

Brain (Encephalon):

Large mass of nerve tissue located within the cranium. The brain consists of five parts. (1) Cerebrum, the largest part of the brain, consists of a right and left hemisphere, each of which is composed of five lobes (temporal, parietal, occipital, frontal, and insula). One hemisphere is functionally dominant. Various functions such as behavior, memory, intelligence, spatial relations, hearing, taste, smell, and sight are regulated within the cerebrum. (2) Cerebellum, functions in muscle coordination and equilibrium. (3) Medulla oblongata, the portion of the brainstem that helps regulate heartbeat, blood pressure, and respiration and influences the autonomic reflexes for swallowing, coughing, sneezing, and vomiting. (4) Pons varolii, the segment of the brainstem in which the trigeminal, abducens, facial, and vestibulcochlear nerves originate. (5) Midbrain, the portion of the brainstem that contains the nerve centers for the oculomotor and trochlear nerves. The brainstem controls and transmits impulses between the brain and spinal cord.

Brain Death:

Currently accepted criterion for biologic death. Two electroencephalograms taken 24 hours apart must demonstrate no electrical activity. There must be no influence from temperature, ventilation, or drugs. The concept of brain death supplants the concept of the cessation of spontaneous ventilation, which may be supported by appropriate mechanical and pharmacologic intervention for long periods. *See* Biologic death.

Brainstem Auditory Evoked Potential (BAEP):

See Auditory evoked potential.

Brass:

Alloy containing copper and zinc in which the zinc content ranges up to 40%.

Brazelton Score:

Elaborate attempt to quantify the behavioral responses of the newborn. First proposed by Brazelton in 1961, the test involves prolonged interaction with the infant and grades responses to stimuli such as noise from a rattle or a bell.

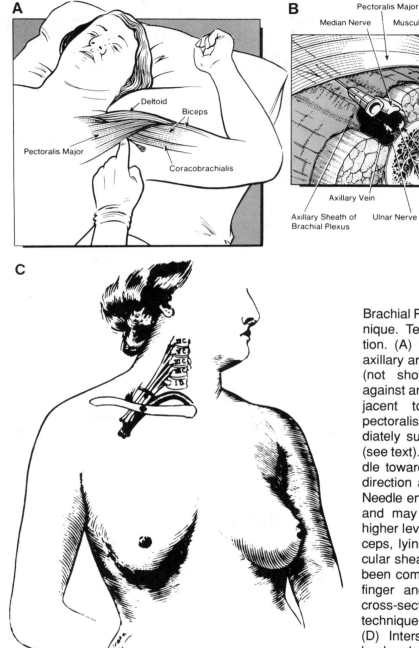

A

Deltoid

Biceps

Pectoralis Major

Coracobrachialis

B

Pectoralis Major

Median Nerve

Musculocutaneous Nerve

Axillary Vein

Radial Nerve

Axillary Sheath of Brachial Plexus

Ulnar Nerve

Axillary Artery

C

Brachial Plexus Block: Axillary technique. Technique of needle insertion. (A) Note forefinger palpating axillary artery. Hand holding needle (not shown) should be braced against arm. Needle insertion is adjacent to coracobrachialis and pectoralis major muscles, immediately superior to tip of forefinger (see text). (B) Note direction of needle toward apex of axilla, in same direction as neurovascular bundle. Needle enters neurovascular sheath and may run inside sheath to a higher level. The medial head of triceps, lying between the neurovascular sheath and the humerus, has been compressed by the palpating finger and is not shown in this cross-section. (C) Supraclavicular technique. Interscalene technique. (D) Interscalene block. Anatomic landmarks. (E) Needle direction in relation to spine from above.

D

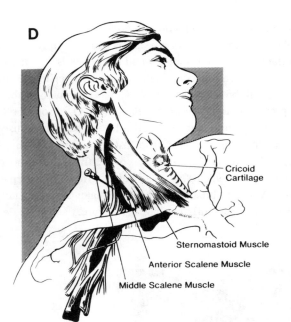

Cricoid
Cartilage

Sternomastoid Muscle

Anterior Scalene Muscle

Middle Scalene Muscle

E

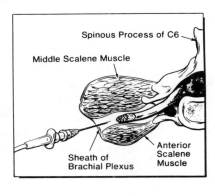

Spinous Process of C6

Middle Scalene Muscle

Anterior
Scalene
Muscle

Sheath of
Brachial Plexus

Breakdown, Electrical:

Sudden, disruptive electrical discharge through an insulator. It proceeds from a state of little or no current flow to a state of massive current flow. The insulation around wires used to conduct electrical current is often rated by breakdown voltage. The higher the breakdown voltage, the better the quality of the insulation.

Breast Feeding Risks:

Possibility that a drug taken by a breast feeding mother will both enter the breast milk and cause infant difficulty. There are four drug categories: Group 1: drugs taken by the mother that *do not* enter the breast milk. Group 2: drugs that *do* enter the breast milk but are not likely to affect the infant. Group 3: these drugs not only enter breast milk but may affect the infant at usual therapeutic doses. Group 4: no information exists for drugs in this category as to whether the drug enters breast milk.

Breath Stacking:

Phenomena of a mechanical breath adding to or stacking on top of a spontaneous breath during intermittent mandatory ventilation. *See* Assisted mechanical ventilation; Ventilator.

Breathing Bag (Reservoir Bag):

Device used to store and conveniently pressurize (by hand squeeze) a volume of gas that will be used to ventilate the lung. There are two types of breathing bags. (1) Self-inflating bag is designed with an internal spring or sponge to return it to its normal volume and configuration after the release of external pressure. It is usually used in combination with a one-way valve that directs exhaled gas to the atmosphere and prevents the negative

115

pressure generated by the expanding spring from affecting the patient's airway. (2) Non-self-inflating bag, also called the rebreathing or anesthesia bag, is simply a rubber sack that is squeezed and then reinflated by fresh gas inflow and the patient's exhaled volume. The non-self-inflating bag is usually used in combination with an overflow device (pop-off valve) to prevent overinflation. Rebreathing of expired CO_2 is prevented by the valve in the self-inflating bag and by proper control of fresh gas flow and CO_2 absorption (when on an anesthesia machine) in the self-inflating bag. The self-inflating bag can be used to administer at most 40–60% O_2 as the bag reexpands too fast for normal O_2 supplies (10–20 L/minute) to fill the bag. (The remaining volume comes from the atmosphere.) The non-self-inflating bag can administer 90–100% O_2 as fresh O_2 flow is augmented by the O_2 returning from the patient. (A patient breathing 40% O_2 exhales approximately 36% O_2.) The Ambu resuscitator is a type of self-inflating bag. *See* Figure.

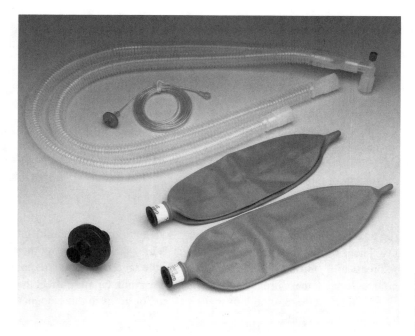

Breathing Bag: Breathing bags (reservoir bag) with other disposable breathing circuit parts.

Bremsstrahlung (Braking Radiation):

Electromagnetic radiation produced when a fast-moving charged particle, usually an electron, decelerates as it approaches an atomic nucleus.

Bretylium (Bretylol):

Drug originally marketed as an oral antihypertensive agent and now accepted for use as an antiarrhythmic agent. It is approved for intravenous or intramuscular administration in patients with life-threatening ventricular arrhythmias that have failed to respond to lidocaine, procainamide, or phenytoin. It tends to decrease the blood pressure.

Brevital:

See Barbiturate.

Bridgeless Mask:

Mask variant designed for a flat face with a nonprominent bridge of the nose. The mask is shallow with an air-filled perimeter.

Brilliant Yellow:

See Indicator dye.

Broca Index:

Calculation used for determining a person's ideal body weight. Insurance companies calculate their tables using this index: ideal weight (kg) = height (cm) – 100. This method is used to correlate overweight versus morbid obesity. *See* Body mass index (BMI).

Bromage Scale:

Scale for estimating motor paralysis caused by epidural and spinal local anesthetic administration: zero 0 = no motor paralysis; 1 = inability to raise an extended leg; 2 = inability to flex knee; 3 = inability to flex the ankle joint.

Bromethol (Avertin, Tribromoethanol):

See Rectal anesthesia.

Bromide:

Ionic form of the element bromine. It was given during the nineteenth century in the form of potassium bromide for the treatment of epilepsy and other seizure disorders. With a long half-life it tends to accumulate in the body if taken daily, which is of concern as it is found in many over-the-counter drugs and preparations. Chronic use may cause depression, confusion, and lethargy. In addition, because bromide is released as a degradation product of halothane, it may be one of the causes of prolonged sedation after extended administration of halothane.

Brompton Mixture—Brompton Cocktail:

Orally administered sedative mixture composed of morphine, cocaine, chloroform water, alcohol, and a flavoring syrup. First popularized at the Brompton Chest Hospital in London during the late nineteenth century. Used for chronic pain relief in cancer patients, it also has been used as an anesthetic in children for short procedures. Various ingredients have been added and subtracted as per individual taste. *See* Lytic cocktail.

Bronchial Blocker:

Device for achieving lung separation and isolation. By use of a bronchoscope, an inflatable blocking device is placed in the bronchus of the lung to be isolated. *See* Double-lumen tube.

Bronchial Intubation:

See Endobronchial intubation.

Bronchiole:

Distinct part of the respiratory tree containing occasional alveoli and connecting the terminal bronchioles (without alveoli) to the alveolar ducts (which are completely lined with alveoli).

Bronchodilation:

Increase in the diameter of the bronchial passageways of the lungs, either by decrease in muscle tone or reversal of tissue swelling.

Bronchodilators:

Drugs that act to increase the diameter of the bronchial passageways in the lung. Generally used for treatment of asthma and asthma-like conditions. *See* Table.

Bronchodilators.

Generic Name	Trade Name	Type of Receptors Stimulated
Racemic Epinephrine	Vaponefrin	Alpha & Beta$_1$
Isoproterenol	Isuprel	Beta$_1$
Metaproterenol	Alupent Metaprel	Beta$_2$
Isoetharine	Bronkosol	Beta$_2$
Terbutaline	Bricanyl	Beta$_2$

1) Beta$_1$: Beta$_1$ receptors along with causing bronchodilation cause tachycardia, palpitations, insomnia and tremor.

2) Beta$_2$: Beta$_2$ receptors mainly cause bronchodilation with little or no effect on the heart.

Bronchography:

Procedure that allows radiographic visualization of the bronchial tree after instillation of a radiopaque material. The procedure can cause bronchial irritation and has a well-recognized morbidity rate.

Bronchomotor Tone:

Continuous state of contraction of the bronchial musculature during respiration. It is apparently affected by vagal impulses as well as by circulating catecholamines.

Bronchopleural:

Abnormal communication between the air passageways of the lung and the pleural cavity. It is most likely to occur after lung surgery, rupture of a lung abscess, or spread of an empyema. It can lead to pneumothorax and severe impairment of respiratory function. If a communication exists between the bronchial tree and the surface of the chest, it is called a bronchopleural cutaneous fistula.

Bronchopleural Cutaneous:

See Bronchopleural.

Bronchoscope, Flexible:

Instrument that allows direct visualization of the bronchi and their distal segments. (It is based on the fiberoptic principle by which an image is transmitted along flexible bundles of coated glass or plastic fibers that have optical properties.) This device can be guided to specific locations directly or using fluoroscopy. The patient is usually mildly sedated and topical anesthetics (e.g., lidocaine) are administered through the bronchoscope. Brush catheters (for obtaining cytologic specimens) and small biopsy forceps are inserted through the scope to sample the lesion(s) visualized. *See* Figures.

Bronchoscope, Rigid:

Firm, hollow stainless steel tube used to directly visualize the interior of the trachea and the mainstem bronchi. General anesthesia is often required during insertion of the scope. With the aid of lenses and a light source within the bronchoscope, the surgeon can readily observe anatomic abnormalities and pathologic conditions. In addition, secretions can be aspirated, foreign bodies removed, and suspicious lesions biopsied through the bronchoscope. *See* Figure. *See* Bronchoscope, flexible.

Bronchospasm:

Sudden, forceful, involuntary contraction of the smooth muscle of the bronchial portion of the respiratory tree. Usually it is a reflex response secondary to the introduction of irritants, including inhalation anesthetics. If mild, bronchospasm can be treated by prompt removal of the irritant; if severe (during anesthesia), it can be treated by (1) providing positive pressure ventilation, (2) deepening anesthesia, and (3) administering a bronchodilating drug. It is a well-observed paradox of anesthesia administration that low doses of some inhalation anesthetics, if introduced too quickly, cause bronchoconstriction, whereas high doses, when administered slowly, cause bronchodilation.

Bronchospirometry:

Determination of the O_2 intake, vital capacity, and CO_2 excretion of a single lung, usually using a double-lumen tube. A differential bronchospirometer can measure the function of each lung separately.

119

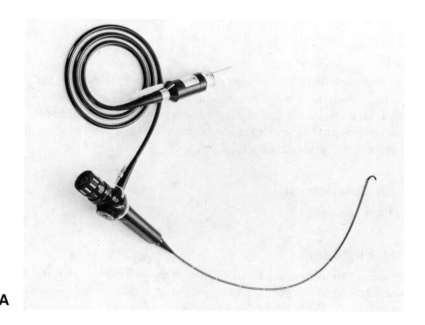

A

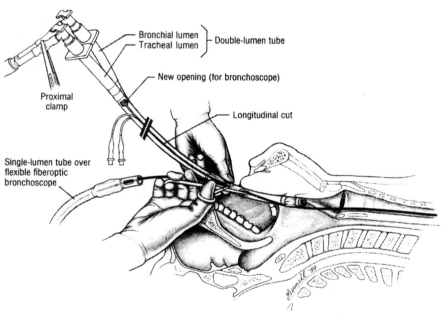

Bronchial lumen
Tracheal lumen } Double-lumen tube

New opening (for bronchoscope)

Proximal clamp

Longitudinal cut

Single-lumen tube over flexible fiberoptic bronchoscope

B

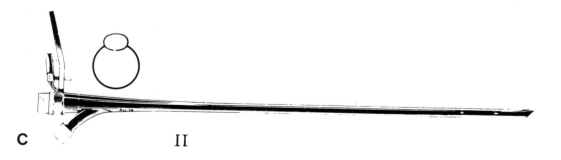

C   II

Bronchus:

One of two main (primary) branches from the trachea that form the major passageways to the lungs. The right main bronchus is more vertical than the left, and foreign objects entering the air passages are more likely to become lodged in it. The primary bronchi are composed of incomplete rings of cartilage and are lined by ciliated columnar epithelium. *See* Conducting airways.

Bronze:

Copper alloy in which the main alloying metal is usually tin.

Brownian Movement:

Random, continuous, irregular motion of small particles when suspended in a liquid. It is a visible demonstration that the molecules of liquids are constantly bombarding the small particles.

Brush Cell:

See Alveolar cell types.

Brush, Electrical:

Specialized electrical conductor, usually made of carbon, which serves to maintain contact with a rotating communication.

Brutaine:

Half-flippant, half-serious name for "anesthetics" that consist primarily of O_2 plus muscle relaxation because the patient is too sick to tolerate a more formal, conventional anesthetic technique. If the patient survives and remembers the proceedings, brutaine can be psychologically damaging. It is primarily a move of desperation.

Bryce-Smith Tube:

See Double-lumen tube.

B-Scan Ultrasonography:

Ultrasound diagnostic technique applied to obstetrics, particularly useful for determining placement of the placenta in the uterus. *See* Ultrasonography.

Bronchoscope, Flexible: (A) Flexible instrument that allows direct visualization. (B) Diagrammatic representation of fiberoptic bronchoscope passed through tracheal lumen of the endobronchial tube and acting as guide for single lumen tube. The bronchial lumen of the endobronchial tube remains in close proximity to the glottic inlet, permitting ventilation of the lungs while the tube's tracheal lumen is freed from the bronchoscope.

Bronchoscope, Rigid: (C) Firm, hollow stainless steel tube for direct visualization of the interior trachea and mainstem bronchi.

Bubble Jar:

Apparatus used for increasing the humidity of fresh gas supplied to a patient by bubbling the gas through a jar of water. Efficiency is contingent on the size of the bubbles, water pathway length, temperature of the jar, and rate of bubble production.

Bubble Oxygenator:

Device used with heart-lung machines in which exchange of gases takes place during cardiopulmonary bypass procedures. It breaks up a stream of supplied O_2 into continually forming bubbles, which diffuse through a column of blood on the bypass machine. Gas exchange occurs on the surface of the bubbles. Rapidity of O_2 transfer to the blood depends on bubble size (surface area) and length of bubble path through the blood. Small bubbles produce a large surface area and thus good oxygenation but are difficult to eliminate before the blood is returned to the patient. Some large bubbles are required for adequate elimination of CO_2. *See* Cardiopulmonary bypass.

Buffer:

Substance that tends to preserve the original hydrogen ion concentration in solution, thereby maintaining the pH despite the addition of quantities of acid or base. It is composed of a weak acid and its salt. The major body buffer systems are bicarbonate, phosphate, nondefined serum proteins, and hemoglobin. Currently, bicarbonate is the only directly measurable buffer system of the body. It is a mixture of carbonic acid and sodium (or magnesium, potassium, or calcium) bicarbonate. *See* Acid-base balance, Acidosis, Alkalosis.

Buffer Base:

Clinical measurement used to evaluate acid-base balance. It indicates the sum of buffer anions in whole blood. This total is divided (approximately) equally between bicarbonate ions and hemoglobin ions. This measurement has become obsolete because its determination varies depending on the pH of the blood specimen at the time of measurement. *See* Base excess.

Bug:

Flaw in a set of instructions to a computer or in the computer circuitry that causes it to provide inappropriate results. (*Debugging* is the process by which errors in computer programming or wiring are eliminated.)

Bunsen Solubility Coefficient:

See Ostwald solubility coefficient.

Buoyancy:

See Archimedes principle.

Bupivacaine:

See Local anesthetic.

Buprenorphine (Tengesic):

Experimental mixed agonist-antagonist narcotic. Approximately 20 times as potent as morphine.

Bus:

Pathway for transmitting information from one location to another. For example, in an electronic typewriter, the impulses generated by the key strokes are carried to the microprocessor by a bus.

Bus Bar:

Conductor that can carry heavy current or connect many points in an electric system.

Bushing:

Type of adaptor used for altering the internal diameter of a system component.

Butabarbital:

See Barbiturate.

Butisol:

See Barbiturate.

n-Butyl p-Aminobenzoate (BAB):

Molecule that is a highly lipid-soluble congener of benzocaine. Used at one time as a local anesthetic, it may have neurotoxic and neurolytic effects.

Butylparaben:

See Preservative.

Butyrocholinesterase:

Enzyme that is found in plasma, liver, and many organs. It is the correct name for nonspecific cholinesterase or pseudocholinesterase. Its physiologic function is unknown. *See* Pseudocholinesterase.

Butyrophenone:

See Antipsychotic agents.

Bypass:

See Cardiopulmonary bypass.

Bypass Capacitor:

Device for providing an alternate path of relatively low impedance (i.e., the total opposition afforded to a flow of alternating current at a specific frequency) for alternating current around a circuit. It effectively prevents alternating current from entering inappropriate parts of a circuit.

C

Caffeine:

White powder alkaloid with the general formula $C_8H_{10}N_4O_2$. It is soluble in alcohol and water and has been used medically as a nonspecific stimulator of the central nervous system.

Caffeine and Halothane Contracture Test (CHCT):

See Malignant hyperthermia.

Caffeine Test:

See Malignant hyperthermia.

Caisson Disease (Bends, Decompression Sickness, Diver Paralysis, Dysbarism):

Disorder that may follow a rapid decrease of air pressure in persons who have been breathing compressed air in hyperbaric chambers, or caissons (pressurized underwater chambers). (Divers may be subject to this condition on ascent.) Under pressure, gases (N_2 in particular) are forced into tissues in direct proportion to the pressure. When this pressure is relieved, as when a diver surfaces, N_2 starts to leave the tissues rapidly. Gas bubbles form in cells and small vessels just as they do in a carbonated beverage first opened to the atmosphere. These bubbles act as occluding plugs, causing ischemia, severe pain, and, in acute cases, rapid elevation of total peripheral resistance and death. The only treatment for caisson disease is repeat exposure to higher pressures with gradual return to normal pressure.

Calcium:

Element vital to multiple body processes. It is a major bivalent cation of the extracellular fluid and is essential for blood clotting (calcium is factor IV). By binding calcium with citrate, as in citrate-phosphate-dextrose (CPD) blood storage, clotting is prevented. More than 90% of body calcium is stored in bone as phosphate or carbonate. Calcium also plays an essential role in muscle contraction and is important in neuromuscular transmission.

Calcium Channel Blocker:

Class of drugs that interfere with cross-membrane transfer of calcium ions. The calcium channel blockers temper the role of calcium in the development of the cardiac action potential and in the coupling of electrical excitation to contraction. The first available intravenous calcium-blocking agent, verapamil, is effective treatment for paroxysmal supraventricular tachycardia. Verapamil and nifedipine (an oral calcium blocker) appear to be effective for treating angina, hypertrophic cardiomyopathy, and chronic atrial fibrillation.

Calcium Chloride:

Inorganic salt, normally administered intravenously, used for its direct inotropic effects on the heart. Irritating to tissues and veins and capable of causing tissue necrosis, calcium chloride contains approximately three times more calcium than two organic salts, calcium gluconate and calcium gluceptate (also used as inotropes). Therefore only one-third to one-half the amount of calcium chloride is necessary when used instead of these other salts. The calcium ion causes the entire plastic blood pathway to clot if it is erroneously injected into the same intravenous line as transfused blood, which has been anticoagulated with citrate (excess calcium overwhelms the citrate.)

Calcium Gluceptate:

See Calcium chloride.

Calcium Gluconate:

See Calcium chloride.

Calcium Tungstate:

See Intensifying screen.

Calibration:

Process of comparing a measuring device to a known standard to determine its accuracy or to devise a new scale. For example, during calibration of an invasive electronic blood pressure monitoring device, a transducer connected to the monitor is opened to room air, which is selected as zero point, and the electronics are set to zero. The transducer is closed, and a mercury column sphygmomanometer in parallel with the transducer applies a set pressure (usually 200 mm Hg). The invasive electronic monitoring device is then adjusted to agree with that pressure. *See* Accuracy.

Calibration Signal:

See Self-test capability.

Calomel Electrode:

Reference electrode, at times employed in pH determinations, consisting of mercury in contact with a solution of potassium chloride saturated with calomel (mercurous chloride). *See* Figure.

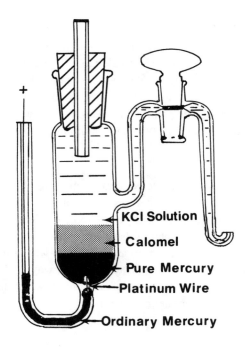

KCl Solution

Calomel

Pure Mercury

Platinum Wire

Ordinary Mercury

Calomel Electrode.

Calorie:

Unit of heat measurement. The large calorie (kilocalorie, or Cal) is the unit used in metabolic studies and is equal to the amount of heat necessary to raise the temperature of 1 kg H_2O 1°C at a pressure of 1 atmosphere. The small calorie (gram calorie, or cal) is 1/1000 of a Cal.

Candela:

Standard international unit of light intensity.

Cannabis:

Ancient drug obtainable from the hemp plant, the sole species of which is Cannabis sativa. All parts of the plant contains psychoactive substances referred to as Cannabinoids. The highest concentration of these products, however, are found in the flowering tops of the plants. The plant synthesizes more than 60 cannabinoids. The most powerful of the psychoactive effects, however, are considered to be caused by tetrahydrocannabinol. Eating or smoking a dose of this agent effects mood, memory, ability to think, perception and motor coordination. Usually there is an increased sense of well-being and euphoria. Time sense is disoriented, and the ability to carry out complex tasks is damaged. This effect on behavior is called "temporal disintegration." At higher doses, cannabis can produce hallucinations and paranoid ideation.

Cannon Wave:

See Central venous pressure.

Cannula:

Tube introduced into a duct or body cavity often with the aid of a trocar. The trocar filling the cannula lumen makes the initial puncture into the space the cannula is to occupy. It is then withdrawn, clearing the lumen of the cannula. The term "cannula" is often used interchangeably with the term "catheter." *See* Catheter.

Cannulization, Arterial; Arterial Line:

See Allen test, Arterial blood pressure, Cardiac catheterization.

Capacitance, Electronic:

Buildup (storage) of electrons on one conductor balanced by the buildup of positive charges on a second conductor separated from the first by an insulator. If the insulator breaks down, current flows to balance and neutralize the charged states. *See* Capacitor.

Capacitance, Fluidic:

Relative ability of a vessel or container to increase linearly in volume without a linear increase in pressure.

Capacitance Vessels:

See Resistance vessels.

Capacitive Coupling:

Process of linking together two portions of a circuit so that energy is transferred from one to the other by means of mutual capacitance. Any two conductors separated by an insulator (even an air gap) can function as a capacitor. Capacitive coupling is one of the ways stray signals may leak between channels. *See* Figure. *See* Capacitor.

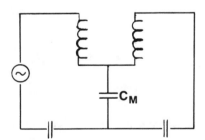

Capacitive Coupling: C_M represents the capacitance seen between the two parallel circuit elements and exists because these two conductors lie in close proximity to each other separated by an air gap which functions as the dielectric in a conventional capacitor.

Capacitor:

Electronic device composed of two conducting plates separated by an insulator. It holds and stores electrical energy, blocks the flow of direct current (blocking capacitor), and allows the flow of alternating current proportional to frequency and capacitance. (Capacitance is measured in farads and is determined by plate material, insulation material, surface area, and distance between the plates.) Cardiac defibrillators, for example, use large capacitors to store electrons. *See* Figure.

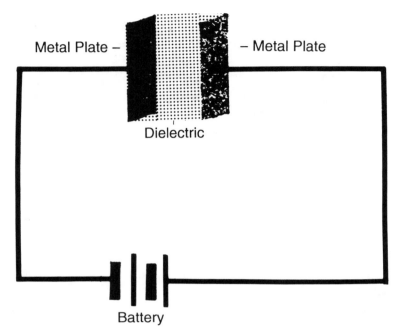

Capacitor: Three elements of a capacitor. They include two conductors separated by an electric insulator called the dielectric. The ability of the capacitor to store charges is related to the area of the two conductors and the relative electric impermeability of the dielectric.

Capillary Blood Flow:

See Microcirculation.

Capnograph:

Alternate name for an infrared CO_2 analyzer. *See* Capnography.

Capnography:

Display and recording of the concentration of end tidal carbon dioxide measured during the respiratory cycle. The display appears on a screen or on paper. *See* Figure.

Capnometry:

Measurement of end tidal carbon dioxide concentration that occurrs during the respiratory cycle.

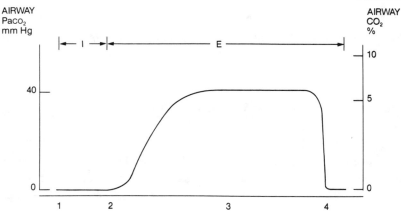

Capnography: Typical airway CO_2 waveform. At point 1, inhalation begins; inspired CO_2 (partial pressure or concentration) is zero. At point 2, exhalation begins; the anatomic dead space is "washed out" of the patient's lungs. Airway CO_2 is thus initially zero, indistinguishable from inhalation. Next, CO_2 rises as gas is exhaled from functional alveoli. At point 3, a flat or gently rising CO_2 plateau is formed as exhaled alveolar gas is measured. At point 4, inhalation begins and airway CO_2 again falls to zero. Carbon dioxide can be measured in units of partial pressure (mm Hg) or concentration by volume (per cent), usually computed as partial pressure divided by dry gas atmospheric pressure: at sea level on a clear day, $760 - 47 = 713$ mm Hg.

Capsaicin:

Natural molecule derived from plants. It appears to render skin insensitive to pain probably by depleting and preventing the reaccumulation of substance P in peripheral sensory nerve endings. *See* Substance P.

Capstan:

Rotating shaft found in the drive mechanism of a tape recorder that controls the speed of tape movement.

Carbachol:

Analog of acetylcholine which is used in the treatment of glaucoma. Solutions of carbachol applied to the conjunctiva decrease intraocular pressure and produce miosis. *See* Methylcholine.

Carbamazepine (Tegretol):

Drug that treats epilepsy, trigeminal neuralgia, bipolar disorders, and related central nervous system problems. Its toxic side effects involve the skin, liver, and bone marrow. It also has been implicated in teratogenic effects. *See* Trigeminal neuralgia.

Carbaminohemoglobin:

Chemical combination of hemoglobin and CO_2. It is one of the principal forms in which CO_2 exists in the blood. The lower the O_2 saturation of hemoglobin, the greater the amount of carbaminohemoglobin that can be found in the blood.

Carbide:

Compound composed of carbon plus one other element (e.g., tungsten, silicon). Silicon carbide is one of the hardest manufactured materials and is frequently used as an abrasive.

Carbocaine:

Trade name for mepivacaine. *See* Local anesthetic.

Carbonated Local Anesthetics:

Technique of adding carbon dioxide to a local anesthetic solution to facilitate more rapid onset and more extensive spread of analgesia. It is based in principle on the manipulation of the pH of the anesthetic solution. Its utility remains controversial. *See* Local anesthesic.

Carbon Black:

Amorphous powdered form of elemental carbon, usually made from the incomplete combustion of a gas. It is mixed with latex in a controlled manner (so the carbon chain connections are not broken) to make conductive rubber products.

Carbon Dioxide (CO$_2$):

Colorless, odorless, noncombustible gas of molecular weight 44, along with water, an end product of metabolism. CO_2 and the carbonates (HCO_3^-) aid in maintaining the neutrality of the blood and tissues. Low concentrations (approximately 5%) of CO_2, alter the pH of the blood and centrally stimulate respiration, whereas high concentrations of CO_2 centrally depress it. In solid form (Dry Ice) CO_2 is used in cryocautery to destroy abnormal tissue. *See* Carbon dioxide absorption; Carbon dioxide combining power; Carbon dioxide response; Carbon dioxide total in blood; Carbon dioxide transport in blood; Carbonic anhydrase.

Carbon Dioxide Absorption:

Elimination of CO_2 from rebreathing systems. It is usually accomplished by allowing exhaled gases to flow through an absorber, normally soda lime or Baralyme, which selectively reacts with the CO_2 from the gas mix. The stages of this reaction for soda lime are as follows: CO_2 combines with H_2O at the surface of the granules to form carbonic acid; carbonic acid combines with sodium and potassium hydroxides to yield sodium and potassium carbonates plus H_2O; the sodium and potassium carbonates then combines with the calcium hydroxide to produce calcium carbonate plus sodium and potassium hydroxides. The chemical reaction of CO_2 with a strong base is exothermic and yields 13,500 cal for each gram-molecular weight of CO_2. Two indicators of absorption ability are effective absorption ability (expressed as the volume of CO_2 absorbed/100 g of absorbent) and effective absorption efficiency (the percent of CO_2 absorbed out of the volume entering a canister). *See* Baralyme; Carbon dioxide absorption canister; Soda lime; To-and-fro carbon dioxide absorption.

Carbon Dioxide Absorption Canister:

Device within the breathing circuit of the patient that removes CO_2 from the recirculating gases. It contains either soda lime or Baralyme as the absorber. The standard canister, uniformly and properly packed with the appropriate absorbent, has a minimal capacity of 8 hours of continuous service in the anesthesia circuit. It should hold approximately 1 kg of absorbent granules. *See* Figures. *See* Carbon dioxide absorption; Soda lime.

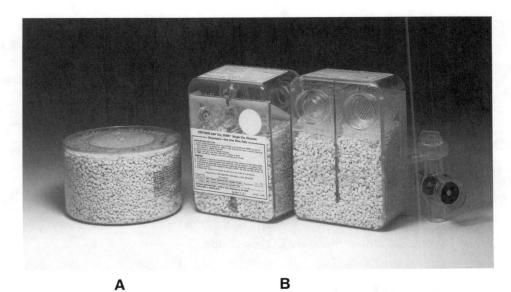

A   **B**

Carbon Dioxide Absorption Canister: Disposable CO_2 Absorbent Canisters. (A) For multiple use. (B) For single use. Front and back view plus cross/directional valve.

Carbon Dioxide Combining Power:

In vitro analysis that measures arterial blood gases to determine the contribution of PCO_2 in pH changes. It is derived by measuring (in millimoles per liter) the total CO_2 (free plus bound) in a plasma sample equilibrated with CO_2 at a pressure of 40 mm Hg at room temperature. (If a sample starts with an elevated CO_2 content, its combining power is less.) This kind of analysis is no longer in general use because it is too dependent on sampling technique.

Carbon Dioxide Dissociation Curve:

Plot that shows the relation between total CO_2 and PCO_2 in the blood. The curve shifts according to the PO_2. *See* Haldane effect.

Carbon Dioxide Electrode:

Element of a blood gas machine that detects and determines CO_2 concentration in a blood sample. It is a modified pH electrode with a semipermeable plastic membrane on one end that comes in contact with the sample. CO_2 diffuses through this membrane and raises the hydrogen ion concentration of the buffer solution contained behind the membrane. The hydrogen ions diffuse through a glass membrane in the electrode and register on a detector as a variation in ion current. The strength of the ion current is registered via appropriate electronics to reflect the CO_2 concentration in the sample. *See* Figure. *See* Oxygen electrode; pH electrode.

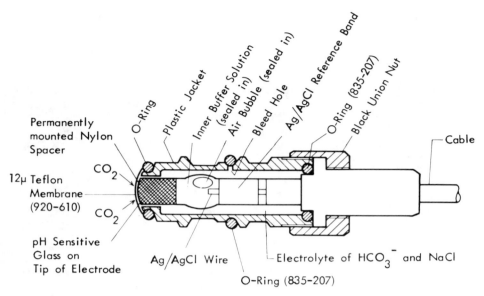

Permanently mounted Nylon Spacer

O-Ring

Plastic Jacket

Inner Buffer Solution (sealed in)

Air Bubble (sealed in)

Bleed Hole

Ag/AgCl Reference Band

O-Ring (835-207)

Black Union Nut

Cable

CO_2

12μ Teflon Membrane (920-610)

CO_2

pH Sensitive Glass on Tip of Electrode

Ag/AgCl Wire

Electrolyte of HCO_3^- and NaCl

O-Ring (835-207)

Carbon Dioxide Electrode: Standard CO_2 electrode.

Carbon Dioxide Method for Determining Alveolar Volume:

Technique based on the fact that gas exchange does not occur in the anatomic deadspace. If exhaled volume is measured and CO_2 concentration in the exhaled volume is also measured along with alveolar CO_2 concentration [approximated well in the healthy individual by arterial partial pressure of carbon dioxide ($PaCO_2$)], a relation can be drawn to determine alveolar volumes. *See* Anatomic deadspace.

Carbon Dioxide Response:

Reaction by the patient to changes in CO_2 concentration. If CO_2 is increased in inspired air, the normal patient increases minute ventilation. Initially depth is augmented followed by the rate. The tension of CO_2 in the arterial blood is one of the most sensitive variables in the body. Normal CO_2 tension in arterial blood is 38–42 mm Hg and venous blood averages 6–7 mm Hg higher. Elevated CO_2 in the arterial blood causes an immediate increase in cerebral blood flow that is almost linear to the increase in CO_2 tension. A decrease in arterial CO_2 causes a proportional decrease in cerebral blood flow. Increased metabolism in the tissues leads to a buildup of CO_2 eliciting local peripheral dilatation. However, this effect may be counteracted by a centrally regulated effect. *See* Cerebral blood flow, Intracranial pressure measurement.

Carbon Dioxide Total in Blood:

Amount of CO_2 in blood or plasma liberated upon acidification of the sample. It is measured in millimoles per liter. A more clinically useful derivative of total CO_2 is actual bicarbonate, which is the total CO_2 minus CO_2 found as carbonic acid and physically dissolved CO_2. Actual bicarbonate can be determined from the Henderson-Hasselbalch equation if pH and PCO$_2$ are determined by multiplying the PCO$_2$ by 0.03 (a factor representing the solubility of CO$_2$ in blood) and subtracting the value from total CO$_2$.

Carbon Dioxide Transport in Blood:

Movement of CO$_2$ in the blood. It is accomplished by three routes. By the first route, CO$_2$ dissolves in the fluid portion of the blood. At a partial pressure of 45 mm Hg, 2.7 ml CO$_2$ dissolves in 100 ml blood (whereas at 40 mm Hg, the amount is 2.4 ml/dl blood). Approximately 7% of the CO$_2$ exhaled per minute is transported to the lungs via this route. By the second route, CO$_2$ is transported in the blood as bicarbonate ions. The reaction is CO$_2$ + H$_2$O $\rightarrow$ H$_2$CO$_3$, which yields H$^+$ + HCO$_3$– (catalyzed by carbonic anhydrase contained in red blood cells). The bicarbonate ions leave the red blood cells (RBCs) to be carried in the fluid portion of the blood. The ions are replaced in the RBCs by chloride ions; therefore the chloride content of venous RBCs is higher than that of arterial RBCs. This phenomenon is called the chloride shift. This route accounts for the transport of 70% of CO$_2$ exhaled. By the third route, CO$_2$ is transported via a loose bonding to hemoglobin as carbaminohemoglobin. A small quantity is also transported joined to other plasma proteins. This route accounts for approximately 20% of CO$_2$ exhaled. Using all three methods, the concentration of CO$_2$ in tissue or blood at a PCO$_2$ of 45 mm Hg is 52 vol%. The concentration falls to 48 vol% when blood is arterialized in the lungs.

Carbonic Anhydrase:

Enzyme found in red blood cells, gastrointestinal mucosa, kidney tubules, and glandular epithelial cells. (Zinc is an integral component of carbonic anhydrase.) The principal function of the enzyme is to catalyze, in both directions, the reversible reaction of CO$_2$ and H$_2$O forming carbonic acid. Normally, the reaction requires several seconds, but carbonic anhydrase allows the reaction to proceed 5000 times faster. Its presence in red blood cells allows huge amounts of CO$_2$ to be transported in blood as bicarbonate, a product of carbonic acid dissociation. In the kidney, the presence of carbonic anhydrase facilitates resorption of bicarbonate. When a carbonic acid inhibitor, such as acetazolamide (Diamox, a mild diuretic) is administered, bicarbonate reabsorption is prevented, and some acidosis occurs in the body as a whole. *See* Carbon dioxide transport in blood.

Carbon Monoxide (CO):

Gas generated by the incomplete oxidation of carbon. Carbon monoxide reacts with hemoglobin (Hb) to form carboxyhemoglobin (COHb), which is highly toxic because it cannot carry O$_2$. Hemoglobin has 210 times more affinity for CO than it does for O$_2$. Carbon monoxide, in very low concentrations, is used to test the diffusion capacity of the lung. *See* Diffusion capacity of the lung.

Carbon Tetrachloride:

Compound first prepared in 1845 and used initially as an anesthetic. Because of its extreme toxicity, however, its use was discontinued. Although it can be decidedly toxic to the heart, causing arrhythmias and marked hypotension, its more deadly effects are on the liver and renal tubular cells.

Carbonyl Chloride:

See Phosgene.

Carcinoid Syndrome:

Complex of signs and symptoms associated with slowly growing malignancies of the enterochromaffin (argentaffin) cell type (found in the gastrointestinal tract, especially the ileum and small intestine, bronchus, and ovary). The tumor cells secrete serotonin (5-hydroxytryptamine, 5-HT), bradykinin, and histamine. These vasoactive substances are responsible for the signs and symptoms associated with carcinoid, including cutaneous flushing, diarrhea, telangiectasia, valvular heart disease, bronchial constriction, and asthma. Anesthetic complications arise from surgical manipulation of the tumor, which releases the vasoactive agents.

Card:

In computer technology, a card is a stiff piece of paper used to record either information or instructions for a computer. The information is recorded on the card by holes punched in it at a particular x-y location; each card has the same number and spacing of sites for holes. The presence or absence of a hole corresponds to the binary code (1 or 0) notation. A card punch or keypunch machine actually makes the holes, and a card-reading machine reads the location and function of the holes accordingly. Now quite obsolescent.

Card Inhaler:

Vaporizer for oral administration of a volatile anesthetic, most frequently used with tri-chloroethylene or methoxyflurane. It has a fixed upper limit of anesthetic concentration, which theoretically makes it safe for self-administration.

Cardiac Assist Device (Aortic Balloon):

See Intraaortic balloon pump.

Cardiac Catheterization:

Diagnostic technique in which a catheter is passed along veins or arteries into the heart to examine the structure of the heart. The catheter may also measure pressures and blood gas values in the heart and visualizes by dye injection, the flow characteristics of the coronary circulation. New catheters can carry visual or ultrasonic imaging modalities. *See* Figure. *See* Swan-Ganz catheter.

Cardiac Cycle:

Electrical and mechanical sequences that begin with the heart at rest, continue through contraction and relaxation of the heart chambers, and return to the heart at rest. *See* Figure. *See* Electrocardiogram.

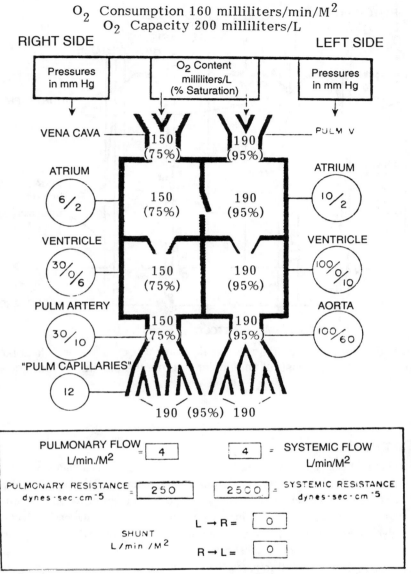

Cardiac Catheterization: Normal circulatory dynamics with O_2 contents, expected pressures, and percent saturations encountered during cardiac catheterization in adults.

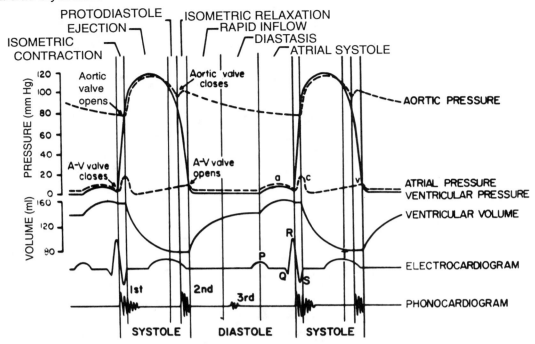

Cardiac Cycle: Events of the cardiac cycle, showing the changes in left atrial pressure, left ventricular pressure, aortic pressure, ventricular volume, the electrocardiogram, and the phonocardiogram.

Cardiac Glycosides:

Group of drugs, derived from the Digitalis or Strophanthus plants, which have a powerful and specific action on the myocardium and circulation. The term *digitalis* is often used to designate all the cardiac glycosides, but generic names of the more commonly used ones are digoxin, digitoxin, ouabain, and deslanoside. Because the basic effect of all the cardiac glycosides is the same, their use in anesthesia is more often determined by rapidity of onset, i.e., the faster the onset, the shorter the duration of action. (The fastest acting is ouabain with an onset of 3–10 minutes. The slowest is digitoxin with an onset of 25 minutes or more.) The cardiac glycosides have a profound positive inotropic effect, i.e., they stimulate the force of myocardial contractions without increasing O_2 demand. The action of the cardiac glycosides on a molecular level is not understood, but it is known to involve facilitation of calcium ion transport. Cardiac glycoside toxicity is enhanced by hypokalemia and hypercalcemia. The cardiac glycosides are most often used for treating congestive heart failure, arterial fibrillation, atrial flutter, and paroxysmal tachycardia. *See* Table. *See* Amrinone.

Cardiac Index (CI):

Relation of the cardiac output to body surface area measured as cardiac output per square meter of surface area. A normal CI for a 70-kg man is 2.5–3.5 L/min/m^2. *See* Cardiac output.

Cardiac Glycosides.

Generic Name (Trade Name)	Onset	Half-Life	Peak Effect	Comments
Digitalis Leaf (Digifortis) (Major active component is digitoxin)	2–6 hrs PO	4–6 days	12–24 hrs	Digitalis leaf is available in a powdered form for oral administration though it has largely been replaced by the purified glycosides. It is only moderately absorbed from the GI tract (20–40%). As with all the digitalis glycosides, its therapeutic indications are for congestive heart failure and various arrhythmias, especially atrial flutter and fibrillation. Side effects mark the onset of toxicity and include GI disturbances (e.g., anorexia, nausea, diarrhea, and pain) and neurologic disturbances (e.g., blurred vision, paresthesias, fatigue, weakness in the extremities, and toxic psychosis). Toxic levels of digitalis also can lead to arrhythmia and increasing heart failure which is worsened by hypokalemia and hypomagnesemia.
Digoxin (Lanoxin)	15–30 min IV	36 hrs	1–5 hrs	Digoxin is becoming the most widely used of the cardiac glycosides due to its intermediate duration of action. GI absorption is fairly good (60–80%) but is affected in patients with malabsorption syndromes and by antacids, kaolin and pectins. It is eliminated from the body via the kidneys.
Digitoxin (Crystodigin)	0.5–2 hr IV	4–6 days	4–12 hrs	Digitoxin is well absorbed from the GI tract (90–100%). It should be used cautiously in patients with liver disease as it is excreted primarily via the hepatic route. It is slowly metabolized in the body.
Deslanoside (Cedilanid-D)	10–30 min IV	33 hrs	1–2 hrs	Deslanoside is used for rapid digitalization. It is eliminated from the body via the kidneys.
Quabain (G Strophanthin)	5–10 min IV	21 hrs	0.5–2 hrs	Quabain is used for rapid digitalization. It has the most rapid onset and shortest duration of action. It is eliminated from the body via the kidneys.

Cardiac Massage:

Technique of directly compressing the heart in order to provide cardiac output. Closed cardiac massage is the type of direct compression administered through the intact chest wall, with cardiopulmonary resuscitation. Open cardiac massage is directly fingering the heart through thoracotomy and rhythmically compressing it. *See* Cardiopulmonary resuscitation.

Cardiac Output (CO):

Volume of blood pumped in 1 minute by either the right or left side of the heart. Because the two ventricles pump in series when healthy, their output must be the same during a given period. In the healthy individual, CO is considered to be the stroke volume (60–90 ml/beat in a 70-kg man × heart rate/minute. There are three principal methods for assessing CO. With the thermal dilution method, which is the most common, a known volume of cold solution is introduced into the circulation over a given time period. The extent and duration of the temperature change in the blood is measured by a thermistor distal to the injection point. If a curve is traced in which the y axis is equal to the temperature difference and the x axis is equal to time, the area under the curve is related to the CO. The thermal dilution method usually employs a Swan-Ganz catheter. With the dye dilution technique, an indicator dye, e.g., Cardio-Green (indocyanine green), is injected in precise quantity into the central venous circulation. Arterial sampling is done by passing the arterial blood through a dye detector. (Here the y axis equals dye concentration, and the x axis equals time.) The dye detector then traces out a curve, the area of which is related to the CO. Aside from requiring samples (which the thermal dilution technique does not), the dye dilution method shows the phenomenon of recirculation (dye that has been returned to the heart and pumped out again). The third method is based on the Fick principle. To be performed properly, it requires the collection of expired gases and right heart catheterization to obtain mixed venous blood. *See* Figure. *See* Area under the curve; Fick principle; Swan-Ganz catheter.

Cardiac Risk in Anesthesia:

Score (first described in 1977) assigned to each preoperative patient (for noncardiac surgery) based on the measurement of nine possible variables. These factors include age over than 70 years, myocardial infarction (MI) during the previous 6 months, an S3 gallop or jugular venous distention, significant valvular aortic stenosis, electrocardiogram rhythm disturbances, major acid-base disturbances or serum electrolyte abnormalities, site of operation, urgency of the operation, and more than five premature ventricular contractions per minute at any time. As an example of the two major risk factors, an MI during the preceding 6 months is worth 10 points, whereas an S3 gallop or jugular venous distention is worth 11 points. A total of 26 points or more (of a possible 53) places the patient in a high-risk category.

Cardiac Risk Index Score:

Scoring system for determining relative risk of general anesthesia based assigning a value for various historical and physical examination findings, the two most significant of which are myocardial infarction within 6 months of surgery and the finding of S3 sound or jugular venous distention on physical examination. The score has been found no more accurate than the cruder but much practiced physical status or ASA score system. *See* Table. *See* Physical status classifications.

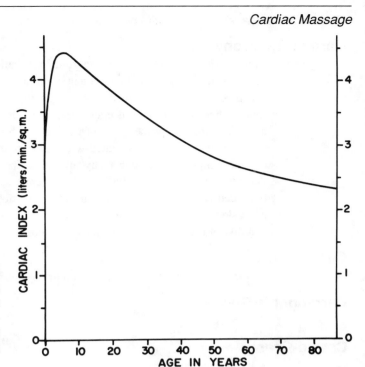

Cardiac Output: Cardiac index is the cardiac output divided by the surface area of the patient in square meters. Note the rise in cardiac index through the age of 10 and then its gradual drop off to old age.

Cardiac Risk Index Score: Multifactorial index of cardiac risk in non-cardiac surgical procedures.

FACTORS	POINTS
1. History: Age > 70	5
MI < 6 months	10
2. Physical exam: S_3 or JVD	11
3. ECG: Any rhythm other than sinus	7
>5 PVCs/min	7
4. General information: pO_2 < 60	
PCO_2 > 50	
K^+ < 3	3
BUN 50	
Creat > 3	
Bedridden	
5. Operation: Emergency	4
Intrathoracic	
Intraabdominal	3
Aortic surgery	
Total	50

Class 1: 0–5 points
2: 6–12 points
3: 13–25 points
4: 26 points or more

Source: Goldman L, et al. Multifactorial index of cardiac risk in non-cardiac surgical procedures. Reprinted by permission of *New Engl J Med* 1977; 297:845–850.

Cardiac Tamponade:

Compression of the heart due to fluid accumulation in the pericardial sac, causing a decrease in cardiac output and potential circulatory failure. Acute cardiac tamponade is a true medical emergency. Its critical state may be reached with as little as 250 ml blood or fluid. When it is chronic, it may take more than 1000 ml of effusion to compromise the heart. Trauma is a prime cause of tamponade; however, tuberculosis, infection, and local tumor growth are also associated with fluid accumulation in the pericardial sac. Signs of cardiac tamponade include tachycardia, decline in blood pressure and pulse pressure, distention of the jugular veins, rapid enlargement of the liver, and equalization of right- and left-sided cardiac pressure. Jugular vein distention is increased during inspiration (Kussmaul sign) or when pressure is applied over the liver (hepatojugular reflux), owing to the inability of the right side of the heart to accommodate the increased inflow of blood.

Carina:

Central ridge formed at the bifurcation of the trachea.

Cardiogenic Shock:

See Shock.

Cardio-Green:

See Indocyanine green.

Cardiokymography:

See Apexcardiography.

Cardioplegia Solution:

See Cardiopulmonary bypass.

Cardiopulmonary Bypass (Extracorporeal Circulation):

Technique of replacing the circulatory and respiratory functions of a patient in order to rest the heart during cardiac surgery. The anticoagulant heparin must be administered to the patient prior to cardiopulmonary bypass. The bypass requires withdrawal of the blood returning to the heart with large-bore cannulas. The blood is then oxygenated, and CO_2 is removed via an oxygenator. The blood is then pumped back to the root of the aorta (via another cannula) where it enters the arterial side of the circulation. The blood can also be heated and cooled by a heat exchanger in line with the heart-lung machine. (The heart-lung machine is operated by a highly trained perfusionist.) The heart is deliberately fibrillated while on bypass, (lowering its intrinsic oxygen demands) usually through the use of cardioplegia solution (placed in the cardiac circulation; a potassium electrolyte mixture). The heart-lung machine may have at least three and as many as six separate pumps. It is capable of maintaining cardiac output in liters per minute at least equal to the output of the patient's heart at rest. It can pump to the coronary arteries (separately if necessary), pump the cryocardioplegia solution, and drain the left ventricle of the blood that flows into it from the thebesian veins. Total bypass eliminates the heart and lungs from the circulation. Partial bypass (in which blood is removed from the femoral vein and returned to the femoral artery) can be used for short periods to assist the failing heart prior to more definitive treatment. *See* Figure. *See* Activated clotting time; Bubble oxygenator; Heparin; Membrane oxygenator; Rotating disk oxygenator; Screen oxygenator.

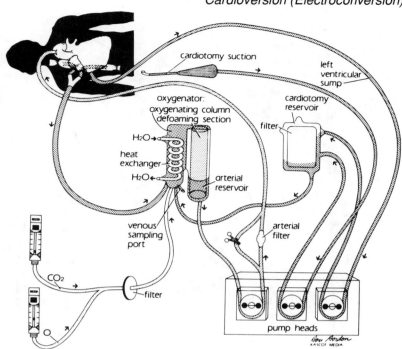

Cardiopulmonary Bypass: Note the following: (1) gravity drainage from venae cavae to oxygenator; (2) heat exchanger with entrance and exit ports for water; (3) separate sources for oxygen and carbon dioxide; (4) left ventricular sump for decompression of left ventricle via right superior pulmonary vein with return of blood to oxygenator via cardiotomy reservoir; and (5) arterial filter bypass in the event of filter obstruction.

Cardiopulmonary Resuscitation (CPR):

Technique for providing respiration and cardiac output for a patient with a failed circulation. There have been efforts to encourage the general population to learn the basic techniques of CPR. (These techniques, termed either the *basic rescue level* or *basic life support* are mouth-to-mouth respiration and closed-chest massage.) Advanced life support techniques usually require specially trained personnel and include such methods as pharmacologic intervention, electrical countershock, and cardiac pacing. Encouragement for basic CPR stems from a recognition that mouth-to-mouth resuscitation can supply all the O_2 necessary for life. (Exhaled breath contains 14–18% O_2 and external cardiac massage can generate one-third the normal cardiac output.) *See* Figure.

Cardiotachometer:

Device for determining heart rate. Primarily used to demonstrate the variability rate in the fetal heart and appropriately plotted on paper or on an oscilloscope screen.

Cardioversion (Electroconversion):

Method that uses electricity to restore normal cardiac rhythm. A shock is given to the heart through the use of external paddles placed against the chest. Commonly, the term cardioversion is interpreted narrowly to mean a technique used to treat any of a number of atrial, junctional, and some ventricular dysrhythmias. The currents used are much less than for ventricular defibrillation. Intravenous administration of barbiturates or diazepam is useful to counteract the pain caused by this procedure. Internal cardioversion is the placing of paddles on the heart through the open chest at the end of open heart surgery to reestablish a normal rhythm when the heart is fibrillating. *See* Defibrillation; Synchronized cardioversion.

141

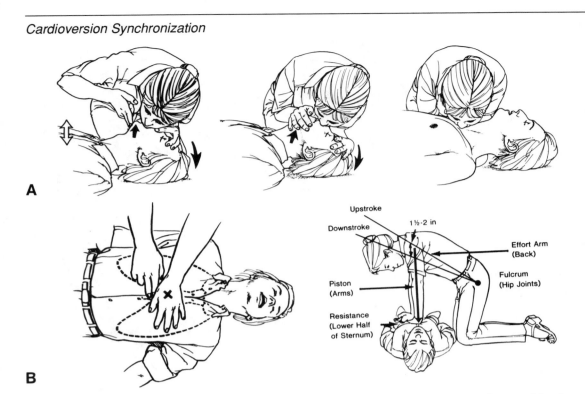

A

B

Cardiopulmonary Resuscitation: (A) Rescue Breathing: Left, Mouth-to-mouth; Center, Mouth-to-nose; Right, Mouth-to-stoma. (B) External Chest Compression: Left, Locating the correct hand position on the lower half of the body; Right, Proper position of the rescuer, with shoulders directly over the victim's sternum and elbows locked.

Cardioversion Synchronization:

See Synchronization mode.

Carlens Tube:

See Double-lumen tube.

Carotid Body:

Small mass of cells located between the origins of the external and internal carotid arteries. The carotid bodies lie adjacent to the carotid sinuses but are different in both function and structure. Their blood supply comes directly from the carotid artery and their basic function is to monitor arterial O_2 tension. Connected by pathways with the respiratory center of the brain (which they stimulate when O_2 tension falls), they have been implicated in the phenomenon known as paradoxical oxygen death. *See* Carotid sinus; Paradoxical oxygen death.

Carotid Shunt:

See Stump pressure.

Carotid Sinus:

Dilated part of the internal carotid artery located above the division of the common carotid artery and its two major branches. The carotid sinus, innervated by the glossopharyngeal (IX cranial) nerve, contains baroreceptors within its walls, which are stimulated by blood pressure changes. *See* Carotid body.

Carrier, Electrical:

Concept used to explain movement of a charge through a solid. Carriers are of two types. The first (and more easily understood) type is the electron, which is the carrier of a negative charge. The second type of carrier is the hole, representing the lack of an electron where one normally would be found. This hole is assigned a positive charge that migrates from one side of a solid to another. The movements of electrons and holes as carriers are the foundation of solid-state electronics, in which charges are moved under precise control through semiconductors.

CAT:

See Computerized axial tomography.

Catalyst:

Material that accelerates or initiates a chemical reaction without entering into that chemical reaction itself. Enzymes, catalysts found in living cells, not only initiate and accelerate reactions, they also enable certain reactions to occur at body temperature that would otherwise require temperatures of many hundreds of degrees.

Catecholamines:

Class of hormones found widely distributed in plants and animals synthesized from the essential amino acid tyrosine. The three prominent catecholamines in humans are dopamine, norepinephrine and epinephrine. Isoproterenol is a wholly synthetic catecholamine. The secretion of the adrenal medulla in humans is 20% norepinephrine, and 80% epinephrine. Both dopamine and norepinephrine are neurotransmitters, and norepinephrine in particular is associated with the sympathetic nervous system. *See* Figure. *See* Autonomic nervous system; Isoproterenol.

Catgut (gut):

String-like material made from the intestines of sheep that is used for suturing. The sheep intestines are soaked and cleaned in an alkali solution, drawn through holes in a plate, sterilized, and graded according to size. Because this material is degradable by various enzyme systems in living tissue, catgut sutures are not permanent. Absorption of the suture can be delayed by adding various minerals that regard degradation, such as chrome (chromic catgut).

Catheter:

Tube used to introduce or remove fluids from a body, channel, or hollow organ. It is made of rubber, plastic, or metal and is usually slender and flexible. The most frequently used is the intravenous catheter. The term "catheter" is often used interchangeably with the term "cannula." *See* Cannula.

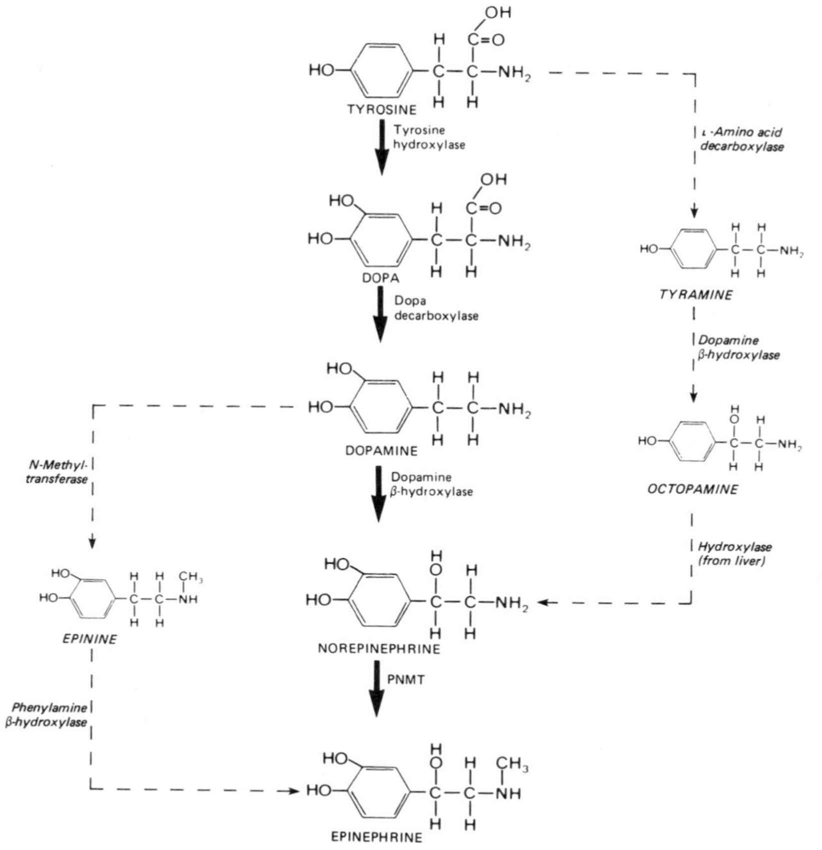

Catecholamines: Biosynthesis of catecholamines. The alternative pathways shown by the dashed arrows have not been found to be of physiologic significance in humans. PNMT, phenylethanolamine-N-methyltransferase.

Catheter Tip Embolism:

Unfortunate complication that occurs when a catheter is withdrawn through a needle and the tip of the catheter is sheared off by the cutting edge. *See* Air embolus.

Cathode:

Negative electrode or source of electrons, (i.e., negative charges) in a battery or vacuum tube.

Cathode-Ray Tube (CRT):

Evacuated glass cylinder, one end of which is coated on the inside surface with a phosphor. (The characteristic of this phosphor is such that it emits light when struck by a stream of electrons.) The other end of the glass cylinder contains a source of electrons, usually a heated wire. The electrons emitted by the heated wire are shaped and directed into a thin beam by either electrical or magnetic fields applied from the outside of the tube. This beam strikes the phosphor, setting it aglow, and can be deflected to draw either pictures, letters, or combinations. CRTs are used in both oscilloscopes and televisions. *See* Figure.

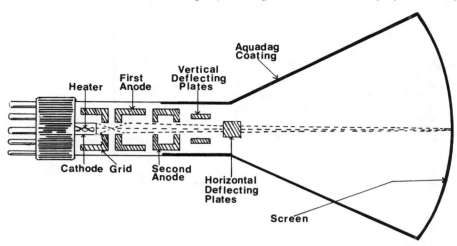

Cathode-Ray Tube: Common elements of the cathode ray tube. The heater provides the electron emission, the first and second anodes concentrate the electron beam, the vertical and horizontal deflecting plates seep the beam across the screen, and the Aquadag coating returns the electrons to ground.

Cation:

Positively charged ion. The principal cations in the body are sodium (Na^+), calcium (Ca^{2+}), potassium (K^+), and magnesium (Mg^{2+}).

Cauda Equina Syndrome:

Lesion of the tail of the spinal cord characterized by urinary retention, loss of sensation in the perineum, and loss of sexual function. It has been reported as a consequence of inadvertent injection of toxic or contaminated drugs during spinal anesthesia. *See* Arachnoiditis.

Caudal Anesthesia:

A type of regional anesthesia produced by injecting local anesthetic agents through the sacral area at the base of the spinal column. Caudal anesthesia is functionally a kind of epidural anesthesia, as the local anesthetic is deposited outside of dura covering the spinal cord. It is a popular technique for rectal and obstetric procedures. *See* Figure. *See* Epidural anesthesia.

Causalgia (Causalgic States; Reflex Sympathetic Dystrophy):

Term now applied to a group of disease states, (e.g., shoulder-hand syndrome, posttraumatic pain syndrome, Sudeck atrophy, and post-frostbite syndrome) that exhibit similar symptomatology, including hyperesthesia, motor disturbances, and skin changes (dryness). The patient suffering from severe causalgia goes to extremes to prevent the affected area from being touched or moved. Causalgia as a single entity was first described after the American Civil War in soldiers who had received injuries to the extremities from projectiles. Causalgia is a controversial entity. It is believed to be due to either peripheral dysfunction or hyperactivity of the sympathetic nervous system. Sympathetic blockade(s) can cause dramatic reversal of the condition, although blockade is less effective if the condition has continued for a year or more.

145

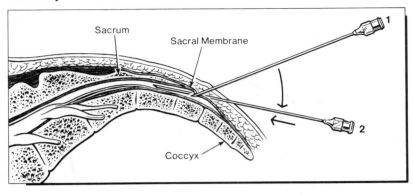

Caudal Anesthesia: Caudal Block: Needle insertion through sacrococcygeal (sacral) membrane.

Causality:

Legal principle stating that every effect is the consequence of an earlier cause(s). Causality can be true even if the antecedent causes are too numerous, too complicated, or too obscure for analysis.

Cauterization:

Process of burning tissue with a caustic drug or heat. Electrocautery, often used in this process, is a metal instrument that is electrically heated and used to burn, cut or coagulate tissue. It is different from an electrosurgery instrument, which uses radiofrequency current for the same purpose but does not necessarily become heated in the process. See Coagulation current.

CC/CNS Ratio:

Ratio between the dosage and the blood level of local anesthetics that cause irreversible cardiovascular collapse versus the dosage and blood level that produce central nervous system toxicity (convulsions).

CCTV:

See Closed circuit television.

CCU:

See Coronary care unit.

Ceiling Effect:

Drug dosing effect in which the desired pharmacologic action of a drug is *not* increased despite increased administration. Most frequently seen with the moderately potent agonist/antagonist opioids.

Celiac Plexus Block:

Regional anesthetic technique in which a local anesthetic is injected into the retroperitoneal area beyond the first lumbar vertebra while the patient is in a prone or lateral position. A

12-cm needle is used. Celiac block is indicated for patients with intractable pain due to acute or chronic pancreatitis or advanced carcinoma of the pancreas, liver, or bladder.

Cellulose:

Polysaccharide in which the basic building block is $C_6H_{10}O_5$ repeated in strands and cross-linkages as many as 2000 times. It is the main constituent of plant cell walls. In medicine, cellulose is often used as a hemostatic agent and as a volume expander for intravenous use.

Celsius Scale:

Temperature scale with the ice point of water at 0° and the boiling point of water at 100°. The Celsius scale (since 1948) is the more correct term for the centigrade temperature scale. One degree Celsius (C) is 1/100th of the temperature differential and is equal in magnitude to the Kelvin (K) scale ($1°K = 1°C$).

Centimeter-of-Water to Millimeter-of-Mercury Conversion:

An equation stating that 1.36 cm water equals 1.0 mm Hg mercury.

Centipoise:

One one-hundredth of a poise. *See* Viscosity.

Central Gas Supply:

System for supplying gas throughout hospital, clinic, or office where the cylinders or tanks are at a remote location from the site at which the gas is being used. The central supply usually consists of a facility for storage of gas, controls to deliver the gas through an in-the-wall piping system (at the appropriate working pressure), and an alarm system that indicates abnormal gas pressure changes. *See* Figure.

Central Nervous System:

Part of the nervous system consisting of the brain and spinal cord that processes information from the peripheral nervous system which is made up of the great nerves with their various end organs such as ganglia and motor endplates. *See* Figure. *See* Amygdala; Brain; Cerebrospinal fluid; Cranial nerves; Respiratory centers.

Central Neurogenic Hyperventilation:

Respiratory pattern seen at times after acute neurologic insult. Hyperventilation can be severe and can lead to an arterial partial pressure carbon dioxide below 20 mm Hg. *See* Apneustic breathing; Biot breathing.

Central Pain (Deafferentation Pain):

Pain that occurs when the nerve tissue that makes up afferent pain pathways has been disrupted and the pain sensation originates within the central nervous system. An example of central pain state is phantom limb pain. It is probably caused by abnormal activity in intermediate neurons along the afferent pain pathway. *See* Phantom limb.

147

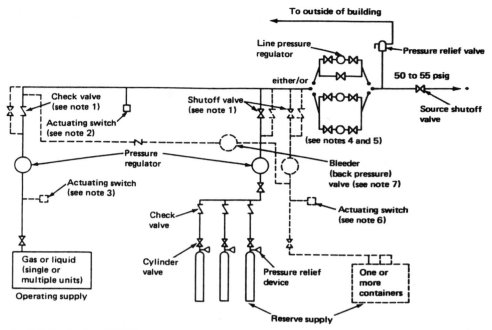

For SI Units: 1 psig = 6.895 kPa gauge.

Central Gas System: Typical bulk supply system (schematic). Bulk supply systems with different arrangements of valves, regulators, and gas supply units are permissible if they provide equivalent safeguards. The reserve supply is shown in the dotted lines.

Central Processing Unit (CPU):

Functional center of any computer that actually performs the mathematic operations necessary to alter input information. Data-processing buffers and temporary storage devices are often used to hold the various batches of information so the CPU can operate on them individually. In parallel processing a single computer uses multiple CPUs, each simultaneously working on a piece of program instruction. *See* Computer; Data-processing buffer.

Central Venous Pressure (CVP):

Pressure measured in the great veins of the thorax. This pressure is considered to be the filling pressure of the right side of the heart and is an indication of both the adequacy of blood return to the heart and the performance of the right ventricle. The normal CVP tracing has five separate wave patterns: *a, c, x, v,* and *y*. (The wave patterns labeled *a, c,* and *v* are positively directed; and the wave patterns *x* and *y* are negatively directed.) The *a* wave is caused by right atrial contraction; the *c* wave is caused by the pushing of the tricuspid valve into the right atrium as the right ventricle contracts. These two waves are followed by the *x* descent, which results from further atrial relaxation and the downward displacement of the tricuspid valve during ventricle contraction. The *v* wave is formed by the filling of the right atrium against the closed tricuspid valve. The *y* descent is caused by the opening of the tricuspid valve as blood begins to flow from the right atrium into the right ventricle. The wave of particular importance is the *a* wave, as it is absent in patients with atrial fibrillation. Enlarged *a* waves occur during conditions of increased resistance to right atrial emptying, such as right ventricular hypertrophy, pulmonary stenosis, tricuspid stenosis, or pulmonary hypertension. A huge *a* wave may be seen when the right atrium contracts with the tricuspid valve closed; it can be seen in nodal rhythms of the heart and results in a "cannon wave." *See* Figure.

Centrifuge:

Machine in which samples of solutions, suspensions, or mixtures may be spun rapidly to separate out the lighter portions (due to centrifugal force).

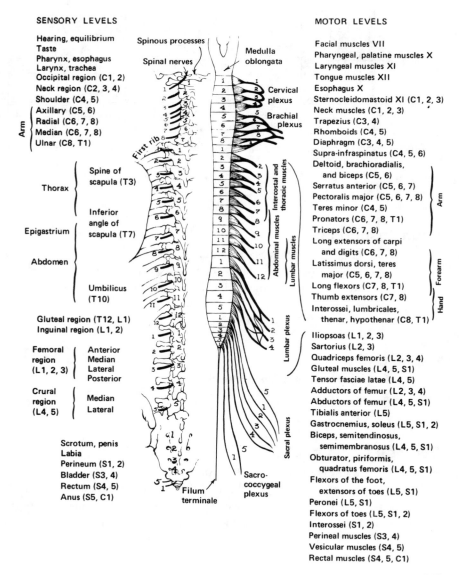

Central Nervous System: The motor and sensory levels of the central nervous system.

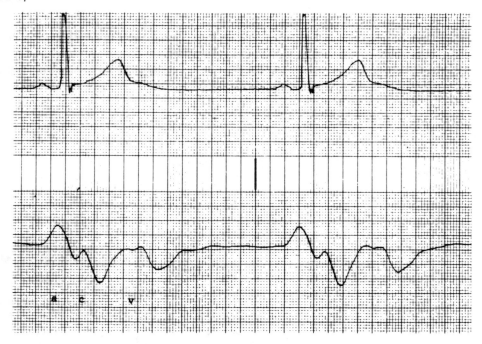

Central Venous Pressure: Tracing of the central venous pressure showing the five waveforms.

Cephalosporins:

Group of antibiotics structurally similar to the penicillins. The antibacterial spectrum of the cephalosporins resembles the broad-spectrum penicillins. A cross-sensitivity reaction between cephalosporins and penicillins exists in some individuals. *See* Table.

Cephalothin:

Cephalosporin. *See* Antibiotics.

Cerebral Angiography:

Radiographic examination of the vascular system of the brain after injection of dye into the carotid artery. Previously the primary technique for the study of neuropathology, it is a relatively safe procedure that has a small but known morbidity and mortality. This procedure is now being replaced or supplemented by computed axial tomography (CAT) scanning and magnetic resonance cerebroplegiaimaging (MRI) techniques. *See* Figure.

Cephalosporins.

Generic Name (Trade Name)	Spectrum of Activity	Comments
Cephalothin (Keflin) IM IV	Active against both G^+ and G^- microbes (especially *Escherichia coli, Proteus mirabilis*) including penicillinase-producing Staphylococcus.	Cephalothin, like other cephalosporins, is the primary agent against *Klebsiella pneumoniae* infections. Side effects include rash, fever, increased SGOT, blood dyscrasias, anaphylactoid reactions, and serum sickness. Severe pain can occur after IM injection and repeated injections can lead to phlebitis.
Cephaloridine (Loridine) IM	Similar to cephalothin plus *Mycobacterium fortuitum. E. coli* and *Clostridium perfringens* are more sensitive to cephaloridine than to cephalothin.	Cephaloridine shows higher and more sustained blood levels and is better tolerated than cephalothin. Side effects include rash, eosinophilia and nephrotoxicity, especially at higher doses.
Cephalexin (Duricef) Monohydrate PO	Similar to cephalothin.	Cephalexin monohydrate is excreted unchanged in urine and is useful in urinary tract infections caused by *E. coli, Pr. mirabilis*, and some Klebsiella.
Cefazolin Sodium (Ancef) IM (Kefzol) IV	Similar to cephalothin thought it is more active against *E. coli, Klebsiella*, some Enterobacter, indolepositive Proteus and *Hemophilus influenzae*.	Cefazolin sodium is recommended for the treatment of urinary tract, skin, respiratory and soft tissue infections. There is less pain after IM injection than with cephalothin. Side effects include rash (uncommon), increased SGOT, and increased alkaline phosphatase.
Cephradine (Anspor) IM (Velosef) IV	Similar to cephalexin though it may be less effective against *E. coli* and *Pr. mirabilis*. It is active against Enterococci.	Cephradine shows excellent absorption after oral administration.
Cephapirin (Cefadyl) IM	Similar to cephalothin though it is more active against *Streptococcus pyogenes* and Pneumococcus.	Cephapirin is not well tolerated IM. Nausea is quite common after administration.
Cefamandole (Mandol) Nafate IM IV	Wider spectrum than cephalothin. Increased activity against Enterobacter, indole-positive Proteus and *H. influenzae*.	Cefamandole is not well tolerated IM. More active than cephalothin against G^- microorganisms. Pseudomonas is resistant.
Cefoxitin (Mefoxin) IM IV	Less active than cefamandole against most G^+ and G^- organisms. Increased activity against indole-positive species of Serratia, Proteus and *Bacillus fragilis*.	Highly resistant to beta-lactamases produced by G^- bacilli.

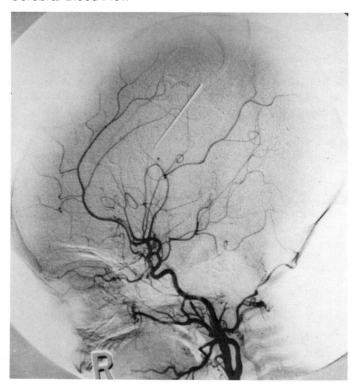

Cerebral Angiography: An angiogram outlining the vasculature of the right side of the brain in a child.

Cerebral Blood Flow:

Amount of arterial blood perfusing the brain each minute. In the normal adult it is about 700 ml/minute, and in the brain as a whole approximately 46–54 ml/100 g/minute. Regional cerebral blood flow is individualized by the structure and function of the brain; it is highest in the gray matter (up to 140 ml/minute in the superior colliculus with the eyes open) and lowest in the white matter (down to 20–25 ml/minute in the corpus callosum). In the past, cerebral blood flow was determined by the Fick principle using N_2O uptake; more recently it has been measured by radioisotope tracer techniques. *See* Figures.

Cerebral Dehydration:

Condition brought about by intravenous injection of drugs, such as mannitol or urea, to increase the osmolarity of the blood. This practice removes water from all cellular structures, particularly the brain, causing the neurons to shrink in volume. It is usually employed as a technique for neurosurgery to "relax the brain" and to allow better access without having to enlarge the incision.

Cerebral Function Monitor:

One of the first clinically available devices for monitoring the electroencephalogram (EEG) intraoperatively. It uses a single pair of electrodes to measure the amplitude of the EEG signal. It also monitors the impedance between those electrodes to show any changes in the

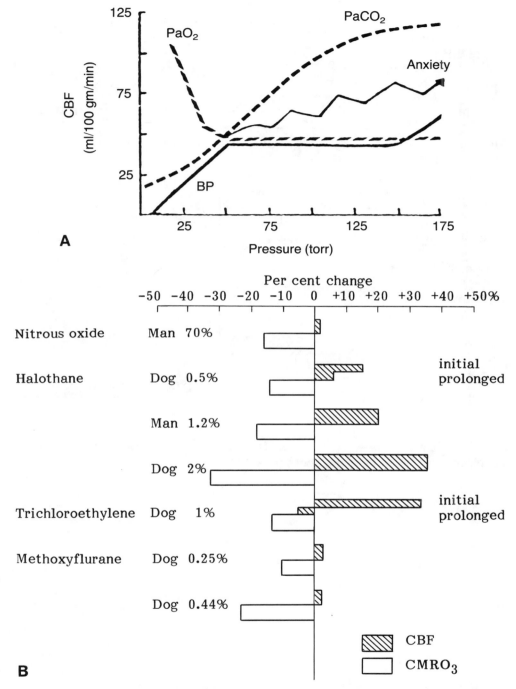

Cerebral Blood Flow: (A) Changes in cerebral blood flow brought about by changes in PaO₂, PaCO₂, and blood pressure, and by the variable effect of anxiety. (B) Effects of the gaseous and intravenous anesthetic drugs on cerebral blood flow and cerebral metabolic rate.

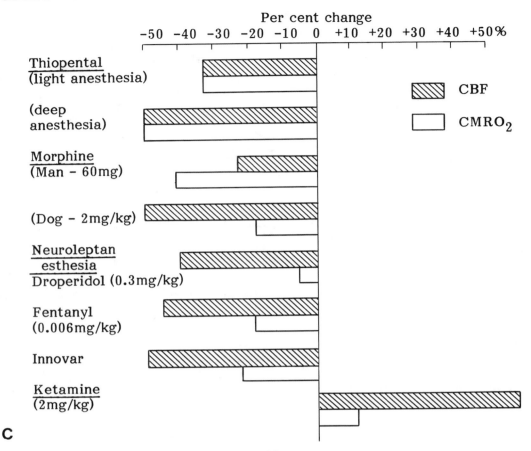

C

Cerebral Blood Flow *(continued):* (C) Effects of the gaseous and intravenous anesthetic drugs on cerebral blood flow and cerebral metabolic rate.

contact between the scalp and the electrodes. The device has not been well accepted in anesthesiology.

Cerebral Metabolic Rate for Glucose (CMR$_g$):

Rate at which the brain uses its major metabolic substrate, glucose, usually listed as milligrams of glucose per 100 grams of brain per minute. Wide regional differences exist in the brain for metabolic use of glucose but averages 5mg/100g/minute. *See* Cerebral metabolic rate for oxygen.

Cerebral Metabolic Rate for Oxygen (CMRO$_2$):

Rate at which the brain uses oxygen for normal metabolic activities (humans average approximately 3.3 cc/100g/minute) usually recorded as cubic centimeters per 100 grams per minute. Multiple regional differences exist in oxygen utilization. The human brain is 2% of the body mass but uses 20% of resting O_2 consumption. *See* Cerebral metabolic rate for glucose.

Cerebral Perfusion Pressure:

Amount of difference between arterial blood pressure and intracranial pressure. In cases of severe trauma, the intracranial pressure can be higher than the systolic blood pressure, completely shutting off arterial blood flow to the brain. *See* Subarachnoid screw.

Cerebroplegia:

Technique for perfusing the brain within an oxygenated crystalloid solution at low temperature, usually 4°C. An experimental technique for brain preservation.

Cerebrospinal Fluid (CSF):

Fluid that bathes and supports the brain. In the normal adult it totals about 140 ml. Measured by lumbar puncture (in the lateral position), CSF pressure is between 10 and 15 cm H_2O. The specific gravity of CSF is about 1.007. This normally clear and colorless fluid is produced by the choroid plexus, a specialized secretory tissue of the lateral third and fourth ventricles, at a rate of about 0.5 ml/minute. The turnover of the entire CSF volume takes about 5 hours. The flow of the CSF is from the lateral ventricles to the third ventricle and then to the fourth ventricle via the cerebral aqueduct. From the fourth ventricle, the CSF enters the subarachnoid space, where it ultimately bathes the brain and spinal cord. It is eventually absorbed by the arachnoid villi, which are specialized tissues projecting into the dural venous sinuses, thereby creating elevations known as arachnoid granulations. *See* Figure.

Certified Registered Nurse Anesthetist:

See American Association of Nurse Anesthetists.

Cervical Plexus Block:

Conduction block of the cervical plexus, which is formed by the first four cervical nerves. The area affected is from the inferior surface of the mandible to the second rib. This block is most often used to provide anesthesia for a conscious patient undergoing carotid endarterectomy.

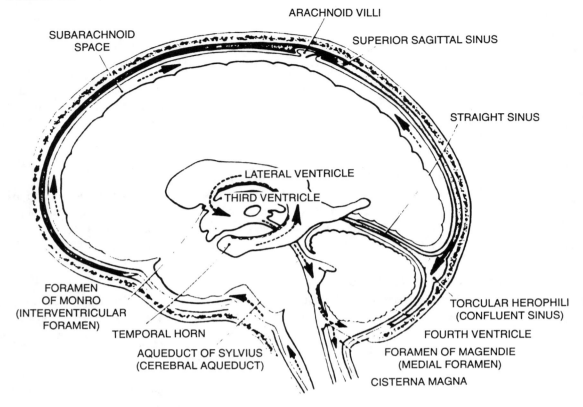

Cerebrospinal Fluid: Circulation.

Cesium-137:

Radioactive element that emits gamma rays with a half-life of 33 years. The gamma radiation energy spectrum is less than that of cobalt 60. It has some medical applications as a radioactive tracer and a radiation treatment modality.

Cetacaine:

Trade name for a liquid topical anesthetic containing tetracaine combined with benzocaine. *See* Local anesthetic.

CFF:

See Critical flicker frequency.

C Fiber:

See Nerve fiber, anatomy and physiology of.

CGS System of Units:

System of measurements in which the centimeter is the unit of length, the gram is the unit of mass, and the second is the unit of time. The CGS system has been superseded by the SI system. *See* SI unit.

Channel:

Defined pathway for information signals. The most obvious example is the channel on a standard television set. Each channel number actually refers to the frequency range of the carrier signal over which the information (the television program) is sent. Biologic membranes also contain channels to facilitate ion transport. *See* Calcium channel blocker.

Charge:

Measurable property of certain elementary particles. The terms *positive* and *negative* are semantic inventions in the most simplified sense. They signify that a particle has either an excess of electrons (negatively charged) or a scarcity of electrons (positively charged).

Charles Law:

Physical law that governs the behavior of an ideal gas. It states that at a constant pressure and 0°C the volume of a fixed mass of gas increases by 1/273 for each degree Celsius rise in temperature. For example, if at constant pressure a gas occupies 1 L at 0°C it will occupy a volume of l L plus 100/273 L (136.3 L) at 100°C.

Chassaignac's Tubercle:

Prominent anterior tubercle of cervical vertebrae VI, which is often used as a landmark for local anesthetic blocks done in the neck. *See* Stellate ganglion block.

CHCT:

Caffeine and halothane contracture test; malignant hyperthermia. *See* Caffeine test.

Chemical Solution:

Liquid mixture in which a chemical reaction has occurred between the solvent and the solute, such that the solute is unrecoverable by physical processes.

Chemiluminescence:

Phenomenon in which bacteria or fireflies produce light without production of heat. It is usually accomplished through oxidation of a species-specific pigment called luciferin promoted by the enzyme luciferase. *See* Anesthesia, pressure reversal of.

Cheng Needle:

See Epidural needle.

Chest Percussion:

See Postural drainage.

Chest Physiotherapy:

Procedure referring to postural drainage in conjunction with chest percussion and vibration. *See* Postural drainage.

Cheyne-Stokes Respiration:

Respiratory pattern in which hyperpnea alternates with apnea. It is seen in various disease states, especially those with damage to the central nervous system. This type of respiratory phenomenon is often demonstrated in patients with uremia and congestive heart failure. *See* Figure. *See* Biot breathing.

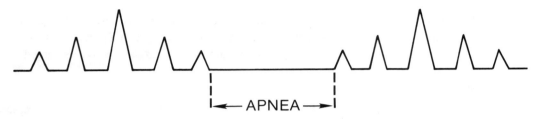

Cheyne-Stokes Respiration: Pattern of Cheyne-Stokes respiration.

CHF:

See Congestive heart failure.

Chip:

Slang term, originally from electronics, for an integrated circuit. *See* Figure. *See* Circuit, integrated.

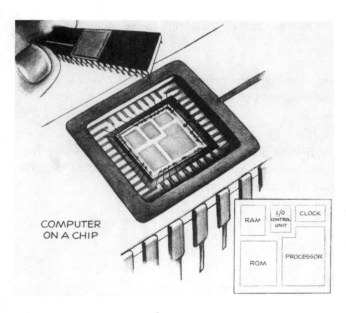

Chip: A chip is a miniaturized electronic circuit. Chips are approximately 1/16th to 1/2 inch square and about 1/30th of an inch thick. They hold from a few dozen to several million electronic components (transistors, resistors, etc). The terms chip, integrated circuit and micro-electronic are synonymous.

Chi-Square Test (χ^2):

Test used to compare frequency distribution and to determine statistical significance of the differences; i.e., a comparison of the observed frequency with the expected frequency. It is useful as an alternative to the Student *t* test on small samples.

Chloral Hydrate:

Sedative-hypnotic drug first used during the 1870s. Most of its effect is believed to be due to its rapid reduction to its active metabolite trichloroethanol. After having been supplanted by the barbiturates, chloral hydrate has again become relatively popular as a children's sedative or as a hypnotic the night before surgery. Combined with ethanol it forms the "Mickey Finn" cocktail. (The power of this cocktail to "knock out" its imbiber is somewhat overrated.)

Chloramphenicol:

Broad-spectrum antibiotic first employed clinically in 1948 and used widely during the 1950s and early 1960s. Its documented tendency to cause serious and often fatal blood dyscrasias, however, has now limited use to the most serious of infections as the drug of last choice. *See* Antibiotic.

Chlordiazepoxide (Librium):

See Benzodiazepine.

Chloride:

Principal extracellular anion in the body. Its normal plasma concentration is given variously as 95–105 mEq/L. Intracellularly, it has low concentration (2 mEq/L). Early technical breakthroughs allowed simple, accurate measurement of chloride in serum and urine before it was possible to measure any other ion (sodium, potassium) correctly. Hypochloremia may be indicative of alkalosis, which is a major consequence of persistent vomiting. Excess chloride appears to be easily excreted by the kidney.

Chloride Shift:

See Carbon dioxide transport in blood.

Chloroform:

General anesthetic first discovered soon after the initial demonstration of ether anesthesia during the 1840s. It has been popular in England and Europe for many decades. Chloroform ($CHCl_3$) is a potent, nonexplosive anesthetic agent that has a fairly rapid induction and emergence time. Associated with severe liver damage and sudden fatal cardiac arrhythmias, it is seldom used in contemporary anesthetic practice. *See* Figure.

$$\begin{array}{c} Cl \\ | \\ Cl-C-H \\ | \\ Cl \end{array}$$

Chloroform.

Chloroprocaine (Nesacaine):

Short-acting, ester-type local anesthetic that is a derivative of procaine. *See* Local anesthetic.

159

Chlorpheniramine Maleate (Chlor-Trimeton):

Commonly used antihistaminic agent, usually administered orally.

Chlorpromazine (Thorazine):

See Phenothiazine.

Cholinergic Crisis:

Medical emergency precipitated by an overdose of an anticholinesterase agent. The crisis shows muscarinic effects (e.g., sweating, miosis, salivation, lacrimation, and bowel hyperactivity) as well as nicotinic effects (e.g., muscle fasciculations and paralysis).

Cholinergic Nervous System:

See Autonomic nervous system.

Cholinergic Receptor:

Proteinaceous structure on the surface of a cell that specifically binds to the neurotransmitter acetylcholine and its congeners. Cholinergic receptors vary in makeup and density at different sites and can be divided into two types by their response to the natural alkaloids, muscarine and nicotine. *See* Receptor.

Cholinesterase (Pseudocholinesterase):

Enzyme that catalyzes the hydrolysis of choline esters. *See* Acetylcholinesterase; Dibucaine number. *See* Pseudocholinesterase.

Chordotomy:

Neurosurgical procedure that diminishes chronic intractable pain. In a chordotomy, the pain pathways on one side of the spinal cord are interrupted by a precise incision. This procedure is in contrast to rhizotomy, in which only the nerve roots of the particularly painful area are sectioned. *See* Rhizotomy.

Christian Science:

System of religious teaching founded in 1866 in the United States. Christian Scientists deny the reality of the world and argue that illness and sin are illusions that can be overcome by the mind. They therefore refuse medical help for illness.

Christmas Disease:

Bleeding disorder due to factor IX deficiency. The disease is named after the family in which it was first diagnosed. *See* Hemophilia.

Chronic Obstructive Pulmonary Disease (COPD) (Emphysema):

Lung disorder seen almost exclusively in heavy smokers and characterized by irreversible airway obstruction associated with emphysema and chronic bronchitis. The emphysematous component results in destruction of the alveolar walls with subsequent abnormal enlargement of the air spaces distal to the terminal nonrespiratory bronchioles. This destruction of alveolar walls causes loss of support and some degree of collapse of the distal nonrespiratory bronchioles, which in turn causes narrowing of their lumens, particularly on expiration. The chronic bronchitis component leads to hyperplasia of mucous glands, inflammation, mucosal edema, bronchospasm, along with impacted secretions. The single most consistent finding in COPD is the loss of the 1-second forced expiratory volume (FEV_1). Practically, it means that the patient with COPD finds it increasingly difficult to expel a given volume of air within a finite period of time. The consequences of COPD are progressive respiratory embarrassment with elevated PCO_2 and decreased PO_2. Treatment of COPD is aimed at providing respiratory support during acute exacerbation and at fighting infection. A genetic predisposition to emphysema has been discovered. Those individuals have a deficiency of α_1-antitrypsin on serum assay. They appear to be uniquely susceptible to autodigestion of pulmonary tissue by the naturally occurring proteases, as the antitrypsin molecule is not present to protect them. These cases may account for as much as 2–3% of all emphysema cases.

Chronotropism:

Ability to influence the cardiac rate via the adrenergic sympathetic nerves. Positive chronotropic drugs increase the heart rate, whereas negative ones decrease it (e.g., acetylcholine).

Ci:

See Curie.

CI:

See Cardiac index.

Cinchocaine (Nupercaine):

British term for dibucaine. *See* Dibucaine; Local anesthetic.

Circadian Rhythm:

Cyclic repetition of certain phenomena that occur on a 24-hour basis. Physiologic functions that seem to follow this periodicity include body temperature, adrenal cortical function, electrolyte concentration, and urine volume. For example, in those people who sleep at night and are awake during the day, adrenal cortisol secretion is at peak levels upon awakening. Its level progressively falls throughout the rest of the day.

Circle of Willis:

Circular formation of arteries at the base of the brain. It is the origin of the six large vessels supplying the cerebral cortex. Composed of the internal carotids and the anterior and posterior cerebral arteries, it is not unusual for the Circle of Willis to be incomplete. *See* Figure.

Circle System:

Assembly of anesthesia hoses and valves that are unidirectional. Theoretically and (for the most part) practically, gas flows through the system in only one direction. The system is considered to be semiclosed or partially rebreathing in type, i.e., part of the gas expired by the patient goes through a CO_2 absorber and forms part of the fresh gas supply of the succeeding inspiration. *See* Figure.

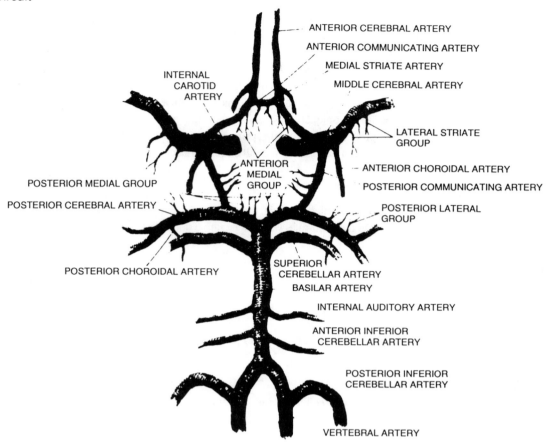

ANTERIOR CEREBRAL ARTERY

ANTERIOR COMMUNICATING ARTERY

MEDIAL STRIATE ARTERY

MIDDLE CEREBRAL ARTERY

INTERNAL
CAROTID
ARTERY

LATERAL STRIATE
GROUP

ANTERIOR
MEDIAL
GROUP

ANTERIOR CHOROIDAL ARTERY

POSTERIOR MEDIAL GROUP

POSTERIOR COMMUNICATING ARTERY

POSTERIOR CEREBRAL ARTERY

POSTERIOR LATERAL
GROUP

POSTERIOR CHOROIDAL ARTERY

SUPERIOR
CEREBELLAR ARTERY

BASILAR ARTERY

INTERNAL AUDITORY ARTERY

ANTERIOR INFERIOR
CEREBELLAR ARTERY

POSTERIOR INFERIOR
CEREBELLAR ARTERY

VERTEBRAL ARTERY

Circle of Willis: (Circulus Arteriosus) Its origins and branches.

Circuit:

System of active and passive electrical components that carry or act on an electrical current. The term usually refers to the smallest combination of two or more electric components that perform a specific function on a current (e.g., amplification, rectification). For example, two diodes can be used to form a circuit that can will change alternating to direct current. *See* Figure.

Circuit Breaker (Overcurrent Protector):

Device used to protect an electric circuit. It interrupts the current flow when the flow exceeds a predetermined limit. A fuse performs the same function; however, it usually can be used only once, as it is destroyed by an overcurrent condition and its destruction interrupts that condition. Circuit breakers are usually mechanical spring-loaded devices that can be reset rather than replaced.

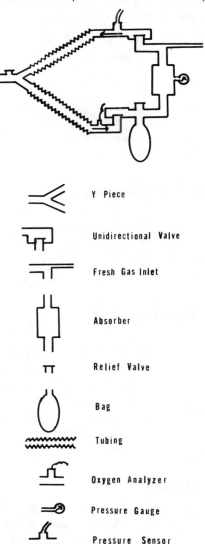

Y Piece

Unidirectional Valve

Fresh Gas Inlet

Absorber

Relief Valve

Bag

Tubing

Oxygen Analyzer

Pressure Gauge

Pressure Sensor

Circle System: One of the many configurations of valves, fresh gas inlet, CO_2 canister, relief valve and breathing bag possible with a circle system.

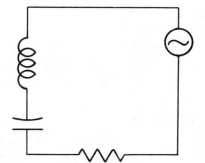

Circuit: Simple circuit showing the symbols for a power source (circle with a sinusoid waveform); resistance (jagged line); capacitance (two lines perpendicular to the current path separated by an air space); and inductance (series of loops).

Circuit, Integrated (IC):

Single unit of semiconductive material that contains thousands of electrically active elements. Integrated circuits are usually made by photo-etchings from photomicrographs. The desired circuit is initially drawn full size and then photographed. The negative is then markedly reduced in size. This negative is used to control a laser, which in turn cuts a layered piece of semiconductive material of the proper electrical characteristics. The end result of this entire process is the IC. Miniaturization is becoming so advanced that limits are being approached that approximate the physical size of electrons. Circuit elements densities can be routinely made greater than 5 million elements/in^3.

Circuit, Solid State:

Set of electrical components that operate on a current in such a way that the current always flows through solid materials. This situation is in contrast to vacuum tube circuitry in which current partially flows through the evacuated glass envelopes of the vacuum tubes. Solid-state circuits (in contrast to vacuum tube circuits) are characterized by small size, low heat generation, and ruggedness.

Circulator, Revell:

Device that uses an external source of power (gas pressure or suction) to move the anesthetic gases continuously around the anesthesia machine breathing circle. This setup reduces the deadspace under the mask by providing fresh gas to this volume even during pauses in ventilation. The circulator, by operating at a flow rate that just "floats the valves," decreases the resistance of these valves, thereby reducing the work needed for spontaneous ventilation. Certain disadvantages have prevented the circulator from gaining wide acceptance, including the need for a power source and the tendency to gas leakage due to the slight increase in pressure during operation. *See* Circle system.

Cirrhosis:

Disease of the liver that causes replacement of hepatic parenchymal cells with collagen. Associated with alcohol abuse, cirrhosis causes a decrease in the number of hepatocytes, which depresses the physiologic functions of the liver. Hepatic blood flow also falls, and the liver is jeopardized during decreases in systemic arterial perfusion pressure or oxygenation. Cirrhosis has an unquantifiable tendency to affect drug metabolism in the individual patient, which leads to a variable lengthened effect for those drugs that depend on liver metabolism for elimination.

Cisapride:

Gastric prokinetic drug that has been shown to reverse morphine induced gastric stasis when given intramuscularly.

Cladding:

Process in which one metal is bonded to the surface of another to prevent corrosion of the protected metal. For example, zinc and nickel are often used to clad iron.

Clark Electrode:

See Oxygen electrode.

Clearance:

Elimination of a biologically active substance from an organism. For example, total body clearance (usually abbreviated as Qb) is a measure of the rate of removal of a given drug from the body.

Click Murmur Syndrome:

See Mitral valve prolapse.

Clock, Electronic:

Device used to precisely time and therefore synchronize the various functions of a multi-purpose circuit. Best device to tell when surgeon is late.

Clorazepate Dipotassium (Tranxene):

See Benzodiazepine.

Closed Anesthesia System:

See Anesthesia system, closed.

Closed Chest Massage:

See Cardiopulmonary resuscitation.

Closed Circuit Television (CCTV):

System usually used for surveillance or security of limited-access areas, e.g., an operating room. All parts of the system, including the cameras, control mechanisms, and the television receiver, are physically linked by cables, eliminating the need to transmit by aerials.

Closed Claims:

Term from the insurance industry that refers to claims, usually for malpractice, that have either been litigated to a conclusion or settled. *See* Closed claims study.

Closed Claims Study:

Investigation of medicolegal cases based upon "closed claims" registered with insurance companies, i.e., claims for malpractice which have been either settled, appropriately defended, or disposed of. *See* Closed claims.

Closing Capacity:

Lung gas displacement at which small airways narrow and close during continuous exhalation. In health, this point should exist at the far end of the expiratory reserve volume but increasing age, smoking, and obesity move it toward the tidal volume (airways close increasingly earlier during exhalation). In general, any reduction of the functional residual capacity shifts the closure of a significant number of small airways from a point in the

165

expiratory reserve volume to a point in the tidal volume. *See* Figure. *See* Absorption atelectasis; Lung volumes and capacities.

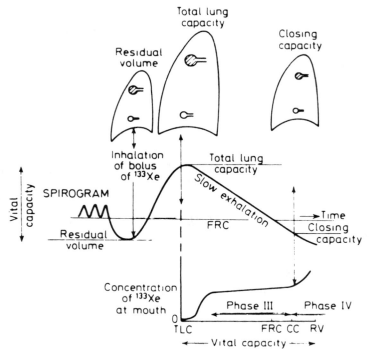

Closing Capacity: Measurement of closing capacity using a radioactive gas as a tracer. The bolus of tracer is inhaled near residual volume and due to airway closure is distributed only to those alveoli with air passages still open (shaded area). During expiration, concentration of the tracer gas becomes constant after the dead space is washed out. This plateau (phase III) gives way to a rising concentration of tracer gas (phase IV) when there is closure of airways leading to alveoli which did not receive the tracer gas.

Clostridium Botulinum Toxins:

Systemic poison elaborated by the bacillus *Clostridium botulinum*, which causes botulism. It prevents release of acetylcholine by cholinergic nerve fibers and gives rise to neurologic symptoms. This toxin is the most potent organic poison ever discovered.

C_m:

See Minimum blocking concentration.

C_{MAX}:

The maximum plasma concentration of a drug achieved after its administration.

CMR_g:

See Cerebral metabolic rate for glucose.

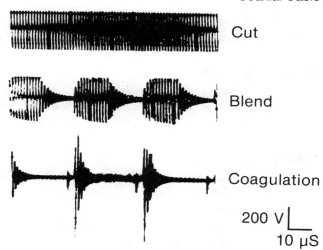

Cut

Blend

Coagulation

200 V

10 μS

Coagulation Current: Oscillographic picture of cutting, blend, and coagulation currents.

CMR$_{O_2}$:

See Cerebral metabolic rate for oxygen.

Co:

See Cobalt.

CO:

See Carbon monoxide.

Coagulation Current:

Type of output available from an electrosurgical instrument that allows maximal coagulability with a minimal incision. The waveform is a damped, intermittent sine wave. *See* Figure. *See* Blend current; Cutting current.

Coarc:

See Coarctation of the aorta.

Coarctation of the Aorta (COARC):

Condition in which there is a stricture or constriction, usually localized, of the aorta. Often seen as a congenital anomaly, it can cause severe cardiac decompensation due to the elevated resistance to left ventricular output. Hyperperfusion occurs below the "coarc" and hypoperfusion above the "coarc." From an anesthetic viewpoint, excessive bleeding may become a problem during the surgical procedure due to the hypertension in the vessels proximal to the stricture.

Coaxial Cable:

Conductor used for the transmission of high-frequency signals. It consists of a central wire surrounded by an insulator with an outer coaxial conducting cylinder. Coaxial cables are more expensive than the usual twin lead cables but do not produce nor are they affected by external electrical fields. Therefore they are used when low noise conditions are required.

Coaxial Scavenger:

Device fitted to the tail of the reservoir bag of the standard Jackson-Rees modification of an Ayre T-piece for pediatric anesthesia. Basically, the device removes undesirable gases via a reservoir that is fitted to the tailpiece of the bag.

Cobalt (Co):

Metallic element with atomic weight 59. Its radioisotope, cobalt 60, has a half-life of 5.3 years and emits highly penetrating gamma rays in the range of 1.1 million to 1.3 million electron volts. Nonradioactive Co is alloyed with chrome to make a number of materials (Vitallium and Tyconium) that are not attacked by body fluids. These materials are used as bone replacements and for making dentures. Depending on the Co/chrome ratios, these materials can be made superhard with tensile strength in excess of 300,000 lb/in$^{2.}$

Cocaine:

First local anesthetic to be discovered and used. This complex molecule is unique in that it produces both anesthesia and local vasoconstriction. These effects are probably due to its ability to block the reuptake of norepinephrine at nerve terminals, thereby prolonging its own action. It is a drug much abused by inhalation of various street forms. It is a true addicting drug with severe abuse potential. Addicts requiring emergency surgery can be combative and psychotic. *See* Local anesthetic.

Code Blue:

In common hospital parlance, the announcement that cardiopulmonary resuscitation is required at a given location.

Codeine:

Weakest of the available narcotics. *See* Narcotic.

Codman, Ernest Amory:

See Anesthesia chart.

Coefficient of Expansion:

Physical characteristic of all materials that represents the percentage of change in a given measurement per degree Celsius.

Coefficient of Variability:

Value indicating the ratio of the standard deviation (SD) to the mean. It is determined by dividing the SD by the arithmetic mean and multiplying by 100. This calculation for two or more data sets allows direct comparison of their frequency distribution without concern for different units of measurement. The data set with the smaller coefficient of variation (read as a percent) has the smaller frequency distribution. For example, if the SD of blood pressure is 15 with a mean of 100, the coefficient of variation is 15%. If the SD of serum sodium is 5 with a mean of 140, the coefficient of variation is 3.5%.

Cogentin:

See Benztropine mesylate.

Cold Saline Injection:

Treatment modality in which large quantities of iced saline are injected under the dura. It is used for relief of intractable pain. It is usually performed during general anesthesia, as the side effects are not pleasant for the patient. It is not a widely used technique.

Cold Spot Imaging:

See Thallium 201.

Collateral Respiration:

Phenomenon seen when lung segments distal to an obstructed small bronchus are inflated via the surrounding tissues. Collateral respiration does not occur if a main bronchus is occluded.

College of Anaesthetists:

The College was originally formed as the second Faculty of Royal College of Surgeons of England in 1948. It achieved college status in 1988. Fellowship of the College is granted upon passing the three-part Fellowship examination. Currently, there are approximately 5500 Fellows. The College is located in Lincoln's Inn Field, London.

Collodion (Collodium):

Highly flammable, colorless, thick solution of gun cotton in ether and alcohol used as a protective dressing for cuts and surgical wounds. [Gun cotton (nitrocellulose or pyroxylin) is produced by reacting cotton with nitric and sulfuric acids.] Collodion is highly flammable.

Colloid Solutions:

Intravenous solutions contain various large molecules plus water and have significant osmotic pressure. Typical solutions are 5% albumin and various starch solutions. *See* Crystalloid solutions; Intravenous solutions.

Colloid Theory of Anesthesia:

An old hypothesis of anesthetic behavior stating that anesthetic agents cause a reversible change in the protoplasm of neurons. This reversible condition interferes with protein function and resembles the physical state known as a colloidal suspension. Currently, this theory is unacceptable, as no physical evidence for this effect exists. (Refer to the major journals for the next few years to see if it makes a comeback.)

Colloidal Osmotic Pressure:

See Oncotic pressure.

Colony Stimulating Factors:

Group of glycoproteins that regulate the production of white blood cells. Depending on their individual compositions, they can be produced by monocytes, fibroblasts, or endothelial cells and other tissues.

Color Flow Doppler Mapping:

Technique for cardiac imaging that separates the amplitude and velocity information obtainable from the doppler ultrasound echocardiogram. Motion toward the transducer is coded *red* (on the CRT) and *blue* when away from the transducer. Various intermediate colors are used to indicate other parameters.

Colorimetric End-Tidal Carbon Dioxide Detector:

Endotracheal tube containing a color indicator that changes from yellow to purple in the presence of carbon dioxide. Although not precise, it gives a rough-and-ready estimate of end-tidal carbon dioxide on a breath-by-breath basis. *See* Figure. *See* End-tidal carbon dioxide measurement.

Colorimetry:

Chemical quantitation method that uses the intensity of color (produced as the result of a test reaction or test sequence) to determine the concentration of a sought-after variable. For example, hemoglobin concentration can be determined by aiming a light source of a frequency known to be absorbed by hemoglobin through an unknown solution at a photocell. The amount of light absorbed by the unknown solution is directly proportional to the amount of hemoglobin present.

Colton, Gardner Quincy:

See Morton, William T. G.

Coma (Comatose):

Condition in which a patient is unaware of his or her surroundings and is unarousable by powerful stimulation. These terms are used relatively indiscriminately, and subcategories such as presence or absence of spontaneous ventilation should be stressed. A method for evaluating the comatose state is the Comascore, which can be used to show patient trends in the intensive care unit. *See* Figures.

Combined Anesthesia:

See Balanced anesthesia.

Combustion:

Rapid and vigorous oxidation of fuel molecules leading to the emission of heat and light. Flames are visible evidence of combustion.

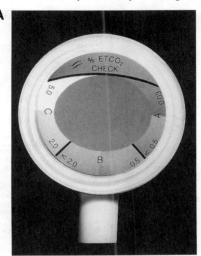

Colorimetric FEF™ End-Tidal CO₂ Detector: (A) The end-tidal CO₂ detector contains a chemically treated membrane that vividly changes color in response to the presence of carbon dioxide. (B) FENEM™ disposable end-tidal CO₂ detector with minimal CO₂ requirements.

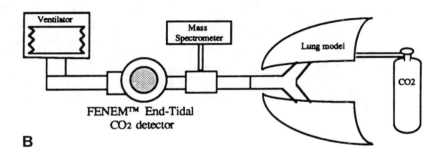

Common Mode Rejection:

Technique for the elimination of electrical artifact. It assumes that artifact is of equal amplitude at two sampling sites. Subtracting the signal amplitude of site one from that site of two rejects the common artifact seen in both sampling signals. Of particular importance in electroencephalography, common mode rejection works only if the electrical impedance of each sampling site is equal.

Comparator:

Electronic or mechanical device that compares two signal inputs. The output of the device depends on some preprogrammed or predetermined relation between the two inputs. For example, the alarm mechanisms on most physiologic monitors use comparators to relate the pulse rate to some internal standard. If the alarm is set to sound at a pulse of 180, the patient's pulse (usually the interval detected between successive R waves) is compared with the alarm time interval (0.33 second). If the patient's pulse is higher, the comparator actuates an alarm. *See* Figure.

Compensatory Damages:

See Punitive damages.

Compensatory Damages

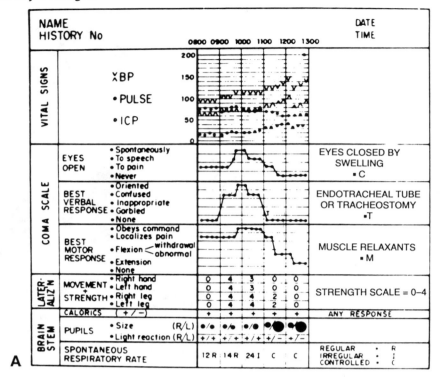

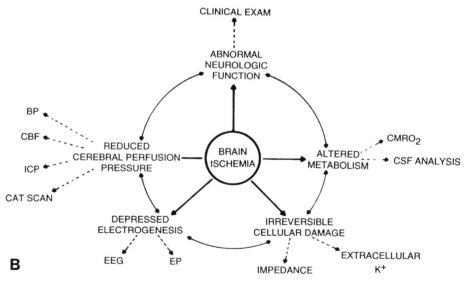

Coma: (A) Example of a neurologic status record. It consists of a vital sign chart, a coma scale, and estimation of lateralization and brain stem function. The patient being followed was initially comatose, emerged from the coma, and then relapsed. (B) Summary of the pathophysiologic consequences of cerebral ischemia and the specialized monitoring involved in detecting them. The outer circle represents the physiologic disorders caused by cerebral ischemia. The dashed arrows indicate the monitoring methods needed to determine these derangements.

Competitive Antagonism (Reversible Inhibition):

Pharmacologic phenomenon seen between two drugs that have affinity for the same tissue receptor site. The number of receptor sites the drugs occupy depends on their concentration. Thus a relative overabundance of one drug can displace the other. Narcotics and narcotic antagonists share a competitive antagonistic relation. The narcotic effect can be terminated with displacement of the narcotic by an antagonist at its tissue receptor sites. *See* Agonist; Antagonist; Noncompetitive antagonism; Receptor/receptor site.

Competitive Inhibition:

See Neuromuscular blocking agent.

Compliance:

Calculation of the elasticity or expandability of the lungs measured when the flow of air into the lungs has ceased, e.g., while holding one's breath. It is best demonstrated in the paralyzed, anesthetized patient. It is the volume change (in liters) divided by the pressure change caused by the expansion to that volume. In normal individuals, the compliance of the lungs and thoracic wall are measured together. It is approximately 100 ml/cm water pressure. For example, if the lungs are inflated to a volume of 1 L in a normal anesthetized patient, a pressure gauge connected to the airway should read about 10 cm H_2O when air movement stops.

Component Therapy:

See Blood storage.

Compound Action Potential:

See Action potential.

Compressed Spectral Array:

Display technique used for interpretation of the electroencephalogram. *See* Fourier analysis.

Compression Nerve Palsy:

Injury often arising during anesthesia due to poor or careless positioning of the patient, thereby affecting the main nerve trunks. The facial, radial, ulnar, and tibial nerves are susceptible to compression nerve palsies.

Compression Volume:

Portion of the tidal volume delivered to a patient by a bag squeeze or ventilator inspiration that functions to distend the hoses leading to the patient. In general, most anesthesia equipment has a compression volume of 3 ml/cm water pressure. Hence if a ventilator delivers a peak pressure of 24 cm H_2O during patient inspiration, 72 ml of the volume pushed by the ventilator does not reach the patient but distends the pliable parts of the ventilator circuit.

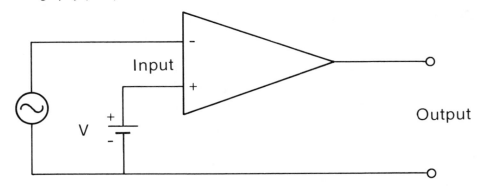

Comparator:
Operational
amplifier
comparator.

Computed Axial Tomography (CAT):

Diagnostic radiology technique using advanced computer methods to form a visual image of a body plane with minimal doses of radiation. The early tomographic x-ray system moved the x-ray head and x-ray film simultaneously, pivoting around an imaginary point within the patient. This point would be in focus while all points above and below it would become blurred. The CAT scanner moves stepwise around the body or segment to be visualized (usually 1 degree per step). The beam that emerges from the body is detected by a photomultiplier tube and is electronically assigned a value, from white to gray to black, in proportion to its energy. (A beam blocked by bone would be greatly attenuated and appear white.) Each point in a plane would be crossed by an x-ray beam multiple times as the x-ray projector steps about the area being examined. The computer adds these densities together and draws a composite picture of the findings on a cathode ray tube. Accurate CAT scanning requires the patient to be immobile. A general anesthetic may be administered to the uncomfortable patient for an extended procedure. *See* Figure.

Computer:

Electronic device that processes information. Most computers, regardless of their complexity, have a number of common subdivisions, including input and output devices, an arithmetic or calculating section (the central processing unit, CPU), temporary and permanent storage facilities, communication units, and a control unit. Large computers handle such sophisticated tasks as weather prediction. The series of orders that direct the computer operations is called the computer program. *See* Analog computer; Central processing unit; Computer logic.

Computer Logic:

Reference to the five functions that any computer can perform: subtraction, addition, division, multiplication, and comparison of results. These processes encompass all necessary functions, as the most complicated equation or process can be separated into these individual steps.

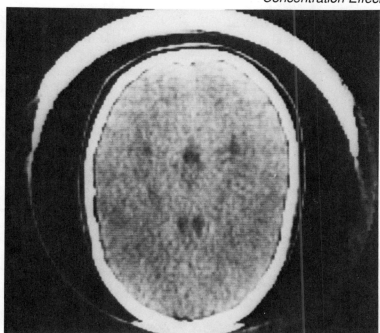

Computerized Axial Tomography: Typical CAT scan of a cross-section of the brain.

Concentration Effect:

Explanation of the observation made during inhalation anesthetic induction that the higher the inspired concentration of an anesthetic, the faster is the relative rise in alveolar concentration. (The alveolar concentration of an agent administered at a 20% concentration rises more than twice as fast as the same agent given at a 10% concentration.) The concentration effect is made up of two parts, the *concentrating effect* and the *increased ventilation effect*. In the latter, gas is drawn down the trachea to replace alveolar gas that has entered the blood. This action tends to augment minute ventilation. For example, if a 70% N_2O/30% O_2 source is connected to a patient, the mix is pulled down the trachea to replace any N_2O taken up in the blood. Because alveolar concentration of N_2O would be less than 70% (due to blood uptake), this action would tend to restore it to the inspired level of concentration. With the concentrating effect, the uptake by blood of an anesthetic changes the alveolar concentration of that agent to a lesser degree if it is in high concentration initially. For example, in an alveolus containing 50% N_2O and 50% O_2, uptake of half the N_2O (O_2 considered in equilibrium with no uptake) leaves more than 25% agent in the alveolus [i.e., old volume 50 parts N_2O + 50 parts O_2 = 100 parts (50% O_2); new volume 25 parts N_2O + 50 parts O_2 = 75 parts (33% N_2O + 67% O_2)]. If we start with 25% agent, uptake of half agent and the new volume is 12.5 parts agent plus 75 parts O_2 = 14.2%. Note that the higher concentration decreased relatively less than the lower concentration. All calculations assume equilibrium of O_2, water vapor, CO_2, and N_2. *See* Diffusion hypoxia; Second gas effect.

175

Conducting Airways:

Passages that start at the trachea, divide into the right and left mainstem bronchi, then into the lobar and segmental bronchi, continue to the terminal bronchioles, and end before the alveoli. There are 23 divisions from the trachea to the terminal bronchioles. These conducting areas contain no alveoli and therefore do not participate in gas exchange. They constitute the anatomic deadspace. *See* Figures.

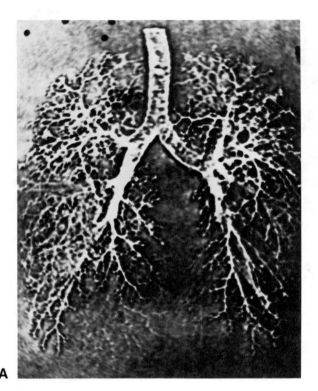

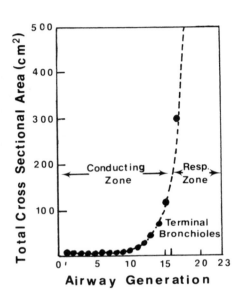

A   **B**

Conducting Airways: (A) Cast of human conducting airways with the alveoli trimmed away. The arborization of the airways from the trachea to the terminal bronchioles is shown. (B) Relationship of cross-sectional area, in square centimeters, to the number of divisions of the airways as they proceed from the trachea. The respiratory zone begins at approximately the sixteenth division soon after the cross-sectional area begins to increase dramatically.

Conduction:

Transmission of some form of energy (heat, electric, or mechanical) from one point to another. It is also used to indicate the transmission of nerve impulses.

Conduction Anesthesia:

Interruption of nerve pathways, particularly sensory pathways, without loss of consciousness. Conduction anesthesia includes local infiltration, local nerve blocks, regional nerve blocks (epidural, caudal, and spinal anesthesia), and nerve blocks by direct pressure and refrigeration. A major conduction block usually refers to spinal, epidural, and regional blocks, whereas all other blocks are called minor conduction blocks.

Conductive Flooring:

Floor that is deliberately rendered conductive to electricity. It is a requirement in enclosed areas, such as operating rooms, where the atmosphere may become flammable or explosive. By being conductive, the floors harmlessly dissipate stray electrical charges that may build up as static electricity on personnel and objects in the room. In order for the flooring to perform its function, a conducting path must be maintained between the floor and the personnel and objects. This path is usually accomplished with conductive shoes, conductive chains hanging from equipment, or deliberate wiring of equipment to the floor.

Conductor:

Material in which resistance to the passage of an electric current is negligible.

Confidence Interval:

See Confidence level.

Confidence Level (Statistics):

Concept that the mean of a group of observations lies within a specified distance of the mean of all possible observations. The choice of confidence level can be any number, but the usual choice is 95%. This choice means that 19 of 20 times the mean of a sample of observations will fall within 2 standard deviations (SD) of the true mean. The mean plus or minus the specified number of SDs is called the confidence level. The confidence level is bounded by the confidence limits.

Congener:

Any discrete object closely related to another. For example, a congener of a drug has similar structure and function to the parent drug.

Congestive Heart Failure (CHF):

Clinical condition in which the heart fails to pump blood adequately, resulting in decreased blood flow to the tissues and congestion in the pulmonary or systemic circulation (or both). Pulmonary and peripheral edema and hepatomegaly develop. Usually CHF is a chronic condition and is associated with sodium and water retention by the kidneys, due to an alteration in renal plasma flow and glomerular filtration. Although the function of one side of the heart may be primarily impaired, the function of the other side is also affected as the two sides work in series. Primary left-sided failure refers to signs and symptoms of increased pressure and congestion in the pulmonary veins and capillaries. Primary right-sided failure refers to signs and symptoms of increased pressure and congestion in the systemic veins and capillaries. The most common cause of right-sided failure is left-sided failure. *See* Figure. *See* Pulmonary edema.

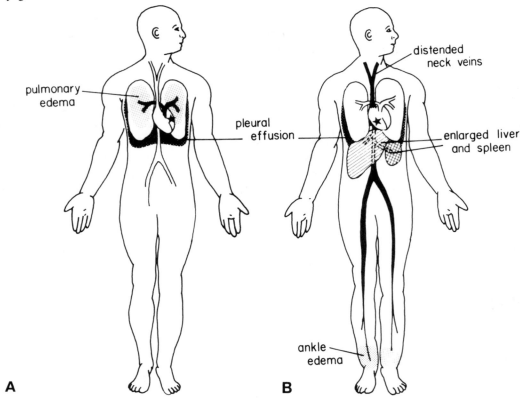

Congestive Heart Failure: Physical findings in (A) left-sided and (B) right-sided congestive heart failure.

Conjugate Pair:

An acid and the base it forms when it gives up a hydrogen ion. For example, carbonic acid (H_2CO_3) forms a conjugate pair when in solution with its conjugate base, the bicarbonate ion HCO_3^-.

Connector:

Device or fitting that joins two or more components.

Conscious Sedation:

Technique of drug administration popular in outpatient procedures. The goal of this technique is to produce a nonanxious, cooperative patient who can respond to commands. The patient's upper airway reflexes remain intact.

Consent Form (Permit Form):

Legal document that is part of a patient's chart and medical record. By signing it, the patient agrees to undergo a specified medical or anesthetic procedure to be performed by specified personnel. Although not completely unimpeachable, a signed consent form shows that an attempt was made to apprise the patient of needed treatment and possible complications before proceeding. *See* Figure. *See* Informed consent.

ROBERT WOOD JOHNSON UNIVERSITY HOSPITAL
New Brunswick, NJ 08901

**CONSENT FOR PHOTOGRAPHY
AND, OR OBSERVERS**

PART 1: <u>CONSENT FOR PHOTOGRAPHY</u>

DATE _____ TIME _____a.m./p.m.

I consent to the taking and publication of any photographs in the course of the performance of the
procedure listed in paragraph 1 of this form on_____
                                                                         (myself or patient's name)

for the purpose of advancing medical education.

_____
(Signature of patient or person authorized to give consent)

_____
(If other than patient, state relationship)

PART 2: <u>CONSENT FOR OBSERVERS</u>

DATE _____ TIME _____a.m./p.m.

For the purpose of advancing medical education, I consent to the admittance of observers to the
operating room during the performance of the procedures listed in part 1 of this form on:

_____
(myself or patient's name)

_____
(Signature of patient or person authorized to give consent)

Consent Form: Consent form used at the Robert Wood Johnson University Hospital in New Brunswick, NJ. (A) Front and (B) Back View.

A

Conservation of Momentum:

Fundamental physical law stating that a body or particle in motion will continue to move unless acted on by an outside force. Best demonstrated when a "slight" push on an anesthesia machine makes it roll over your foot.

Continuity Test:

In electrical terms, a test to determine whether a pathway for electric current exists between two points of the circuit. In terms of gas piping, a continuity test is performed to ensure that only the gas designated by the label on an outlet is present at the outlet.

Continuous Anesthesia:

Technique of introducing a catheter into a body space for intermittent injection of local anesthetics over an extended period in order to maintain an anesthetic response. Continuous spinal, epidural, and caudal techniques have been used since the 1920s.

ROBERT WOOD JOHNSON UNIVERSITY HOSPITAL
New Brunswick, NJ 08901

**REQUEST FOR OPERATIVE OR
PROCEDURAL INTERVENTION**

PATIENT NAME _____ DATE _____ TIME _____ a.m./p.m.

PART I: PROPOSAL FOR OPERATIVE OR PROCEDURAL INTERVENTION

As the physician(s) responsible for the care of the above-named patient, I/we Dr.(s)_____
propose to perform the following operation or procedure:

a) IDENTIFICATION OF OPERATION OR PROCEDURE (in scientific terms):

_____
_____

b) DESCRIPTION OF OPERATION OR PROCEDURE (in layman's language):

_____
_____
_____

c) PHYSICIAN CERTIFICATION. I, _____ have counseled this
patient as to the nature of the procedure which I have proposed. I have specifically discussed the more
common risks of this procedure, the nature and purpose of this procedure, and the possible alternative
methods of treatment. In proposing this treatment, I have told this patient that it is my opinion based upon
my knowledge of the case and upon my training and experience, that the potential benefits of this
procedure outweigh the potential risks, but I have also acknowledged that other opinions may exist and
have offered to facilitate obtaining such "second opinions" for the patient if he/she so requests. I have
also indicated that the possible complications which I have discussed are those which I consider to be the
most common ones, and that other, less common complications may occur, to which I have not
specifically referred.

PART II: PATIENT REQUEST FOR SURGERY OR PROCEDURE

I, the undersigned hereby request and authorize Dr. (s)_____
(and whomever he/she may designate as his assistants) to perform the operation or procedure proposed
and described above in sections 1(a) and 1(b).

I have read the physician's certification above, and agree that the information referred to in it has been
discussed with me, and that I have been given the opportunity to ask further questions about any areas
which were not clear to me.

I acknowledge that no guarantees have been made or implied to me regarding the expected results of the
operation or procedure.

I understand that medicine is not an exact science and that additional operations or procedures may be
found to be necessary during the course of the proposed procedure. I request and authorize the
performance of such additional procedures except for_____
(if none, write "NONE").

PATIENT SIGNATURE _____

PHYSICIAN SIGNATURE(S) _____

B   PA-30

Consent Form
(continued)

Continuous Flow Anesthesia Machine:

Complete name for the standard anesthesia delivery system. It is found in operating rooms worldwide. Flow from the machine continues regardless of changes caused by patient respiration. Gas issues from the common outlet, mixed according to the setting on flowmeters for each separate gas, and moves from the common outlet into the patient's circuit at all times, so long as the flowmeter is functioning. Gas leaves the common outlet at a pressure of 2–10 lb/in^2. Continuous flow machines are also currently available that use a single control for both O_2 and N_2O rather than two separate needle valves. *See* Figures. *See* Intermittent flow machine.

Continuous Monitoring for Pollution:

Constant use of a detector for trace anesthetic gases in an operating room. This can immediately determine leaks or faulty techniques.

180

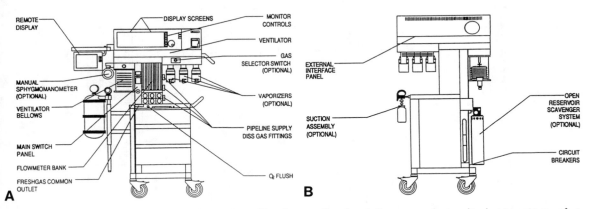

REMOTE DISPLAY
DISPLAY SCREENS
MONITOR CONTROLS
VENTILATOR
GAS SELECTOR SWITCH (OPTIONAL)
EXTERNAL INTERFACE PANEL
MANUAL SPHYGMOMANOMETER (OPTIONAL)
VENTILATOR BELLOWS
VAPORIZERS (OPTIONAL)
SUCTION ASSEMBLY (OPTIONAL)
OPEN RESERVOIR SCAVENGER SYSTEM (OPTIONAL)
MAIN SWITCH PANEL
PIPELINE SUPPLY DISS GAS FITTINGS
CIRCUIT BREAKERS
FLOWMETER BANK
FRESHGAS COMMON OUTLET
O₂ FLUSH
A
B

Continuous Flow Anesthesia Machine: Total anesthesia delivery and monitoring system of a NARKOMED 4. (A) Front view, (B) Back view.

Continuous Positive Airway Pressure (CPAP):

Method of spontaneous or mechanical ventilation by which the pressure of the upper airways is not allowed to decrease to atmospheric pressure (zero). (CPAP is also referred to as continuous positive pressure breathing, CPPB.) It is particularly useful in patients whose distal airways would collapse if not kept continuously inflated by greater-than-atmospheric pressure. CPAP is frequently employed for treatment of infants with respiratory distress syndrome. *See* Figure. *See* Infant respiratory distress syndrome.

Continuous Positive-Pressure Breathing (CPPB):

Synonym for continuous positive airway pressure (CPAP). *See* Continuous positive airway pressure.

Continuous Wave Doppler Ultrasonography:

Technique for determination of cardiac output. It uses a probe placed in the suprasternal notch that is directed toward the ascending aorta and broadcasting ultrasonic waves. The velocity of the blood is known because of doppler shift, and the cross sectional area of the aorta can be determined from a table knowing the patient's physical parameters. The two values are then compiled into a cardiac output number. This technique has not gained wide clinical acceptance. *See* Thoracic bioimpedance.

Contract:

Agreement between two or more persons that sets up a binding legal relationship. For an agreement to be a legal contract it must include the following elements. (1) The persons involved must be legally capable of making binding agreements. (2) They must be in some agreement as to the meaning of the contract. (3) The agreement must contain at least one promise and a consideration (something of value) that has to be either delivered, promised, or given. A contract exists when the promises and obligations are clear, well defined, and understood by all parties. Expressed contracts can be either verbal or written. An implied contract is not sharply delineated for the parties involved but flows from the circumstances of the individual case, e.g., a patient, by seeking out a physician for a physical examination, has implied a contract with that physician to pay for the service.

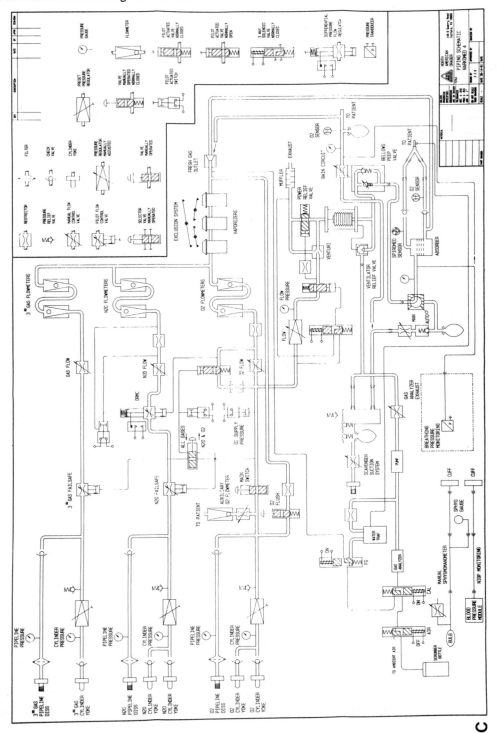

Continuous Flow Anesthesia Machine *(continued)*: (C) Piping diagram for the NARKOMED 4 continuous flow anesthesia machine.

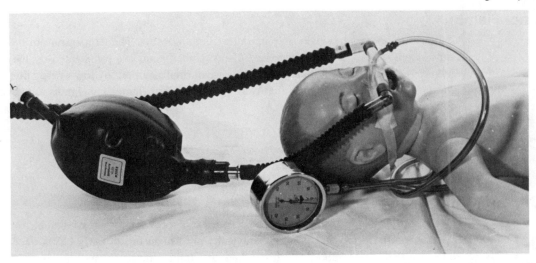

Continuous Positive Airway Pressure: Nasotracheal tube attached to a modified Jackson-Rees apparatus with a pressure gauge for the administration of continuous positive airway pressure as set up for an infant.

Contrast Echocardiography:

Technique employing echocardiography augmented by injected microbubbles placed at the aortic root proximal to an aortic occlusion clamp. The bubbles travel with the cardiac circulation and allow greater resolution of the echocardiogram. Currently an experimental technique only.

Contrast Medium:

See Barium sulfate.

Controlled Hypotension (Induced Hypotension):

Deliberate reduction of the blood pressure (particularly the mean arterial pressure) to some predetermined level and maintenance at that level to decrease bleeding during surgery.

Controlled Mechanical Ventilation:

See Ventilator.

Controlled Oral Word Association Test:

Verbal test for fluency consisting of time trials, asking the patient to repeat all words he or she can think of starting with a particular letter (usually C, F and L). Damage to any part of the brain tends to lower these fluency scores.

Converting Enzyme:

See Renin.

Cool Flame:

Combustion process in which only partial oxidation occurs. The temperature of the cool flame is only a few hundred degrees Celsius. Cool flames are propagated by the most reactive fragments of fuel molecules. They are normally ignited by low-energy points of ignition and can occur only in fuel-rich mixtures. Cool flames can ignite a detonable mixture.

COPD:

See Chronic obstructive pulmonary disease.

Copper Kettle:

Device used for vaporization of a liquid anesthetic in a controlled and predictable manner. Invented by Dr. Lucian Morris at The University of Iowa during the early 1950s, the copper kettle is a "universal vaporizer." It can take any liquid anesthetic and vaporize it into a stream of O_2, the quantity of vapor being proportional to the vapor pressure at a given temperature. The underlying principle of the copper kettle is as follows: As finely divided bubbles of O_2 are allowed to rise through a standing volume of liquid, vapor penetrates them and reaches equilibrium. *See* Figure.

Core Memory:

Type of information storage device often seen in large computers. Information is kept in binary form. In a magnetic core memory, microscopic metal areas become the storage media. Magnetized in one direction they correspond to a 0; in the other direction they correspond to a 1.

Core Temperature:

Temperature of the blood measured at the level of the left atrium or, alternately, the temperature of the heart and brain.

Corneal Abrasion:

Irritation, scratch, or wearing away of the external layer of the eye by a foreign body or object. Corneal abrasions are a potential hazard in the anesthetized or unconscious patient because the eyelid reflex, which normally protects the cornea, does not function in the anesthetized patient.

Corneal Reflex (Eyelid Reflex; Eye Blink):

Automatic closing of the eyelids when the eyelashes or cornea are touched. This reflex is often tested to demonstrate the onset of general anesthesia. The reflex path involves the corneas, ophthalmic branch of the trigeminal nerve, synapse in the the main sensory nucleus of the trigeminal nerve, medial longitudinal bundle, synapse in the main motor nucleus of the facial nerve, and efferent impulses via the facial nerve to the orbicularis oculi. *See* Cranial nerves.

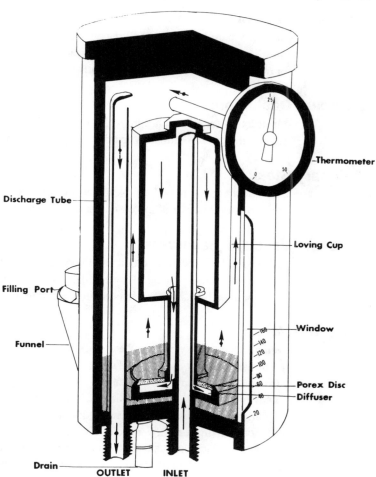

Discharge Tube

Filling Port

Funnel

Drain

OUTLET   INLET

Thermometer

Loving Cup

Window

Porex Disc
Diffuser

Copper Kettle Vaporizer: The redesigned version with the filling port at the back to prevent overfilling.

Coronary Arteries:

Arterial supply of the myocardium. The left coronary artery arises from the portion of the ascending aorta, which protrudes between the main pulmonary artery and the left atrium. The left coronary artery runs under the left atrium and divides into the anterior descending (interventricular) and circumflex branches. The anterior descending artery supplies oxygenated blood to the ventricular walls, whereas the circumflex artery supplies the walls of the left ventricle and left atrium. The right coronary artery arises from the ostium of the right aortic sinus or right sinus of valsalva of the ascending aorta in approximately 50% of patients and runs into the right atrioventricular sulcus. It then divides into the posterior interventricular and marginal branches. The posterior interventricular artery supplies oxygenated blood to the walls of both ventricles, and the marginal branch supplies the myocardium of the right ventricle and right atrium.

185

Coronary Care Unit (CCU):

Specialty care hospital ward for patients with recent or incipient myocardial infarctions. Increased monitoring and vigilance in the unit is aimed directly at reducing the incidence of myocardial electrical instability (arrhythmia).

Coronary Occlusion:

Obstruction (acute or chronic) of blood flow in a coronary vessel that prevents adequate flow to the portion of the myocardium supplied by that vessel. *See* Myocardial infarction.

Coronary Steal:

Absolute decrease in blood flow to one area of myocardium that depends on collateral flow for perfusion in favor of increased perfusion in a normally perfused area.

Coronary Vascular Reserve:

Difference in myocardial blood flow between the total flow when autoregulation is intact subtracted from the maximally vasodilated flow where autoregulation is lost. It is critically dependent on baseline cardiac perfusion pressure and oxygen utilization.

Coronary Veins:

Venous drainage system of the myocardium. There are three systems of coronary veins: thebesian, anterior cardiac, and coronary sinus and its tributaries. The thebesian veins (the smallest system) are located mostly in the septa of the right atrium and right ventricle. (They may be seen in the left side as well but less commonly.) The anterior cardiac veins, which provide most of the venous drainage of the right ventricle, are formed over the anterior wall of the right ventricle. Their branches drain in the direction of the anterior right atrioventricular sulcus and empty into the right atrium. The coronary sinus and its branches are the largest system of coronary veins. They are responsible for the venous drainage of the left ventricle.

Cor Pulmonale:

Condition characterized by enlargement of the right ventricle secondary to malfunctioning lungs. Cor pulmonale is always associated with pulmonary hypertensive heart disease and is frequently associated with chronic obstructive pulmonary disease (bronchitis, emphysema). Severe pulmonary alveolar proteinosis may lead to cor pulmonale. *See* Pulmonary alveolar proteinosis.

Corticosteroid:

General term for the steroids produced by the adrenal cortex and having 21 carbons. They are further classified as mineralocorticoids and glucocorticoids. The mineralocorticoids (aldosterone being the most significant) are responsible for sodium retention (preventing excessive loss in the urine) and potassium excretion. Cortisol (hydrocortisone, compound F) is the most abundant and physiologically important glucocorticoid. (Corticosterone, compound B, is another glucocorticoid.) Glucocorticoids exert diverse effects on the body. (1) They stimulate gluconeogenesis (the biosynthesis of glucose from amino acid precursors), thereby influencing carbohydrate and protein metabolism. (2) They help store body fat. (3) They help the body resist and react to a range of stresses, such as fright, temperature extremes, high altitude, bleeding, and infection. (4) They exert an antiinflammatory effect. Therapeutically, the glucocorticoids are used for myriad disease conditions, such as Addison disease, bronchial asthma, rheumatoid arthritis, adrenocortical insufficiency, systemic lupus erythematosus, sarcoidosis, allergic conjunctivitis, and acquired hemolytic anemia. Transient beneficial effects are seen when they are used to treat acute leukemia and multiple myeloma. It is important to recognize that for the most part, steroids do not provide a cure but only symptomatic relief to the patient. The administration of glucocorticoids represents replacement therapy only in the treatment of Addison disease and adrenocortical insufficiency. Small doses of glucocorticoids for a short period rarely cause adverse effects. However, chronic use (at a higher than physiologic level) may result in severe complications for the patient, relating to either abrupt withdrawal of the steroid or prolonged use. (The dosage regimen must be reduced gradually to prevent acute adrenal insufficiency.) Common side effects include those characteristic of Cushing disease: "moon face," hirsutism, fatty deposits on the back, and amenorrhea. Other adverse effects are osteoporosis, hypokalemia, myopathy, aggravation of diabetes mellitus and peptic ulcer, psychotic disorders, and increased susceptibility to infections. Those patients whose bodies have been accustomed to high levels of circulating steroids are poor surgical risks and should be protected by corticosteroid supplementation prior to, during, and after surgery. *See* Table.

Corticosteroid: Comparison and dosage forms of various steroids.

Steroid	Anti-Inflamitory potency	Sodium retention	Dosage Forms (mg)
Cortisone (Cortone)	0.8	0.8	T: 5-25; 1: 25, 50
Hydrocortisone (Cortef, Hydrocortone)	1	1	T, 5-20; 1: 25, 50*
Prednisone (Orasone, others)	2.5	0.8	T: 1-50; S: 5
Prednisolone (Cortalone, others)	3	0.8	T 5; S: 15; 1: *
Methylprednisolone (Medrol)	4	0	T: 2-32; 1: *
Triamcinolone (Aristocort, Kenacort)	5	0	T: 1-8; S: 2, 4; 1; *
Dexamethasone (Decadron)	20	0	T: 0.25-6; S: 0.5; 1: *
Paramethasone (Haldrone)	6	0	T: 1, 2
Betamethasone (Celestone)	20	0	T 0,6; S: 0.6; I: *
Desoxycorticosterone (DOCA, Percorten)	0	10-25	I: 5; P: 125; RI: 25
Fludrocortisone (Florinef)	12	100	T: 0.1
Aldosterone	0.2	250	
For oral Inhalation			
Beclomethasone (Beclovent, Vanceril)			A: 0.042
Dexamethasone (Decadron)			A: 0.084
Flunisolide (AeroBid)			A: 0.250
Triamcinolone (Azmacort)			A: 0.100
For nasal Inhalation			
Beclomethasone (Beconase, Vancenase)			A: 0.042
Dexamethasone (Decadron)			A: 0.084
Flunisolide (Nasalide)			A: 0.025

A, Aerosol or spray (approximate dose per actuation); *I*, Injection (per millimeter), *P*, pellets for subcutaneous Implantation, *RI*, repository injection (per milliliter); *S*, syrup elixir, or oral solution (per 5 ml); *T*, tablet.
Various salts are available for injection by various routes

Cortisol:

See Corticosteroid.

Corundum:

Extremely hard crystalline mineral found in nature. It is composed of aluminum oxide and is used as an abrasive. The ruby and the sapphire are corundums colored with oxides.

Cost-Effectiveness:

Measurement of performance that analyzes the monetary cost of a device, process, or system in relation to the tangible benefits produced.

Coulter Counter:

See Automated cell counter.

Coumarin:

See Anticoagulant.

Council on Accreditation of Nurse Anesthesia Educational Programs:

Autonomous group that is housed within the offices of the American Association of Nurse Anesthetists. Members include physicians, CRNAs, public members, and students. The Council formulates or adopts standards and guidelines, and it accredits nurse anesthesia programs. National headquarters is Park Ridge, Illinois.

Counter:

Device that detects and counts individual particles and photons. *See* Geiger counter; Photomultiplier.

Coupling:

Spatial or electrical connection between two circuits that allows power or signal information to be transferred from one to the other. *See* Capacitance electronic; Inductance.

CP50:

Index of anesthetic potency for intravenous drugs. At steady state, the plasma drug concentration that prevents a somatic response to skin incision in 50% of test subjects.

CPAP:

See Continuous positive airway pressure.

CPD Blood:

See Blood storage.

CPD Blood Preservation:

Method of storing blood in a solution of citrate-phosphate-dextrose to prolong shelf life. It is also a better preservative than ACD. *See* 2,3-DPG (diphosphoglycerate). *See* Blood storage.

CPK:

See Creatine phosphokinase.

CPPB:

See Continuous positive-pressure breathing.

CPR:

See Cardiopulmonary resuscitation.

CPT:

See Current procedural terminology.

CPU:

See Central processing unit.

Cranial Nerves:

Twelve pairs of large nerves that directly exit from the brain. *See* Table.

Craniosacral Division:

See Parasympathetic division.

Craniosacral Outflow:

See Parasympathetic division.

Crash Induction:

See Induction.

Crawford Needle:

See Epidural needle.

Creatine Phosphokinase (CPK):

Series of similar enzymes found in skeletal muscle, heart, gastrointestinal tract, and brain. CPK catalyzes the transfer of phosphate between different energy-storing molecules. The serum level of this enzyme rises in patients with progressive muscular dystrophy, and other primary diseases of skeletal muscle, and cerebral infarcts, and after injuries to the heart or skeletal muscles. Serum samples of cardiac specific CPK are helpful for determining the presence of myocardial tissue necrosis. Elevated serum levels of CPK are found in patients with malignant hyperthermia. There are many innocuous reasons for raised CPK levels. *See* Malignant hyperthermia.

Cranial Nerves: Twelve cranial nerves and their components: (BM) brachial motor, (GSS) general somatic sensory, (SM) somatic motor, (SSS) special somatic sensory, (VM) visceral motor, and (VS) visceral sensory.

Nerve	Components	Primary Cell Body	Course	Peripheral Termination
I Olfactory	SSS	Olfactory epithelium	Through roof of nasal cavity	Olfactory epithelium
II Optic	SSS	Ganglionic layer of retina	Orbit → optic chiasm → optic tracts	Bipolar cells of retina rods and cones
III Oculomotor	SM	Oculomotor nucleus	Orbit	Rectus superior, inferior, medial; obliquus inferior; levator palpebrae muscles
	VM	Edinger–Westphal nucleus	Ciliary ganglion ↑ ciliary nerves	Constrictor pupillae and ciliary muscles of eyeball
IV Trochlear	SM	Trochlear nucleus	Orbit	Obliquus superior muscle
V Trigeminal	BM	Masticator nucleus	With mandibular	Muscles of mastication
	GSS	Semilunar ganglion	Ophthalmic, maxillary, mandibular branches	Face, nose, mouth
	GSS	Mesencephalic nucleus	With mandibular and maxillary branches	Proprioceptive to jaw muscles and tooth sockets
VI Abducens	SM	Abducens nucleus	Under pons, into orbit	Rectus lateralis
VII Facial	BM	Facial nucleus	Temporal bone, side of face	Muscles of expression, hyoid elevators
	VM	Superior salivatory nucleus	a) Greater superficial petrosal to spheno-palatine ganglion	a) Glands of nose, palate, lacrimal gland

No.	Nerve	Type	Nucleus / Ganglion	Course	Distribution
		VS	Geniculate ganglion	b) Chorda tympani to submaxillary ganglion	b) Submaxillary and sub-lingual glands
				Chorda tympani	Anterior taste buds
VIII	Vestibular	SSS	Vestibular ganglion	Internal acoustic meatus	Cristae of semicircular canals, maculae of utricle and saccule
	Cochlear	SSS	Spiral ganglion	Internal acoustic meatus	Organ of Corti
IX	Glosso-pharyngeal	BM	Nucleus ambiguus	Jugular foramen → side of pharynx	Superior constrictor, stylopharyngeus muscles
		VM	Inferior salivatory nucleus	Lesser superficial petrosal → otic ganglion → auriculotemporal nerve	Parotid gland
		VS	Petrous ganglion	Side of pharynx	Taste buds of vallate papillae
		GSS	Superior ganglion	Side of pharynx	Auditory tube
X	Vagus	BM	Nucleus ambiguus	Recurrent and external branch of superior laryngeal nerve	Pharyngeal and laryngeal muscles
		VM	Dorsal motor nucleus	Along carotid artery, esophagus, stomach	Viscera of thorax and abdomen
		VS	Nodose ganglion	With motor	Viscera of thorax and abdomen
		GSS	Jugular ganglion	Auricular branch	Pinna of ear
XI	Accessory	BM	Accessory nucleus	Side of neck	Sternocleidomastoid
XII	Hypoglossal	SM	Hypoglossal nucleus	Side of tongue	Muscles of tongue

Creatinine:

Breakdown product of protein detectable in urine. High levels of creatinine may indicate kidney disease or malfunction.

Cremophor El:

See Althesin.

Cricoid Cartilage:

Shaped like a signet ring, the cricoid cartilage is the only supporting element of the larynx that completely extends around the air passageway. It supports the lower portion of the laryngeal wall. Because of a tendency to perichondritis and possible stenosis, classic tracheostomies are done below the cricoid cartilage. It is united with the thyroid cartilage by the cricothyroid ligament. It is through this ligament anteriorly that the conventional emergency tracheostomy is performed. *See* Larynx.

Cricotracheotomy:

See Tracheostomy.

Critical Coronary Stenosis:

Stenosis of a coronary vessel that prevents reactive hyperemia in response to demand but that does not effect the resting blood flow. The vascular bed, which is distal to the critical coronary stenosis, is maximally dilated and its reserve exhausted.

Critical Frequency:

See Tetanic contraction.

Critical Flicker Frequency (CFF):

Threshold used to evaluate the effects of acute oral doses of psychotropic drugs. Stimulants tend to increase CFF, whereas hypnotics decrease it. The patient reports his or her perception of a change in the flicker of a light source with constant intensity but varying frequency.

Critical Opening Pressure:

Pressure that must be exceeded in a system, such as a collapsed arteriole, before any flow can begin. *See* Pulmonary perfusion, zones of.

Critical Path Method (Critical Path Analysis):

Method of temporal analysis based on the relations between parts of a complex process. The critical path is the longest process in a multiprocess task. The entire complex task cannot take less time than the critical path task. For example, during orthopedic replacement of a joint, the critical path is the length of time it takes bone cement to adhere and harden. Anesthesia induction, patient preparation, completion of the surgery, and emergence from anesthesia are all variable; the cement setting time is a physical constant that is difficult to change.

Critical Pressure:

Minimum pressure necessary to liquefy a gas at its critical temperature or, conversely, the saturated vapor pressure of a liquid when it is at its critical temperature.

Critical Temperature:

Temperature above which a gas cannot be liquefied by increase of pressure. For example, the critical temperature of N_2O is 36.5°C.

Critical Velocity:

Velocity at which the motion of a fluid changes from laminar (parallel) to turbulent (erratic) flow. *See* Laminar flow; Turbulent flow.

Cross-Filling:

See Transfilling.

Cross-Infection:

Infection in one patient that can be identified as having come from another patient.

Crossmatch to Transfusion Ratio (CT):

Term from blood banking that refers to the ratio between the number of units crossmatched to the number of units actually transfused. It is an indicator of the appropriate use of banking facilities. Blood banks currently attempt to maintain a ratio of about 2.5 units for each unit that is actually used.

Crossover Network:

Type of filter circuit designed to pass high frequencies through one path and low frequencies through another. (The frequency at which these two pathways divide is known as the crossover frequency.) This particular type of network is often used in multispeaker systems for high-fidelity reproduction of sounds.

Crossover of Gases, Crossover Accident:

Grave consequence of having incorrect connections between either separated gas piping systems (e.g., O_2, N_2O) or filling a gas piping system by using a wrong source supply such that the gas appearing at an outlet does not correspond to the gas label on the outlet.

Cross-Filling:

See Transfilling.

Cross-Talk:

Term first used in regard to telephone circuits and now expanded to relate to circuits in general. It indicates undesirable signals (caused by direct or indirect coupling) that degrade a normal circuit signal. *See* Capacitive coupling.

CRT:

See Cathode-ray tube.

Cryocardioplegia:

See Cardiopulmonary bypass.

Cryocautery:

Technique for tissue destruction using extreme cold, also called "cold cautery."

Cryogenics:

Science of the production and effects of very low temperatures.

Crystal-Controlled Clock (Crystal-Controlled Oscillator):

Electrical circuit that oscillates at a precise frequency and is controlled by the piezo effect of a quartz crystal. *See* Crystal, Piezoelectric effect.

Crystalloid Solutions:

Intravenous solutions that contain water plus various mineral ions without large osmotically active molecules. *See* Colloid solutions; Intravenous solutions.

Crystal, Piezoelectric:

Piece of natural quartz or other crystal that vibrates at a desired frequency when placed in an appropriate electrical circuit. It is used as an electromechanical transducer. *See* Crystal-controlled clock; Piezoelectric effect.

CSF:

See Cerebrospinal fluid.

CT:

See Computed tomography; Crossmatch to transfusion ratio.

Cuirass Ventilator:

Obsolete, shell-like, airtight device that fits onto the thorax and abdomen and aids in respiration. Suction is applied under the cuirass to lift up the ribs and abdomen and cause inspiration. An advance over the "iron lung," it allows some degree of mobility but is uncomfortable and heavy.

Cuneiform Cartilages:

Variably found in humans, a pair of small isolated cartilages found in the aryepiglottic folds. *See* Cricoid cartilage; Larynx.

Curare:

See Muscle relaxant; Neuromuscular blocking agent; Tubocurarine chloride.

Curie (Ci):

Unit used to measure the number of disintegrations of a radioactive substance per second. One curie is equivalent to 3.7×10^{10} disintegrations/second.

Current Density:

Ratio of the current or electron flow to the cross-sectional area of the conductor.

Current Procedural Terminology (CPT):

System of terms and codes (five digits) used to describe medical services for a patient. It provides a uniform language for reliable communication. CPT coding is a requirement of most third-party carriers for billing purposes.

Curve Fitting:

Mathematic technique used to formulate an equation that describes a line drawn through plotted data points. The equation may then be used to predict new data points.

Cushing, Harvey:

See Anesthesia chart.

Cushing Syndrome:

See Corticosteroid.

Cushing Triad (Cushing Response):

Consequences of elevated intracranial pressure (ICP) named for neurosurgeon Harvey Cushing. The Cushing response or reflex is an elevated arterial pressure accompanied by bradycardia as pressure on the brain increases. Respiratory irregularity is added to these two to form the triad. Other signs and symptoms associated with elevated intracranial pressure (but not part of the triad) are headache, vomiting, and papilledema. *See* Intracranial pressure measurement.

Cutdown:

Surgical technique for gaining entry to a large vessel of a patient when percutaneous puncture has failed or is impossible.

Cutoff Frequency:

Frequency at which the attenuation of a signal rapidly changes from a small value to a much higher one. For example, the input amplifiers of an electroencephalograph (EEG) usually have cutoff frequencies well below 60 cycles/second, the frequency of line current, which must never intrude on the EEG signal.

Cutting Current (Pure Cut):

Selected output of an electrosurgery machine designed to maximize incision-making ability and minimize coagulation. The waveform of this modality is of constant amplitude with a fundamental frequency between 1 and 3 MHz. *See* Blend current; Coagulation current.

CVP:

See Central venous pressure.

Cyanosis:

Bluish discoloration, usually of the skin and mucous membranes, indicative of a high concentration of reduced (deoxygenated) hemoglobin in the blood. Blueness of the skin is a subjective evaluation that depends on the observer, the patient's complexion, the lighting intensity, and so on. It is generally thought to be seen consistently when reduced hemoglobin is at a level of 5g/dl.

Cybernetics:

Study of human, animal, and mechanical control and communication systems and their capabilities for handling, processing, and routing information. (The central nervous system can be compared to a mechanical-electrical control system).

Cyclopropane:

Simple cyclic hydrocarbon (C_3H_6) gas that is colorless, sweet-smelling, flammable, and explosive. It was introduced as a general anesthetic in 1933 by Waters and coworkers. Cyclopropane was the anesthetic agent of choice in certain circumstances because of its effects, which include rapid induction of anesthesia, wide safety margin between the anesthetic and lethal dose, and support of cardiovascular stability (maintains blood pressure and increases cardiac output). Cyclopropane is excreted almost entirely by the lungs and approximately half is removed from the body within 10 minutes of discontinuing its use. Frequently arrhythmias occur during induction. *Cyclopropane shock* is a term used to explain the sudden hypotension sometimes observed during emergence from deep cyclopropane anesthesia. The hypotension and collapse were thought to be due to the sudden withdrawal of the sympathetic actions of cyclopropane. Cyclopropane was widely used until the 1960s.

Cyclopropane Shock:

See Cyclopropane.

Cylinder Connections:

See American standard compressed gas cylinder valve outlet connections.

Cylinder, Gas:

Container for compressed gas. Medical gas cylinders are usually constructed of steel, with walls between 5/64 and 1/4 inch thick; they must meet the standards of the U.S. Interstate Commerce Commission to be transported across state lines. The size of the tank is commonly letter-coded; contents are color-coded. *See* Table.

Cylinder Pressure Gauge:

Gauge that records and displays the pressure remaining in a gas cylinder.

Cylinder, Gas: Common medical gases and their color code.

Gas	Formula	United States	International	70° Service Pressure in psig (kPa × 100)	State in Cylinder	Filling Density
Oxygen	O_2	Green	White	1900–2200 (130–150)*	Gas†	
Carbon dioxide	CO_2	Gray	Gray	838 (57)	Liquid <88°	68%
Nitrous oxide	N_2O	Blue	Blue	745 (50)	Liquid <98°	68%
Cyclopropane	C_3H_6	Orange	Orange	75 (5)	Liquid	55%
Helium	He	Brown	Brown	1600–2000 (110–136)*	Gas	
Nitrogen	N_2	Black	Black	1800–2200 (122–150)*	Gas	
Air		Yellow‡	White & black	1800 (122)	Gas	

* Depending on type of cylinder.

† Special containers for liquid oxygen are discussed in Chapter 2.

‡ Air, including mixtures of oxygen with nitrogen containing 19.5–23.5% oxygen, is color-coded yellow. Mixtures of nitrogen and oxygen other than those containing 19.5–23.5% oxygen are color-coded black and green.

Cylinder Valve:

Device that allows controlled access to the contents of a gas cylinder. Each valve consists of: (1) the body (the basic structure); (2) the port (exit point for the gas); (3) the stem or shaft (when open allows the gas to flow to the port); (4) the handle or handwheel (turns the valve stem); (5) the safety relief device (allows discharge of cylinder contents) for preventing cylinder explosion if internal pressure goes above a preset maximum; (6) the conical depression (on small cylinder valves, receives the retaining screw of the yoke); and (7) the noninterchangeable safety systems (prevent attachment of an incorrect cylinder to the yoke or regulator). The most common safety system is the Pin-Index Safety System. Two types of cylinder valve design exist: (1) the packed type (also called the direct-acting valve), in which the stem is sealed by a resilient, compressible packing material such as Teflon; and (2) the diaphragm type, which acts indirectly so that turning the stem raises or lowers a metal diaphragm. The latter valve operates better under low-temperature conditions and does not cause a great deal of wear to the valve seat.

Cyprane Inhaler:

See Penthrane analgizer.

Cystic Fibrosis (Fibrocystic Disease of the Pancreas):

Congenital disease of the exocrine glands (especially those that secrete mucus) that affects many organ systems. It is transmitted as a recessive trait. Among the important clinical manifestations are (1) pancreatic insufficiency; (2) dysfunction of the mucous glands of the entire gastrointestinal tract; and (3) susceptibility to heat, in which excessive sweating may result in loss of fluids and electrolytes, leading to hypochloremia, hyponatremia, and dehydration. The most disabling pathologic changes affect the lung. The patient may suffer from chronic bronchitis and emphysema and is susceptible to bronchial pneumonia. Patients usually succumb to progressive respiratory failure as the bronchi become obstructed by viscid mucous secretions. Diagnosis is usually made by a "sweat test," which measures the sodium and chloride concentrations in sweat. Appropriate respiratory care enables patients with moderate cases to live longer. These patients, however, should always be considered to have a compromised respiratory tract, and manipulation of the respiratory tract should be done only with extreme care and precautions taken against infection.

Cytochrome P-450 System:

Complex of pigmented hemoproteins and enzymes found in the liver that cause most oxidative and some reductive biotransformations. The term comes from the fact that when the heme-containing pigments are reduced by carbon monoxide, they have an absorption spectrum at the 450 nm wavelength. The system itself is incorporated into the smooth endoplasmic reticulum of the hepatocytes. Cytochrome P-450 is also found in the kidneys, lung, gut and skin but in much less significant amounts. *See* Enzyme induction.

Cytopathology:

Study of cells in disease states. It is a recognized subspecialty of pathology, and its practitioners often rely on the expertise of trained cytotechnologists. Working together, these individuals are capable of diagnosing benign, atypical, premalignant, and malignant processes in cellular samples obtained from different body sites. Becoming increasingly more sophisticated and widespread, the technique of fine-needle aspiration biopsy allows cytopathologists and cytotechnologists to render a diagnosis on limited samples. The aspirates may be performed: (1) preoperatively (in some cases eliminating the need for surgery and in others altering the extent of the surgery, depending on the diagnosis); (2) intraoperatively (to diagnose a possible metastatic nodule not visualized by other techniques beforehand); or (3) postoperatively (as a follow-up). Frequently, the cytotechnologists are in attendance during the aspiration so as to prepare and fix the slides, they then return to the laboratory to stain and examine the cellular material microscopically. Using a quick-stain technique, it is possible to arrive at a diagnosis within a few minutes. This technique is the cytopathologic equivalent of a frozen section. If the sample is inadequate, the procedure can be repeated in most cases. Cellular samples obtained by other methods, such as exfoliation, direct scraping, endoscopic brushing, or centesis, are examined by cytopathology personnel as well.

Cytoplasm:

Protoplasm of the cell that is not contained within the nucleus. It consists of a viscous, semitransparent fluid that contains the cellular organelles. It is the site where most of the chemical activities of the cell take place.

D

DADL:

Modestly selective "sigma" agonist used to investigate opioid receptor interactions in the spinal cord. *See* Opioid receptor.

DAGO:

Highly selective mu enkephalin agonist currently used to determine opioid actions on the spinal cord. *See* Opioid receptor.

Dalmane:

See Flurazepam.

Dalton's Law of Partial Pressures:

Principle that the total pressure of a mixture of gases is the sum of the partial pressures of the individual gases.

Damages:

Monetary compensation paid to an individual for loss or injury, usually as a result of a legal determination of negligence. *See* Punitive damages.

Damping:

Progressive reduction of mechanical or electric oscillations due to the expenditure of energy by viscosity, resistance, friction, or other work. When the damping is such that the oscillations stop rather than continue, the oscillations are "critically damped." In "overdamped systems" the oscillations are attenuated rapidly (more than is necessary for critical damping). In "underdamped systems" damping never reaches critical proportions; the oscillations continue although they may undergo shape changes. A water manometer connected to a central venous pressure line is an example of damping. The viscosity of the water in the column and the subsequent friction against the inside glass surface damp rapid oscillations in the central venous pressure but allow trends to be discerned.

Dantrolene (Dantrium):

Hydantoin derivative that appears to act on skeletal muscle beyond the neuromuscular junction. Although primarily used in athetosis and dystonia, it is also considered to be the only specific clinical treatment for malignant hyperthermia. *See* Figure.

Dantrolene.

Darvon:

See Propoxyphene.

Data, Analog:

See Analog.

Database (Database Management):

Compilation, management, and use of the fundamental facts or parameters of a particular case or class of individuals. For example, a patient's laboratory results represent a database. The way this information is stored, retrieved, and disseminated constitutes database management.

Data-Processing Buffer:

Device used in electronics or computer engineering to alter, prevent, or temper the interaction of two other devices. For example, a user may insert information into a small computer at a faster rate than it can be processed. The overflow insertions are stored in a buffer (often called a buffer register), which then feeds them to the processor at a slower rate. On large computers, buffers may be used to temporarily store an intermediate result, which can then be reinserted into the processor as required. *See* Central processing unit.

DBS:

See Double burst stimulation.

Deadspace:

See Alveolar deadspace; Anatomic deadspace; Physiologic deadspace.

Deadspace Equation:

See Bohr equation.

Deadspace Ventilation Per Minute:

Volume of gas in each tidal volume that fills the respiratory passageways (but not the alveoli where changes in gas composition take place) times the number of breaths per minute. *See* Anatomic deadspace; Single-breath test; Ventilation/perfusion abnormality.

DEAE:

See Diethylaminoethanol.

Deafferentation:

Interruption or elimination of afferent nerve impulses by destruction of nerve pathways.

Death:

See Biologic death.

Debug:

See Bug.

Decadron:

See Dexamethasone.

Decamethonium (Drug C-10):

Depolarizing neuromuscular blocking agent used for brief anesthetic procedures. Phase II block is reported to be relatively frequent with large doses. Succinylcholine is frequently used instead of decamethonium bromide. *See* Neuromuscular blockade, assessment of; Neuromuscular blocking agent; Phase II block.

Decelerations:

See Fetal monitor.

Declarative Memory:

See Long-term memory.

Decompression Sickness:

See Caisson disease.

Decremental Conduction:

Phenomenon that occurs in the partially anesthetized region of a nerve in which activation of the nerve at one node of Ranvier initiates at the next node an impulse of smaller magnitude. This action results in the impulse and the speed of conduction progressively decreasing during propagation until they may, in fact, be extinguished.

Defamation:

Dissemination of false or objectionable information about an individual.

Defibrillation:

Termination of ventricular fibrillation and restoration of a normal cardiac rhythm by means of an externally applied powerful direct current (DC). (It is also referred to as external defibrillation.) Defibrillators are the devices that deliver the DC current. Most defibrillators are portable and battery-powered to allow easier access to the patient. In simplified form, a battery supplies power to an electronic circuit, which boosts the battery voltage dramatically and uses this voltage to accumulate electrons on a large capacitor. This charge is then fired across the patient's chest between two paddles (very large electrodes). The paddles are usually covered with a gel to break down resistance between the paddles and the skin. In modern designs, discharge occurs when the individual holding the paddles simultaneously presses a button on each paddle. Modern defibrillators can deliver energy in the range of 510 joules over a few thousandths of a second, which is the equivalent of at least 2/3 hp. This large current or flow of electrons should, in theory, completely depolarize all polarizable membranes in the heart, which allows those areas that repolarize quickly (i.e., the normal specialized tissue that maintains the cardiac rate) to begin discharging in a normal fashion. Internal defibrillation, usually done after heart repair with cardiopulmonary bypass, is done by paddles placed directly on the myocardium. Very low currents are used. *See* Figure. *See* Cardiopulmonary bypass; Cardiopulmonary resuscitation.

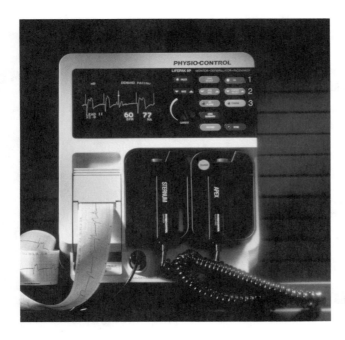

Defibrillation: Modern Lifepak® 9P defibrillator/monitor/pacer with paper-charting capacity.

Deflagration:

Combustion of a fuel/air or fuel/O_2 mixture accompanied by a self-propagating flame. Once ignited, the flame continues to burn any new fuel even if the original source of ignition is removed.

Degaussing:

Magnetic neutralization by current-conducting coils to prevent stray magnetic fields from interfering with electrical phenomena, such as the display on a cathode ray tube.

Dehydration:

Loss of body fluids to the point that signs of fluid deprivation occur. Dehydration is termed isonatremic when the serum sodium levels remain normal (130–150 mEq/L), hyponatremic when serum sodium levels are less than 130 mEq/L, and hypernatremic when serum sodium levels are above 150 mEq/L. In infants and young children the percent weight loss is evaluated to determine the degree of dehydration: 5% weight loss is mild, 10% is moderate, and 15% is severe. *See* Figure.

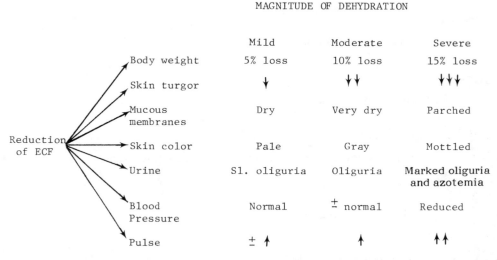

MAGNITUDE OF DEHYDRATION

	Mild	Moderate	Severe
Body weight	5% loss	10% loss	15% loss
Skin turgor	↓	↓↓	↓↓↓
Mucous membranes	Dry	Very dry	Parched
Skin color	Pale	Gray	Mottled
Urine	Sl. oliguria	Oliguria	Marked oliguria and azotemia
Blood Pressure	Normal	± normal	Reduced
Pulse	± ↑	↑	↑↑

(Reduction of ECF)

Dehydration: Correlation between the intensity of clinical findings with the magnitude of dehydration. It is specifically applicable to isotonic dehydration in an infant. Age and hypertonic or hypotonic dehydration may cause some variations.

Delay Line:

Transmission line or circuit element that introduces a known delay in signal transmission.

Delee Trap:

Device used for suctioning the airway of newborn infants. Concerns of infection transmission arise in its use.

Delirium:

Mental disturbance characterized by illusions, confusion, hallucinations, disordered speech, restlessness, and incoherence.

Delirium Tremens:

Mental disturbance related to alcohol withdrawal in the alcoholic. It is characterized by profound confusion, hallucinations, delusions, muscle tremors, anxiety, agitation, and gastrointestinal symptoms. It is usually accompanied by increased activity of the autonomic nervous system exemplified by tachycardia, hypertension, and profuse perspiration. Delirium tremens is fatal in approximately 15% of patients due to cardiovascular collapse or hyperthermia. Treatment involves correction of fluid, electrolyte, and metabolic abnormalities, appropriate sedation, and cardiovascular and respiratory support.

Delta (Δ):

Greek alphabet letter usually written as a triangle. It stands for "change in" or "deviation from" some resting or standard condition.

Delta-Cortef:

See Corticosteroid; Prednisolone.

Deltasone:

See Corticosteroid; Prednisone.

Demand Flow Machine:

See Continuous flow anesthesia machine; Intermittent flow machine.

Demerol:

See Meperidine; Narcotic.

Dendrite:

Nerve cell process that carries an impulse toward the cell body. *See* Axon.

Denervation:

Removal of nervous control of a structure, particularly muscle; alternately, it is the destruction of the neurons or neuronal tract that supply a structure.

Denervation Hypersensitivity:

Condition in which denervated muscle fibers become responsive to externally applied acetylcholine shortly after denervation. Prior to denervation, only the muscle motor endplate region is sensitive to acetylcholine. It is thought that new acetylcholine receptors develop as a consequence of denervation.

Denitrogenation:

Elimination of N_2 from the body by breathing a gas mixture free of N_2, allowing no rebreathing of exhaled gas. It is often done deliberately when beginning inhalation anesthesia to saturate the body with 100% O_2 in order to gain as large a margin of safety as possible in case of decreased ventilation, e.g., airway obstruction or airway instrumentation. With normal lungs and normal alveolar ventilation, lung O_2 concentration reaches inspired O_2 concentration (100%) in approximately 3 minutes.

Density:

Mass per unit volume of substance. The relative density (i.e., the density of the substance divided by the density of water) is known as the specific gravity.

Density Modulated Spectral Array:

Display technique used for interpretation of the electroencephalogram. *See* Electroencephalogram; Fourier analysis.

Depolarization:

Neutralization or elimination by redistribution of electrical charges found in a state of polarity. Depolarization is one of the most fundamental processes during nerve conduction. The membrane of the resting nerve is polarized; i.e., the inside is negatively charged, and the outside is positively charged (70–90 mV). When the nerve conducts an impulse, the nerve membrane becomes depolarized, and the difference in electrical charge effectively goes from –70 mV to 0 mV. In fact, it is transiently repolarized in the opposite direction to approximately +40 mV. The membrane returns to the resting state with the accumulation of positive charges inside and negative charges outside the membrane. *See* Action potential; Polarization; Sodium.

Depth of Anesthesia:

Inexact term referring to the progressive attenuation of the patient's response to painful stimuli as increasing quantities of anesthetics are administered. *See* General anesthesia; Stages and planes of anesthesia.

Depth of Field:

Zone in which an image is acceptably sharp when observed through a camera lens.

Dermatome:

Skin segment in which innervation is supplied by afferent nerve fibers from a single spinal cord level. It is also an instrument for cutting thin layers of skin for grafting procedures. *See* Figure.

Dermatomyositis:

Inflammation of the skin, subcutaneous tissues, and underlying muscles with necrosis of muscle fibers. The etiology of the disease is obscure, but it appears to be associated with an autoimmune reaction. When the disease is confined to the musculature it is known as polymyositis. Patients with dermatomyositis or polymyositis may be particularly sensitive to muscle relaxants, and approximately half the adult patients have an underlying malignancy.

Desensitization Block:

See Phase II block.

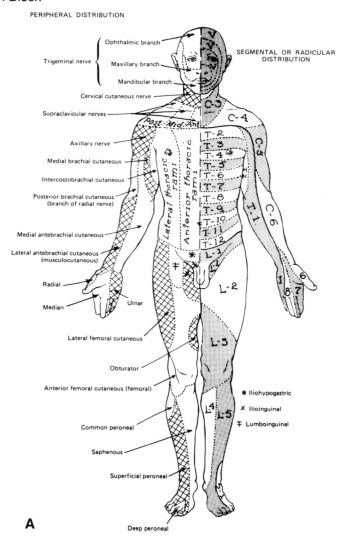

PERIPHERAL DISTRIBUTION

SEGMENTAL OR RADICULAR
DISTRIBUTION

Trigeminal nerve {
Ophthalmic branch
Maxillary branch
Mandibular branch

Cervical cutaneous nerve

Supraclavicular nerves

Axillary nerve

Medial brachial cutaneous

Intercostobrachial cutaneous

Posterior brachial cutaneous
(branch of radial nerve)

Medial antebrachial cutaneous

Lateral antebrachial cutaneous
(musculocutaneous)

Radial

Median

Ulnar

Lateral femoral cutaneous

Obturator

Anterior femoral cutaneous (femoral)

Common peroneal

Saphenous

Superficial peroneal

Deep peroneal

❋ Iliohypogastric

✕ Ilioinguinal

‡ Lumboinguinal

A

Dermatome: Distribution of the various dermatome levels on the (A) anterior and (B) posterior surfaces of the body.

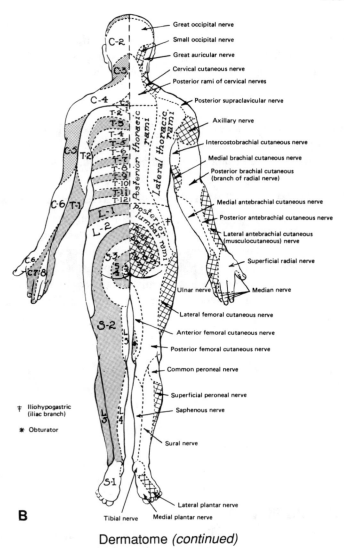

Great occipital nerve
Small occipital nerve
Great auricular nerve
Cervical cutaneous nerve
Posterior rami of cervical nerves
Posterior supraclavicular nerve
Axillary nerve
Intercostobrachial cutaneous nerve
Medial brachial cutaneous nerve
Posterior brachial cutaneous
(branch of radial nerve)
Medial antebrachial cutaneous nerve
Posterior antebrachial cutaneous nerve
Lateral antebrachial cutaneous
(musculocutaneous) nerve
Superficial radial nerve
Median nerve
Ulnar nerve
Lateral femoral cutaneous nerve
Anterior femoral cutaneous nerve
Posterior femoral cutaneous nerve
Common peroneal nerve
Superficial peroneal nerve
Saphenous nerve
Sural nerve
Lateral plantar nerve
Medial plantar nerve
Tibial nerve

‡ Iliohypogastric
(iliac branch)

✳ Obturator

B

Dermatome *(continued)*

Desflurane:

New inhalational anesthetic derived by fluorine substitution for a chlorine in the isoflurane molecule. It has both rapid onset and recovery. Studies suggest that it undergoes little or no metabolism, indicating minimal biodegradation potential.

Desiccation:

Process during which water is removed from an object. Electrodesiccation (a technique of electrosurgery) involves the destructive drying of cells and tissues by short, high-frequency electrical sparks, which evaporate the intracellular water.

Desmopressin Acetate (1-desamino-8-D-arginine vasopressin):

Drug that is a synthetic analog of arginine vasopressin, the normally occurring antidiuretic hormone (ADH). It has a prompt onset of action with a longer duration than the natural hormone. A single dose produces an antidiuretic effect that may persist 8–20 hours. Its primary indication is to treat central diabetes insipidus. It also has been used extensively to improve hemostasis and reduce postoperative blood loss in those patients who have various platelet disorders. The platelet disorder seen after cardiopulmonary bypass appears to respond to desmopressin. *See* Antidiuretic hormone.

Desoxycorticosterone:

Naturally occurring mineralocorticoid. It is useful for treating electrolyte abnormalities associated with adrenal insufficiency. *See* Corticosteroid.

Detergent:

Substance that decreases the surface tension of a liquid and allows it to spread further. Detergents are used in respiratory therapy aerosols to break down fixed secretions. *See* Surface tension.

Determinants of Fluid Flow:

Physical parameters that modify flow in a conduit. Doubling the diameter of an infusion line or a needle increases the flow rate of a fluid 16 times (because the rate varies to the fourth power of the radius of a tube). Because of this relation, it is more important to start with a large intravenous line if rapid flow is required, rather than adding pressure to the administration system or raising the bottle (or bag) to achieve a greater pressure gradient.

Detonability, Limits of (Limits of Explosiveness):

Combinations of fuel and O_2 above and below the ratios that produce a powerful shock wave. At the lower limit, not enough heat is liberated; at the upper limit, too much fuel exists for the O_2 available. Between the limits of detonability, the speed of detonation varies over a narrow range; practically, detonations are equally destructive throughout the range of detonability. For practical purposes, anesthetic agents and air mixtures (ether/air, cyclopropane/air), though highly flammable, do not detonate because of the physical characteristics of the flame front generated.

Device:

Manufactured implement, usually mechanical or electrical in nature, used for a single purpose or related set of purposes.

Dew Point:

Highest temperature of a surface at which water vapor condenses from a humid atmosphere.

Dexamethasone (Decadron):

Potent glucocorticoid and often the drug of choice for steroid therapy in acute situations. It has been used to treat acute and chronic aspiration pneumonia, increased intracranial pressure, and shock-like states.

Dexmedetomidine (DMED):

Drug that is a novel α_2-adrenergic-agonist. It has approximately eight times the α_2-receptor activity of clonidine. In animal studies, this agent appears to be a complete anesthetic. Its initial clinical use appears to be as an anesthetic adjuvant.

Dextran:

Any of numerous polysaccharides that yield glucose upon hydrolysis. Partial hydrolysis and cleavage have produced two forms of dextran solution for intravenous use: one with an average molecular weight of 75,000 and one with an average weight of 40,000. They are useful for expanding plasma volume; however, the newer, smaller molecule product is claimed to have some advantage over the older, higher-weight product. A single infusion in appropriate quantities can improve the hemodynamic status for 24 hours. Marked allergic reactions can occur with both products. At higher doses, some dextran preparations have been noted either to have a deleterious effect on coagulation or to interfere with some techniques of blood typing and crossmatching. *See* Albumin; Hetastarch.

Dezocine:

Agonist-antagonist opioid that is slightly more potent with a shorter duration of action and a more rapid onset than morphine. It appears to be more effective as an anesthetic supplement than other agonist-antagonists.

Diabetes Insipidus:

Relatively rare disease marked by excessive thirst and excretion of a large volume of dilute urine. It is usually due to inadequate production or release of vasopressin, the antidiuretic hormone (ADH) that is produced by the posterior pituitary. It can also be produced by renal resistance to ADH. This condition is termed nephrogenic diabetes insipidus. The patient with diabetes insipidus is the converse of the patient with inappropriate ADH secretion syndrome; however, both can occur with central nervous system trauma. *See* Table. *See* Inappropriate antidiuretic hormone (ADH) secretion syndrome.

Diabetes Insipidus: Differences between pituitary diabetes insipidus and nephrogenic diabetes insipidus.

Pituitary Diabetes Insipidus	Nephrogenic Diabetes Insipidus
Idiopathic	Congenital
Familial	Familial
Brain tumor	Acquired
	Amyloidosis
Head trauma	Chronic renal failure
	Hyperthyroidism
Postneurosurgical	Multiple myeloma
	Nephrocalcinosis-hypercalcemia
Infection disorder (e. g., encephalitis)	Obstructive uropathy
	Potassium deficiency
Vascular disorder (e. g., postpartum necrosis)	Sickle cell anemia
	Sjögren's syndrome
	Drugs
Systemic disorder (e. g., Hand-Schüller-Christian disease, sarcoidosis, tumor metastasis)	Demeclocycline
	Lithium carbonate

Diabetes Mellitus (DM):

Chronic systemic disease marked by disorders of the metabolic utilization of the pancreatic hormone insulin, which in turn deranges carbohydrate, protein, and fat metabolism. Diabetes is divided into type 1 and type 2. Type 1 is immune-mediated, and type 2 is non-immune mediated. The key laboratory finding is a high fasting concentration of glucose in the blood. The diagnosis, however, is firm only if this value can be repeated in the absence of factors that might influence this measurement, such as drugs, exercise, or diet. For the DM patient about to be anesthetized, the appropriate timing of exogenous insulin administration in conjunction with the patient's last nourishment before surgery is important. Insulin injection, in particular, can lead to severe hypoglycemia, which in the acute situation is associated with a much higher morbidity than the hyperglycemia that may result from withholding insulin.

Diabetic Ketoacidosis:

Condition that occurs when a patient is hyperglycemic but does not have enough functioning insulin to prevent the mobilizing and circulation of organic acids (ketone bodies) as alternate energy sources. These patients demonstrate a large "anion gap," decreased circulating volume, and decreased potassium. *See* Anion gap; Diabetes mellitus.

Diacetylmorphine:

See Heroin; Narcotic.

Diagnostic Related Groups (DRG):

A system for hospital health care reimbursement based on a predetermined list of human diseases. Developed initially at Yale University, the program is an attempt to group patients based on the cost of care required rather than the length of hospital stay. Currently, all diseases are grouped into approximately 500 categories.

Dialysis:

See Hemodialysis.

Diameter Index Safety System (DISS):

System that provides removable, noninterchangeable connections for low-pressure gas lines. These connections act as a safeguard against the incorrect coupling of gas supplies with the anesthetic equipment. Each type of gas has a specifically sized receptacle and attached nipple for its gas line. *See* American standard compressed gas cylinder valve outlet connections; Pin index safety system.

Diaphoresis (Sweating):

Exudation of fluid onto the surface of the skin in response to elevated heat production. The evaporation of sweat from the skin's surface cools the body. The sweat glands are innervated by cholinergic fibers of sympathetic origin. Sweating by the anesthetized patient is considered to be a sign that anesthesia is too light. By contrast, sweating by a patient being resuscitated indicates that effective circulation is taking place and resuscitative efforts should therefore continue. *See* Autonomic nervous system; Insensible loss and insensible water loss.

Diaphragm:

Large, thin membranous muscle that separates the abdominal and thoracic cavities and is chiefly responsible for respiration (approximately 70% of inspired respiratory volume). The diaphragm is supplied by the left and right phrenic nerves, which arise from the cervical plexus at C2, C3, and C4 levels. The downward contraction of the diaphragm creates a slight negative pressure in the thorax. This action is aided by contraction of the intercostal muscles, which expands the rib cage. This negative pressure causes inspiration as air moves down the upper airway along the pressure gradient from atmospheric to subatmospheric areas.

Diaphragmatic Hernia:

Disorder in which the intestines, and often the stomach and spleen, protrude into the thoracic cavity through the diaphragm wall (on the left side in 90% of the cases). It may be either congenital or acquired. It is a surgical emergency in newborns. The lung on the affected side is often hypoplastic. Because the abdominal viscera occupy the thoracic cavity, the mediastinum is shifted toward the unaffected side, disrupting cardiovascular dynamics. Death may occur rapidly owing to the respiratory distress caused by the hypoplastic lung. Newborns who develop severe respiratory distress within the first 24 hours of life have a 50% mortality rate. Infants who survive on their own for more than 72 hours have survival rates approaching 100%.

Diastolic Pressure:

Arterial pressure when the ventricles are at rest and filling.

Diathermy:

Use of high-frequency electromagnetic radiation to generate heat within a body part. *See* Cauterization.

Diathesis:

Condition in which there is enhanced susceptibility to disease. For example, hemophilia is a bleeding diathesis in which the propensity to hemorrhage is increased.

Diatomaceous Earth:

See Gas chromatography.

Diazepam:

See Benzodiazepine.

Diazoxide (Hyperstat IV):

Derivative of the thiazides (but devoid of diuretic effect). It is used as an intravenous agent for the prompt treatment of hypertensive crisis. Diazoxide causes marked salt and water retention, and therefore its clinical effect directly opposes many diuretic antihypertensive drugs.

Dibenzyline:

See Phenoxybenzamine.

Dibucaine:

See Local anesthetic.

Dibucaine Number:

Quantification of the inhibition of plasma cholinesterase activity (in breaking down succinylcholine) by dibucaine. At least two types of plasma cholinesterase (pseudocholinesterase) enzyme exist: normal and atypical. (There is more than one subtype.) The difference between them is evident clinically only after injection of succinylcholine. A person with the normal enzyme is able to hydrolyze the succinylcholine rapidly, whereas the one with the atypical enzyme cannot. (A heterozygous individual, i.e., one with a normal and an atypical enzyme gene, hydrolyzes the drug much less efficiently than do normal individuals.) With the dibucaine test, if a plasma sample has a high normal enzyme content, it is inhibited by dibucaine and has a high dibucaine number. Patients with a low dibucaine number have low levels of normal plasma cholinesterase; however, patients with low levels of normal plasma cholinesterase do not necessarily have a low dibucaine number. The low enzyme level may be due to malnutrition and liver damage, not to an atypical gene. If the presence of an atypical gene is verified, however, other family members may be prone to the same response to succinylcholine and should be forewarned. Evidence exists for a second gene, a fluoride gene, which also determines plasma cholinesterase activity. The fluoride number and the dibucaine number may differ in individuals, i.e., one may be normal and the other abnormally low. An abnormal homozygous fluoride gene (low fluoride number) gives a moderately prolonged response to succinylcholine. A third gene, the "silent gene," which also determines plasma cholinesterase activity, has been identified. Patients with this gene show total plasma cholinesterase inhibition and therefore have a prolonged response to succinylcholine. *See* Acetylcholinesterase; Pseudocholinesterase; Succinylcholine.

DIC:

See Disseminated intravascular coagulation.

Dichloroacetylene (C_2Cl_2):

A toxic breakdown product of the obsolete anesthetic trichloroethylene (Trilene, $2C_2HCl_3$). Trilene decomposes in the presence of elevated temperatures and soda lime, and therefore should never be used in rebreathing circuits. Dichloroacetylene causes cranial nerve damage and decomposes into phosgene and CO. *See* Phosgene.

Dichlorodifluoromethane:

See Freon.

Dicrotic Notch:

Cleft seen in the descending portion of the aortic blood pressure trace caused by a sharp deceleration of blood flow and abrupt closure of the aortic valve. If observed in a radial artery tracing, the notch seen is an artifact of pressure wave reflection from the arterioles. *See* Peripheral vascular resistance; Pulse pressure tracing.

Dielectric:

Medium that acts as an insulator between the two plates of a capacitor.

Dielectric Heating:

Technique for heating an insulator by compressing it between two conducting plates, or electrodes, and applying a high-frequency current.

Dielectric Strength:

Measurement of the maximal electrical difference an insulator can withstand without breakdown.

Diethylaminoethanol (DEAE):

One of the two major metabolites of procaine, the other is paraaminobenzoic acid. DEAE has many of procaine's actions, including analgesia, antiarrhythmia, and impulse blockade.

Diethyl Ether (Ether):

Highly flammable general anesthetic. It has a slow induction and emergence period, and its vapors are respiratory irritants that induce copious secretions. It provides excellent cardio-vascular stability. At low concentrations it is a good analgesic agent. A wide margin of safety exists between the anesthetic and toxic doses. Major contraindications of diethyl ether include postoperative nausea and vomiting and its potential flammability.

Differential Block:

Phenomenon that occurs when a local anesthetic is injected close to a nerve trunk contain-ing many differently sized nerve fibers. Differential blockade occurs because of the varia-tions in fiber diameter, myelin covering, and position in the mixed nerve. Some fibers are completely or partially blocked, whereas others are not blocked at all. There is a general order in which differential blockade occurs: B fibers, then A-delta fibers, then C fibers. The A-alpha fibers may be totally unaffected. Clinically, therefore, there is analgesia to a pinprick, but motor activity may be preserved. (The large fibers also convey touch and light pressure sensations, which may be misinterpreted by the patient as pain.) An alternate (and possibly equally valid) explanation of the differential blockade phenomenon is that local anesthetic agents first block those nerves that carry the heaviest number or the highest frequency of action potentials. Pain sensation is a high-frequency transmission, which may explain why it is blocked before the low-frequency motor nerves are blocked. It is thought that high-frequency transmission keeps more sodium channels open for longer periods, allowing rapid entry of the local anesthetic molecule, which acts on the inside opening of the sodium channel. Differential blockade may be deliberately induced by using a low concentration of local anesthetic to block sympathetic fibers without blocking sensory or motor fibers. *See* Nerve fiber, anatomy and physiology of.

Diffusion:

Process by which gases, fluids, and solids intermingle owing to the kinetics of their constituent atomic particles. Mixing is complete unless one set of particles is much heavier than the other; in this case gravitational effects cause sedimentation of the heavier particles.

Diffusion Block:

See Alveolar end-capillary difference.

Diffusion Capacity of the Lung:

Measurement of the ability of the lung to transfer alveolar gas to capillary blood without significant delay during passage of the gas through the alveolar capillary membrane. Diffusion capacity is affected by the area, thickness, and diffusion properties of the alveolar membranes and the solubility (in the alveolar membrane) of the gas concerned. Carbon monoxide (CO) is used to measure diffusion capacity because its transfer from the alveolus into the blood is diffusion-limited rather than perfusion-limited, i.e., combination of hemo-globin with CO occurs so readily that all CO in low concentrations is absorbed into blood even if blood flow past the alveolus is slowed to nearly zero. Measurements of diffusion capacity using CO (D_{CO}) can be made by the single-breath method, steady-state method, rebreathing technique, and fractional CO uptake technique. The D_{CO} is affected by many variables. It increases with increasing lung volume and exercise. Body position affects the D_{CO}: It is highest if the body is in a supine position and higher sitting rather than standing. The D_{CO} varies in direct proportion to body size. Within the physiologic range of O_2, diffusion capacity decreases insignificantly with inspired O_2 tension and increases with increased CO_2 tension. The normal value (at rest) for D_{CO} is approximately 17–25 ml/min/mm Hg of P_{CO}.

Diffusion Constant:

Specific quantity necessary to determine accurately the transfer of gas across a membrane. The constant is directly proportional to the solubility of the gas in the membrane and is inversely proportional to the square root of the molecular weight of the gas. *See* Figure.

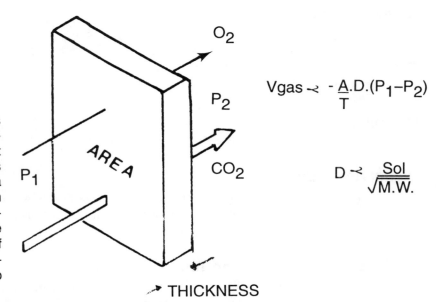

Diffusion Constant: Gas diffusion through a tissue sheet. The amount of gas transferred is proportional to the area of the tissue, a diffusion constant, and the difference in partial pressure across the surfaces of the tissue, and inversely proportional to the tissue thickness.

$$Vgas \approx \frac{- A.D.(P_1 - P_2)}{T}$$

$$D \approx \frac{Sol}{\sqrt{M.W.}}$$

Diffusion Hypoxia:

Phenomenon that can be produced after prolonged anesthesia with high concentrations of N_2O/O_2. If the patient is allowed to breathe room air at the termination of the anesthetic, the outflow of N_2O from blood dilutes the O_2 in the alveolus, lowering its partial pressure below the 21% normally seen in room air. This event can cause some arterial O_2 desaturation. Although this phenomenon is of little significance in the normal patient, it may become highly important in the patient with marginal oxygenation. The anesthetist may avoid this occurrence by flowing high concentrations of O_2 instead of room air at the termination of anesthesia. *See* Concentration effect.

Diffusion Limitation:

Concept that a barrier to diffusion across the alveolar capillary membrane can limit uptake of alveolar gas by the blood (alveolar-capillary block). *See* Alveolar end-capillary differences; Diffusion capacity of the lung.

Diffusion Resistance:

Relative impedance by a given membrane to gas transfer. *See* Diffusion capacity of the lung.

Diffusion Respiration:

See Apneic oxygenation.

Digital Block (Finger Block):

See Digital nerve block.

Digital Computer:

See Analog computer.

Digital Data:

See Binary code; binary number system.

Digitalis:

See Cardiac glycosides.

Digital Nerve Block:

Direct injection with local anesthetic of the digital nerves, which supply fingers and toes. It is important that there be no added vasoconstrictor in the local anesthetic solution, as marked vasoconstriction of a digit can cause gangrene.

Digital Symbol Substitution Test:

Test of cognitive ability used after an outpatient procedure to evaluate a recovering patient. It requires substituting symbols for numbers in an orderly, prescribed fashion. *See* Trieger dot test.

Digitoxin:

See Cardiac glycosides.

Digoxin:

See Cardiac glycosides.

Dihydrohydroxymorphinone; Oxymorphone (Numorphan):

Semisynthetic morphine derivative. *See* Narcotic.

Dilantin:

See Diphenylhydantoin.

Dilatation:

Stretching of an orifice or tube in cross section beyond its normal dimensions.

Dilaudid (Dihydromorphinone):

See Narcotic.

Dimethyl Tubocurarine Chloride (Tubarine):

See Tubocurarine chloride.

Dimethyl Tubocurarine Iodide (Metocurine):

Synthetic derivative of d-tubocurarine (curare) that is two to three times as potent. *See* Neuromuscular blocking agent; Tubocurarine chloride.

Dinamap™:

See Automatic blood pressure device.

Diphenhydramine (Benadryl):

Antihistamine useful in oral and parenteral form. It antagonizes the action of histamine at its receptors and may cause some central nervous system depression. *See* Antihistamine.

Diprivan:

See Propofal.

Diphenylhydantoin; Phenytoin (Sodium Dilantin):

Anticonvulsant drug used to treat epileptic and psychomotor seizures. It appears to exert specific antiepileptic actions without causing general depression of the central nervous system. Its therapeutic effectiveness and toxicity may be correlated with the plasma concentration of the drug: Low levels are ineffective, and high levels produce neurotoxicity. Common side effects of the drug are ataxia, nystagmus, double vision, excitement, tremors, and gingival hypertrophy. Diphenylhydantoin is also useful for treating digitalis-induced tachyarrhythmias.

Dipole:

Object with two equal and opposite charges located close to each other. For example, a small magnet constitutes a magnetic dipole.

Direct Fetal Electrocardiography:

Technique for recording fetal heart activity during labor by placing an electrode onto a presenting part. The electrode contains a stainless steel coil that penetrates the skin. Sterile technique is required.

Disk Float:

Type of indicator used in early flowmeters. It consists of a thin horizontal disc with a long protruding stem. The disk and the stem are pushed upward in the tapered tube as in modern flowmeters; however, the disk is the only portion of the float that acts as an obstructs flow. The tip of the stem moves upward behind a calibrated scale to indicate the amount of flow.

Disintegration Scheme:

Line drawing showing the products of decay of a radioactive atom including the forms of energy released, types of particles released, and final stable nucleus.

Dispersive Electrode (Ground or Indifferent Electrode):

Electrode by which radiofrequency energy is returned to an electrosurgery machine (unit). It must provide a wide area of contact with the patient's skin so the density of radiofrequency energy over any particular square centimeter of tissue is below the level that can heat the tissue. Factors in the design or development of the dispersive electrode include the area of the electrode, medium for maintaining contact (i.e., gelled or ungelled), and geometric shape of the electrode. Even with the best contact and optimal pattern, current flow under the surface of the electrode is not uniform due to skin variations. *See* Figure. *See* Cutting current.

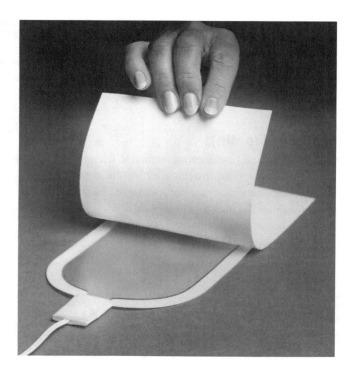

Dispersive Electrode: Bovie® adult-size disposable conductive adhesive pads. Smaller, pediatric pads are designed to conform to children between one and twelve years old.

DISS:

See Diameter index safety system.

Disseminated Intravascular Coagulation (DIC):

Clotting disorder that is almost invariably catastrophic. Seen in trauma patients or obstetric patients after amniotic fluid embolization; it is characterized by the continuous consumption of clotting factors and platelets, formation of fibrin thrombi, decrease in platelet count, and activation of the fibrinolytic system. This process is diffuse, occurring throughout the body. The patient with DIC may present either with massive bleeding (bleeding from every needle stick), which is the more usual presentation, or with thrombotic symptoms (or a combination of the two). No single laboratory test can diagnose DIC. It has been suggested that the test criteria are lengthened prothrombin time, low platelet count, and low fibrinogen level. While heparin has been used to treat DIC, the underlying cause(s) should be treated first. *See* Table. *See* Primary fibrinolysis.

Disseminated Intravascular Coagulation: Diagnostic criteria for disseminated intravascular coagulation (DIC).

1. Decrease in platelet count
2. Abnormal serial thrombin test
3. Normal clot lysis time
4. Decrease in fibrinogen
5. Positive test for split products of fibrinogen, i.e., positive protamine test, positive Fi test (fibrinogen degradation products)

Dissociation Constant (pK$_a$):

The pH at which a given acid or base is 50% ionized and 50% nonionized. The pK$_a$ of a drug is important because in most biologic systems it is only the nonionized drug that can cross cell membranes easily (the lower the pK$_a$ of a drug, the stronger the acid; the higher the pK$_a$ of a drug, the stronger the base). *See* Table. *See* Henderson-Hasselbalch equation; Local anesthetic.

Dissociation Constant (pK$_a$): Dissociation constants of local anesthetics.

Agent	pK$_a$	% base at pH 7.4	Approximate onset of action (min)
Mepivacaine	7.6	40	2 to 4
Etidocaine	7.7	33	2 to 4
Articaine	7.8	29	2 to 4
Lidocaine	7.9	25	2 to 4
Prilocaine	7.9	25	2 to 4
Bupivacaine	8.1	18	5 to 8
Tetracaine	8.5	8	10 to 15
Chloroprocaine	8.7	6	6 to 12
Procaine	9.1	2	14 to 18

From Cohen S, Burns RC: Pathways of the pulp, ed 4, St Louis, 1987. The CV Mosby Co.

Dissociative Anesthesia:

Pharmacologic state in which the patient does not lose consciousness but is emotionally detached from and disinterested in the environment. The patient shows no desire to change position or move about. The term is often used interchangeably with neuroleptanesthesia. The only difference between the two seems to be that neuroleptanesthesia is caused by drugs such as droperidol and fentanyl in combination (Innovar), whereas dissociative anesthesia is induced by ketamine. Because increasing the dosage of these agents or adding the proper concentrations of N_2O produces a state indistinguishable from general anesthesia, these terms are somewhat arbitrary.

Dissolved Oxygen:

O_2 that is dissolved in blood. The O_2 obeys Henry law, which states that the solubility of a gas in a liquid solution is proportional to the partial pressure of the gas. Normal arterial blood with a PaO_2 of 100 mm Hg contains 0.3 ml O_2/dl blood.

Distortion:

Change, usually undesirable, in the shape of a waveform caused by either mechanical or electrical interference. On an electrocardiograph displayed on a poorly adjusted oscilloscope, for example, the upstroke of the electrical complexes may be overextended enough to indicate nonexistent ventricular hypertrophy. *See* Electrocardiogram.

Diuresis:

Increased excretion of urine. Diuretics cause diuresis.

Diurnal Rhythm:

See Circadian rhythm.

Diver Paralysis:

See Caisson disease.

Divinyl Ether:

Early general anesthetic. *See* Diethyl ether.

DM:

See Diabetes mellitus.

DMED:

See Dexmedetomidine.

Dobutamine:

Synthetic catecholamine that is a modification of isoproterenol. It acts directly on β-adrenergic receptors but has a much weaker β_2-action than does its parent isoproterenol. It produces a positive inotropic effect. The drug has a brief half-life and hence is controllable.

Dolophine:

See Methadone.

Domperidone:

Pharmacologic agent that is a dopamine receptor blocking agent, like metoclopramide. It has the advantages of its action being longer in duration and acting primarily peripherally. It antagonizes atropine effects on the lower esophageal sphincter and increases gastric emptying. It may be a useful agent in the prophylaxis against aspiration pneumonia.

Dopamine Hydrochloride (Intropin):

Naturally occurring precursor of epinephrine and norepinephrine that is used as a chemical messenger in certain parts of the central nervous system. When given as a continuous infusion for cardiovascular support (depending on dosage), cardiac contractility, cardiac output, and renal blood flow increase. Dopamine is useful for management of various types of shock. It may cause serious cardiac arrhythmias.

Dopar:

See L-dopa; Levodopa.

Doping:

Technique for creating semiconductors. Alternately, filling a medical student with misinformation. *See* Semiconductor.

Doppler Blood Pressure Measurement:

See Doppler effect.

Doppler Effect:

Apparent shift in the frequency of sound or light waves when the wave source is moving in relation to the observer. The classic example of this phenomenon concerns a train with a constant-pitch whistle. As it approaches the stationary observer the pitch of the whistle is perceived as higher (up doppler) than it is, and lower (down doppler) as the train recedes. The amount of observed change is proportional to the speed of the train. A doppler device can be used to determine blood pressure. Arterial wall movement changes the frequency of the sound wave produced by a transmitting crystal. This change is detected by a receiving crystal and is used with a known cuff pressure to determine arterial pressure. *See* Figure.

Dose-Response Curve:

Graphic representation of the relation between the amount of an administered drug and the biologic effect observed. (The x-axis represents the drug amount; the y-axis represents the effect.) A flat response curve indicates that major changes in dosage produce little biologic effect, whereas a steep response curve demonstrates that minor changes have a significant effect.

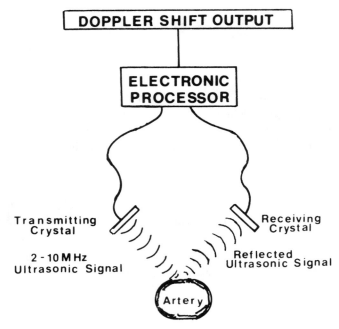

DOPPLER SHIFT OUTPUT

ELECTRONIC PROCESSOR

Transmitting Crystal

Receiving Crystal

2 - 10 MHz Ultrasonic Signal

Reflected Ultrasonic Signal

Artery

Doppler Effect: Mechanism for determining arterial wall movement and subsequent measurement of blood pressure by means of the Doppler effect. Sudden vibrations in the arterial wall when the cuff pressure falls slightly below systolic pressure cause variations in the reflected ultrasonic signal frequency. An electronic processor compares the transmitted and reflected frequencies and from their differences generates a Doppler signal.

Dosimetry:

Measurement technique for quantitating a radiation dose. The x-ray film badge, worn by those occupationally exposed to radiation, is analyzed by dosimetry.

Double Burst Stimulation (DBS):

Alternative means of accessing neuromuscular blockade. It consists of a burst of three 200-μs impulses at a frequency of 50 Hz, followed 750 ms later by an identical burst. It is modified as $DBS_{3,2}$ which has three 200-μs bursts followed by two such bursts 750 ms later. DBS appears to have a high degree of linear correlation with the train-of-four neuromuscular blockade assessment technique. *See* Figure. *See* Train-of-four.

Double-Lumen Tube:

Type of tube available for selective control of either lung during anesthesia. Each lung can be ventilated separately or blocked off from the other. Because these tubes have two lumens, the cross-sectional area of each is small and resistance is high. There are many types of double-lumen tube: Carlens, Bryce-Smith, and Robertshaw. Each has a tracheal cuff and a cuff to be inflated in the intubated bronchus. The latter two tubes come with either right or left configurations depending on the mainstem bronchus to be intubated. *See* Figure. *See* Bronchial blocker; Endobronchial intubation; Intubation.

	During induction			During operation			In the recovery room
	Thiopental	Supramaximal stimulation	Tracheal intubation	Intense blockade	Moderate blockade	Reversal	
Single twitch		1.0 Hz	0.1 Hz				
TOF							?
PTC							
DBS							

Double Burst Stimulation: This diagram shows when the different modes of electrical nerve stimulation can be used during clinical anesthesia. Dark dotted areas indicate appropriate use; light dotted areas, less effective use. Modes of nerve stimulation: TOF, train-of-four stimulation; FTC, post-tetanic count; and DBS, double burst stimulation. The "?" means that TOF is less useful in the recovery room.

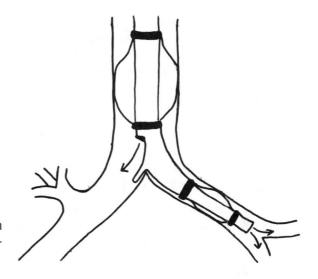

Double-Lumen Tube: Carlens double-lumen tube seated in the trachea. The arrows indicate the direction of gas flow.

Down Time:

Period during which a system, particularly a computer, is malfunctioning and cannot meet its operational requirements. It also refers to the period when an operating room is not functioning.

Doxacurium Chloride (Nanomex):

A new long-acting muscle relaxant.

Doxapram (Dopram):

Respiratory stimulant used to treat postoperative respiratory depression. It tends to activate carotid chemoreceptors and has a wide margin of safety.

dP/dT:

Rate of change of pressure (P) in the ventricle (usually measured in the left) with respect to time (t). The maximum dP/dt is reached at the same time as the peak positive deflection in an apexcardiogram. It has been advocated as a measurement of cardiac contractility.

DPDPE:

Manufactured enkephalin that is a selective sigma agonist in the spinal cord. It is used to investigate opioid receptor interactions. *See* Opioid receptor.

2,3-DPG (Diphosphoglycerate):

See CPD blood preservation; Oxygen-hemoglobin dissociation curve.

Dramamine (Dimenhydrinate):

See Antihistamine.

Draw-Over Vaporizer:

Device that vaporizes liquid anesthetic into a stream of gas being drawn or pulled over the surface of the anesthetic, usually by spontaneous respiration of the patient. Although a wick may be used to increase surface area, no attempt is made to regulate vaporization except that the process of rapid vaporization cools the liquid anesthetic, thereby lowering its vapor pressure and inhibiting further vaporization. It is often confused with a flow-over vaporizer, which vaporizes anesthetics into a gas stream pushed by a machine rather than the patient. *See* EMO inhaler; Vaporizer, draw-over, flow-over, bubble-through.

DRG:

See Diagnostic Related Groups.

Driver:

Electrical circuit in which the output is used to provide input for one or more other circuits. Commonly, the amplifier stage immediately preceding the output stage of a transmitter or receiver "drives" the speakers.

Dromoran:

See Levorphanol tartrate.

Dronabinol:

Derivative of a major ingredient of marijuana. This drug is a centrally acting antiemetic used for treating chemotherapy-induced nausea and vomiting. *See* Cannabis.

Droperidol (Inapsine):

Butyrophenone related to haloperidol. It is used in combination with the potent narcotic fentanyl to produce neuroleptanesthesia. Used alone as a premedicant for its antianxiety effect, it is also employed clinically for its antiemetic and antinausea actions. *See* Dissociative anesthesia; Innovar.

Drowning:

Suffocation by submersion, especially in water. For medical purposes (because drowning implies death), two further categories are defined: near-drowning with aspiration and near-drowning without aspiration. It is estimated that approximately 10% of drowning victims die without aspirating water. It appears that death in these patients is caused by laryngospasm and acute asphyxia. Animal studies have shown that in acute asphyxia arterial O_2 tension drops from a control value of approximately 100 mm Hg to 40 mm Hg in 1 minute, 10 mm Hg in 3 minutes, and 4 mm Hg in 5 minutes. It is this hypoxia that causes death as an increase in CO_2 tension high enough to cause death could not take place in such a short period. With aspiration, a distinction is made between those individuals who aspirate fresh or salt water. With fresh water (hypotonic compared to plasma) aspiration, the water is rapidly absorbed into the circulation, causing dilution of the blood (hemodilution). With sea water (hypertonic compared to plasma) aspiration, plasma water leaves the circulation, further filling the alveoli and simultaneously causing hemoconcentration. Although these two conditions both lead to derangement in serum ion concentration, they are rarely of sufficient magnitude to cause death.

Drug Dependence:

State of tolerance or psychological or physiologic need for a drug as a result of periodic or continued use of that drug. The specific characteristics of dependence vary for different drug classifications. Whereas psychological dependence may be altered by subjective and behavioral factors, physiologic dependence and tolerance are pharmacologically based in that normal body functions are maintained only in the continued presence of the drug. Abrupt withdrawal of the agent results in the adverse physiologic changes of withdrawal syndrome. *See* Tolerance.

Drug Distribution:

Concept that drugs introduced into the body tend to accumulate in or avoid various locations depending on dose, tissue absorption, blood flow, and time. *See* Figure.

Drug Interaction:

Change in the performance of one drug when combined with the administration of another. Most drug interactions involve one drug changing the rate of excretion or metabolism of another drug or its tissue binding. Major drug interactions are rare and may involve physical incompatibilities between two or more compounds. For example, injectable diazepam cannot be added to many common intravenous solutions because it precipitates. *See* Synergism.

Drug Level Monitoring in Serum:

Laboratory determination of the amount of drug present in a sample of the patient's blood. This measurement is particularly useful for evaluating drug levels that cannot be readily monitored by clinical observation. Because patients' responses vary to specific drugs owing to concurrent illnesses or conditions and drug tolerances, dosages may have to be adjusted for each patient in order to achieve the desired response. Serial serum level measurements are more accurate than a single determination.

225

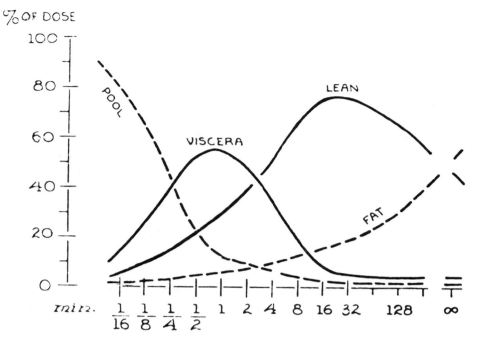

Drug Distribution: Distribution of thiopental in different body tissues and organs at various times after its intravenous injection.

Drunken Sailor Effect:

Metaphor for intermittently controlling ventilation such that the $PaCO_2$ drifts back and forth around the normal level. First the patient is hyperventilated by the anesthetist and becomes alkalotic. Then controlled respiration is stopped, and the patient becomes acidotic as $PaCO_2$ builds up until spontaneous respiration begins again. Controlled ventilation is then resumed. The drunken sailor effect is also a metaphor describing an inexperienced anesthetist trying to establish the proper required depth of anesthesia. He or she acts much like a drunken sailor trying to navigate a straight line and lumbering first to one side and then to the other, overcorrecting at each extreme.

d-Tubocurarine:

See Tubocurarine chloride.

Dual Block:

See Phase II block.

Duality of Pain Transmission:

Two systems for the transmission of pain sensation that appear to occur side by side in humans. One transmission pathway is comparatively fast and comprises the myelinated A-delta fibers. The other pathway is made up of the slow-conducting nonmyelinated C fibers. The A-delta fibers and the C fibers are roughly equally sensitive to local anesthetics. *See* Gate theory of pain; Nerve fiber, anatomy and physiology of.

Dubowitz Score:

System for evaluating gestational age of premature infants. Its scores neurologic signs primarily related to muscle tone that are dependent on the maturation of the nervous system. *See* Early neonatal neurobehavioral scale.

Duke Inhaler:

See Penthrane analgizer.

Dupaco Incorporated:

A manufacturing company of many anesthesia-related items including blood-warming devices and varied respiratory equipment. They are now located in Oceanside, California.

Dural Puncture:

Penetration of the dura, the covering over the spinal cord and brain, usually with a needle. It is a prerequisite for the induction of spinal anesthesia.

Dust Cell:

See Macrophage.

Duty:

Legally enforced obligation that requires one person to act in a particular way with respect to another person.

Dye Dilution:

See Cardiac output.

Dynamic Compression:

Condition of airway resistance that occurs during forced expiration. High intrapleural pressure is applied to the alveoli and to the outside walls of the airways as a forced effort is made to empty them. This pressure can cause the airways to collapse. This paradoxical situation flattens expiratory flow rate despite increased respiratory effort. (With a greater effort, more of the airways collapse, thereby impeding flow.)

Dynamometer (Torque-Meter):

Device for measuring the rotational force of an engine or motor.

Dyne:

Unit of force in the centimeter-gram-second (CGS) system. It is equal to the force acting on a 1-g mass to give it an acceleration of 1 cm/sec^2. One dyne is the equivalent of 10^{-5} newton.

Dyrenium:

See Triamterene.

Dysbarism:

See Caisson disease.

Dysesthesia:

Sensation that is both unpleasant and abnormal, usually pertaining to the sense of touch.

Dysgeusia:

Distortion in the perception of taste. For example, what should taste salt tastes sweet. It differs from ageusia, which is the inability to detect the qualities of the four main taste parameters: sweet, salt, bitter or sour.

Dysphoria:

Distressed emotional state that can be manifested by malaise, restlessness and depression.

Dyspnea:

Condition in which there is difficult or labored breathing. It may be a subjective sensation in the patient. It is usually defined as an awareness of respiration that is distressful. It should not be confused with shortness of breath, as the latter is usually explained by physical causes, e.g., exercise.

Dystocia:

Condition of difficult or abnormal labor and delivery. It can occur because of multiple antecedent conditions but is usually seen as a result of cephalopelvic disproportion (CPD) (a generalized term for a mismatch between the cross-section measurement of the fetal head and the cross-section diameter of the pelvic outlet).

E

E:

Unit charge of an electron. It is equal to 1.60210×10^{-9} coulomb.

Early Neonatal Neurobehavioral Scale (ENNS):

Neonatal test to determine lingering effects of anesthetic drugs. *See* Brazelton score; Neurologic and adaptive capacity score.

ECG, EKG:

See Electrocardiogram.

Echothiophate Iodide (Phospholine):

Topically applied ophthalmic drug used to treat glaucoma. It is a cholinesterase inhibitor of the organophosphorus class. It is possible for enough Phospholine to be absorbed, via the cornea, into the systemic circulation to seriously depress serum cholinesterase activity, which in turn can significantly prolong neuromuscular blockade caused by succinylcholine. *See* Cholinesterase.

Eclampsia:

Disease process that occurs in a pregnant woman usually after the 24th week. It is often referred to as "toxemia of pregnancy." The initial triad of symptoms: maternal hypertension, proteinuria, and generalized edema is called preeclampsia. When grand mal seizures occur, the entire constellation is called eclampsia. Magnesium sulfate is the long-standing drug of choice for the central nervous system (CNS) effects. Because it is a depressant, it is synergistic to general anesthetics and other depressants. Its effect on the motor junction makes the patients on magnesium sulfate more sensitive to muscle relaxants. *See* Preeclampsia.

ECMO:

See Extracorporeal membrane oxygenation; Membrane oxygenator.

ECRI:

Originally an acronym for Emergency Care Research Institute, ECRI has now become the official name of a large, not for profit organization based in Plymouth Meeting, Pennsylvania. It tests and publishes results on a wide variety of health care equipment. Of particular interest to individuals in anesthesia is *Technology for Anesthesia,* ECRI's monthly publication summarizing health care technology issues for the field.

ECT:

See Electroconvulsive therapy.

ED$_{50}$ (Effective Dose 50%):

Dose of a pharmacologic substance that produces an effect in 50% of the subjects given the substance. The greater the difference between the ED$_{50}$ and the LD$_{50}$ (lethal dose 50%), the safer is the substance. *See* LD$_{50}$; Therapeutic index.

Edecrin:

See Ethacrynic acid.

Edema:

Accumulation of excessive amounts of fluid in the interstitial spaces. Edema may be due to congestive heart failure, venous obstruction, inadequate lymphatic drainage, and renal or hepatic disease. Generalized massive edema is known as anasarca, whereas the accumulation of fluid in lung tissue and air spaces is known as pulmonary edema. *See* Pulmonary edema.

Edit:

To modify, rearrange, delete, or expand data or information. (Why this book looks the way it does.)

EDRF:

See Endothelium-derived relaxing factor.

Edrophonium (Tensilon):

Cholinesterase inhibitor that, in appropriate dosages, is shorter acting than neostigmine or pyridostigmine. In the patient who is not receiving anticholinesterase therapy, a small dose of edrophonium can be used as a diagnostic test for myasthenia gravis. (The disease is strongly suspected if muscle strength improves after drug therapy.) Edrophonium is also a potent antagonist to curare-like agents. *See* Myasthenia gravis; Neostigmine; Pyridostigmine.

Educated Hand:

Concept that the hand of the trained anesthetist could, by feeling the breathing bag, detect beginning attempts at respiration, bronchospasm, breath holding, and, in general, any changes in lung compliance, and could thereby monitor indirectly the depth of anesthesia. The further idea that the "educated hand" could, breath after breath, deliver the same tidal volume over a prolonged period of time has been discredited.

EEG:

See Electroencephalogram

Effacement:

Process by which the cervix is progressively thinned and the os dilated (during the first stage of labor) until only the thinned, external os remains.

Effective Absorption Ability:

See Carbon dioxide absorption.

Effective Absorption Effeciency:

See Carbon dioxide absorption.

Efferent:

Going or moving away from the center. For example, efferent motor nerves transmit signals away from the central nervous system to muscles causing contractions.

Efficacy:

Relative ability of a drug to cause a specific biologic effect. For example, barbiturates are more efficacious than narcotics for decreasing cerebral electrical activity. Efficacy depends on uptake and distribution, receptor site availability, and the development of intolerable side effects.

Efficiency:

Ratio (in mechanical terms) of energy output to input, usually expressed as a percentage.

Eicosanoids:

Large group of compounds related because their common precursors are 20-carbon eicosanoic fatty acids. The eicosanoids include the prostaglandins, thromboxanes, hydroxyeicosatetraenoic acid (HETEs), and leukotrienes (some of which participate in anaphylactic responses, e.g., "the slow reacting substances," the lipoxins).

Einthoven Triangle:

Conventional way of describing the skin surface projections of the electrical activity of the heart, named after the first electrocardiographer. The triangle is drawn from right shoulder to left shoulder, to left leg, and back to right shoulder. Lead I connects left shoulder to right shoulder, lead II connects left leg to right shoulder, and lead III connects left leg to left shoulder. Each lead records the difference in potential between the two connected limbs. If these points are connected, the electrical axis of the heart lies parallel to lead II, which means that in the normally positioned heart lead II has the highest QRS voltage. Lead II is equal to the sum of the corresponding complexes in leads I and II (Einthoven law). *See* Figure. *See* Electrocardiogram; QRS complex.

Eisenmenger Syndrome:

Congenital heart condition characterized by pulmonary hypertension with reversed or bidirectional shunt through either a ventricular or atrial septal defect or a patent ductus arteriosus. There is an elevation of the pulmonary vascular resistance. Signs and symptoms of this syndrome include dyspnea, feeding difficulty, fatigue, cyanosis, and failure to gain weight. *See* Atrial septal defect; Patent ductus arteriosus; Tetralogy of fallot; Ventricular septal defect.

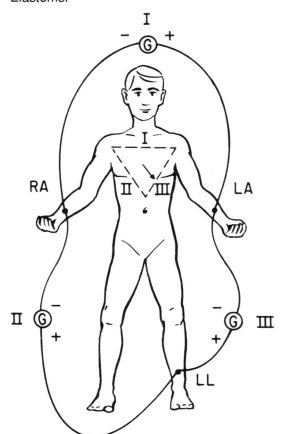

Einthoven Triangle: So-called Einthoven equilateral triangle as shown on the anterior chest wall indicating the relationship of the first three leads of the electrocardiograph.

Elastomer:

Huge variety of materials distinguished from other "plastics" because of their extensibility. To be officially classified as an elastomer, a material must be able to be stretched to at least twice its initial length at room temperature and return quickly to its original length on release. Elastomers are also categorized as synthetic rubbers. A common brand name is Neoprene. Elastomers are capable of resisting chemical attack, extremes of use, and abrasion.

Electrically Vulnerable Period:

See Synchronized cardioversion.

Electroanesthesia:

See Electronarcosis.

Electrocardiogram (ECG, EKG):

Recording, by means of electrodes or leads, of the electrical activity of the heart. Conventionally, three electrode lead systems are used in which standard positions for electrode placement exist: (1) three limb leads in which lead I connects right and left arm; lead II, the right arm and left leg; and lead III, the left arm and left leg; (2) three augmented unipolar limb leads, aVR (right arm), aVL (left arm), and aVF (left leg); and (3) six precordial leads, that connect different areas on the anterior chest to a limb and are known as leads V_1–V_6 according to the specific placement along the intercostal spaces. Each of these leads shows the electric activity of the heart on the side nearest the respective limb. The American Heart Association recommends a frequency band width of 0.5–100 Hz for diagnostic ECG recording. A much narrower band width of 1–50 Hz is adequate for monitoring purposes. *See* Figure. *See* Einthoven triangle; Electrocardiography, His bundle.

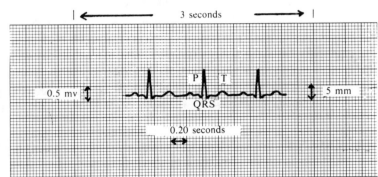

Electrocardiogram: Some of the standard parameters of the ECG shown in lead II.

Electrocardiographic Frequency Spectrum:

Sum of the individual electrical oscillations that make up the clinical electrocardiogram. They extend from 0.5 to 100 Hz when heart rates below 200 beats/minute are considered. *See* Fourier analysis.

Electrocardiography, His Bundle:

Method of recording heart electrical activity, specifically that of atrioventricular conduction. An electrocardiograph lead is placed through an intravenous catheter into the right side of the heart.

Electrocautery:

See Cauterization.

Electroconversion:

See Cardioversion.

Electroconvulsive Therapy (ECT); Electroshock Therapy:

Treatment modality used in psychiatry for severe depressive disorders. The endpoint of the technique is creation of an artificial grand mal seizure that causes (as yet poorly explained) a decrease in the degree of depression. Frequently, a patient may receive a series of ECT treatments, and the only overt effect is some loss in recent memory function. ECT has replaced the older pharmacologic convulsive therapies such as intravenous (IV) atropine, scopolamine (in a dosage range of 50–100 mg IV push), or insulin. (Insulin causes deliberate hypoglycemic shock and convulsions, promptly terminated by glucose.) Modern ECT machines generate a voltage greater than 150 V, have a frequency range of 50–70 Hz, and have a current output ranging from 200 to more than 1500 mA. General anesthesia, a requirement for this therapy, is usually intravenous barbiturate plus succinylcholine, the latter being given to prevent stress fractures, particularly of the vertebral column, due to the tremendously strong muscle contractions that accompany the generated seizures. *See* Defibrillation; Electronarcosis.

Electrode:

Device that emits, collects, or deflects electrical charge carriers. An anode is an electrode carrying a positive charge, and a cathode is an electrode carrying a negative charge.

Electrodental Anesthesia:

Technique for inducing anesthesia in and around the teeth using an electrical current administered by means of a modified transcutaneous nerve stimulator. It is controversial technique that has not gained wide acceptance in dentistry.

Electroencephalogram (EEG):

Recording, by means of electrodes (usually placed on the scalp), of the electrical activity generated by the brain during its normal functioning. (Normal EEG signals recorded on the scalp are on the order of 10–100 μV.) The standard EEG is usually measured in at least eight separate channels, which record the activity of the brain in its many subdivisions. *See* Figure. *See* Fourier analysis.

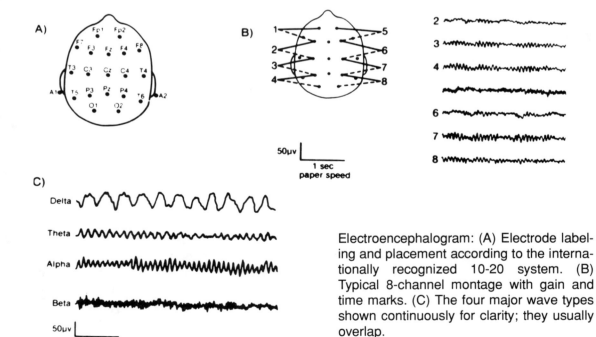

Electroencephalogram: (A) Electrode labeling and placement according to the internationally recognized 10-20 system. (B) Typical 8-channel montage with gain and time marks. (C) The four major wave types shown continuously for clarity; they usually overlap.

Electrolyte Balance:

Concept that the ion content of the body has ideal levels. Specific disease processes, such as kidney failure or bowel obstruction, cause an electrolyte imbalance by selectively eliminating or concentrating various ions. For example, loss of gastric contents by vomiting results in hypochloremia. *See* Anion gap.

Electromagnet:

Coil of wire that produces a magnetic field when an electrical current is passed through it. The strength of the magnet depends on whether a metallic core is placed within the windings, the number and spacing of the turns, and the current flow.

Electromagnetic Flowmeter:

See Blood flow, methods for measuring.

Electromagnetic Radiation:

Form of energy generated by the acceleration of charged particles. It consists of electrical and magnetic fields vibrating transversely, longitudinally, and at right angles to the direction of motion and to each other. The waves require no medium for propagation and can therefore traverse a vacuum at a uniform velocity of $2.997\ 925 \times 10^8$ m/second (i.e., the velocity of light). The characteristics of electromagnetic radiation depend solely on the frequency of the wave motion. Most phenomena connected with electromagnetic radiation, such as reflection or refraction, can be explained by wave motion. Certain other effects, however, require that electromagnetic radiation be explained as particles. The latter concept is the basis for the quantum theory, in which electromagnetic radiation consists of particles or quanta (photons) that travel at the speed of light and have zero rest mass.

Electromagnetic Spectrum:

Range of frequencies over which electromagnetic radiation can be propagated. The order of frequencies (from lowest to highest) are radio waves, infrared radiation, light, ultraviolet radiation, x-rays, and gamma rays. *See* Figure.

Electromechanic Systole (EMS):

See Systolic time intervals.

Electromyogram (EMG):

Recording, by means of electrodes (surface or needles), of the electrical activity of contracting skeletal muscle.

Electron:

Elementary particle usually found orbiting the nucleus of an atom. It has a negative charge of $1.602\ 192 \times 10^{-19}$ coulomb and a mass of $9.10\ 956 \times 10^{-31}$ kg. A moving electron (i.e., a free electron, one not circling a particular nucleus) constitutes an electrical current. *See* Carrier, electrical.

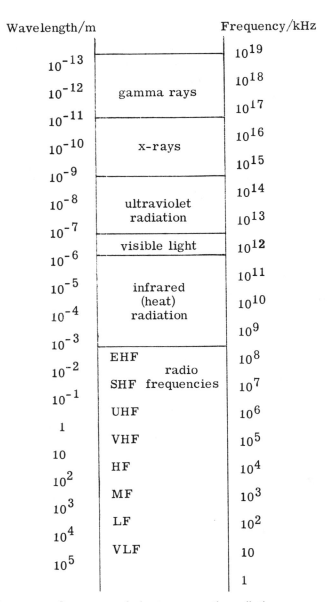

Wavelength/m   Frequency/kHz

Electromagnetic Spectrum: Spectrum of electromagnetic radiation.

Electron Gun:

Device used to produce a beam of electrons. The beam is usually created by heating a wire (emitter), which causes emission of electrons in all directions. These electrons are then focused and formed into a beam by magnetic or electrical fields surrounding the emitter. The electron gun is called a cathode because it is the source of negative charges. *See* Cathode-ray tube.

Electron Multiplier:

Electron tube that amplifies single-electron effects. The original electron hits an electrode, which in turn releases more electrons (secondary emission) on impact. The resulting electrons are then accelerated to another electrode, where the process is repeated. Electron multipliers are the basis for various instruments, such as scintillation counters and night vision scopes. *See* Figure.

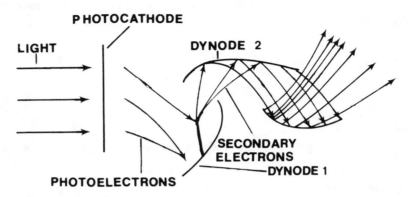

Electron Multiplier: Operating principle of the electron multiplier. Light rays approach from the left and strike the photocathode. The photocathode emits electrons which strike the first dynode. This dynode emits more than one electron for each electron hitting it. Magnetic fields direct these electrons to dynode 2, which has the same characteristics as dynode 1. The process continues with an ever larger cascade of electrons being reflected from dynode to dynode.

Electron Volt:

Energy unit employed in atomic physics. It signifies the energy acquired by an electron while falling freely through a potential difference of 1 V. It is equal to 1.602×10^{-19} joule.

Electronarcosis:

Technique for producing anesthesia by passing an electrical current through the brain via electrodes placed on the temples. The current is clearly below that which would produce convulsions. The efficacy of this technique is questioned in the United States, but it is reported to be used widely in the former Soviet Union.

Electro-Optical Counter:

See Automated cell counter.

Electrophoresis:

Movement of small particles suspended in a liquid or gel when an electric field is applied across the liquid. This technique is used extensively in laboratory work to separate serum proteins. Each protein migrates at a different rate owing to minor differences in electrical charge.

Electrophrenic Respiration:

Diaphragmatic respiration of a patient caused by electrically induced rhythmic stimulation of the phrenic nerves. This technique is most often used on patients who have suffered high cervical injuries and who would otherwise be apneic.

Electroplating:

Process of coating, by means of ion deposition, the surface of one metal with another for protection.

Electroshock:

See Electroconvulsive therapy.

Electrospinogram:

Recording, by means of electrodes, of the electrical activity of all or part of the spinal cord.

Electrostatic Unit:

Measurement of electrostatic charge in the centimeter-gram-second (CGS) system. It is defined as the charge that, if concentrated at one point in a vacuum, would repel with a force of 1 dyne a similar charge placed 1 cm away. *See* Dyne.

Electrosurgery:

See Coagulation current.

Elementary Particle (Fundamental Particle):

Any bit of matter that is a fundamental building block of the universe and cannot be subdivided into smaller particles. The only stable elementary particles are photons, electrons, neutrinos, and protons. (The neutron, another elementary particle, is stable only when it is bound in a nucleus.) All other subatomic particles ultimately decay into combinations of these particles.

Elimination, Drug:

Processes that terminate the action of a drug in the body. Drugs may be eliminated or excreted unchanged, or they may undergo biotransformation, i.e., a change in molecular structure.

Embolism:

Sudden obstruction of a blood vessel by an abnormal clot, air, or foreign material circulating in the blood. The major target for embolization is the lungs, as it is the only organ to receive the total cardiac output per minute. *See* Air embolus.

238

Emergence:

Period between the termination of an anesthetic (particularly a general anesthetic) and an appropriate patient response to direct commands. It is a particularly dangerous time as there may be a tendency on the part of the anesthetist to relax vigilance because anesthetic administration is complete and the patient may appear to have adequate upper airway reflexes when, in fact, he or she does not.

Emesis:

See Antiemetic.

EMG:

See Electromyogram.

EMLA:

Topical anesthetic formulation composed of a eutectic mixture of 5% lidocaine and prilocaine. It must be applied under an occlusive bandage for 45 to 60 minutes in order to be effective for skin anesthesia. *See* Table. *See* Azeotrope.

EMLA: Various preparations intended for topical anesthesia.

Anesthetic Ingredient	Concentration (%)	Pharmaceutical Application Form	Intended Area of Use
Benzocaine	1–5	Cream	Skin and mucous membrane
	20	Ointment	Skin and mucous membrane
	20	Aerosol	Skin and mucous membrane
Cocaine	4	Solution	Ear, nose, throat
Dibucaine	0.25–1	Cream	Skin
	0.25–1	Ointment	Skin
	0.25–1	Aerosol	Skin
	0.25	Solution	Ear
	2.5	Suppositories	Rectum
Cyclonine	0.5–1	Solution	Skin, oropharynx, tracheobronchial tree, urethra, rectum
Lidocaine	2–4	Solution	Oropharynx, tracheobronchial tree, nose
	2	Jelly	Urethra
	2.5–5	Ointment	Skin, mucous membrane, rectum
	2	Viscous	Oropharynx
	10	Suppositories	Rectum
	10	Aerosol	Gingival mucosa
Tetracaine	0.5–1	Ointment	Skin, rectum, mucous membrane
	0.5–1	Cream	Skin, rectum, mucous membrane
	0.25–1	Solution	Nose, tracheobronchial tree

EMMA:

See Engstrom multigas monitor.

EMO Inhaler (Epstein, Macintosh, Oxford):

Sophisticated draw-over vaporizer used to administer diethyl ether. The inhaler contains a waterbath to prevent sudden temperature changes in the anesthetic, has an integral bellows for intermittent positive-pressure ventilation, and can be equipped to vaporize a small amount of halothane initially before switching to ether in order to speed induction. It is a particularly useful anesthesia administration device for hospitals where limited facilities exist. *See* Figure.

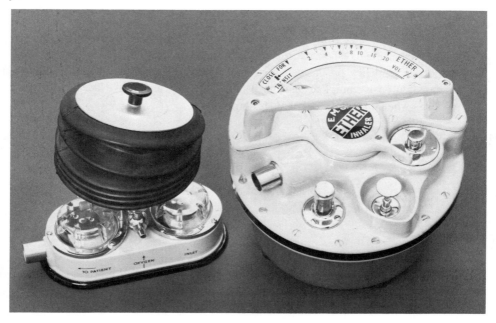

EMO Inhaler: Up-to-date version of this famous anesthetic device with attachment for assisted ventilation.

Emphysema:

See Chronic obstructive pulmonary disease.

Empyema:

Infection of the pleural space, usually leading to abscess. It may be local or generalized.

EMS:

See Electromechanic systole.

Emulsifier:

See Surface-active agent.

Encephalitis:

Inflammation of the brain. When possible, encephalitis is classified by naming the causative agent (e.g., measles encephalitis or herpes encephalitis).

Encephalocele:

Congenital malformation in which a portion of the brain substance is contained in an outpocketing of the meninges which protrude through a skull defect. It is a midline lesion.

Encephalon:

See Brain.

Encephalopathy:

Any disease of the brain.

Endless Loop Tachycardia:

See Pacemaker-mediated tachycardia.

Endobronchial Anesthesia:

See Bronchial blocker; Double-lumen tube.

Endobronchial Intubation:

Deliberate or inadvertent insertion of a tube into the bronchus. When deliberate, bronchial intubation is performed therapeutically to deflate or lavage one lung (as for pulmonary alveolar proteinosis). When inadvertent, it is the unfortunate placement of the tip of the endotracheal tube into a bronchus (usually the right). This accident may occur when altering the position of the head and may lead to obstruction of the other bronchus and ultimately to collapse of the nonventilated lung, a shift of the mediastinum, and progressive embarrassment of both respiratory and circulatory functions. *See* Double lumen tube; Endotracheal tube; Pulmonary alveolar proteinosis.

Endocardial Cushion Defect (Persistent Common Atrioventricular Canal):

Congenital cardiac abnormality characterized by an atrial septal defect of the ostium primum type resulting from imperfect fusion of the endocardial cushion. *See* Atrial septal defect.

Endogenous Pyrogen (EP):

Polypeptide manufactured by, among others, monocytes and macrophages in response to toxins from bacteria and commonly called interleukin-1 (IL-1). This agent enters the brain and produces a fever by directly acting on the preoptic area of the hypothalamus. It also acts on lymphocytes to activate the immune system directly. Other endogenous pyrogens may exist.

Endorphins:

Group of chemical entities found in the central nervous system thought to be endogenous opiate-like compounds. At least three endorphins have been isolated: alpha (α), beta (β), and gamma (γ), each having a specific amino acid sequence. β-endorphin is the most potent, being 10 times as active as morphine. These specific functions of endorphins are still speculative; however, in vivo, β-endorphin, which is broken down slowly, acts as a modifier of neuronal activity and alters responsiveness for hours. The endorphins display analgesic activity and seem to play a role in temperature homeostasis and muscle tonus. It appears that endorphins possess the same addictive potential as narcotics, and all effects are abolished (in vivo) by administration of a narcotic antagonist. Enkephalins comprise

241

another group of opiate-like compounds somewhat similar to endorphins. Both groups are indistinguishable from morphine in opiate-binding bioassays. *See* Enkephalins.

Endoscopy:

Visual inspection of the interior of a body organ or canal with the aid of a light-carrying instrument inserted within it. Examples are laryngoscopy, bronchoscopy, esophagoscopy, colonoscopy, and cystoscopy.

Endothelium-Derived Relaxing Factor (EDRF):

Molecule synthesized and released from endothelial cells when they are stimulated by a number of agents, such as ADP and acetylcholine. It diffuses into the vascular smooth muscle, where it activates an enzyme cycle that leads to vascular smooth muscle relaxation.

Endothermic:

Process that requires external heat in order to continue.

Endotracheal Tube:

Semiflexible plastic catheter used to deliver anesthetic gases directly into the trachea of a patient. By proper sizing or by means of an inflatable cuff, the tube protects the airway against foreign matter when protective airway reflexes are obtunded. The tube also decreases anatomic deadspace by traversing the oropharynx and nasopharynx, which contribute to the deadspace. Most tubes currently in use are single-use disposable items made out of polyvinylchloride. The uncuffed type is simply a tube of semiflexible polyvinylchloride that is supplied in a sterile package and most frequently used in pediatric anesthesia. The cuffed endotracheal tube has a balloon or cuff approximately 1 cm from the distal end that can be inflated by a pilot line running down in the sidewall of the tube, topped by a one-way valve and a pilot or indicating balloon. Cuff inflation permits a tight fit, preventing gas escape around the tube. Two subcategories of cuffed tubes are available. One is the high-volume, low-pressure cuff that when inflated, is generally sausage-shaped and has a large contact area with the tracheal mucosa and a low pressure per unit area of tracheal contact. The other is a low-volume, high-pressure cuff that, when inflated, is elliptical in shape, has a small area of contact with the tracheal mucosa, and exerts relatively high pressures on the area of the trachea it contacts. As a generality, the high-volume, low-pressure cuffs may cause more postoperative sore throats within a short period of time but can be left in place much longer than the high-pressure, low-volume cuffs. The latter cause fewer sore throats postoperatively but, when left in place for a long time, cause moderate to severe mucosal erosion. Tubes can also be manufactured from Silastic, which has a high degree of tissue compatibility but is expensive. Most commonly, the size of an endotracheal tube is designated by its inside diameter. (The French system assigns each tube a number derived from the external diameter measured in millimeters and multiplied by 3. This system is no longer used.) The distal end of the endotracheal tube is beveled and rounded to cause the least amount of trauma. Specific tube modifications exist, such as the Kamen-Wilkinson tube in which a foam rubber cuff is deflated for insertion by applying a negative pressure to the pilot line. Murphy endotracheal tubes have a hole through the tube wall opposite the beveled end. Tubes that do not have this accessory hole are Magill tubes. Two special tubes, which are found most frequently in pediatric practice, are the Cole tube, which has a tapered end, and the Rae® tracheal tube, which has a fixed curvature to facilitate access to the head and neck during surgery. Although most single-use endotracheal tubes look alike, the degree of curvature of the tube may be used to designate it orotracheal or nasotracheal depending on the intended route of entry. The nasotracheal tube has more of a curve. *See* Figures, Table.

Endotracheal Tube: Common numbering systems for endotracheal tubes.

Age	Weight	Tracheal Tube Size			Anatomic Distance		
		Diameter		Length (cm)* Orotracheal	Teeth to Cords (cm)	Teeth to Carina (cm)	Sagittal Diameter Trachea (mm)
		ID (mm)	French				
Premature	<5 lbs	2.5	12	10	7	11	
Term infant–3 mo	8	3	14	11	8	12	4
3–12 mo	10–20	3.5	16	12	8.5	13	7
2 yr	20–25	4	18	14	9	14	8
3 yr	30–35	4.5	20	15	9	14	
4 yr	35–40	5.0	22	16	9		
6 yr	40–45	5.5	24	16	9.5	15.5	9
8 yr	55–60	6	26	18	9.5	16	9
10 yr	65–70	6.5	28	18	10	17	
12 yr	80–90	6.5	28	20	10	17	
14 yr	90–140	7	30	22	11	18	10
16 yr	100–150	7.5	32	24	12	20	11–15
Adults	130–200	F 8	34	24	14		
		M 8.5	36	24	15		13–23
60+		F 8.5	38	24		22	
		M 9	40	24			

*Add 2–3 cm for nasotracheal tube.
Abbreviation: ID, Inside diameter.

Endotrol® Tracheal Tube:

Endotracheal tube with an embedded guide stylet that acts as a cable such that when pull is exerted on the cable the curvature of the tube changes. *See* Figure.

Endplate:

See Neuromuscular blockade, assessment of.

End-Systolic Pressure-Length Relation (ESPLR):

Close derivative of the end-systolic pressure volume relation and used as an index of myocardial contractility. It appears to be most useful measured in the isolated heart for studying regional contractility.

End-Systolic Pressure-Volume Relation (ESPVR):

Index of myocardial contractility that appears to be sensitive, linear, and relatively afterload-independent as a measure of intrinsic inotropic state, certainly in the isolated heart. Use in the intact heart has been controversial.

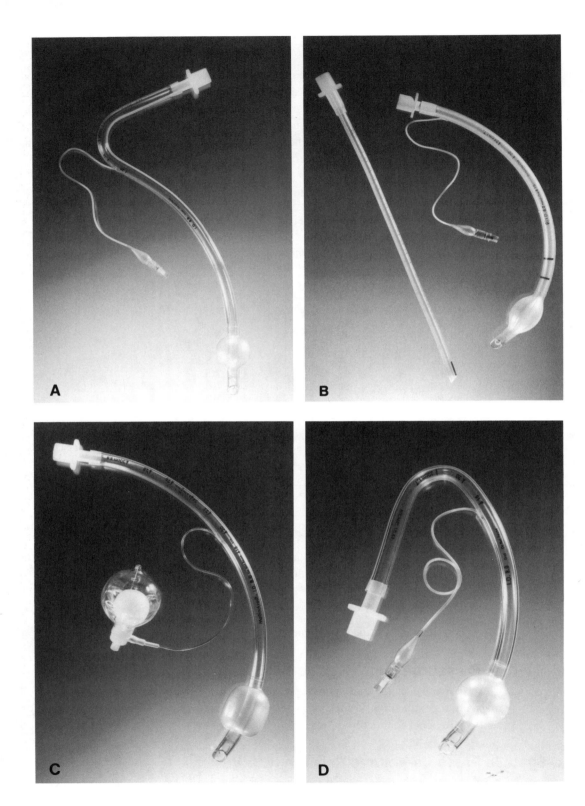

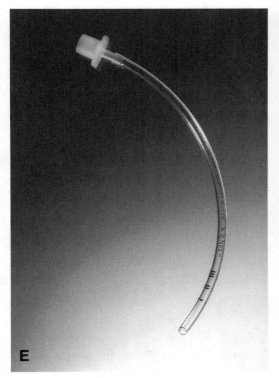

E

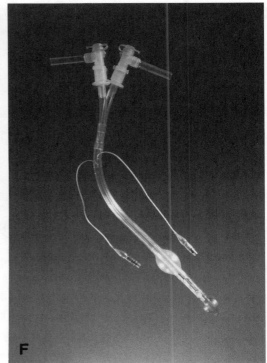

F

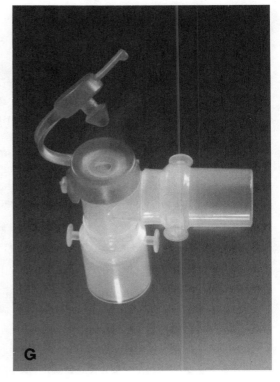

G

Endotracheal Tube: (A) A Nasal RAE® Tracheal Tube designed for oral and maxillofacial procedures. May be temporarily straightened to insert suction catheter. (B) Reinforced Tracheal Tube maintains a patent airway when patient is placed in a compromising position or during long-term intubation. Above the cuff are reference marks which aid proper placement of tube tip. (C) HiLo® Tracheal Tube with Lanz® Pressure Regulating Valve which reduces the risk of tracheal damage during long-term intubations when intracuff pressure is especially critical. (D) Oral RAE® Tracheal Tube proves improved surgical access during nasal, ophthalmic and facial surgery. May be temporarily straightened to insert suction catheter. (E) Uncuffed Tracheal Tube has distal tip reference lines and depth marks to assist placement. (F) Broncho-Cath® Endobronchial Tube has color-coded cuffs, pilot balloons and proximal lumens which help identify bronchial and tracheal lumens. When independent ventilation of either lung is indicated, the double lumen design permits an airtight seal of the trachea and one bronchus. (G) Opti-Port™ right angle double-swivel connector that has free-moving double-swivel joints which allow connector to move with the circuit (if pulled) to reduce tissue trauma or tracheal tube dislodgment.

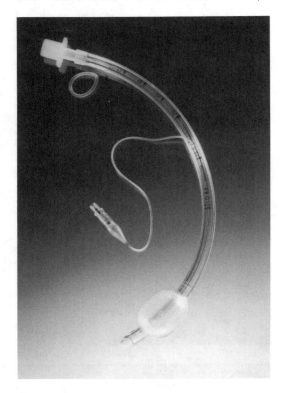

Endotrol® Tracheal Tube: An endotracheal tube which has an embedded guide stylet that acts as a cable such that when a pull is placed on the cable, the curvature of the tube changes.

End-Tidal Carbon Dioxide Measurement (FET CO$_2$):

Technique of measuring the CO$_2$ content just as air movement ceases during expiration. A sample taken at this time is considered to come from the alveoli, as the deadspace gas has been swept past the detectors. It is used clinically as a technique for detecting air embolization in the pulmonary circulation. The principle involved is that before embolization has become florid enough to cause blood pressure changes, a significant portion of the pulmonary vessel may become blocked, increasing the deadspace volume and diluting expired CO$_2$ with deadspace air. *See* Colorimetric end-tidal carbon dioxide detector.

Energy:

Capacity for performing work (actual or potential). Energy is quantified in joules.

Enflurane (Ethrane):

Nonflammable liquid that is one of the most frequently used inhalation agents for general anesthesia. It is stable chemically and does not require a preservative. Postoperative side effects, such as nausea, shivering, and vomiting, may occur but to a lesser extent than with other agents (e.g., halothane). High concentrations of enflurane, however, are associated with respiratory and circulatory depression and may produce seizure-like activity even in the neurologically normal patient. The vapor pressure of enflurane (2-chloro-1,1,2-trifluoroethyldifluoromethyl ether) at 20°C is 175 mm Hg. *See* Figure.

Enflurane.

Engine:

Machine for turning heat energy into mechanical work.

Engstrom Multigas Monitor (EMMA):

Device for measuring the concentration of halogenated agents in a breathing circuit. It works on the principle that halogenated hydrocarbons are absorbed into oil, which is used to coat a crystal that is part of a resinating electrical circuit. Absorption by the oil of the halogenated agent increases the mass of the crystal, changing its frequency of oscillation. This change, in turn, is proportional to the concentration of agent. The instrument can be affected by water vapor, and it cannot distinguish the various halogenated agents.

Enhancement:

Increase in value or in quantity. Radiographs taken with low levels of x-rays can be enhanced by a computer, sparing patients an increased radiation dose.

ENIAC:

Acronym for Electronic Numerical Integrator and Calculator. It was a computer that was designed and developed by scientists at the University of Pennsylvania during World War II and considered by many to be the first computer. A prior claim to developing the first computer, however, belongs to a British code-cracking group who built an electronic machine during the early 1940s to break the German Ultra Code. It is interesting to note that the capabilities of ENIAC were essentially duplicated in a hand-held calculator in 1976.

Enkephalins:

Group of endogenous opiate-like compounds. Composed of pentapeptides such as met-enkephalin and leu-enkephalin, they are synthesized in brain tissue and appear to function as neurotransmitters. They display a weak analgesic action and are broken down rapidly. The enkephalins are somewhat similar to endorphins, and both are indistinguishable from morphine in opiate-binding bioassays. *See* Endorphins.

ENNS:

See Early neonatal neurobehavioral scale.

Enterohepatic Recirculation:

Pathway by which drugs excreted in bile return to the body by being reabsorbed further along in the intestine. This pathway is clinically significant when it involves drugs with toxic effects that remanifest after a period of apparent recovery as the initial drug or its active metabolites return to the circulation from the intestine.

Enthalpy:

Heat content of a system.

Entropy:

Measure of the disorder of a system. The human body can, under normal circumstances, be considered to have low entropy. As the body ages and control mechanisms become less precise, entropy is increased; as random or uncontrolled activity increases, so does entropy.

Enzyme Induction; Enzyme Inhibition:

Enhancement or retardation of an enzymatically mediated drug breakdown. For example, the drug phenobarbital (and to some extent other barbiturates) increases the effectiveness of liver enzymes for metabolizing a broad spectrum of other drugs. Cytochrome P-450, often involved in drug metabolism, is one of the enzyme systems most frequently affected by phenobarbital. Enzyme inhibitors that decrease drug metabolism include such drugs as chloramphenicol and some of the phenothiazines.

EP:

See Endogenous pyrogen.

Ephedrine:

Naturally occurring compound known to Chinese medicine for thousands of years and introduced to Western clinical practice during the 1920s. Ephedrine is classified as a sympathomimetic drug. It stimulates both alpha and beta receptors and is used for those conditions in which both central and peripheral cardiovascular stimulation is desired. It has a positive inotropic effect on the heart while at the same time constricting peripheral vasculature. In anesthetic practice it is often used as the drug of choice to counteract the pressure drop seen with epidural and spinal anesthetics.

Epidermolysis Bullosa (Acantholysis Bullosa):

Rare hereditary disorder of the skin. The disease is characterized by blistering, with fluid formation due to a separation within the epidermis. The blisters occur when lateral shearing forces are applied to the skin. Clinical history is important for the anesthetist, and extreme care must be taken because rapid obstruction of the airway may follow any manipulation of the area during anesthesia.

Epidural Anesthesia (Peridural Anesthesia):

Type of regional anesthesia induced by injection of a local anesthetic agent into the epidural (extradural) space, thereby blocking the spinal nerve trunks. The block occurs by diffusion of the drug through the dura and by direct contact with the nerves as they exit the dural sleeves. The percentage contribution from each pathway is controversial. Compared to subdural (spinal) anesthesia, epidural anesthesia (1) requires greater volumes of anesthetic agent (5–10 times more depending on the effect desired); (2) is not as dependable; (3) has a slower onset; and (4) is associated with a greater incidence of differential blockade. *See* Differential blockade; Spinal anesthesia.

Epidural Narcotics:

Administration of narcotics into the epidural space or part of a pain management regiment can be patient-controlled. *See* Epidural anesthesia; Patient-controlled analgesia.

Epidural Needle:

Needle used to place either a catheter or a dose of local anesthetic into the epidural space. Many types of epidural needle exist. *See* Figure. *See* Hustead epidural needle; Spinal needle.

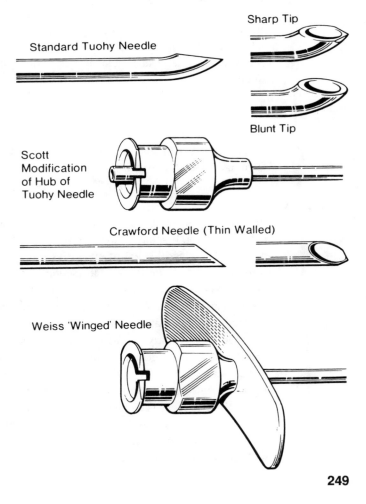

Epidural Needle: Various epidural needles.

249

Epidural Patch (Blood Patch):

Technique for relieving of severe spinal headache. A fluid, usually autologous blood, is injected at the same vertebral level as the previous puncture site in the dura. Relief of the headache is accomplished by sealing this hole, thereby preventing leakage of cerebrospinal fluid (CSF). Because the brain normally floats in and is supported by CSF loss of this fluid may produce headache. This proposed mechanism does not explain a number of clinical cases in which the patient experiences immediate relief after placement of the patch, long before CSF pressure could have been built up. Although essentially without major morbidity, back pain and signs of meningeal irritation have been noted in the patient using this technique. *See* Spinal headache.

Epidural Plica Mediana Dorsalis:

Connective tissue band that divides the epidural space at the dorsal midline. Its existence is somewhat controversial, but it is clear that it occurs in some individuals and not in others.

Epidural Pressure Switch:

Pressure-sensing device used to detect changes in intracranial pressure (ICP). It is applied to the dura through a burr hole in the skull and generates a signal proportional to the pressure of the dura against the tip of the switch. This technique lacks long-term stability and has a poor response speed; it does not, however, require a dural puncture and therefore is theoretically safer than other ICP detection techniques. *See* Intracranial pressure measurement.

Epiglotitis:

Life-threatening inflammation of the epiglottis that is fairly frequent in children ages 2 to 7. Currently, it is treated by nasotracheal intubation under anesthesia by a well-prepared team in an operating room.

Epilepsy:

Recurrent disorder of brain function affecting either the entire central nervous system or only a part of it. It is manifested by altered consciousness and abnormal motor and sensory activity. The classification of epilepsies now distinguishes primary generalized epilepsy from partial (focal) epilepsy. Malfunction of the poorly understood central, brain-integrating mechanism is the direct cause of primary generalized seizures (centrencephalic epilepsy). The terms *petit mal* and *grand mal* are imprecise and are no longer used to describe a seizure. Approximately 10% of seizure patients have primary generalized epilepsy, which is a specific hereditary disease. Seizures of this type consist of: (1) typical absence attacks (true petit mal); (2) generalized convulsive seizures (true grand mal); and (3) myoclonic and akinetic seizures. Typical absence attacks are precipitated by repetitive flashes of bright light and by forced hyperventilation (the latter being a diagnostic test because primary generalized epilepsy is the only seizure disorder precipitated this way). The patient, usually a young child, does not respond to stimuli or verbal commands during an attack. Rapid eye blinking, blank stares, and upper extremity muscle twitching may be present as well. These attacks may last only a few seconds and may go unnoticed. They are followed by a complete return to consciousness and the patient may deny the entire episode. Generalized convulsive seizures usually develop during adolescence or young adulthood. The attacks occur without warning as the patient suddenly becomes unconscious and falls. During the tonic phase of this seizure, the patient is rigid for approximately 30 seconds, the face is contorted, and the skin appears purplish. The tongue may be severely bitten during this phase. As the seizure progresses, the tonic phase is followed by repetitive symmetric clonic jerks of the arms and legs. As the patient recovers and takes some breaths, the cyanotic appearance disappears. This phase is followed by a confused, restless state, and then sleep. The patient has no memory of the events. Myoclonic and akinetic seizures consist of small, symmetric, rhythmic jerking movements of the upper extremities. The patient does not lose consciousness. The other type of seizure disorder, partial (focal) epilepsy, occurs in nearly 90% of patients with seizures. The etiology is usually related to trauma, anoxia, infection, vascular disease, tumor, or some specific metabolic disease; the seizures are merely symptoms of the underlying brain abnormality. The manifestation of the focal seizure depends on the site of brain damage, not the pathologic process that caused it. The ultrashort-acting barbiturate Brevital is a specific provoking agent for psychomotor seizures, a subcategory of partial seizures. Airway maintenance may be critical during seizure activity. *See* Status epilepticus.

Epinephrine:

Naturally occurring catecholamine that is one of the most potent vasopressors and cardiac stimulants known. It is normally produced by the adrenal medulla and reaches its sites of action through the circulation. It stimulates metabolism and promotes blood flow to skeletal muscles to prepare the body for the "flight-or-fight" response. Because of its powerful effects, it is the drug of choice during resuscitation because it increases cardiac contractility and peripheral resistance. It can also be used under less extreme circumstances as an intravenous drip to support circulation. At times it is used in local anesthetic preparations to promote vasoconstriction, thereby prolonging anesthetic action.

Epistaxis:

Nosebleed.

Epoxy Resin:

Class of synthetic resin compounds that have a highly reactive ring consisting of an oxygen atom bonded to two adjoining carbon atoms. Epoxy resins are used as adhesives and coatings.

Epsom Salts (Hydrated Magnesium Sulfate):

See Magnesium sulfate.

EPSP:

See Excitatory postsynaptic potential.

Equalization:

Electronics term that refers to the use of various circuits to compensate for a known distortion.

Equipotential:

Term referring to a surface or body on which all points are at the same electrical potential.

Equivalent System of Measurement (Milliequivalent):

System for quantitating an ionic solution by the number of electrical charges contained per unit volume. The unit of measurement is the milliequivalent per liter (mEq/L), which is derived from the weight measurement of milligrams per liter (per ion) by the following equation: milliequivalents per liter = milligrams per liter × valence of the ion ÷ by the atomic weight of the ion. *See* Table.

Equivalent System of Measurement: Conversion of milligrams percent to milliequivalents.

		To Convert mg% to Milliequivalents per Liter		To Convert Milliequivalents per Liter to mg%	
		Multiply by:	Divide by:	Multiply by:	Divide by:
Sodium	Na^+	0.435	2.30	2.30	0.435
Potassium	K^+	0.256	3.91	3.91	0.256
Magnesium	Mg^{++}	0.820	1.22	1.22	0.820
Calcium	Ca^{++}	0.500	2.00	2.00	0.500
Chloride	Cl^-	0.282	3.55	3.55	0.282
Bicarbonate	HCO_3^-	0.164	6.10	6.10	0.164

Erythropoiesis:

See Anemia.

Escape Velocity:

Velocity an object must achieve in order to escape a gravitational field. Speed of a resident escaping the observation of the clinical director on Friday afternoon.

Eschmann Endotracheal Tube Introducer:

Woven fiber glass stylet used to probe an in-place endotracheal tube. If the tube is in the trachea, the probe is stopped by the corona or the cartilage of the main stem bronchus. If the tube is in the esophagus, the introducer passes unopposed into the stomach. Used to determine proper placement of the endotracheal tube.

Eserine:

See Physostigmine.

Esmolol:

Beta-blocker unique because of its rapid degradation. It is cardioselective and has little or no effect on bronchial or vascular tone at doses that effectively lower cardiac rate.

Esophageal Atresia:

See Tracheoesophageal fistula with esophageal atresia.

Esophageal Detector Device:

Device (based on use of a syringe) attached to the distal end of the endotracheal tube that is used to determine if the tube has been correctly placed in the trachea or incorrectly placed in the esophagus. *See* Eschmann endotracheal tube introducer.

Esophageal Lead:

Electrocardiograph lead inserted into the esophagus. It records electrical activity posterior to the heart. This lead is particularly important for establishing the relative timing of atrial contractions. It is also useful for obtaining additional information concerning individual atrial conduction.

Esophageal Reflux (Stomach Reflux):

Reverse flow of gastric contents into the esophagus. This flow is usually a passive process whereas vomiting is an active process that involves contraction of gastric and esophageal smooth muscle. With both processes, however, the esophageal sphincter must open for the liquid and solid matter to pass out of the stomach. In the normal individual, the lowest limit of pressure necessary to open the esophageal sphincter is approximately 15 cm H_2O.

ESPLR:

See End-systolic pressure-length relation.

ESPVR:

See End-systolic pressure-volume relation.

Essential Hypertension:

Elevation of arterial blood pressure with little or no symptomatology and no discernible etiology. Hypertension can be called essential after all known causes of elevated arterial pressure, (e.g., restricted kidney blood flow, hormone-secreting tumors, inappropriate drug administration) are ruled out. A resting diastolic pressure of 90 mm Hg is considered the threshold of disease in an adult when determined on multiple occasions.

Estradiol (E₁):

Estrogen variant produced by the placenta during pregnancy.

Estriol (E$_2$):

Estrogen variant produced by the placenta during pregnancy from a fetal precursor. Tested for in either plasma or a 24-hour urinary collection, it is used as a measure of fetal well-being.

ESU:

Electrosurgical unit. *See* Coagulation current.

ESWL:

See Extracorporeal shockwave lithotripsy.

Ethacrynic Acid (Edecrin):

Potent diuretic believed to exert its major action in the loop of Henle. Overdosage can lead to circulatory collapse and severe hypokalemia.

Ethanol (Ethyl Alcohol):

Chemical name for alcohol. Although it may be the most popular molecule in history, its medicinal uses are severely limited. Intravenously, it has been used to control premature labor. Its use as a general anesthetic is restricted because of the proximity of its therapeutic and lethal doses. *See* Tocolytic.

Ether:

See Diethyl ether.

Ether Dome:

See Morton, William T. G.

Ethinamate (Valmid):

Minor short-acting hypnotic-sedative drug.

Ethrane:

See Enflurane.

Ethyl Alcohol:

See Ethanol.

Ethyl Carbamate (Urethan):

Ester of ethanol used occasionally as an anesthetic in animals. It has no human anesthetic clinical use.

Ethyl Chloride:

Simple organic molecule used for many years as a rapid-induction, short-duration general anesthetic. Because of its tremendous rate of evaporation at room temperature, it is also used as a topical anesthetic to cool and numb the skin rapidly. Ethyl chloride use as a general anesthetic is now obsolete because of its hepatotoxicity and the small difference between its therapeutic and toxic doses.

Ethylene:

Organic molecule, gaseous at room temperature, formerly used as a substitute for N_2O in balanced anesthesia. Considered to be slightly more potent than N_2O, its chief disadvantages are that: (1) it is explosive in clinical concentrations; (2) it is lighter than air (floating in the atmosphere of an operating room it may be detonated by the electrical wiring in the ceiling); and (3) it has a slightly sick-sweet odor. Its major uses outside the medical field are as a raw material for the manufacture of plastics and as an agent to ripen tomatoes on the way to market, which has led to an unusual number of conflagrations at vegetable depots around the country.

Ethylene Oxide Sterilization:

Method used to sterilize heat- or moisture-sensitive hospital equipment. Ethylene oxide (ETO), a highly toxic gas, penetrates some materials well, allowing items to be prepackaged in polyethylene or paper prior to sterilization. Long-term storage is then possible after the aeration process, which removes the residual ETO. The disadvantages of the ETO technique include (1) the extended period needed for sterilization (up to 12 hours in some circumstances); (2) the possible complications of skin reactions and laryngotracheal inflammation (due to inadequate aeration of the sterilized items); and (3) the rigid controls necessary to keep ETO concentrations low in the work place.

Ethyl Ether:

See Diethyl ether.

Ethyl Orange:

See Indicator dye.

Ethylparaben:

See Preservative.

Ethyl Vinyl Ether (Vinamar):

Obsolete variant of diethyl ether and vinyl ether no longer used in clinical anesthesia.

Ethyl Violet:

See Indicator dye.

Ethyl Yellow:

See Indicator dye.

Etidocaine (Duranest):

Amide-type local anesthetic. *See* Local anesthetic.

Etomidate:

Intravenous anesthetic agent that is chemically unrelated to any others. It is used primarily as an induction agent and demonstrates excellent patient cardiovascular stability upon injection. It is painful when used intravenously, and patients frequently complain postoperatively of this side effect.

Etorphine:

One of the most potent narcotics ever synthesized. *See* Lofentanil.

Eutectic Mixture:

Mixture of two or more substances that has the lowest melting point of any combination of its constituents.

Eutonyl:

See Pargyline.

Evaporation:

Conversion of a liquid to its vapor at a temperature below its boiling point. This process causes cooling of the liquid because the fastest molecules escape the surface, thereby lowering the average kinetic energy of those remaining. *See* Vapor pressure.

Evipal:

See Barbiturate; Hexobarbital.

Evoked Potential (Evoked-Related Response):

Adaptation of electroencephalographic monitoring used to test the functional integrity of the brain. A stimulus is presented to the brain by visual, auditory, or somatosensory means, repeatable in intensity and time interval as often as necessary. The changes in neuroelectrical activity occur in two parts. The first part, the primary or specific complex, occurs after each stimulus with a latency of less than 15 ms and is made up of a 10- to 15-ms surface-positive deflection followed immediately by a negative deflection. The combined positive and negative deflections last for less than 30 ms. The specific complex is followed by smaller, diffusely distributed positive and negative oscillations. Anesthetic agents have a minimal effect on the specific complex but greatly affect the late-occurring, diffusely distributed deflections. Primary or specific complex disappearance is more closely correlated with irreversible hypoxic cellular damage, although under certain circumstances it can be elicited when the spontaneous electroencephalogram is absent. To be of value, evoked potential monitoring must have the capability of recording and displaying a number of evoked potentials in series for comparison. *See* Figure. *See* Far-field potential; Near-field potential; Signal averaging.

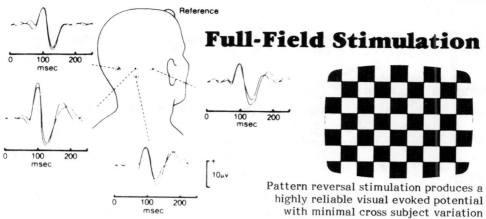

Full-Field Stimulation

Pattern reversal stimulation produces a highly reliable visual evoked potential with minimal cross subject variation

Evoked Potential: Visual evoked potential showing the signal recorded from various locations on the back of the head.

Excitability:

State in which a tissue is capable of a rapid response to a stimulus. Nerve tissue and muscles, by their nature, are excitable. The threshold of excitability can be raised or lowered by various methods.

Excitatory Postsynaptic Potential (EPSP); inhibitory postsynaptic potential (ipsp):

Effects (excitatory and inhibitory) at synaptic junctions of the release of single quanta of neurotransmitters. The postsynaptic membrane is changed slightly to either facilitate or prevent the initiation of an impulse. Usually this change in potential is too small to cause postsynaptic membrane depolarization or the initiation of an action potential. *See* Neuro-muscular transmitter, quantal release of.

Excitotoxin Concept:

Postulate that the excitatory neurotransmitters glutamate and aspartate contribute to the mechanism of hypoxic-ischemic neuronal damage. Experimental data appear to show that under normoxic conditions glutamate and aspartate are harmless. However, during condi-tions of hypoxia and reoxygenation, neuronal function decreases with rising levels of the two neurotransmitters.

Excretion:

Elimination of a substance from the body, e.g., in saliva, bile, urine, feces, or sweat.

Exhaust System:

See Scavenger system.

Exosurf:

Newly approved artificial surfactant for treatment of newborns with surfactant deficiency syndromes.

Experimental Neurosis:

Technique of conditioning a test subject with stimuli so nearly identical that they cannot be distinguished. The subject soon becomes upset, fails to cooperate, and tries to escape. [Note similarity to residency training.]

Expiration:

Expelling of air from the lungs, usually due to the elastic recoil of the lungs and the thoracic wall. Although it can be aided by forceful contraction of the abdominal muscles, expiration is usually a passive process. Some older ventilators placed a negative pressure in the airway during the expiratory phase to aid and speed up expiration. (The reverse is the physiologic state in which airway pressure is slightly positive in relation to atmospheric pressure during expiration.) This procedure is no longer widespread, however, as negative pressure in the airway tends to promote the closure of small air passageways, thereby trapping air.

Expiratory Center:

See Respiratory centers.

Expiratory Retard:

Setting on a ventilator that can variably increase the duration of expiration. The purpose of expiratory retard, or its modification expiratory plateau, is to maintain positive pressure in the airways for as long as possible to prevent small-airway collapse and to improve ventilation perfusion. Expiratory retard is a step away from positive end-expiratory pressure (PEEP), which has replaced it in ventilation therapy. *See* Continuous positive airway pressure; Positive end-expiratory pressure.

Explosimeter:

Device for measuring the combustion capabilities of a gas/air or gas/O_2 sample. It must be calibrated for individual gas mixtures.

Explosion:

Detonation that occurs in gaseous mixtures when the flame (propagating outward from the point of ignition) moves so rapidly there is no time for the heat generated by the passage of the flame to be dissipated into the surroundings. The pressure in the flame front rises to high values. This pressure wave interacts with the adjoining layer of fresh gaseous mixture and heats it by compression, which in turn raises the adjoining layer to well above its ignition temperature. If enough fuel/gas mixture is available, a narrow zone of high pressure traveling at supersonic speed is created, called a shock wave. With a true explosion, the shock wave and the accompanying flame front behind it can reach speeds of 2000–3000 m/second. The maximum temperature is in excess of 2500°C, and maximum pressure is in excess of 20 atmospheres.

Explosion Limits:

See Detonability, limits of.

Explosion-Proof:

See Intrinsically safe device.

Expressed Consent:

Legal term denoting the expressed (either oral or written) permission by a patient for the performance of a procedure. *See* Implied consent.

External Jugular Vein:

See Jugular veins.

Extra Alveolar Vessel:

Blood vessel that is not exposed to alveolar gas, although it is part of the pulmonary circulation. The caliber of the extra alveolar vessels is greatly affected by lung volume, as they are supported, and entirely surrounded by lung parenchyma.

Extracorporeal Circulation:

See Cardiopulmonary bypass.

Extracorporeal Membrane Oxygenation (ECMO):

Technique for performing the respiratory functions of the lungs by removing blood from the body, running it through a membrane oxygenator, and returning it. It can be used to maintain life in severe but potentially reversible lung damage or can be used as a cardio-pulmonary bypass technique. *See* Figure. *See* Membrane oxygenator.

Extracorporeal Shockwave Lithotripsy (ESWL):

Technique for disrupting kidney stones by generating shockwaves outside the body and transmitting them through a water or other fluid to the skin and then through the tissue. The shockwave is capable of fragmenting the stone, allowing for passage through the ureters and eliminating the need for an operative procedure.

Extrapolation:

Estimation of a value for a variable from outside the range of those values already known.

Extrinsic Pathway:

Mechanism for activating blood coagulation. It is initiated by the blood contacting extra-vascular structures. The prothrombin time (PT test) laboratory test evaluates this pathway. *See* Blood coagulation; Intrinsic pathway.

Extubation:

Process of removing an endotracheal tube. Never a casual process, extubation must be preceded by patient evaluation, as removal of the endotracheal tube immediately increases

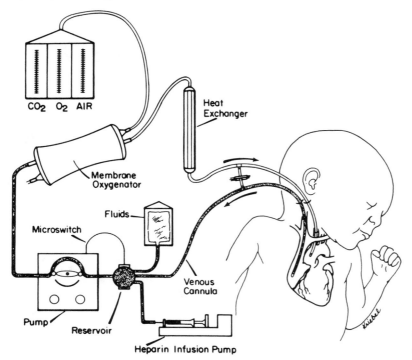

CO_2 O_2 AIR

Heat
Exchanger

Membrane
Oxygenator

Fluids

Microswitch

Venous
Cannula

Pump

Reservoir

Heparin Infusion Pump

Extracorporeal Membrane Oxygenation: The ECMO circuit.

the deadspace and, in many instances, leaves the patient with some vocal cord incompetence. The degree of incompetence is related to the length of time the tube was in place. *See* Endotracheal tube.

Eye Signs During Anesthesia:

Attempt to monitor depth of anesthesia by evaluating eyelid reflex, pupillary size, response to light, and eyeball activity. Of great value during ether anesthesia (with no premedication), it is considered to be unreliable with more rapidly acting agents, particularly when multiple premedications have been given. *See* Stages and planes of anesthesia.

F

Face Mask:

Device used for breathing anesthetic gases and vapors. It is designed to maintain and form a gas-tight seal over the nose and mouth. Qualitative variations include shape, type of seal around the border, and opacity or clarity of the mask material itself. *See* Figure.

Facial Nerve:

Seventh cranial nerve. *See* Cranial nerves.

Faculty of Anaesthetists Royal College of Surgeons of England (FARCS):

British counterpart of the American Board of Anesthesia. Faculty of Anaesthetists was founded in 1948 as the second Faculty of the College of Surgeons. Fellowship in the Faculty is granted after an examination. There are now approximately 4300 individuals who have the full title of Fellow, Faculty of Anaesthetists Royal College of Surgeons of England (FFARCS). FARCS is located in Lincoln's Field, London.

Fade:

See Neuromuscular blockade, assessment of.

Fahrenheit Scale:

Temperature scale in which the ice or freezing point of water is 32° and the steam or boiling point is 212°. In scientific usage it has been replaced by the Celsius scale.

Fail-Safe Device:

Device so designed and constructed that it cannot malfunction in a damaging or detrimental manner when it or the apparatus it controls exceeds design limits. The most frequently encountered fail-safe system in anesthesia is the anesthesia machine valve that prevents the delivery of any gas other than O_2 when the pressure of the O_2 supply falls below a preset point. Fail-safe devices can be defeated by improper maintenance and inadequate understanding of their limits. *See* Figure.

Falling Column:

Technique for determining interpleural catheter placement. A syringe with the plunger removed, filled with saline, is attached and directed into the interpleural space. The column of fluid in the syringe is seen to fall away as the saline is pulled into the interpleural space by negative pressure.

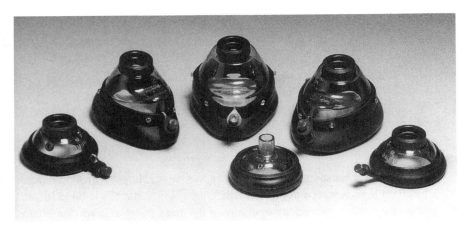

Face Mask: Series of transparent face masks specifically designed to create a tight seal with the face. Sizes range from the pediatric to the adult.

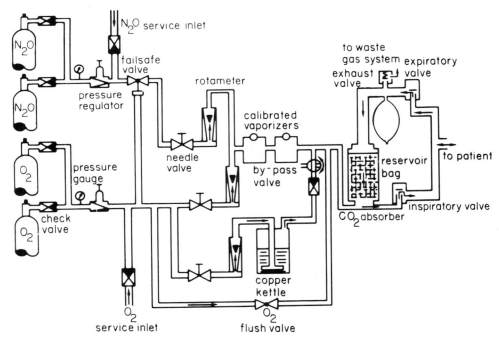

Fail-Safe Device: Circuitry of a modern anesthesia machine showing oxygen and nitrous oxide entering the machine from cylinders or from the hospital service supply. The fail-save valve presents flow of nitrous oxide if the oxygen supply fails.

Familial Dysautonomia (Riley-Day Syndrome):

Inherited disorder of the central nervous system that shows disturbances of autonomic sensory, motor, and psychic function. These patients can have sudden alterations in blood pressure. A characteristic of the syndrome is the failure of heart rate to increase in response to a reduction in blood pressure. The disease is almost exclusively seen in children of eastern European Jewish ancestry. These patients also demonstrate erratic temperature control, and pain sensation can be dramatically lacking.

Familial Periodic Paralysis:

Rare type of muscle disease that has a definite, though obscure, genetic basis. At least three distinct types have been described; hypokalemic, hyperkalemic, and normokalemic. The hypokalemic attack can be precipitated by large carbohydrate-containing meals and stress of any kind, including infection, surgery, or trauma. Paralysis is variable and may be asymmetric. The cardiac effects of hypokalemia can be demonstrated by electrocardiography. Muscles are unresponsive to even direct electrical stimulation, and the attack can be of such severity that the patient dies from respiratory insufficiency. For anesthetic purposes, patients who are so diagnosed must be exquisitely managed for fluid and electrolyte levels, and muscle relaxants are relatively contraindicated. The hyperkalemic form of the disease appears unrelated to high-carbohydrate meals with attacks occurring spontaneously after exercise or stress. This form is marked by a rise in serum potassium, and administration of potassium can provoke an attack. The cardiac effects of hyperkalemia can be demonstrated by electrocardiography. This form of the disease appears to exaggerate the action of depolarizing muscle relaxants. With normokalemic periodic paralysis the serum potassium remains unchanged during an attack, although cardiac arrhythmias do occur. Attacks may be precipitated by stress or may occur spontaneously. Anesthetic management is aimed at preventing respiratory embarrassment, maintaining serum fluid and electrolyte balance, and avoiding neuromuscular blocking agents.

Family Centered Maternity Care:

Concept of the psychology of childbirth that advocates a direct interaction between mother, father, and child during the first few minutes of life, believing that it will greatly influence a child's future relationship with his or her environment.

Farad (F):

Standard international unit by which to measure capacitance. One farad is the capacitance of a capacitor that acquires a charge of 1 coulomb when a potential difference of 1 V is applied. This unit is far too large to be used handily, as most common capacitors are in the pico-, nano-, micro-, and millifarad ranges. *See* Capacitance, electronic.

FARCS:

See Faculty of Anaesthetists Royal College of Surgeons of England.

Far-Field Potential:

Electrical potentials recording by electrodes (particularly during evoked potential monitoring) that are at some distance from the neurogenerator causing the electrical signal. *See* Evoked potential; Near-field potential.

Fasciculation:

Random contraction of part of a muscle mass due to uncoordinated stimulation of the motor endplates. Most commonly seen in the normal individual with extreme muscle fatigue, fasciculations are also seen after administration of a depolarizing muscle relaxant. These agents first stimulate and then block the motor endplate. This action does not occur over the whole muscle simultaneously because of local circulation differences. Because the external muscles of the eyes are the most highly innervated muscles in the body (thus having the most motor endplates), they fasciculate strongly when a depolarizer is administered. This action elevates intraocular pressure transiently, which is of no consequence in the normal eye but can be catastrophic if the eye is disrupted by injury. The abdominal muscles can also fasciculate strongly which may cause a transient rise in intragastric pressure. This pressure rise can theoretically cause esophageal reflux and can increase the danger of aspiration of gastric contents. Fasciculations caused by a depolarizing neuromuscular blocker can be prevented almost totally by giving a small dose of nondepolarizing drug first, but this effect is not 100% reliable.

Fasting:

Abstinence from all food intake for a specified period of time.

Fat Emboli Syndrome:

Occurring in traumatized patients, this type of embolism occurs because of the circulation of marrow fat from fractured bones. Deposited in lungs, it can cause a rapid decrease in pulmonary circulation and hypoxia, either through occlusion and/or toxic chemical interaction. Fat globules in urine and sputum (not always present) are diagnostic signs. As with any embolic phenomenon, it is possible for material to get into the arterial circulation and directly affect the brain. Stabilization of the fracture and circulatory and ventilatory support are nonspecific treatment measures.

Fault Current:

Flow of electrons in an unintentional path resulting from a complete breakdown of the normal separation of circuit parts or current-carrying wires. A fault differs from a leak in that a fault activates an overcurrent protector, whereas a leak usually does not. For example, a nail bridging two conductors is a fault, whereas a gradual degradation of insulation allowing a small current flow is a leak.

FBM:

See Fetal breathing movements.

FDP:

See Fibrinogen degradation products.

Feedback:

Process of returning a part of the output of a machine or system to the input as a means of control. Negative feedback indicates that input energy is decreased, whereas positive feedback indicates that input energy is increased. *See* Hormone.

Felypressin:

Totally synthetic polypeptide related to vasopressin. Its pharmacologic use is as a vasoconstrictor and it may be substituted for epinephrine in local anesthetic combinations. It appears to have fewer systemic effects than epinephrine.

Fenoterol:

β_2-adrenergic agonist under investigation as a bronchodilating agent.

Fentanyl (Sublimaze):

Popular synthetic narcotic that is approximately 80 times more potent than morphine. Onset of action is rapid when administered intravenously. Combined with droperidol (a butyrophenone) and marketed as Innovar, it is useful as an adjunct to N_2O/O_2 administration to produce neuroleptanesthesia. Sufentanil and alfentanil, synthesized derivatives of fentanyl, have different potencies and half-lives. *See* Alfentanil; Narcotic; Neuroleptanesthesia.

Fentanyl Lollipop:

See Oral transmucosal fentanyl citrate.

Fetal Alcohol Syndrome:

Syndrome seen in infants born to women who are chronic alcoholics. These infants demonstrate both prenatal and postnatal growth retardation and various craniofacial anomalies. Later in life they can demonstrate hyperactivity and mental retardation.

Fetal Biparietal Diameter (BPD):

Measurement that can be determined by ultrasonography. Used to determine fetal gestation when dates are uncertain.

Fetal Breathing Movements (FBMs):

Motion of respiration imaged by ultrasonography seen in the fetus. FBMs can be used as an indicator of fetal distress. Diminished fetal breathing motions is an indicator of fetal compromise.

Fetal Circulation:

Specialized system of blood flow in utero comprising the fetal heart, umbilical arteries and vein, foramen ovale, ductus arteriosus, and placental villi. The fetus must receive O_2 and excrete CO_2 through the placenta because the lungs are collapsed and nonfunctioning. With the first breath after birth, the lungs begin to expand, and the pulmonary vascular resistance decreases. More blood goes to the lungs and is returned to the left atrium, causing left atrial pressure to increase and the foramen ovale to close. Semiindependently, the umbilical vessels begin to close. The functioning lungs effectively raise the Po_2 in the aorta, and the ductus arteriosus also begins to close. *See* Figure.

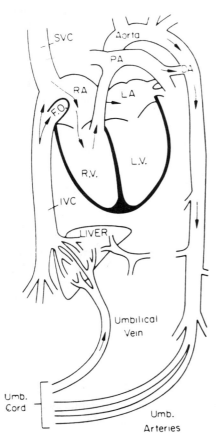

Fetal Circulation: Diagram of fetal circulation and circulatory changes at birth. The pulmonary vessels open up as the lungs expand; umbilical vessels close; foramen ovale closes when left atrial pressure exceeds right atrial pressure; ductus arteriosus closes as pulmonary artery resistance falls.

Fetal Heart Rate (FHR) Terminology:

When monitoring the fetal heart rate, many periodic changes can be demonstrated in association with uterine contractions: (1) *Early* decelerations, which occur concomitantly with each uterine contraction. These decelerations are smooth and are mirror images of the contractions. They are mild in nature and never drop the fetal heart rate more than 20 beats/minute below baseline. (2) *Late* deceleration occurs after resolution of the contraction, usually delayed 10–30 seconds. (3) *Variable* decelerations differ in duration, extent, and appearance from contraction to contraction. They are usually abrupt in onset and offset and reflect a reflex, probably of vagal origin. (4) Excelerations of the fetal heart rate are sometimes seen with contractions; they have not been associated with fetal compromise. Fetal heart rate patterns are further divided into a stress pattern and a sinister pattern. These two phrases now replace the older term "ominous," which is falling out of use. *See* Tables, Figure.

Fetal Heart Rate (FHR) Terminology: Characteristics of Normal (Above) and Abnormal (Below) Fetal Heart Rate Patterns

Baseline rate	120–160 bpm
Baseline variability (amplitude range)	>6 bpm
Periodic pattern	Absent or early decelerations or accelerations
Fetal outcome	Vigorous; Apgar score >7 at 5 min
Scalp sampling	Not useful
Treatment of fetus	Not necessary

	Stress Pattern		Sinister Pattern
	Acute	Prolonged (Decompensatory)	
Baseline rate	Normal or abnormal	Normal or abnormal	Normal or abnormal
Baseline variability	>6 bpm	<6 bpm	Absent
Periodic pattern	Late or variable decelerations	Late or variable decelerations or absent	Severe late or variable decelerations or absent
Fetal outcome	Apgar score >7 at 5 min	Possibly depressed	Usually depressed
Scalp sampling	Not necessary if abnormality is abolished	Mandatory for management	Rapid delivery preferred
Treatment of fetus	Vigorous treatment necessary	Vigorous treatment necessary while evaluating fetus	Rapid delivery preferred

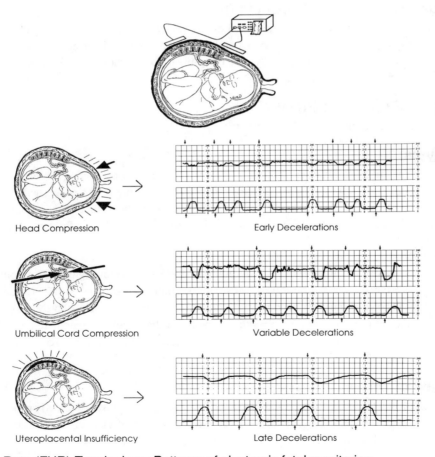

Head Compression → Early Decelerations

Umbilical Cord Compression → Variable Decelerations

Uteroplacental Insufficiency → Late Decelerations

Fetal Heart Rate (FHR) Terminology: Patterns of electronic fetal monitoring.

Fetal Monitor:

Device used to evaluate and record continuously the effect of labor on the fetus. A gauge attached to the abdomen of the mother follows the force of uterine contractions and the pulse rate of the fetus by tracing fetal heart movement via doppler ultrasonography. Some sophisticated monitors record both fetal (by a scalp electrode) and maternal electrocardiograms.

FEV₁:

See Forced expiratory volume.

Fiberoptics:

Transmission of an image by means of coated glass fibers that have special optical properties. Light, transferred by internal reflection along the length of the fibers, can traverse long distances with minimal attenuation. This process facilitates endoscopic examinations. *See* Figures. *See* Endoscopy.

Fibrillation, Ventricular:

See Ventricular fibrillation.

Fibrinogen Degradation Products (FDP):

Substances produced by the action of fibrinogen (plasmin) on fibrin and fibrinogen called "split products." Measured by laboratory test and used to determine the activity level of the clotting processes in the body. The more breakdown products of fibrinogen that are found, the more clotting has occurred.

Fibrinogen-Fibrin Split Products:

See Fibrinogen degradation products.

Fibrinolysis:

Enzymatic breakdown of fibrin. During this process the circulating protein (plasminogen) is activated to plasmin by tissue factors. Plasmin destroys fibrin, fibrinogen, and clotting factors V and VIII. The plasmin activation system appears to be the method by which the body disposes of intravascular clots. *See* Disseminated intravascular coagulation; Primary fibrinolysis.

Fick Principle:

Means of calculating cardiac output and blood flow to an organ. The amount of a given substance taken up by a tissue or organ per unit time is equal to the arterial level of that substance minus the venous level multiplied by the blood flow to the tissue or organ in question. Using O_2 uptake as the variable, cardiac output is calculated as follows: CO = oxygen consumption ÷ arterial oxygen content minus venous oxygen content X 100, or $\dot{V}O_2/CaO_2 - C\dot{V}O_2 \times 100$.

Fick's Law of Diffusion:

Principle stating that the amount of gas moving across a tissue is directly proportional to the tissue area and the difference in the partial pressure of gas between the two sides of the tissue. It is inversely proportional to the tissue thickness.

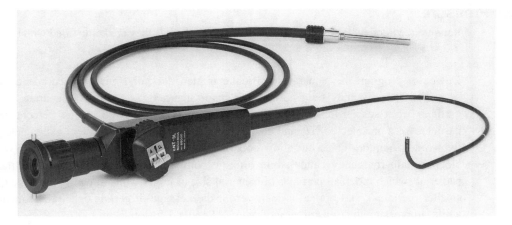

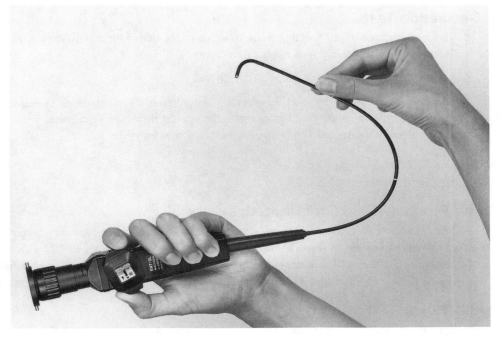

Fiberoptics: Types of fiberoptic laryngoscope.

Field Block:

Type of anesthesia technique by which a series of injections are used to encircle the operative site. It can be used in combination with any regional technique. *See* Block.

Fifteen/Twenty-Two Standard:

Connectors with a 15-mm inner diameter and a 22-mm outer diameter that join anesthesia equipment, particularly hoses, bags, masks, and endotracheal tubes.

Filling Pressure:

Pressure recorded in the various chambers of the heart while they are being filled with blood.

Filter:

Device or program that separates particular matter, data, or signals in accordance with selected criteria. It may be a porous membrane that acts as a sieve to separate minute particles from suspension. The efficiency of a filter is measured by the percentage of particles (of a preselected size and characteristic) trapped. Types of filters include electric (which stop random noise but allow coherent signals to get through), frequency (which block certain frequency bands while offering comparatively little resistance to others), bacterial (which block all particles of bacterial size or larger while allowing the passage of smaller particles), and optical (which permit the passage of certain spectral frequencies while suppressing the transmission of others). *See* Transfusion filter.

Finger Oscillation Test:

Test to determine motor speed and coordination of the dominant and nondominant hands. Below-normal scores can indicate brain impairment.

Finipres:

Blood pressure device that uses a variation of oscillometrics to determine systemic blood pressure with a minicuff continually inflated around a digit. *See* Oscillometry method of taking blood pressure. *See* Penaz continuous blood pressure method.

Fink Valve:

See Nonrebreathing valve.

First Order Process (First Order Kinetics):

Manipulation of a constant fraction or percentage of a particular molecular group per unit of time. For example, glomerular filtration (passive process) may filter 10% of a given drug per hour. If 100 mg of this drug circulates to the glomeruli in 1 hour, 10 mg is filtered; during the next hour, of the 90 mg available, 9 mg is filtered. *See* Zero order process.

Fishmouth Valve:

Type of gas flow flat valve that is primarily unidirectional. Flaps meet in the midpoint of the valve. Flow of gas in one direction blows the flaps open. Flow of gas in the other direction slaps the flaps closed.

Fistula:

Abnormal passage between two internal organs or that leads from an internal organ to the surface of the body. It is named according to the organs or parts with which it communicates, such as tracheoesophageal, bronchocutaneous, or bronchopleural.

Fixed Acid (Nonvolatile Acid):

Acid molecule that does not have a significant vapor pressure at body temperature. It must be metabolized or excreted in order to be eliminated from the body. Lactic acid is an example of a fixed acid.

Flagg Can:

Crude draw-over vaporizer that was often used to administer diethyl ether. This vaporizer is a can with several openings on the top. A mask or endotracheal tube is attached to the can by a hose and the ether vapor is picked up as air is blown back and forth by the patient's respiratory movements. This vaporizing method is obsolete. *See* Vaporizer, draw-over.

Flail Chest:

Traumatic condition characterized by multiple rib fractures. A paradoxical motion of the chest wall with respiration is evident. There is inadequate pulmonary ventilation and frequently the patient requires mechanical ventilatory support with positive-pressure respiration.

Flame Photometer:

Instrument for measuring the light emitted by a substance when made incandescent by a flame. It is useful for determining the concentration of sodium, potassium, and calcium ions in biologic solutions. Flame photometry is based on the principle that when an atom is exposed to a hot flame its orbiting electrons are excited, causing light emission at a specific frequency. Light intensity is proportional to ion concentration.

Flame Speed:

Speed at which a self-propagating flame travels in a fuel/air or fuel/O_2 mixture. If the flame speed is too slow, there is no deflagration in the mixture. *See* Deflagration.

Flammability:

Capability of a substance or material to support combustion. A self-propagating flame may lead to deflagration. *See* Deflagration.

Flammability Limits:

Upper and lower limits of the ability of a gas or liquid to support combustion, i.e., a lean or rich fuel/air or fuel/O_2 mixture. Generally, the upper and lower limits of flammability for a given fuel are much higher with O_2 than with air.

Flash-Lamp Pumped 585-nm Tunable Dye Laser:

Laser that produces a yellow (585-nm) pulse that is passed through the skin and absorbed by oxyhemoglobin. It is particularly effective to photocoagulate the abnormal blood vessels responsible for a port wine stain.

Flashover (Sparkover):

Destructive formation of an arc or spark between two electrical conductors.

Flash Point:

Lowest temperature at which the vapors of a volatile combustible substance ignite when exposed to flame.

Flaxedil:

See Gallamine triethiodide.

Fleisch Pneumotachograph:

> *See* Pneumotachograph.

Flexometallic:

> *See* Armored endotracheal tube.

Flight-or-fight Response:

> *See* Epinephrine.

Flow Compartments:

> Subsections of organs that are characterized by the rate of blood flowing through them.

Flow Control Valve (Needle Valve; Pin Valve):

> Basic device used to adjust the amount of gas entering a flowmeter. It is usually located in the base of the flowmeter. As its stem is turned counterclockwise, it moves a pin, which allows gas to escape into the flow column. A flow control valve is a precision device easily damaged by misuse, especially if it is overclosed; thereby wearing out the pin. *See* Figure. *See* Flowmeter.

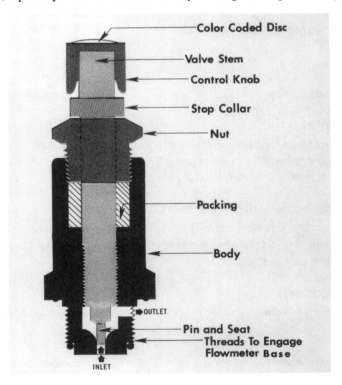

Flow Control Valve: The valve is shown in the closed position. Turning the stem creates a leak between the pin and seat so that gas flows to the outlet. The stop collar prevents overtightening of the pin in the seat.

Flow-Limited Ventilator:

See Ventilator.

Flowmeter:

Device for measuring the flow rate (usually in milliliters or in liters per minute) of a gas passing through it. Modern anesthesia machines use flowmeters or flow columns of the variable orifice type (Thorpe tube). A Thorpe tube is a transparent, tapered tube that has a smaller internal diameter at the bottom than at the top. The tube contains an indicator (also called a ball, float, or bobbin) that floats freely inside the tube. When the flow control valve at the base of the tube is opened, gas entering at the bottom flows upward and lifts the float. Because the tube is tapered, the cross-sectional area of the opening between the float and the inner walls of the tube increases in size as the float goes higher in the tube. The float is buoyed in the gas flow when the pressure drop caused by the gas flowing past the float (which acts as a restriction to flow) equals the weight of the float. This pressure drop across the float tends to remain constant, irrespective of the location of the suspended float in the tube. When the needle valve is turned outward, more gas passes up the flowmeter tube; and for a very short period of time a larger pressure drop occurs across the float. This pressure drop is greater than the weight of the float so the float moves higher until the pressure drop just equals the weight of the float again. Flowmeter tubes can be of a single-taper type (in which the internal diameter increases by uniform amounts from bottom to top) or the dual-taper type (in which the taper of the lower end increases more slowly than that of the upper part of the tube). *See* Figure. *See* Bernoulli law; Poiseuille law.

Flow-Over Vaporizer:

See Draw-over vaporizer.

Flow Sheet (Flowchart):

Method of data recording and display that illustrates one or more parameters in relation to each other and to time. An example of a flow sheet would be recordings of arterial blood gases at 30-minute intervals on a patient with concurrent recordings of respiratory function. A flow sheet can also indicate alternate or progressive pathways for routing messages or materials.

Fluid:

All-encompassing term for liquids and gases.

Fluidics:

Technique of using pressurized jets of fluid in specially designed circuits performing tasks such as switching or amplifying, which are usually carried out by electronics. For example, a fluidic anesthesia ventilator used in the operating room is powered by high-pressure O_2 switching between inspiration and expiration cycles.

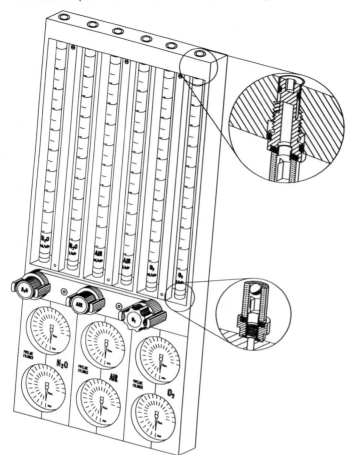

Flowmeter: Schematic diagram of a
bank of flowmeters.

Flumazenil (RO 15-1788, Anexate, Mazicon):

Specific short-acting competitive benzodiazepine antagonist. Flumazenil antagonizes the
amnestic, anxiolytic, and anesthetic effects of the benzodiazepines.

Fluomar:

See Fluroxene.

Fluorescence:

Emission of light or electromagnetic radiation by a substance as a result of the absorption of
energy of shorter wavelengths. When the material on the inside surface of a fluorescent tube is
excited by ultraviolet (UV) radiation that has been generated when current passes through
mercury vapor contained within the tube, it dissipates the UV energy by emitting visible light.

Fluorescent Lamp:

Device that efficiently converts electrical energy to light energy. It may consist of a glass
cylinder that contains mercury vapor at low pressure. The inner surface of the lamp is

coated with a phosphor. When an electrical current is passed through the vapor, ultraviolet radiation is produced, which in turn causes visible radiation as it strikes the phosphor. The circuitry that provides high voltage across the ends of the lamp in order to initially ionize the gas is referred to as a ballast.

Fluorescent Screen:

Screen coated with a phosphor that fluoresces as a result of electron excitation. This type of screen is used on cathode-ray and television picture tubes. *See* Fluorescence.

Fluoride:

Ionic form of fluorine. Fluoride ion is one of the degradation products of fluorinated hydrocarbon anesthetics, and its production in the body has been implicated in renal toxicity, particularly with the drug methoxyflurane. *See* Methoxyflurane.

Fluoride Number:

See Dibucaine number.

Fluorinated (Halogenated) Hydrocarbons:

Class name for the stable, nonflammable inhalation anesthetic agents (introduced during the 1950s) characterized by different halogen atoms added to a short carbon chain. Fluorine is frequently used for this purpose, being present in halothane, methoxyflurane, enflurane, and isoflurane. *See* Enflurane; Halothane; Isoflurane; Methoxyflurane.

Fluorocarbon:

Diverse group of chemically inert compounds containing both carbon and fluorine atoms as basic parts of the molecule. *See* Freon.

Fluosol-DA:

See Blood substitutes.

Fluotec Mark II:

See Vaporizer, fluomatic.

Fluothane:

See Halothane.

Flurazepam (Dalmane):

Benzodiazepine derivative used as a nighttime sedative. *See* Benzodiazepine.

Flurothyl:

Volatile liquid with a mild, pleasant odor administered by inhalation to cause convulsions. It is an alternative to electroshock therapy but has little clinical use at the present time.

Fluroxene; Trifluoroethyl Vinyl Ether (Fluromar):

Halogenated hydrocarbon, liquid at room temperature, that was introduced into clinical practice during the early 1950s as a general anesthetic. It is unique in that it is a flammable substance even though it is fluorinated. Because of this flammability the use of fluroxene was discontinued during the 1970s.

Flutter:

Defect in the reproduction of high-fidelity sound characterized by changes of more than 10 Hz in frequency.

Foam Test, Shake Test:

Simple procedure to determine surfactant activity in amniotic fluid.

Focal Cortical Seizure (Jacksonian Epilepsy):

Type of seizure seeming to emanate from a single site in the brain. There is no loss of consciousness. Single arm or leg jerking may be the only manifestations. *See* Epilepsy.

Forane:

See Isoflurane.

Forced Expiratory Volume (FEV_1):

Volume a patient exhales maximally following a complete inspiration. The amount exhaled in the first second is the FEV_1, whereas the total volume exhaled is the vital capacity (VC). In healthy individuals, the FEV_1 is approximately 80% of the VC. The FEV is a fairly sensitive pulmonary function test to detect obstructive diseases of the air passageways, in which a marked reduction of the FEV_1 is noted.

Force-Velocity Relations (Force-Velocity Curve):

Basic method for investigating myocardial contractility. An inverse relation exists between the force and the velocity of the contractions of cardiac muscle. The velocity decreases as the total load increases. The maximum velocity at which the muscle shortens is called the V_{max} and is considered a good measurement of contractility. Theoretically, at zero load V_{max} is optimal. Because these measurements are easily made only in a suspended intact papillary muscle, it is not a clinically applicable technique; however, it is useful for developing and testing inotropic agents. *See* Figure.

Foregger Company:

Division of Puritan-Bennett Corporation (since 1978) that manufactured anesthesia machines and equipment. Originally founded by Richard Foregger in 1914.

Formaldehyde (CH_2O):

Colorless, pungent, irritant gas. It is routinely used as a tissue specimen preservative at 10% concentration. These aqueous solutions of formaldehyde contain some methanol and are known as formalin. Formaldehyde has many industrial uses.

276

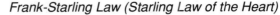

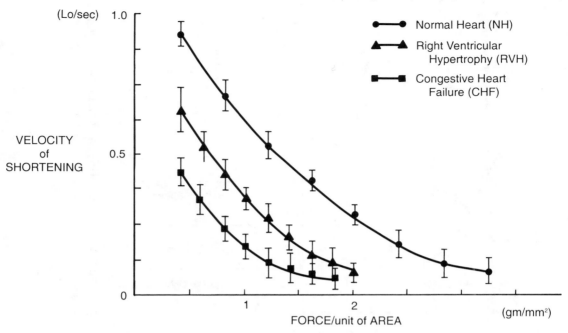

Force-Velocity Relations: Mean force-velocity curves obtained from isolated papillary muscles in the cat. Y axis: velocity of shortening expressed as a fraction of initial muscle length per second; X axis: force per unit of cross-sectional area in grams per square millimeter.

Four-Maximal Breath Preoxygenation Technique:

Technique for preoxygenating a patient in which a mask is tightly fitted to the face and the patient voluntarily takes four maximal breaths rapidly. *See* Preoxygenation.

Fourier Analysis:

Expression of a complex waveform as the summation of sine wave components. For example, both the electrocardiogram (ECG) and the electroencephalogram (EEG) can be broken down into sine wave components of various frequencies. The human EEG can be shown to represent the summation of multiple sine waves with frequencies ranging between 0 and 32 Hz. With fast Fourier analysis, a complex waveform is devolved into its components on line by a computer. This allows display of an EEG as an analyzed waveform a few milliseconds after its detection by scalp electrodes. *See* Figures. *See* Compressed spectral array; Electroencephalogram.

Fractional Receptor Occupancy (FRO):

See Receptor reserve.

Frangible Disk:

See Safety release device.

Frank-Starling Law (Starling Law of the Heart):

Principle stating that the force of cardiac contraction is related to the presystolic length of the muscle fibers (and end-diastolic volume). The clinical significance of this observation

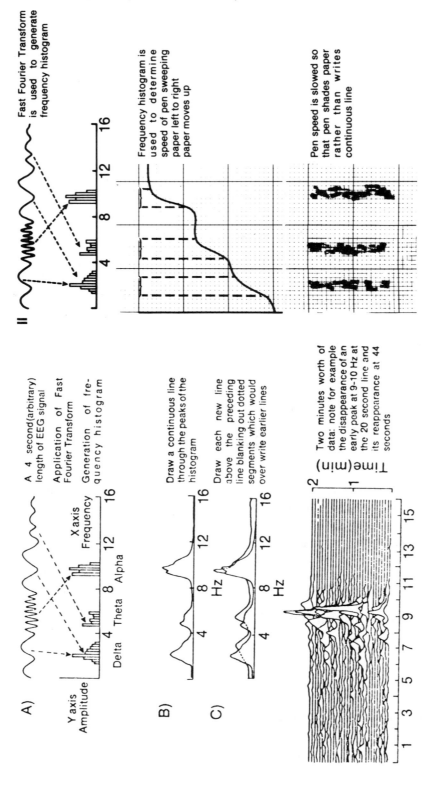

Fourier Analysis: Use of the fast Fourier transform to generate a frequency histogram from an EEG signal. (I) The frequency histogram is used in turn to generate a compressed spectral array. (II) The Fourier transform is used to generate a density modulated spectral array.

is that the larger the volume at the beginning of systole, the larger is the volume ejected. Practical limits exist regarding the ability of this mechanism to cope with increased filling volume, and therefore this relationship progressively attenuates in the failing heart.

Free Electron:

Electron that is not permanently attached to an atom or molecule and can move under the influence of applied electrical or magnetic fields.

Free (Unbound) Drug:

Portion of a drug that is not bound to plasma or tissue protein following administration. Typically, it is this unbound (free) drug that is pharmacologically active and is available for metabolism and excretion.

Freeze Trace:

See Shift register.

Freezing Point:

Temperature at which the liquid and solid phases of a substance exist in equilibrium at a defined pressure.

French Numbering System:

See Endotracheal tube.

Freon:

Trademark for a group of halogenated hydrocarbons that contain fluorine. They are widely used as refrigerants and propellants for aerosols. The most common is Freon 12 (dichloro-difluoromethane), which is inflammable in normal usage.

Frequency:

Number of complete oscillations or cycles in a unit of time (usually a second). The frequency is measured in hertz.

Frequency Curve:

Method of presenting data in which each data point is plotted on a graph and is then joined by a continuous line. The curve most often encountered in biologic data is the bell-shaped curve (also called the symmetric, normal, or Gaussian distribution curve), in which data points on opposite sides of the central maximum point and equidistant from it have the same magnitude. Curves displaced to the left or the right are called skewed curves and are not symmetric. *See* Figure.

Frequency Distribution:

Technique for organizing a complex signal into a series of components based on the frequency of the component. *See* Fourier analysis.

Fresnel Lens:

Type of lens that uses a series of cuts (or steps) to gain the magnifying qualities of a much thicker and heavier conventional lens.

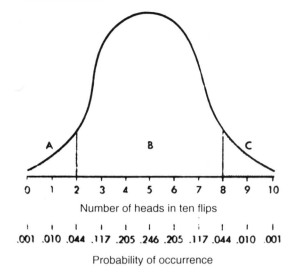

Number of heads in ten flips

.001 .010 .044 .117 .205 .246 .205 .117 .044 .010 .001

Probability of occurrence

Frequency Curve: Frequency curve showing the distribution of heads and tails when a coin is flipped 10 times and the probability of any particular outcome.

Frozen Section:

Pathology laboratory technique in which part of a tissue sample taken during surgery is flash frozen, rapidly stained and examined for abnormality while the patient waits in the operating room. *See* Cytopathology.

Frumin Valve:

See Nonrebreathing valve.

Fuel Cell:

Device or machine that converts a chemical process, usually oxidation or reduction, into a flow of electricity. The requisite substrates or reagents are introduced continually from outside the cell and react together with the aid of a catalyst.

Fuel, Rich/Lean Mixture of:

Evaluation of quantity of fuel mixed with O_2 or air. Fuel concentration is greater in a rich mixture than in the stoichiometric mixture. Combustion is not complete; i.e., there is some fuel remaining. With a lean mixture all the fuel is consumed, but O_2 remains and appears with the final products. *See* Stoichiometric mixture.

Functional Residual Capacity:

Volume of gas remaining in the lungs after a normal expiration. It comprises the residual volume and the expiratory reserve volume. *See* Lung volumes and capacities.

Furosemide (Lasix):

Sulfonamide related to the thiazides. It is, however, a more potent diuretic. Excessive diuresis with this agent can lead to severe hypokalemia and cardiovascular collapse.

Fusible Plug:

See Safety release device.

G

GABA:

See Gamma-aminobutyric acid.

Galanthamine:

Compound that acts as an antagonist to the nondepolarizing relaxants. It does not appear to be as potent as neostigmine in terms of anticholinesterase activity.

Gallamine Triethiodide (Flaxedil):

Nondepolarizing competitive muscle relaxant and vagal blocker. The actions of gallamine are similar to those of tubocurarine, although they may be of slightly shorter duration. The effects of gallamine are dose-dependent. Gallamine is inappropriate for patients with poor renal function. It is metabolized poorly by the body and excreted unchanged by the kidney. Gallamine also tends to produce tachycardia. *See* Tubocurarine chloride.

Galvanic Sensor:

See Oxygen analyzer.

Galvanometer:

Instrument that measures or detects small currents.

Game Theory:

Mathematic analysis of conflicting interests to determine the best possible strategy to reach a particular outcome.

Gamma-Aminobutyric Acid (GABA):

Inhibitory neurotransmitter of the central nervous system. Experiments show that drugs such as the benzodiazepines and barbiturates enhance the inhibitory effects of GABA. *See* Receptor/receptor site.

Gamma Camera:

Large, expensive gamma ray detection device for visualizing the distribution of radioactive compounds in the body. A radioisotope that is known to emit gamma radiation is administered to a patient. Abnormal concentrations are then detected by the gamma camera, which scans the body. The particular radioisotope used depends on its affinity for different body tissues. For instance, phosphorus is used to outline the skeletal system, and iodine is used to examine the thyroid gland.

Gamma-Endorphin:

See Endorphins.

Gamma-Hydroxybutyric Acid:

Intravenous anesthetic agent introduced for clinical use in 1960. It has a slow onset but in appropriate doses deepens into an unarousable anesthetic-like state after which rapid awakening occurs. It does not appear, however, to be a true analgesic as, even during its deepest effects, surgical stimulation causes tachycardia, hypertension, and sweating. It is not currently in clinical use.

Gamma Ray:

Electromagnetic radiation spontaneously emitted from the nucleus of a decaying radio-active substance. Gamma rays constitute the extreme shortwave end of the electromagnetic spectrum. They are not deflected in magnetic or electrical fields and have great penetrating power. *See* Alpha particle; Beta particle.

Ganglion:

Collection of nerve cell bodies located outside the central nervous system. Ganglia are unmyelinated nerve cell bodies and are therefore masses of gray matter. A network of nerves is known as a plexus. Nerve fibers coming into a ganglion and synapsing with neurons contained within are preganglionic fibers. The fibers that leave a ganglion and are anatomically part of the ganglionic neurons are postganglionic fibers. Ganglia can multiply or amplify signals received from the preganglionic fibers, when those fibers synapse with many neurons.

Gargle:

Technique for agitating a solution in the throat with air from the lungs (keeping the glottis closed). It is used for topical anesthesia of the upper airway in the cooperative patient.

Gas Chromatography:

Technique for analyzing of liquid or gas mixtures and for identifying components. The heart of the gas chromatograph is a glass or stainless steel tube, usually several feet long with an outside diameter of an one-eighth to a one-fourth inch. This tube is filled with a separating medium such as diatomaceous earth. The column is mounted inside an oven. The column is perfused by a steady flow of an inert carrier gas such as argon. The mixture to be analyzed is injected at the front of the column. The various parts of the sample are swept through the column and separated by retardation according to their affinities for the column packing. The gas chromatograph is calibrated using standard sample mixtures.

Gas Cylinder:

See Cylinder, gas.

Gaseous Anesthetic Agent (Anesthetic Gas):

Pharmacologic agent that is a gas at room temperature and pressure. Included among these are N_2O, cyclopropane, and ethylene. These agents are in contrast to the volatile anesthetics that are liquids at room temperature and pressure, such as diethyl ether, halothane, and trichloroethylene.

Gasserian Ganglion Blockade:

Direct local anesthetic block of the trigeminal nerve. When successful, it blocks all three branches of the fifth cranial nerve and is recommended for treatment of severe trigeminal neuralgia. It has multiple side effects and should be attempted only by experts under good conditions.

Gas Trap:

See Scavenger system.

Gastroschisis:

Congenital defect of the abdominal wall that allows the intestines to protrude. The intestines are not covered by the peritoneal sac as they are in an omphalocele. The defect in the abdominal musculature is usually much smaller than with omphaloceles, and therefore the musculature can usually be stretched to admit the extruding loop of intestine. The intestine usually takes several weeks to heal because of exposure to the irritating amniotic fluid in utero. Intravenous hyperalimentation is necessary for nutritional maintenance during this recovery period. *See* Omphalocele.

Gate:

Electronic circuit with one output and two or more inputs. Whether an output signal is emitted depends on the combination of inputs. There are four basic gates: "and," "or," "nand," and "nor." These terms refer to the possibilities in which either 1 and 2 = x, 1 or 2 = x, 1 but not 2 also = x, or neither 1 nor 2 = x. For example, an operating room has two thermostats, one in the room and one in the corridor. The two thermostats feed into an "and" gate. Both thermostat 1 and thermostat 2 must detect a critical temperature before the "and" gate energizes a heater. If the two thermostats operate an "or" gate, a signal from either thermostat operates a heater. *See* Figure.

Gate Theory of Pain:

Theory that an area of the central nervous system exists that acts like a "gate," i.e., it can block pain sensation from reaching the conscious levels of the brain when activated or "closed." Two observations have led to formulation of the gate theory of pain control. (1) Stimulation of large sensory fibers from peripheral mechanoreceptors greatly depresses pain transmission in the spinal cord from either the same area of the body or from areas located many segments away. (2) Corticifugal signals (which begin in the cortex where the pain pathway terminates) decrease pain sensitivity by a feedback loop. The common action point of these two mechanisms appears to be in the substantia gelatinosa, a group of small neurons located near the tip of the dorsal horn of the spinal cord. This point is where pain fibers terminate after they enter the spinal cord and pass into the tract of Lissauer. It is believed to be in the substantia gelatinosa that the peripheral mechanoreceptor and corticifugal pathways can greatly suppress or prevent the upward travel of pain sensation in the spinal cord. *See* Figure.

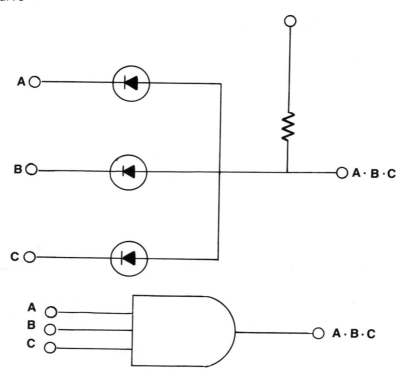

Gate: Electronic gate (top) made of three diodes called an AND gate along with the circuit symbol (bottom) for this gate. An output signal only occurs when inputs A, B, and C occur simultaneously.

Gaussian Curve:

See Frequency curve.

Geiger Counter:

Device for detecting and measuring charged particle emission or electromagnetic radiation.

General Anesthesia:

Physiologic altered state classically containing four progressive components: (1) analgesia, (2) amnesia, (3) muscle relaxation, and (4) unconsciousness. Areflexia (particularly of the autonomic nervous system) is now considered a goal of general anesthesia as well. The agents capable of producing these conditions may be administered by inhalation, intramuscularly, intravenously, or via the gastrointestinal tract. Light general anesthesia implies anesthesia with an absolute minimum depression of bodily functions from which the patient returns to normal as rapidly as possible. Deep general anesthesia implies total body depression to just before the point of deleterious reduction of vital signs requiring intervention and support. Light to deep anesthesia is a continuum that depends on levels of surgical stress as well as dose of anesthetic. *See* Anesthesia, awareness during; Balanced anesthesia; Depth of anesthesia.

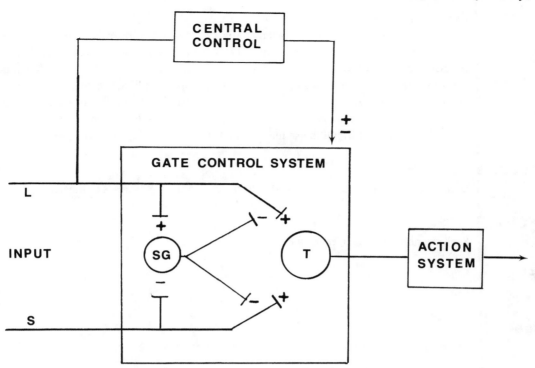

Gate Theory of Pain: Schematic of gate control of pain mechanisms: Small-diameter fibers (S); large-diameter fibers (L). The fibers project to the substantia gelatinosa (SG) and the first central transmission (T) cells. The inhibitory effect exerted by SG on the afferent fiber terminals is increased by activity in L fibers and decreased by activity in S fibers. The central control trigger is represented by a line running from the large-fiber system to the central mechanisms; the mechanisms, in turn, project back to the gate control system. The T cells project to the entry cells of the action system. +, excitation; −, inhibition.

Generator:

Device for converting mechanical energy into electrical energy.

Generic Drug:

Drug not protected by patent or trademark. The name usually describes the chemical structure of the agent. Most medications may be sold less expensively in the generic form.

Gentamicin (Garamycin):

Aminoglycoside antibiotic that inhibits protein synthesis in microorganisms. It has been implicated in augmenting neuromuscular blockade during anesthesia and is useful for treating serious gram-negative infections. It can be both nephrotoxic and ototoxic. *See* Antibiotic.

285

Georgia Valve:

Low-pressure relief valve found on breathing systems. When open, it allows for passive escape of excess gas, but it closes rapidly when the pressure jumps to a high level as the bag is squeezed to assist ventilation. This action is in contrast to that of the more common high-pressure relief valve (pop-off valve), which opens only when the preset limit of pressure on the system is exceeded. Both types of valve rid the system of excess gas, and both have been used in a circuit at the same time. In general, the low-pressure relief valve is considered more difficult to use than the high-pressure one. *See* Pop-off valve.

Geriatrics:

Branch of medicine that is concerned with the problems and diseases of the aged.

GFCI; GFI:

See Ground fault circuit interrupter.

GFR:

See Glomerular filtration rate.

Giga-:

Prefix meaning 1 billion (10^9). It may be abbreviated G or B. *See* SI unit.

Glasgow Coma Scale:

Evaluation of patients with severe central nervous system dysfunction that relies upon various independent patient observations and responses to determine the level of brain injury performed serially, it is a reasonable predictor of efficacy of therapeutic measures and prognosis. *See* Table.

Glass:

Amorphous inorganic substance consisting of silicates combined with borates or oxides of boron and phosphorus. Ordinary glass transmits 85–90% of the light striking it, whereas the best optical glass (highly refined with closely controlled impurities) can transmit up to 99%. Borosilicate glass (Pyrex) is known for its resistance to heat and thermal shock and for its low coefficient of thermal expansion.

Glaucoma:

Disease of the eye characterized by increased intraocular pressure as high as 70 mm Hg (normal range 10–30 mm Hg). The rise in pressure is due to the blockage of aqueous humor flow from the anterior chamber. Glaucoma leads to blindness due to atrophy of the optic nerve. Two types of primary glaucoma exist: chronic open-angle (wide-angle) (95% of cases) and acute or chronic angle-closure (narrow-angle) (5% of cases). These terms describe variations in the anatomy of the anterior chamber of the eye, which appears normal in chronic open-angle glaucoma or, by contrast, shallow in acute or chronic angle-closure glaucoma. In the latter type, excess dilatation of the pupils may precipitate worsening of the glaucoma condition. Large systemic doses of scopolamine or atropine may produce this effect.

Glasgow Coma Scale.

Glasgow Coma Scale[a,b]		
Eye opening	Spontaneous	E4
	To speech	3
	To pain	2
	None	1
Best motor response	Obeys commands	M6
	Localizes	5
	Withdraws	4
	Abnormal flexion	3
	Extension	2
	None	1
Verbal responses	Orientated	V5
	Confused conversation	4
	Inappropriate words	3
	Incomprehensive	
	sounds	2
	None	1

Reactivity and size of pupils
 May be affected by drugs or trauma to eye or cranial
  nerves

Eye position and movements

Other cranial nerves

Spinal cord function
 Level of paralysis
 Level of sensory deficit

Level of reflexes

[a] From Jennett B, Teasdale G: Aspects of coma after severe head injury. Lancet 1:879, 1977.
[b] Add E, M, and V; 15 is normal; <7 after 6 hours indicates severe head injury.

Glenn Shunt:

Anastomosis of the superior vena cava to the right pulmonary artery. It is usually performed on older pediatric patients with tricuspid atresia in order to increase pulmonary blood flow.

Glomerular Filtration Rate (GFR):

Quantity of glomerular filtrate (similar to plasma but containing no significant amount of protein) formed per minute in the nephrons of both kidneys. In the glomeruli of the kidney, the filtrate passes through the walls of the glomerular capillaries into the renal tubules. In the tubules, some reabsorption of water and some secretion of solutes change this glomerular filtration fluid into urine. In order to measure the GFR, a substance, such as inulin, is required that is be freely filtered in the glomeruli and neither reabsorbed nor secreted in the tubule. The GFR in an average-sized adult man is approximately 125 ml/minute, which is the equivalent of 180 L/day. The normal urine volume is approximately 1 L/day, indicating that more than 99% of the glomerular filtrate is reabsorbed in the tubules. It also means that in 1 day the kidney filters an amount of fluid equal to 4 times the total body water, 15 times the extracellular fluid volume, and 60 times the plasma volume.

Glottis:

Portion of the larynx consisting of the true vocal cords and the opening between them. *See* Larynx.

Gluconeogenesis:

See Corticosteroid.

Glycolysis:

Splitting of sugars into simpler compounds, such as pyruvate and lactate, usually for the purpose of energy production.

Glycopyrrolate (Robinul):

Long-acting atropine-like agent used for anesthesia to dry the mouth and respiratory passageways. It also decreases the acidity and absolute quantity of gastric secretions and acts as an antispasmodic. Because its actions last longer than those of atropine or scopolamine, it can be matched with the longer acting anticholinesterases to reverse neuromuscular blockade.

Gold:

Yellow metal, regarded as precious for thousands of years. Its tarnish resistance is used in plating electrical conductors. *See* Oxygen analyzer.

Goldman Vaporizer:

Universal flow-over vaporizer that does not contain a wick and can be used in or out of a breathing system. It has no temperature compensation and volatilizes many agents. The Goldman vaporizer is controlled by changing a variable bypass. It was originally designed for use in dentistry in conjunction with intermittent flow machines. *See* Boyle bottle.

Gold Standard:

Concept found in equipment or drug testing in which a new entity is compared to an older entity considered to be as close to the ideal as heretofore practical. For example, a new monitor for determining cardiac dysfunction would be compared to the electrocardiogram, which would be considered the "gold standard."

Grab Sample:

See Instantaneous sample.

Graham's Law of Diffusion:

Pinciple stating that the rate of transfer of different gases through a fine membrane (when the gases are at the same temperature and pressure) is inversely proportional to the square roots of their densities.

Gram-Atomic Weight (Gram-Atom):

Atomic weight of an element measured in grams.

Gram-Molecular Weight (Gram-Molecule; Mole):

Amount in grams of an element or compound that is numerically equivalent to its molecular weight.

Grand Mal Seizure:

Type of seizure disorder that is characterized by psychomotor movements. They are usually proceeded by a sensory or motor aura, consciousness is lost, anal and bladder sphincter tone is lost, and respiratory activity is arrested. Arterial hypoxemia ensues; a tonic phase can last 20–40 seconds and is followed by the clonic phase, which lasts a variable period of time. Following the seizure during the postictal period the patient may be severely depressed. *See* Epilepsy.

Graticule:

Network of fine lines set on a cathode-ray tube or the eyepieces of a microscope or telescope that are in simultaneous focus with the object being viewed. They act as a convenient scale with which to measure the object.

Ground (Earth):

Conducting body, of no resistance (usually the earth) used to transmit electrical current and act as a reference. The electrical potential of the ground is arbitrarily set at zero. Conveniently, the ground is usually a stake or cold water pipe directly thrust into the earth. *See* Grounding.

Ground Electrode:

See Dispersive electrode.

Ground Fault Circuit Interrupter (GFCI; GFI):

Device that interrupts the current flowing in a circuit when there is a discrepancy in the flow through the grounded and nongrounded conductors of that circuit. If the currents differ, the GFI opens the circuit so that current flow stops. The GFI acts as a safety device to prevent current from returning to ground through an unplanned path.

Grounding:

Concept referring to the connection of electrical equipment to an external common conductor. It provides a harmless pathway for electrical current to flow. For instance, the grounding of an electrocardiography machine is accomplished by connecting its case through the ground wire in its power cord to a conductor beyond the wall socket. This grounding provides for a current path in case the hot side of the power line makes contact with the case due to insulation breakdown or instrument malfunction. If the case is not grounded, the next individual touching the case and ground simultaneously would become the path to ground for the hot side and be shocked. *See* Ground; Hot versus cold electrical circuits.

Ground Loop:

Unwanted feedback of signal or current through the common ground of two or more instruments. Ground loops can be broken by not grounding the instrument sensitive to the ground loop, although this alternative is unsafe . Ground loops may also be broken by connecting the sensitive equipment different parts of a common ground. The nature of the unwanted feedback signal can be determined and a specific remedy applied, such as inserting an appropriately sized blocking capacitor into the path to ground.

G Suit:

Inflatable garment that can be wrapped around or zipped onto a patient. To achieve the greatest benefit, the suit must be adapted to the patient from the upper chest to the toes. When inflated, the suit places external pressure against the skin of the chest wall, abdominal cavity, and large muscle masses in the legs. The suit counteracts peripheral dilatation and has been found useful for transporting or maintaining patients with low circulating blood volumes or poorly responding sympathetic nervous systems.

Guanethidine (Ismelin):

Antihypertensive agent that appears to block postganglionic adrenergic receptor sites and deplete the store of catecholamines. It is useful for management of severe hypertension. Its actions are similar to those of reserpine but the advantage of guanethidine's is that it does not cross the blood-brain barrier. *See* Reserpine.

Guillain-Barré Disease:

See Acute idiopathic polyneuritis.

Gyve:

Shackle or restraint, particularly for the leg.

290

H

H:

See Henry.

Habituation:

(1) Diminished response to a drug, particularly evident with central nervous system agents when given repeatedly. (2) Diminished response to a neural stimulus, particularly less electrical response, it is considered to be a simple form of learning. Sensitization is another simple form of learning that is usually considered the opposite reaction in which a repeated stimulus produces an ever greater response if it is coupled in the mind with an unpleasant or, for that matter, a pleasant response. A common example of this type of learning is known as the arousal response, which is best exemplified by the busy intern eating dinner, paying no attention to the overhead page noise until his own name is mentioned, whereupon he leaps up, scattering food in every direction.

Haldane Apparatus:

Device used for measuring CO_2 in a sample. It works by measuring the volume change in a solution that is known to expand upon absorption of CO_2.

Haldane Effect:

Phenomenon in which the deoxygenation of the blood increases its ability to transport CO_2. The binding of O_2 with hemoglobin (Hb) tends to displace CO_2 from Hb. When Hb combines with O_2 it becomes a stronger acid than in its uncombined form. The increase in hydrogen ions from the stronger acid drives the reaction of hydrogen and bicarbonate ions toward the formation of carbonic acid, which in turn dissociates to CO_2 and H_2O. Thus, the Haldane effect causes increased removal of CO_2 from the periphery owing to O_2 being removed from Hb. In the lungs, CO_2 release is enhanced by Hb binding with O_2. The Haldane effect is more important to CO_2 transport than the Bohr effect is to O_2 transport. *See* Bohr effect, Carbon dioxide dissociation curve.

Haldol:

See Haloperidol.

Half-Life:

Duration of time in which the original quantity of a radioactive isotope decays to half its original amount. Decay rates are constant for a given radioactive nuclide. Half-life also refers to the time required for the serum concentration of a particular drug to be reduced by 50%.

Half-Value Thickness (Half-Thickness):

Thickness of a uniform sheet of material that reduces the intensity of radiation passing through it by one-half. The term is commonly used when comparing the ability of various materials to shield against radiation.

Hallucination:

Perception of stimuli, whether visual, auditory, or tactile, that do not actually exist. *See* Anesthesia, awareness during.

Halogen:

Atomic group made up of the elements fluorine, chlorine, bromine, iodine, and astatine. In elemental form, halogens can be toxic to tissues. When organic molecules are combined with halogens, they become stabilized; and their susceptibility to flame, degradation, and metabolism is decreased.

Haloperidol (Haldol):

Antipsychotic agent of the butyrophenone series. Its pharmacologic actions are similar to those of the phenothiazines. *See* Butyrophenone; Phenothiazine.

Halopropane:

Experimental halogenated hydrocarbon anesthetic. Clinical studies on halopropane revealed its tendency to cause myocardial irritability, and its use was therefore abandoned.

Halothane (Fluothane; C₂HBrClF₃):

Halothane (Fluothane; $C_2HBrClF_3$):

First halogenated hydrocarbon to find wide clinical acceptance as an anesthetic. It is currently the most popular inhalation anesthetic agent worldwide. Both a cardiovascular and central nervous system depressant, overdose usually leads to cardiovascular collapse. Induction and recovery are relatively rapid with this agent. Halothane is readily vaporized. It has been implicated in the condition known as halothane hepatitis, progressive liver failure seen in a small percentage of patients who receive halothane. The incidence of this disease is given variously as 1:50,000 or 1:14,000 halothane administrations. Usually seen following the second or third exposure, the disorder, however, has occurred in some individuals after their first exposure. Halothane hepatitis is associated with a high mortality rate when florid, and no specific treatment has been found. An aphorism in the anesthesia world states that before the invention of halothane there were many causes of postoperative jaundice. After the drug was introduced into clinical practice, only one cause remained. *See* Figure.

F—C—C—H

Halothane.

Halothane Analyzer:

Device for the quantitative measurement of halothane vapor concentration. There are two principal types. One relies on ultraviolet light and the other on infrared light. Both depend on the fact that halothane absorbs ultraviolet and infrared rays, thereby decreasing the intensity of a light beam in proportion to its concentration. The ultraviolet device is less expensive, has a slower response time, and is accurate to approximately 0.1%. The device measures only halothane. In contrast, the infrared analyzer is rapid and accurate; but it is sensitive to the presence of N_2O and other halogenated agents and is considerably more expensive. Other methods to detect halothane exist. *See* Gas chromatography; Mass spectrometer; Narkotest.

Halothane Hepatitis:

See Halothane.

Halstead, William (Surgeon):

Early pioneer in anesthesia research. He was the first person to describe nerve blocks of the sensory nerves of the face and arms.

Hand Grip Strength:

Crude test for determining residual neuromuscular blockade. The patient grips the examiner's hand and the strength of grip is estimated. The efficacy of the examination depends on the experience of the examiner.

Hanging Drop Technique:

Manipulation done during placement of an epidural needle to verify that the needle orifice is in the epidural space. A drop of fluid in the hub of the needle is usually sucked back into the needle upon patient inspiration because of negative pressure in the epidural space communicated from the pleural space.

Hard Copy:

Any information recorded in some permanent manner that can be directly read by individuals.

Hard Radiation:

Type of ionizing radiation that has a high degree of penetration. This designation is most commonly applied to x-rays (of short wavelength) and gamma rays.

293

Hardware, Computer:

Physical components of a computer system.

Hb:

See Hemoglobin.

Head Raise Test:

Sensitive test to determine recovery from neuromuscular blockade. The supine patient is asked to lift and hold up his or her head. Inability to sustain the head raise indicates incomplete recovery.

Heart, Conduction System of:

Intrinsic regulating system of the heart composed of specialized muscle tissue. It is responsible for initiating and conducting the electrical stimuli that trigger myocardial contraction. These structures are the sinoatrial (SA) node, atrioventricular (AV) node, AV bundle (His bundle), internodal atrial pathways, and Purkinje fibers. The SA node, known as the cardiac pacemaker, has the most rapid rate of depolarization. (Its rate of discharge determines the heart rate.) It is located in the right atrium inferior to the opening of the superior vena cava. Once an electrical impulse is initiated by the SA node, the impulse spreads outward over both atria causing them to contract, which depolarizes the AV node. The AV node is located near the inferior portion of the interatrial septum and is one of the last portions of the atria to be depolarized. The internodal atrial pathways (anterior, middle, and posterior) conduct impulses from the SA node to the AV node. Projecting from the AV node is the His bundle which descends along the posterior margin of the membranous interventricular septum. The His bundle continues as the right and left bundle branches. It distributes electrical impulses over the medial surface of the ventricles. The actual contractions of the ventricles are stimulated by the Purkinje fibers that emerge from the bundle branches and enter the myocardium.

Heart Synchronized Ventilation:

Technique of controlling respiration to synchronize breathing with the heart rate (high frequency ventilator techniques being used), in an attempt to minimize kidney stone movement during lithotripsy.

Heat:

Amount of energy (measured in joules) associated with the random movement of the atoms and molecules that make up a substance. When a material contains no heat energy, the molecules are theoretically at rest. This point is used as a zero point in the Kelvin temperature scale.

Heat Exchanger:

Device for transferring heat from one fluid to another. For example, to rapidly cool a patient during extracorporeal circulation, the blood is pumped through tubes sitting in a cold waterbath, and heat is dissipated to the water in the bath. The important principle of any heat exchanger is that the two substances exchanging heat do not come into direct contact with one another.

Heat Exhaustion:

See Heatstroke.

Heating or Cooling Blanket:

See Temperature blanket.

Heat Sink:

Device employed to dispose of unwanted heat, thereby preventing a damaging rise in temperature. Most often used in electronics, heat sinks are usually passive, multifinned metal mounts with a large surface area.

Heatstroke (Heat Hyperpyrexia; Sunstroke):

Condition marked by the cessation of sweating, extremely high body temperature, and collapse. A breakdown of the body's heat regulatory system occurs after prolonged exposure to excessive temperatures. Internal body temperatures higher than 43°C have been recorded. Clinical signs of heatstroke are an increased bounding pulse; hot, dry skin; and rapid, weak respirations. Heatstroke is a threat to life, and immediate reduction of body temperature is necessary. An ice-water bath and vigorous massage to increase circulation are indicated. Heatstroke should be differentiated from the less dramatic heat exhaustion, the symptoms of which are cold, sweaty skin; weak, rapid pulse; shallow respirations; and no discernible elevation in body temperature (in fact, it may be subnormal). Heat exhaustion patients are treated with appropriate electrolyte and fluid administration.

Heat Transfer:

Movement of heat energy from one body to another. It can occur by any of the following methods: (1) conduction (heat energy is transferred directly from one molecule to another); (2) convection (heat energy in a fluid is transferred by the movement of the fluid itself); and (3) radiation (heat energy is transferred by means of electromagnetic waves in the infrared range emanating from the body).

Helium:

Light, colorless, nonflammable gaseous element. It is difficult to liquefy even at temperatures of −195°C. It lowers the specific gravity of any gas(es) with which it is mixed. Therapeutically, a mixture of O_2 and helium can be beneficial in cases of partial respiratory obstruction. In this situation, the mixture decreases the work of breathing and oxygenation improves. However, the use of O_2/helium combinations has been nearly eliminated owing to the current practice of tracheal intubation to manage respiratory obstruction.

Helium Dilution Technique:

Measures functional residual capacity or residual volume using helium, a nearly blood-insoluble gas. A patient breathes in and out of the spirometer, which contains a known volume of helium and air. After a few breaths (to reach equilibrium), the helium concentration is measured in the spirometer. From this concentration, the volume into which the helium has been diluted in the lung can be calculated.

Hellp Syndrome:

Acronym for "hemolysis of red blood cells, elevated liver enzymes and low platelet count." It is associated with high maternal morbidity and mortality. Usually noted with pre-eclampsia or eclampsia.

Hematocrit:

Percent volume of erythrocytes (packed by centrifugation) in a given volume of whole blood. The normal hematocrit value differs between males and females; and it is highly labile during the immediate postoperative period owing to ongoing fluid shifts.

Hematoma:

Mass of blood, usually clotted, in an organ, space, or tissue.

Hemicholinium:

Experimental drug that blocks acetylcholine synthesis by interfering with the transport of choline across the neuronal membrane.

Hemoconcentration:

See Hemodilution.

Hemodialysis (Dialysis):

Procedure for removing certain unwanted products from the blood. These substances may include (1) natural metabolic end products that have accumulated because of renal disease; (2) ingested toxins; and (3) drug overdoses. The technique requires creation of an artificial shunt between a large artery and a vein. Blood is diverted from the artery into a long coil of semipermeable tubing, which is bathed in a dialysate solution into which the undesirable blood constituents migrate. For anticoagulation purposes, heparin is added as the blood leaves the artery, and the heparin effect is reversed by protamine as the blood is returned. With peritoneal dialysis, the dialyzing solution is introduced either continuously or intermittently into the peritoneal cavity. The dialyzing membrane is the gut wall itself. After a period of time the dialysate containing the noxious products is withdrawn. Peritoneal dialysis is often the technique of choice for treating acute poisoning because it requires less time and technology.

Hemodilution:

Increase in the volume of the blood plasma with a resulting decrease in red blood cell (RBC) concentration. Hemodilution is most frequently seen in clinical practice when non-RBC-containing volume expanders have been administered to counteract blood loss. Hemoconcentration, in contrast to hemodilution, is a decrease in plasma volume resulting in increased RBC concentration.

Hemoglobin (Hb):

O_2-carrying pigment of the erythrocytes that is formed in the bone marrow. It is a conjugated protein: heme is an iron-porphyrin compound joined to the protein globin that consists of four polypeptide chains. Differences in the amino acid sequences of the polypeptide chains give rise to variations in human Hb. Normal adult Hb is called type A; fetal Hb is called type F and is gradually replaced during the infant's first year by type A. In Hb S (sickle), glutamic acid replaces valine in the polypeptide chains. With this rather minor change, the deoxygenated Hb form becomes poorly soluble and crystallizes within the red blood cell at low O_2 tension. Changing red cell shape from biconcave to crescent greatly increases fragility. Normal Hb A contains iron in its ferrous (Fe^{2+}) form. Drugs such as some local anesthetics (prilocaine and benzocaine), nitrates, and a number of the sulfonamides oxidize the (Fe^{2+}) of Hb to the ferric (Fe^{3+}) form. In this state, Hb cannot carry O_2 and is known as methemoglobin. Hemoglobin level in the blood is measured in grams per deciliter. The normal range is 12–16 g/dl; women usually have lower Hb levels than do men.

Hemolysis:

Destruction of red blood cells resulting in liberation of hemoglobin into the surrounding fluid. It can be caused by changes in osmolarity and by numerous toxins and drugs.

Hemolytic Jaundice:

Inherited chronic disease characterized by a yellow appearance to the skin, increased fragility of red blood cells (leading to their destruction), absence of bile pigment in urine, and splenomegaly. Elements of this condition may also be seen following massive red blood cell destruction in a mismatched transfusion.

Hemophilia:

Bleeding disorder, almost invariably occurring in males, caused by an inherited (sex-linked recessive) deficiency of at least one blood-clotting factor. It is characterized by spontaneous or traumatic intramuscular and subcutaneous hemorrhages. Classic hemophilia is a deficiency of factor VIII. Christmas disease (pseudohemophilia), a deficiency of factor IX, resembles classic hemophilia in terms of the clinical features. *See* Blood coagulation.

Hemoptysis:

Expectoration of blood or blood-stained sputum originating from the bronchi, trachea, or lungs.

Hemopump (HP):

Miniature left ventricular assist device (LVAD), which is a pump mounted on a catheter that can be introduced quickly via peripheral vascular access. It can provide nonpulsatile blood flow in the range of 3 L/minute. *See* LVAD.

Hemorrhage:

Heavy loss of blood.

Hemostasis:

Process by which bleeding is stopped. It may be accomplished by vasoconstriction, coagulation, or surgical methods. *See* Tables. *See* Blood coagulation.

Henderson-Hasselbalch Equation:

Formula for calculating the fundamental relation of buffer systems such as bicarbonate-carbonic acid. For the bicarbonate-carbonic acid buffer system the equation is $pH = pK + log (HCO_3^-/H_2CO_3)$. The pK for the bicarbonate-carbonate acid buffer system is 6.1. Thus the equation becomes $pH = 6.1 + log (HCO_3^-/H_2CO_3)$. In 1916 Hasselbalch changed the Henderson equation of 1909 into logarithmic form. The Henderson-Hasselbalch equation is used clinically when the pH and the $PaCO_2$ are determined. The equation can then be solved for bicarbonate and the value can be used to correct acid-base abnormalities. *See* Dissociation constant.

Henry (H):

Standard international unit of inductance. When a current variation of 1 ampere/second induces in a circuit an electromotive force of 1V, the inductance of that circuit is said to be 1 Henry. The milliHenry (mH = one one-thousandth of a Henry) is the subunit frequently used in electronics. *See* Conduction.

Hepa Filter:

Efficient air filter often used in operating room heating and cooling systems. HEPA is an acronym for high-efficiency particulate air. It actually increases in efficiency as it accumulates dirt. HEPA filters are used in laminar flow hoods. *See* Laminar flow hood.

Heparin:

Naturally occurring group of molecules (molecular weight 3,000–30,000 daltons of the glycosaminoglycans class) produced by the mast cells that are found in connective tissue, especially around the lungs and liver, and in blood vessels. Although the normal physiologic functions of heparin are in dispute, it is used in large, nonphysiologic doses (source: bovine lung on porcine gut) to prevent clotting and platelet aggregation. The anticoagulation effect of heparin is caused by enhancement of the action of antithrombin III, the major natural inhibitor of coagulation in the blood. (Heparin is the standard drug used to render blood nonclottable for extracorporeal circulation.) *See* Figure. *See* Anticoagulant; Protamine sulfate.

Heparinoids:

Class of small molecules that are considered nonheparin glycosaminoglycans formed as a by-product of heparin production. They may prove useful as agents to replace heparin in patients who have severe side effects to the letter.

Heparin Rebound:

Phenomenon seen after protamine reversal of the heparin effect. It includes worsening bleeding. It may be due to body heparin depots. *See* Activated clotting time; Heparin.

Hemostasis: (A) Primary (Screening) Tests of Hemostasis.

1. Activated coagulation time (ACT)	Can be done in OR. Observe for clot retraction and lysis.
2. Fibrinogen level	Depressed in DIC.
3. Prothrombin time (PT)	Prolonged in liver disease, vitamin K deficiency, coumarin anticoagulation, DIC.
4. Partial thromboplastin time (aPTT)	Prolonged in Factors V, VIII deficiency (massive transfusion), the hemophilias, or the presence of heparin.
5. Platelet count	

These are the initial tests used to confirm the presence of a disorder of hemostasis.

Hemostasis: (B) Secondary Tests of Hemostasis.

1. Bleeding time	Widely accepted clinical test of platelet function.
2. Platelet aggregation	A more refined test of platelet function using various agents to determine the responsiveness of the platelets.
3. Protamine titration	Definitive test used to confirm/disprove presence of heparin.

Hemostasis: (C) Characteristics Desirable in the Ideal or Test of Hemostasis.

1. Only simple maneuvers are necessary to obtain reproducible results.

2. Minimum equipment, which is compact, inexpensive, and operates quietly, is required.

3. Result is available quickly, even with abnormally prolonged bleeding time.

4. Test is performed on whole blood rather than plasma.

5. Test reagents are stable indefinitely.

6. Test must not require prolonged attention away from operator's usual duties.

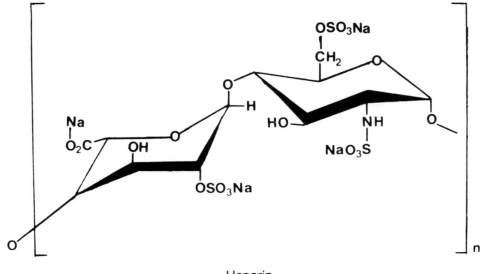

Heparin.

Heparin Resistance:

Decreased sensitivity to the anticoagulation effect of heparin. *See* Heparin.

Hepatitis:

Inflammation of the liver usually caused by viral or toxic agents. Subcategories of hepatitis are viral (type A, type B, and type C), toxic (as in carbon tetrachloride poisoning), alcoholic, and halothane-induced. Viral hepatitis is often associated with multiple transfusions (type B and C) or the ingestion of infected shellfish (type A). Populations at increased risk for hepatitis B include drug addicts, renal dialysis patients and personnel, dentists, and other health workers in general. A vaccine is available that provides a high level of protection against hepatitis B.

Hepatojugular Reflux:

See Cardiac tamponade.

Hepatotoxicity:

Property of a substance to damage or destroy liver cells. Carbon tetrachloride is the classic example of a hepatotoxin. Exposure to this volatile chlorinated hydrocarbon in significant concentrations causes direct liver damage proportional to the dose.

Hepcon:

Device from Hemotec, Inc., Englewood, CO, that measures heparin levels in blood.

Hering-Breuer Reflex:

Mechanism that starts inspiration after lung deflation and then initiates deflation after inflation. The action is mediated by the vagus nerve in response to the stimuli of stretch receptors in the lungs. Of the two opposing effects, the one preventing overinflation is stronger. (In humans, the inherent rhythmicity of the respiratory center appears more important than these reflexes in controlling respiration.)

Heroin (Diacetylmorphine):

Powerful narcotic that is physically and psychologically addictive. One of the most abused drugs of this century, it was originally synthesized for use as an antitussive. Produced by a simple chemical alteration of morphine, its relative potency is 2.5 times that of morphine. *See* Narcotic.

Herpetic Neuralgia (Postherpetic Neuralgia):

Pain syndrome seen usually in older patients in which varicella zoster virus dormant for decades in posterior root ganglia begins to multiply and invades corresponding sensory nerves causing painful cutaneous lesions. Much local pain therapy such as direct injections or phenol intercostal nerve blocks, are not effective. Relief seems to be possible, at least in the early stages, by appropriate sympathetic nerve blocks.

Hertz (Hz):

Unit of frequency measurement equal to 1 cycle/second.

Hetastarch; Hydroxyethyl Starch (Hespan, Volex):

Synthetic colloidal polymer used as a plasma expander to replace circulating volume after large blood loss. It is administered by infusion as a 6% solution in 0.9% sodium chloride. Hetastarch has been associated with bleeding difficulties, interference with type and cross-match, and a low incidence of anaphylactoid reaction. *See* Dextran.

HETE (Hydroxyeicosatetraenoic Acid):

See Eicosanoids.

Heterologous Desensitization:

Type of desensitization that occurs when the continuous stimulation of a cell receptor with an agonist agent causes a decrease in the responsiveness of the cell to other agonists, as well as to the administered agent. *See* Homologous desensitization.

Hexachlorophene:

Phenol derivative (e.g., pHisoHex) that was popular as a skin antiseptic. Toxicity studies however, have cast enough doubt on the long-term use of hexachlorophene that its clinical use has been curtailed.

Hexadimethrine:

Drug that is clinically effective as a heparin antidote. It is not currently available for clinical use in the United States, although it has been used successfully as a protamine substitute when protamine is contraindicated.

Hexafluorenium (Mylaxen):

Skeletal muscle relaxant of the competitive (neuromuscular blocking) type that also inhibits plasma cholinesterase and prolongs the action of succinylcholine. It is given as an adjunct to succinylcholine to increase the duration of muscle paralysis and decrease the fasciculations. Its current use is limited.

Hexamethonium (C-6):

Ganglionic blocking agent originally used to decrease sympathetic tone, thereby lowering blood pressure. The drug is now considered obsolete and is used for experimental purposes only.

Hexobarbital (Evipal):

Intravenous barbiturate anesthetic that is more potent than thiopental. It is used as an ultrashort-acting sedative and hypnotic. *See* Barbiturate.

HFV:

See High-frequency ventilation.

Hiccup:

Involuntary spasm of the diaphragm associated with closure of the glottis. Its etiology is obscure but it appears to occur frequently during light anesthesia. Many methods have been proposed for terminating hiccups, as they can interfere with proper ventilation. The spasm can best be eradicated by deepening the anesthesia, less satisfactorily by increasing muscle relaxation.

High-Efficiency Particulate Air Filter:

See HEPA filter.

High-Frequency Ventilation (HFV):

Ventilation of the lungs at respiratory rates in excess of 60 times/minute. Experimentally, respiratory rates upward of 600 times/minute have been attempted. At such high rates tidal volume is dramatically decreased, almost invariably, to below deadspace volume. Despite this fact, researchers have reported excellent gas exchange and maintenance of arterial blood O_2 and CO_2 concentrations. It is believed that HFV causes a negligible increase in airway pressures and therefore does not produce the circulatory depression that can occur with conventional techniques. It is claimed that it is possible to impose HFV onto spontaneous respiration so it can assist ventilation without having to paralyze the patient. The three subcategories of HFV (delineated by the mechanical means used for ventilation) are high-frequency positive-pressure ventilation (HFPPV), high-frequency jet ventilation

(HFJV), and high frequency oscillation (HFO). One proposed mechanism of action for HFV is that it works by oscillating the air column in the tracheobronchial tree, thereby facilitating diffusion of O_2 downward and CO_2 upward without the actual mass movement of gas.

High Pressure Gas Nebulizer:

See Nebulizer.

High Threshold Mechano Receptors:

See Somatic pain.

High Voltage:

Term denoting voltage in excess of 650 V, usually used in reference to electric power generation or distribution.

Hi-Low Jet Tube:

Endotracheal tube with three lumens. The main lumen conventionally ventilates the patient. The second lumen is a clear one and is used for jet ventilation and administration of oxygen during suctioning and bronchoscopy. The third lumen is usually opaque and may be used for tracheal gas sampling and tracheal irrigation.

Hippocampus:

Stratified, curved structure bulging into the inferior horn of the lateral ventricle of the brain. The hippocampus, one of the deep structures of the limbic system, plays a primary role in olfaction and feeding behavior.

His Bundle:

See Heart, conduction system of.

His Bundle Electrocardiography:

See Electrocardiography, His bundle.

Histamine:

Naturally occurring substance widely distributed in the body. It can be found in high concentrations in blood (particularly within basophils and mast cells), skin, intestinal mucosa, and lungs. Although its functions are not well understood, it may act as a neurotransmitter. There appear to be at least two types of receptor for histamine: H_1 and H_2. H_1 receptors are located in the smooth muscles of the intestine, bronchi, and blood vessels. The classic antihistamines bind with this receptor. H_2 receptors are located in the smooth muscle of some blood vessels and in gastric parietal cells. Useful antagonists are cimetidine and ranitidine. Stimulated H_1 receptors generally cause contraction of small muscles and an increase in vascular permeability, whereas stimulated H_2 receptors cause an increase in gastric acid secretion and some vasodilatation. *See* Table. *See* Antihistamine.

303

Histamine: Structure of Histamine and Distribution of Histamine Receptors in the Body.

$$HC\!\!=\!\!C\!-\!CH_2\!-\!CH_2\!-\!NH_2$$

Histamine Receptor	Tissue	Antagonist
H_1	Smooth muscle of intestine, bronchi, blood vessels.	Classic antihistamines (diphenhydramine).
H_2	Gastric parietal cell. Smooth muscle of some blood vessels. Guinea pig atria. Rat uterus.	Cimetidine Metiamide Burimamide

Histiocyte:

See Macrophage.

Histogram (Frequency Histogram):

Graphic representation using a set of rectangles on an x-y axis to present a mass of data in a summarized and easily understandable form. Histograms are most often used to demonstrate the relative contribution of individual frequencies to a complex signal. *See* Figure.

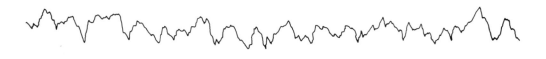

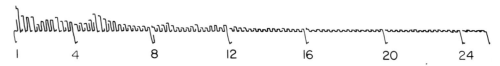

Histogram: Frequency histogram generated by fast Fourier analysis of an EEG signal.

Hives:

See Urticaria.

Hofmann Elimination:

Major means of terminating the neuromuscular blockade of specific muscle relaxants. The quaternary ammonium rings, on which the blockade depends, spontaneously rupture as the pH and temperature of the drug molecules equilibrate with the body. (A muscle relaxant, such as atracurium, is at refrigerated temperatures when administered and undergoes nonenzymatic degradation when its pH and temperature are equilibrated with the body.) *See* Atracurium.

Hole, Electrical:

See Carrier, electrical.

Homologous:

See Autologous.

Homologous Desensitization:

Type of desensitization in which stimulating a cell receptor with an agonist drug causes the cell to become more unresponsive to the administered drug only. *See* Heterologous desensitization.

Hormone:

Chemical substance that has a specific regulatory body function. In general, rapid adaptation to stimuli is mediated by the nervous system whereas slower adaptation to stimuli is mediated by hormones. A hormone may stimulate changes in the "target" organ or may directly affect the activities of all cells in the body. The major endocrine glands and the hormones they produce are as follows. (1) The anterior lobe of the pituitary (adenohypophysis) secretes human growth hormone, adrenocorticotropic hormone, thyroid-stimulating hormone, follicle-stimulating hormone, luteinizing hormone, prolactin, and melanocyte-stimulating hormone. (2) The posterior lobe of the pituitary (neurohypophysis) secretes but does not synthesize antidiuretic hormone and oxytocin. (3) The adrenal cortex secretes glucocorticoids, mineralocorticoids, and, in insignificant amounts, estrogen and androgen, the female and male sex hormones. (4) The adrenal medulla secretes epinephrine and norepinephrine. (5) The thyroid secretes thyroxine, triiodothyronine, and thyrocalcitonin. (6) The pancreas secretes insulin and glucagon. (7) The parathyroid secretes parathormone. (8) The testes secrete testosterone and limited amounts of estrogen. (9) The ovaries secrete estrogen, progesterone, and androgen. (10) The placenta, considered a temporary endocrine gland, secretes human chorionic gonadotropin, estrogen, progesterone, and human placental lactogen. The adrenal medulla and the adenohypophysis differ from the other endocrine glands in that they appear to secrete their hormones under direct nervous system control. For example, the adrenal medulla can be said to function like a secretory ganglion of the central nervous system, as the actions of epinephrine and norepinephrine are broad and the duration of their action is short.

Horner Syndrome:

Effects seen when the cervical sympathetic chain is successfully blocked by anesthetic injection (stellate ganglion block) or destroyed by disease (apical lung tumors). Miosis, ptosis, and exophthalmos are present on the affected side and comprise the original triad of

Horner syndrome. Other changes seen on the affected side are reduced sweating, blockage of the nose due to congestion of the nasal mucosa, and flushing of the skin.

Horsepower (HP):

Unit of power in the foot-pound-second system in which 1 HP is equal to moving 550 lb 1 foot vertically in 1 second. One horsepower also equals 746 watts.

Hospital Oxygen Supply:

Overall term for bulk oxygen storage and delivery in the hospital environment. Small institutions use banks of G or H oxygen cylinders, whereas larger institutions use liquid oxygen bulk storage in a single location external to the building. *See* Liquid oxygen.

Hot Spot Imaging:

See Technetium 99(^{99}Tc); Technetium 99m (^{99m}Tc) pyrophosphate.

Hot Versus Cold Electrical Circuits:

Convention used fpr describing electrical power circuits. The cold side of the circuit (connected to a ground) is the conductor distal to the equipment using the electrical power. The hot side is the conductor proximal to the equipment. The conductors are usually in a single cord separated by an insulator. *See* Ground; Grounding.

Hot Wire Respirometer:

See Anemometer, hot wire.

Howard Jones Solution (Jones Solution):

Proprietary solution of dibucaine that was commonly used for hypobaric spinal anesthesia.

Howland Lock:

Device that fits between the handle and the blade of a laryngoscope. It changes the angle between the handle and the blade. It is worthwhile in patients with a receding mandible or other abnormalities of the head and neck.

HP:

See Horsepower.

Huffman Prism:

Plastic lens-like device that attaches to the proximal end of the Macintosh laryngoscope blade, allowing better vision of those structures near the tip of the blade.

Hum:

Unwanted tone or series of tones heard in the output of an audio circuit. It is caused by extraneous alternating currents generated by the coupling of the audio circuit with nearby power lines. It is an example of incidental capacitance or inductance.

Human Immunodeficiency Virus:

See AIDS.

Human Immune Response:

Vastly complicated series of cellular and molecular responses whose purpose is to distinguish "self" from "nonself" and to clear the "nonself" foreign material or antigens from the body. "Nonself" entities include bacteria, viruses, transplanted organs or cancer cells. The precise mechanisms are still incompletely understood. However, there are two major components of the immune system response: the nonspecific and the specific. These components are further divided into cellular and humoral. The nonspecific immune response can detect a wide range of entities. The specific components seek out specific targets and require prior sensitization to work appropriately. Anesthetic agents have been implicated as interfering with the human immune system at various stages. *See* Figures.

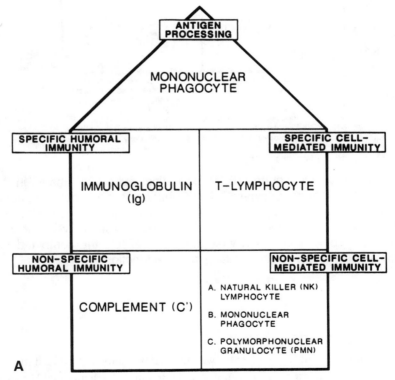

Human Immune Response: (A) Five functional components of the immune response: antigen processing, specific humoral immunity, specific cell-mediated immunity, nonspecific humoral immunity, and nonspecific cell-mediated immunity.

307

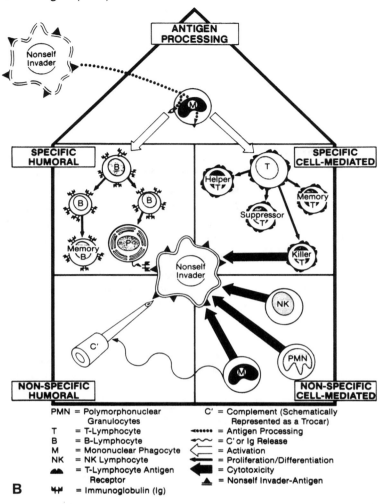

B

PMN = Polymorphonuclear Granulocytes
T = T-Lymphocyte
B = B-Lymphocyte
M = Mononuclear Phagocyte
NK = NK Lymphocyte
= T-Lymphocyte Antigen Receptor
= Immunoglobulin (Ig)

C' = Complement (Schematically Represented as a Trocar)
= Antigen Processing
= C' or Ig Release
= Activation
= Proliferation/Differentiation
= Cytotoxicity
= Nonself Invader-Antigen

Human Immune Response *(continued):* (B) Participating leukocyte subsets in the overall immune response: mononuclear phagocytes; B,T, NK phagocytes; and polymorphonuclear granulocytes (PMN). (C) Principal activities of biological response modifiers (BRM), including their leukocyte subset sources. (D) Effects of anesthetic agents (primarily halothane) on in vitro function of immune components. The in vivo summary reflects the combined effects of both anesthetic agents and surgery on postoperative immune function.

Human Placental Lactogen (HPL):

Protein hormone of low molecular weight (21,600 daltons) produced in large amounts by the placenta. It has a half-life of less than 30 minutes. High and low HPL levels have been documented to be associated with various obstetric syndromes and complications, and it appears to correlate with placental function and possibly be a predictor of placental fetal risk.

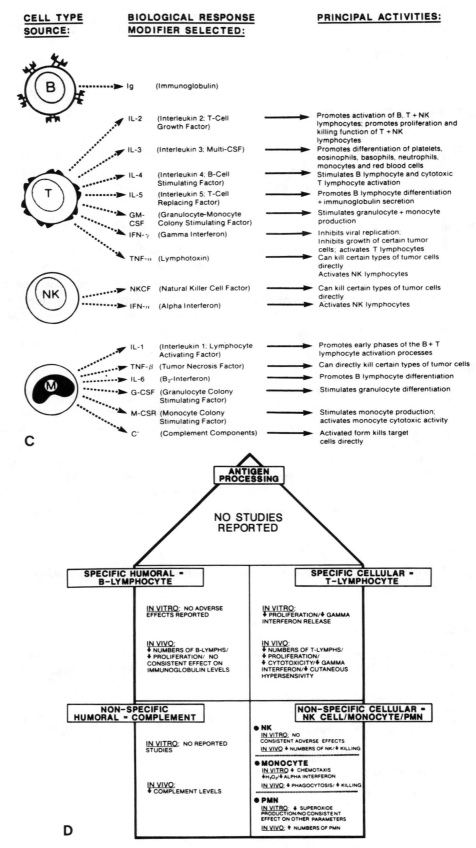

CELL TYPE SOURCE:	BIOLOGICAL RESPONSE MODIFIER SELECTED:		PRINCIPAL ACTIVITIES:

B ····> Ig (Immunoglobulin)

T
- IL-2 (Interleukin 2; T-Cell Growth Factor) → Promotes activation of B, T + NK lymphocytes; promotes proliferation and killing function of T + NK lymphocytes
- IL-3 (Interleukin 3; Multi-CSF) → Promotes differentiation of platelets, eosinophils, basophils, neutrophils, monocytes and red blood cells
- IL-4 (Interleukin 4; B-Cell Stimulating Factor) → Stimulates B lymphocyte and cytotoxic T lymphocyte activation
- IL-5 (Interleukin 5; T-Cell Replacing Factor) → Promotes B lymphocyte differentiation + immunoglobulin secretion
- GM-CSF (Granulocyte-Monocyte Colony Stimulating Factor) → Stimulates granulocyte + monocyte production
- IFN-γ (Gamma Interferon) → Inhibits viral replication; Inhibits growth of certain tumor cells; activates T lymphocytes
- TNF-α (Lymphotoxin) → Can kill certain types of tumor cells directly; Activates NK lymphocytes

NK
- NKCF (Natural Killer Cell Factor) → Can kill certain types of tumor cells directly
- IFN-α (Alpha Interferon) → Activates NK lymphocytes

M
- IL-1 (Interleukin 1; Lymphocyte Activating Factor) → Promotes early phases of the B + T lymphocyte activation processes
- TNF-β (Tumor Necrosis Factor) → Can directly kill certain types of tumor cells
- IL-6 (B₂-Interferon) → Promotes B lymphocyte differentiation
- G-CSF (Granulocyte Colony Stimulating Factor) → Stimulates granulocyte differentiation
- M-CSR (Monocyte Colony Stimulating Factor) → Stimulates monocyte production; activates monocyte cytotoxic activity
- C' (Complement Components) → Activated form kills target cells directly

C

ANTIGEN PROCESSING

NO STUDIES REPORTED

SPECIFIC HUMORAL – B-LYMPHOCYTE

IN VITRO: NO ADVERSE EFFECTS REPORTED

IN VIVO: ↓ NUMBERS OF B-LYMPHS/ ↓ PROLIFERATION/ NO CONSISTENT EFFECT ON IMMUNOGLOBULIN LEVELS

SPECIFIC CELLULAR – T-LYMPHOCYTE

IN VITRO: ↓ PROLIFERATION/↓ GAMMA INTERFERON RELEASE

IN VIVO: ↓ NUMBERS OF T-LYMPHS/ ↓ PROLIFERATION/ ↓ CYTOTOXICITY/↓ GAMMA INTERFERON/↓ CUTANEOUS HYPERSENSIVITY

NON-SPECIFIC HUMORAL - COMPLEMENT

IN VITRO: NO REPORTED STUDIES

IN VIVO: ↓ COMPLEMENT LEVELS

NON-SPECIFIC CELLULAR – NK CELL/MONOCYTE/PMN

● NK
IN VITRO: NO CONSISTENT ADVERSE EFFECTS
IN VIVO ↓ NUMBERS OF NK/↓ KILLING

● MONOCYTE
IN VITRO: ↓ CHEMOTAXIS ↓H₂O₂/↓ ALPHA INTERFERON
IN VIVO: ↓ PHAGOCYTOSIS/↓ KILLING

● PMN
IN VITRO: ↓ SUPEROXIDE PRODUCTION/NO CONSISTENT EFFECT ON OTHER PARAMETERS
IN VIVO: ↑ NUMBERS OF PMN

D

Human Immune Response *(continued)*.

Human Review Committee:

See Human Subjects Review Committee.

Human Subjects Review Committee:

Internal group of individuals in a health care institution who must review all human research protocols to verify that no standards of humane research are violated. It has its counterpart in the Animal Research Review Committee, which does the same thing for research projects concerning animals.

Humidifier:

Apparatus that both supplies and maintains desired water vapor levels in the air. It is used in operating rooms to maintain a minimal relative humidity of 50–60% (a level that ensures continuous discharge of built-up static charges). It is also used on anesthesia machines and ventilators to add water vapor to the dry fresh gas flow, keeping the respiratory tract moist and secretions loose and preventing the patient (particularly small children) from losing moisture from the respiratory tract. *See* Nebulizer; Vaporizer.

Humidity:

Measure of the degree of dampness in the form of water vapor found in room air or in a breathing circuit. Relative humidity is the ratio of the amount of water vapor present in the air to the maximum amount possible at the same temperature. Humidity depends on temperature, i.e., the warmer a gas mass the more water vapor it can hold. If the gas mass is saturated with water vapor and suddenly cooled, water droplets form. Fully saturated air at 37°C contains 44 mg water vapor/L which exerts 47 mm Hg partial pressure. Fully saturated air at room temperature contains water at approximately 24 mg/L, which means that 20 mg of water must be added to each liter of inspired gas to saturate it fully.

Hunting:

Continuous attempts made by automatic control mechanisms to find and maintain a desired equilibrium.

Hustead Epidural Needle:

Needle with a rounded point used for epidural anesthesia. The point directs a catheter up or down the epidural space depending on needle position. *See* Epidural needle; Spinal needle.

HVR:

See Hypoxic ventilatory response.

Hyaline Membrane Disease:

See Infant respiratory distress syndrome.

Hyaluronidase:

Soluble enzyme found in some animal tissues (and in some malignant human tissues). Hyaluronidase for injection, prepared from mammalian testes, is reported to promote drug absorption and diffusion, by breaking down intracellular sibstrate.

Hydrate Crystal Theory of Anesthesia (Clathrate Theory):

Theory stating that an anesthetic effect is produced by anesthetic molecules organizing water molecules to form hydrated microcrystals (clathrates), which interfere with the excitability of neurons. No experimental evidence exists to confirm this action of anesthetics, and the theory remains unproved.

Hydrocephalus:

Excessive or abnormal accumulation of cerebrospinal fluid (CSF) in the ventricles of the brain. The skull may become enlarged, and the brain may atrophy. Hydrocephalus, which may be congenital or acquired, can be classified as either communicating or noncommunicating, depending on whether the CSF in the lateral ventricles is in communication with the lumbar subarachnoid space. With communicating hydrocephalus the ventricles are not obstructed and the CSF passes out of the brain into the spinal canal but is not absorbed by the subarachnoid villi. With noncommunicating hydrocephalus, there is an obstruction of the aqueduct of Sylvius to the fourth ventricle caused by scarring, malformation, or posterior fossa hemorrhage. It can also occur because of obstruction of the foramens of Magendie and Luschka (Dandy-Walker syndrome) blocking flow to the subarachnoid space. Hydrocephalus is treated in an attempt to prevent brain damage caused by progressive encroachment of the ventricles on the brain mass. It requires insertion of a Silastic shunt from the ventricles to the peritoneal cavity or, infrequently, to the right atrium. Prognosis is favorable for those infants without brain deformities who have shunts placed prior to brain damage. The shunt becomes a permanent part of the patient; it must be replaced if it becomes infected and lengthened as the patient grows. *See* Figure.

Hydrocortisone:

See Corticosteroid.

Hydrogen:

Colorless, odorless, tasteless gas that is the lightest chemical element. It is flammable and explosive when combined with air. The hydrogen ion concentration is an index of the relative acidity of a solution. Hydrogen, which has an atomic number of 1, is a constituent of water and of nearly all organic compounds. The three isotopes of hydrogen—protium, deuterium, and tritium—are all naturally occurring. *See* Acid-base balance.

Hydrometer:

Flotation instrument for determining the relative density or specific gravity of a liquid.

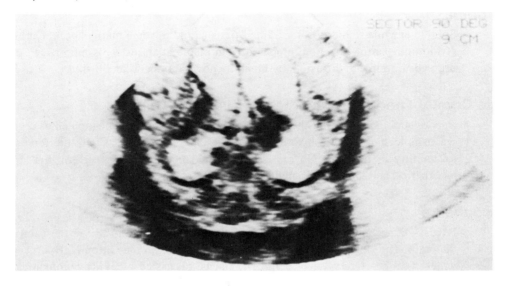

Hydrocephalus: Ultrasound demonstration of the enlarged ventricles of hydrocephalus.

Hydromorphone (Dilaudid):

Semisynthetic derivative of morphine used as a narcotic analgesic. It is approximately 10 times more potent than morphine.

Hydrophilic:

See Lipophilic.

Hydroxydione (Viadril):

Mildly potent steroid preparation used as a general anesthetic. It is not currently available for clinical use in the United States.

5-Hydroxytryptamine (5-HT):

See Serotonin.

Hydroxyzine (Atarax, Vistaril):

Synthetic compound closely related to the antihistamine drugs. It is an antianxiety drug with antiemetic properties and produces drowsiness. It is a useful preanesthetic medication.

Hyoscine:

See Scopolamine.

Hyperalgesia:

Phenomenon that occurs when a pain pathway becomes excessively and easily excitable. It may be primary, such as reimpacting a stubbed toe or secondary, usually from lesions in the spinal cord or thalamus.

Hyperalimentation:

See Amigen.

Hyperbaric Chamber:

See Hyperbaric oxygen therapy.

Hyperbaric Oxygen Therapy:

Treatment modality using high-pressure O_2. The patient is placed in a chamber of great structural strength within which O_2 pressure can be contained at two to three times atmospheric pressure. At high pressure more O_2 dissolves in blood and tissue, so its content increases. The driving pressure differential for O_2 is raised, allowing it to reach into areas of low PO_2. Current indications for hyperbaric O_2 therapy include gas gangrene, CO poisoning, and acute arterial insufficiency.

Hyperbaric Solution:

Hypertonic solution used in spinal anesthesia. Its specific gravity is greater than that of cerebrospinal fluid. *See* Hypobaric solution.

Hyperbaric Technique:

See Hyperbaric oxygen therapy.

Hyperbarism:

Deleterious condition resulting from exposure to atmospheric pressures that are higher than the pressures within the body.

Hypercapnia (Hypercarbia):

Excessive amount of CO_2 in the blood. It refers to an increase in CO_2 arterial tension above 44 mm Hg. *See* Hyperpnea; Hypoxic ventilatory response.

Hypercapnic Ventilatory Response (HCVR):

Reflexive response causing a rise in minute ventilation when there is a rise in inspired carbon dioxide. *See* Hypoxic ventilatory response.

Hyperesthesia:

Abnormal increase in sensitivity to sensory stimuli.

Hyperglycemia:

Excess glucose in the circulating blood. Can be due to relative insulin resistance, insulin lack, or overenthusiastic short-term intravenous therapy. Stress and trauma cause body mechanisms to tend toward hyperglycemia. Acute changes caused by hyperglycemia are osmotic in nature and result in, for example, osmotic diuresis. *See* Diabetes mellitus.

Hyperinsulinemia:

Excess of insulin in the blood. The condition can be caused by islet cell tumors, injection of excess insulin, or ingestion of sulfonylureas (which stimulate the islet tissue to secrete insulin). Hyperinsulinemia almost invariably leads to hypoglycemia.

Hyperosmolar Nonketotic Coma:

Cause for obtundation, usually in the elderly when remarkably high blood glucose levels and profound dehydration cause CNS disturbances partially by osmotic changes.

Hyperpathia:

Exaggerated subjective response to noxious or painful stimuli. The patient may incorrectly localize or identify a stimulus and perceive the pain as radiating from nonstimulated areas.

Hyperpnea:

Ventilatory increase that is proportional to an increase in CO_2 production. It is seen in moderate exercise states. Can also be rapid deep breathing due to brain injury. *See* Cheyne-Stokes respiration.

Hyperpolarization:

Brief increase in electrical charge across excitable membranes. This period of greater than normal polarization follows membrane depolarization, which in turn is followed by the return to normal polarization. *See* Action potential; Depolarization.

Hyperpyrexia:

Extreme elevation of body temperature. *See* Malignant hyperthermia.

Hyperstat:

See Diazoxide.

Hypertension:

Condition in which the arterial blood pressure (particularly diastolic pressure) is higher than the norm for the age of the patient. It may be idiopathic or may be associated with other diseases (e.g., pheochromocytoma or renal parenchymal disease). *See* Arterial blood pressure.

Hypertension, Essential:

See Essential hypertension.

Hypertonic Solution:

In biologic terms, a fluid having an osmotic pressure that is greater than that of another standard solution, usually blood. For spinal anesthesia (cerebrospinal fluid [CSF]) is the standard solution. When cells are surrounded by a hypertonic solution, a net flow of water out of the cells results.

Hypertrophic Cardiomyopathy:

Genetically transmitted increase in the mass of the ventricle that can result in obstruction of left ventricular outflow. It is often referred to as idiopathic hypertrophic subaortic stenosis (IHSS), which manifests as asymmetric hypertrophy of the interventricular septum. This type of obstruction tends to be malignant as the left ventricular outflow tract becomes progressively occluded, and ultimately left ventricular failure occurs.

Hyperventilation:

Augmented ventilation disproportionate to CO_2 production. An increased amount of air enters the alveoli resulting in a decrease of CO_2 tension and ultimately alkalosis. Prolonged voluntary hyperventilation is often used as a test for epilepsy or tetany. *See* Epilepsy.

Hypervolemia:

Abnormally increased volume of body fluids.

Hypnosis:

Altered state of consciousness in which an individual accepts suggestions. An alternate view states that the individual's power to criticize is either partially or fully suppressed during hypnosis. It is postulated that the power of criticism is largely a function of the conscious mind and is therefore bypassed in the hypnotic state. Hypnosis theoretically deals with the unconscious mind (that portion of the mind which constantly influences thought and behavior, although an individual is normally unaware of its presence). In many ways, the state of clinical anesthesia and the state of hypnosis are similar in that both deal with the brain, can be easily demonstrated and described, and are poorly understood. It is a demonstrable fact, however, that in certain individuals deep hypnotic states can completely replace pharmacologic anesthesia for the suppression of noxious stimuli. In clinical terms, it is important to remember that practical hypnosis and pharmacologic anesthesia can be used as adjuncts to one another. For example, the induction of general anesthesia by inhalation can be made smoother in all patients if it is accompanied by a hypnotic state suggesting concentration on quiet, even respirations.

Hypnotic Drug:

Compound that produces central nervous system depression resembling normal sleep. *See* Table.

Hypobaric Solution:

Hypotonic solution used for spinal anesthesia. The specific gravity of the drug is less than that of cerebrospinal fluid. *See* Hyperbaric solution.

Hypnotic drugs: Approximate serum half-lives of sedative hypnotic drugs.

Generic Name	Trade Name	Half Life (Hours)
Barbiturates		
Amobarbital	Amytal	8–42
Amobarbital Na	Amytal Sodium	8–42
Aprobarbital	Alurate	14–34
Butabarbital Na	Butisol Sodium	34–42
Butalbital	Sandoptal	
Hexobarbital	Sombulex	2.7–7
Mephobarbital	Mebaral	11–67
Pentobarbital	Nembutal	15–48
Pentobarbital	Luminal, Sodium	80–120
Secobarbital	Seconal Sodium	15–45
Talbutal	Lotusate	
Benzodiazepines		
Chlordiazepoxide	Librium, others	5–15
Clorazepate (dipotassium)	Tranxene, others	50–80
Diazepam	Valium, others	30–60
Flurazepam HC1	Dalmane, others	50–100
Lorazepam	Ativan, others	10–20
Oxazepam	Serax, others	5–10
Temazepam	Restoril, others	10–17
Triazolam	Halcion	2–4

Hypocapnia (Hypocarbia):

Deficiency of CO_2 in the blood. It refers to a decrease in arterial CO_2 tension below 36 mm Hg.

Hypoesthesia:

Diminished sensitivity to stimulation of the skin or sense organ.

Hypoglossal Nerve:

See Cranial nerves.

Hypoglycemia:

Condition in which the glucose concentration in the blood is below normal. The patient may exhibit hyperactivity, sweating, skin pallor, confusion, bizarre behavior, or obtundation.

Hypokalemic Periodic Paralysis:

See Familial periodic paralysis.

Hypophysectomy:

Surgical removal of the pituitary gland. It is commonly performed through an oral incision, a procedure that causes mild chronic anxiety on the part of the anesthetist because of the proximity of the surgical site to the endotracheal tube.

Hypotension:

Arterial blood pressure that is lower than normal for the age and level of physical activity of the patient. It may be seen during shock. Hypotension per se is not a disease and is not considered harmful unless it leads to inadequate tissue perfusion, which can be demonstrated by the onset of metabolic acidosis or, more subtly, by derangement of central nervous system function. The conventional treatment includes position change to increase cardiac return, fluid administration to increase circulating volume, and administration of vasoconstrictors to decrease peripheral blood pooling.

Hypothalamus:

Deep part of the brain forming the floor and part of the lateral wall of the third ventricle. It includes the mamillary bodies, tuber cinereum, infundibulum, and optic chiasm. Through the autonomic nervous system, the hypothalamus appears to control or regulate visceral functions (mostly related to homeostasis), such as systemic temperature control, food and fluid intake, heart rate, movement of food through the digestive tract, and stimulation or inhibition of the anterior pituitary gland.

Hypothermia:

Subnormal body temperature. This condition may be either deliberately induced or accidental, e.g., environmental. Hypothermia lowers metabolism and the need for O_2 (helpful during cardiac surgery). Under these circumstances, the blood pressure is reduced and bleeding is minimal. At 28°C the basal metabolic rate is reduced by approximately 50%; at 18°C the basal metabolic rate is reduced by approximately 87%. However, below 30°C spontaneous ventricular fibrillation becomes an increased hazard. As the body cools, the electroencephalogram shows a less active pattern. At 30°C, the O_2 consumption of the brain is decreased by 50%; at 25°C the O_2 consumption is reduced by 75%. At 15°C the brain can go without circulation for approximately 45 minutes. Hypothermia can be accomplished by surface cooling (which is inefficient) or by extracorporeal circulation (heart-lung machine) of the blood volume through a heat exchanger. Anesthesia must be deep enough so shivering is inhibited. Deliberate or inadvertent lowering of body temperature below 15°C is called supercooling (profound hypothermia). *See* Cardiopulmonary bypass; Heat exchanger.

Hypothermic Subarachnoid Irrigation:

See Cold saline injection.

Hypotonic Solution:

The opposite of hypertonic solution. *See* Hypertonic solution.

Hypoventilation:

Ventilation reduced enough to be insufficient in rate or total volume to maintain alveolar O_2 tension and eliminate CO_2 (PaO_2 falls, and $PaCO_2$ rises).

Hypovolemia:

Abnormally diminished volume of body fluids, particularly in the intravascular space.

Hypovolemic Shock:

See Shock.

Hypoxia:

Relative lack of O_2 transported to or used by the tissues. Often used interchangeably with the term "anoxia." There are four classical types of hypoxia: (1) Anemic hypoxia is a relative lack of O_2 in the tissues due to a reduction of the O_2-carrying capacity of the blood. It is usually caused by an insufficient amount of hemoglobin (Hb) in red blood cells. (2) Anoxic hypoxia is a relative lack of O_2 delivered to the tissues due to insufficient oxygenation of Hb in the lungs. (3) Histotoxic hypoxia is a relative lack of O_2 due to impaired ability of the tissues to use O_2, e.g., cyanide toxicity. (4) Stagnant (ischemic) hypoxia is a relative lack of O_2 due to a too-slow delivery of oxygenated blood to the tissues, which does not compensate for O_2 uptake and usage. *See* Figure.

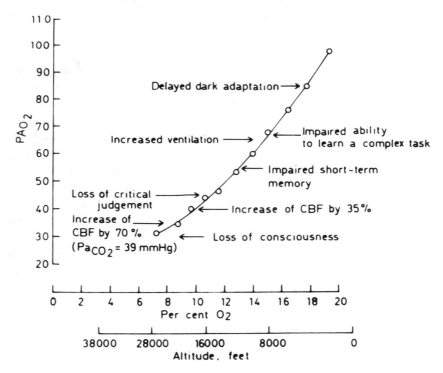

Hypoxia: Influence of inspired O_2 concentration on PaO_2 in humans as well as on some symptoms of and physiologic responses to hypoxia.

Hypoxic Pulmonary Vasoconstriction:

Homeostatic mechanism that occurrs in the lungs in areas that have reduced oxygen tension. The pulmonary vessels in these areas constrict which diverts blood to areas with greater oxygen tension and therefore tends to reduce arterial hypoxemia. This hypoxic pulmonary vasoconstriction is inhibited by inhalational anesthetics. *See* Figure. *See* Hypoxic shunt.

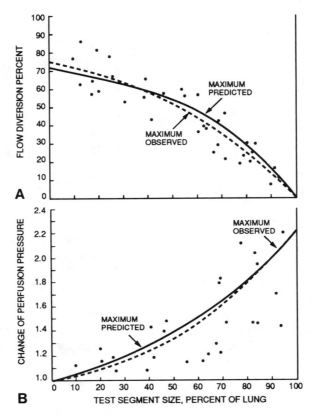

Hypoxic Pulmonary Vasoconstriction: Influence of fraction of lung hypoxia on HPV in canine lung. The dual response of: (A) flow diversion and (B) perfusion pressure change is shown when different size lung segments are stimulated with maximum hypoxia while the rest of the lung receives 100% oxygen. In both figures, the solid circles are the values for individual dogs and the dashed lines represent the best fit curves for these observations.

Hypoxic Shunt:

Physiologic response of normal lung tissue triggered by a sharp decrease in inspired O_2 tension. This effect is best seen experimentally when a hypoxic gas mixture is administered to only one lung. The pulmonary vascular resistance of the hypoxic lung rises, thereby shunting blood to the normal lung. The effect may occur in small areas of the lung after regional airway obstruction. The shunted fraction of pulmonary blood flow may rise for many hours before peaking. The peak is reached faster in younger individuals with healthy lungs. *See* Hypoxic pulmonary vasoconstriction.

Hypoxic Ventilatory Response (HVR):

Increase in minute ventilation seen as a response to decreased oxygen content in inspired gas. *See* Figure. *See* Hypercapnia; Hyperpnea.

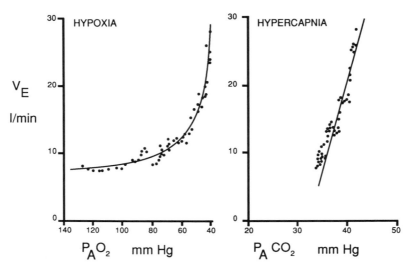

Hypoxic Ventilatory Response: Normal ventilatory responses to hypoxia and hypercapnia are displayed with each data point representing mean value for end-tidal gas tension and ventilation for three successive breaths. Goodness of fit can be seen by noting relationship between observed data points and computed curve.

Hyskon:

A brand name for a 32% solution of Dextran 70. *See* Dextran.

Hysteresis, Lung:

Demonstration of the effect of lung surfactant. It is a phenomenon seen in the laboratory in an isolated lung that is first degassed, then inflated with air to its maximum volume, and then deflated. The relation between pressure and volume is different on the inflation curve from what it is on the deflation curve. For a given pressure, the volume of the lung is greater during deflation than inflation. This separation of the curves of inflation and deflation is termed hysteresis. Hysteresis is caused by surface forces at the air-liquid interface that exist in the air-filled lung. Evidence for this explanation is that when the degassed lung is filled and emptied with a liquid hysteresis is negligible. *See* Figure. *See* Surfactant.

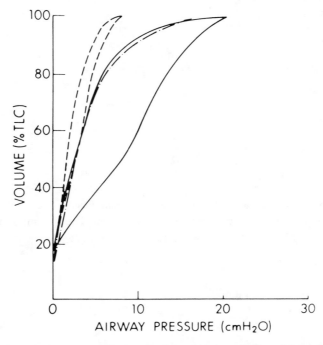

Hysteresis, Lung: Pressure-volume relation in the adult lung inflated from Vmin by air (solid line) and by liquid (dashed line).

H Zone:

See Actomyosin.

I

I²R Loss:

Form of power loss measured in watts and dissipated as heat because of the flow of current (I) through a conductor, e.g., machine or transformer. The amount of heat generated within a machine may be calculated if the current and resistance (R) are known.

IABP:

See Intraaortic balloon pump.

IARS:

See International Anesthesia Research Society.

Iatrogenic:

Term applied to any adverse condition that occurs as the result of treatment by a health care worker. A sore throat after intubation of the trachea is an example of an iatrogenic complication.

IC:

See Circuit, integrated.

ICD:

See International Classification of Diseases.

ICT:

See Isovolumic contraction time.

ICU:

See Intensive Care Unit.

Ideal Gas:

Theoretic entity that perfectly obeys the Boyle law, Charles law, Joule law of internal energy, Dalton law of partial pressure, and Avogadro hypothesis. Actual gases obey these laws only as their pressure approaches toward zero.

I/E Ratio:

Ratio of the time for inspiration versus expiration. Because it is a slow, passive process (particularly in the patient on a ventilator), expiration should be given as much of the breathing cycle time as possible. The minimum expiratory time should be equal to the inspiratory time. Many ventilators have an I/E ratio control that can be preset at 1:1, 1:2, or 1:3. As the respiratory rate increases, the time available per minute for expiration decreases. High ventilatory rates are often precluded by the requirement that expiration time be (at least) equal to inspiration time.

Idiopathic Hypertrophic Subaortic Stenosis (IHSS):

See Hypertrophic cardiomyopathy.

Ignition Temperature:

Temperature to which a fuel/air or fuel/O_2 mixture must be raised to start deflagration.

IHSS:

See Idiopathic hypertrophic subaortic stenosis.

Image Intensifier:

Device that combines the capabilities of x-rays and television (TV) to produce an image with minimal radiation exposure to the patient. With conventional x-ray techniques, a relatively large amount of radiation must be used to "expose" an x-ray plate. With an image intensifier, only a low dose of radiation is necessary to penetrate the patient and then strike a fluorescent screen. This screen is scanned by a television camera, the signal output of which is amplified, increased in contrast, and displayed on a TV monitor. The key to the technique is the electronic amplification provided by the TV technology.

Impedance:

See Bypass capacitor.

Impedance Plethysmography:

Measurement of cardiac output or tissue volume changes of a body part based on the detected alterations in electrical impedance between two surface electrodes. A constant difference in voltage is maintained between the electrodes. As the impedance of tissue varies, owing to the ingress and egress of blood, current flow changes between the electrodes and is related to cardiac output or volume changes. *See* Ohm law.

Implant Tested (IT):

See Z-79.

Implied Consent:

Legal term relating to the inferred approval by a patient for medical intervention during emergency situations. Although the patient is unable to communicate, it is assumed that he or she would agree to the necessary treatment. In addition, a patient may imply consent by his or her actions, e.g., by extending an arm, consent is given for palpating the pulse.

Implied Contract:

See Contract.

Impurities, Electrical:

Naturally occurring or deliberately implanted foreign atom found in semiconductors. Impurities fundamentally affect basic electrical conductivity. The technique of implanting impurities is called doping. *See* Doping.

IMV:

See Intermittent mandatory ventilation.

Inactivated Channel:

See Ion channel.

Inappropriate Antidiuretic Hormone (ADH) Secretion Syndrome (also Syndrome Of Antidiuretic Hormone Secretion, or SIADH):

Disorder in which an abnormal amount of ADH is excreted, leading to water retention with respect to body fluid osmolality. It is frequently associated with small cell carcinoma (oat cell variant) of the lung, or a variety of pulmonary and central nervous system disorders, or it may be idiopathic. *See* Antidiuretic hormone.

Inapsine:

See Droperidol.

Incandescence:

Emission of visible radiation from a substance at high temperatures.

Independent Lung Ventilation:

Sophisticated form of mechanical ventilation in which a double-lumen tube allows two ventilators to be used on one patient with each ventilating one lung. Coordination of the two ventilators can be difficult, and problems include mechanical movement of the intrathoracic contents if the lungs are significantly different in resistance and compliance. *See* Compliance; Ventilator.

Independent Variable:

Quantity the value of which bears no direct relation to any other variables of concern. For example, the time of day is an independent variable when plotting a patient's pulse rate.

Inderal:

See Propranolol.

Indicator Dye:

pH-sensitive chemical used to determine the exhaustion point of CO_2 absorbers. Some indicators are phenolphthalein, ethyl violet, ethyl yellow, ethyl orange, mimosa Z, brilliant yellow, and MN extra dye concentrate. *See* Absorption indicator.

Indifferent Electrode:

See Dispersive electrode; Electrostatic unit.

Indirect Monitor:

See Noninvasive monitor.

Indocyanine Green (Cardio-Green):

Dye injected for the measurement of cardiac output by the dye dilution technique. *See* Cardiac output.

Inductance:

Resistance a coil offers to an alternating current because of the creation of a magnetic field surrounding the coil. Capacitance, simple resistance, and inductance together constitute electrical impedance. *See* Capacitance, electronic; Impedance.

Induction:

Period during anesthetic administration that starts at the time the first drug is administered until the desired depth of the anesthetic state is reached. Various subcategories of induction exist. Inhalation induction refers to the steady increase of anesthetic vapor concentration delivered to a patient's airways. Intravenous (IV) induction is the IV administration of an anesthetic agent in a stepwise or continuous infusion. Routine induction implies that the drug administration occurs in a controlled and incremental manner. Crash induction (rapid sequence induction) involves the administration (usually IV) of a single overwhelming dose of anesthetic, commonly with a neuromuscular blocking agent, in order to gain control of the patient's respiration and reflexes as rapidly as possible. Crash induction is indicated in a patient with a full stomach in whom regurgitation and aspiration of gastric contents would be a possibility with prolonged induction. However, it is important to remember that crash induction involves increased risk, as there is a concurrent stepwise change in the vital signs. *See* Sellick maneuver.

Induction Heating:

Method of producing heat in a conducting material by passing a high current through it.

Inductive Coupling:

Transfer of signal or electrical current by the magnetic field created by current passing through a coil impinging on another electrical conductor. A transformer is the simplest example of this electrical phenomenon.

Infant Apnea Syndrome:

See Sudden infant death syndrome.

Infant Respiratory Distress Syndrome (IRDS; Hyaline Membrane Disease):

Major cause of death in premature infants. The immature lung does not manufacture sufficient quantities of surfactant to reduce alveolar fluid surface tension in order to stabilize the alveoli. The air sacs collapse on expiration producing atelectasis, and the infant becomes cyanotic and hypoxic. Prediction of whether a premature infant will develop IRDS is based on the ratio of lecithin, a major component of surfactant, to sphingomyelin in the amniotic fluid. If the ratio is higher than 2:1, the probability that the infant will have IRDS is less than 10%. Infants with severe IRDS require long-term intensive care. *See* Adult respiratory distress syndrome; Surfactant.

Infarct:

Area of tissue necrosis caused by local obstruction of the arterial blood supply. This obstruction is usually an embolus or thrombus, and the actual cause of the tissue necrosis is insufficient oxygenation. *See* Myocardial infarction.

Inferior Vena Cava Syndrome:

See Aortocaval syndrome.

Inflow Occlusion:

Technique used during myocardial surgery. A snare is placed around the superior and inferior vena cavae and the pulmonary veins to prevent flow of blood into the heart. At normal body temperature, approximately 3 minutes of surgical time is available before cardiac damage occurs; at 30°C, 8 minutes is available. The technique has generally been abandoned in favor of extracorporeal circulation, which provides more surgical time and better operating conditions. *See* Cardiopulmonary bypass.

Information Theory:

Mathematic technique concerned with the analysis of parameters involved in information acquisition and handling.

Informed Consent:

Legal doctrine that every patient must understand the potential complications of any procedure before it is performed. To give informed consent for anesthesia, a patient must be aware it is conceivable that the anesthetic process could result in debility, disfigurement, or death. *See* Consent form; Lay standard rule.

Infraclavicular Axillary Vein:

The main return from the upper extremities to the central circulation and is proposed as an easy access site for central venous pressure monitoring.

Infrared Analyzer:

Device for measuring the content of a particular gas in a gaseous mixture. It is most useful for the quantification of N_2O and CO_2, as both of these gases absorb infrared light of a specific band proportional to their concentration with correctable overlap. *See* Halothane analyzer.

Infrared Radiation (IR):

Part of the electromagnetic spectrum that transfers heat energy from its source to its surroundings. *See* Electromagnetic spectrum.

Infrasound:

Automated device for determining arterial blood pressure. The principle involves detection and amplification of sounds (in a frequency range below human hearing) created by turbulent blood flow past a deflating cuff. It is favored for pediatric and low arterial pressure situations. *See* Arterial blood pressure; Sound.

Inhalation Anesthesia:

Administration of volatilized pharmacologic agents via the respiratory tract for the purpose of producing anesthesia. The outstanding advantage of administering drugs in this manner is that they can be retrieved by the same route so long as respiration is maintained. It, of course, presupposes that the drugs are neither metabolized nor excreted via another route in the body. Inhalation administration allows drugs to reach the central circulation rapidly and appear on the arterial side of the circulation faster than by intravenous injection. Significant disadvantages of inhalation anesthesia include the necessity of complex and sophisticated equipment to ensure controlled administration. Inhalation anesthesia also requires manipulation of the upper airway. In addition, if the agent used is a liquid, it must have a vapor pressure at room temperature high enough to ensure administration of a therapeutic dose. *See* Halothane.

Inhaler:

Apparatus for vaporizing liquids that will be inhaled. When used for analgesia, it is a simple device with a fixed upper limit of output and can therefore be safely used for self-administration. *See* Goldman vaporizer.

Inhibition of Oxidation:

Theory that attempts to explain the action of general anesthetics. It states that anesthetics primarily inhibit the utilization of O_2. (The theory is more an observation than an explanation of the anesthetic mechanism.)

Inhibitor:

Agent that slows or stops a chemical reaction or a biologic process.

Inhibitory Postsynaptic Potential (IPSP):

See Excitatory postsynaptic potential.

Initial Segment:

Nonmyelinated part of an axon hillock from which the axon arises. It is the area of a neuron in which the threshold for depolarization is lowest.

Initial Volume of Distribution (Central Volume of Distribution V_c or V_1):

Volume that, when a drug is first administered to the body, it instantaneously appears to be mixed with (*before* flow, mixing, and diffusion and before it is disseminated throughout the remainder of its distribution volume). *See* Volume of distribution.

Ink Space Cuff (Dural Sleeve) Region:

Thin area of the dura surrounding the nerve trunk that may be the site for transdural anesthetic transfer from the peridural space to the perineural region. This area has been found to permit passage of colloidal carbon particles, and it is therefore presumed to permit passage of crystalloid particles and local anesthetic agents. *See* Epidural Anesthesia.

Innervation:

Supply of nervous pathways (or the conveyance of nervous impulses) to or from a body part or organ.

Innovar:

Proprietary combination of droperidol and fentanyl in a 50:1 ratio (by weight). It is useful as both a preoperative medication and as a supplement to N_2O/O_2 anesthesia. Innovar produces neuroleptanesthesia. *See* Neuroleptanesthesia.

Inotropism:

Ability to influence muscular contraction either negatively or positively. Propranolol is a negative inotropic agent in relation to myocardial contractility, whereas isoproterenol is a positive one.

Input-Output (I/O):

Term that generally refers to the equipment used to communicate with a computer and to receive its results. For example, a cathode-ray tube terminal is an I/O device. *See* Cathode-ray tube.

Insensible Loss and Insensible Water Loss:

Water lost directly through the skin due to evaporation of sweat plus water lost from the lungs due to the exhalation of 100% water saturated gas, plus any fluid lost from the GI tract. Insensible water loss is approximately 100–400 ml/day in adults depending on environmental conditions. *See* Urinary output.

Inspiratory Center:

See Respiratory centers.

Inspiratory Hold:

Technique of respiratory therapy used to expand atelectatic areas of lung tissue. The lungs are held for a few seconds in the inflated state either by hand pressure on a breathing bag or by inhibition of the expiratory cycle on a ventilator.

Instantaneous Pulmonary Blood Flow:

Measurement of pulmonary blood flow taken while a patient is in a body plethysmograph (air-tight chamber). The patient breathes a mixture of N_2O and O_2 from a rubber bag inside the chamber. The N_2O is absorbed into the pulmonary blood, which decreases the total amount of gas in the chamber and reduces its volume. The blood flow can be calculated by measuring (1) the small, stepwise drops in pressure and volume in the chamber; (2) the N_2O concentration in the alveoli; and (3) knowing the solubility coefficient of N_2O in the blood. *See* Body plethysmograph.

Instantaneous Sample (Grab Sample):

Single sample of atmospheric gas taken in a leak-free and nonabsorbent container to spot-check for trace anesthetic gas contamination.

Institutional Review Board (IRB):

See Human Subjects Review Committee.

Insufflation:

Act of blowing a gas, powder, or vaporized drug into a body cavity. *See* Insufflation, intraperitoneal.

Insufflation Anesthesia:

Technique by which a high flow of anesthetic gas is delivered via an "ether" hook inserted at the corner of the mouth. The patient breathes spontaneously. Although insufflation anesthesia is simple to administer, it has been largely replaced by more sophisticated delivery systems that do not waste gas, dry the airways, or pollute the operating room environment.

Insufflation, Intraperitoneal:

Technique by which CO_2 is introduced into the abdomen via a trocar through a small infraumbilical incision. CO_2 is the gas of choice, as N_2O may combine with bowel gas released by an inadvertent puncture of the intestines to form a flammable or explosive mixture. Insufflation with CO_2 enlarges the abdominal cavity, thereby facilitating direct visual examination of the organs with a laparoscope. The technique is often used for electrosurgical tubal ligation and for investigation of possible abdominal or pelvic disease or trauma (where a conventional laparotomy is contraindicated because of the patient's condition). *See* Laparoscopy.

Insulin:

Essential hormone secreted by the islets of Langerhans in the pancreas. It is important for the proper control of plasma glucose levels. Interference with or nonproduction of insulin results in a constellation of abnormalities collectively referred to as diabetes mellitus. *See* Diabetes mellitus.

Insult:

Action or event that decreases the functional integrity of an organism or system.

Intensifying Screen:

Plate or screen, coated with a material such as calcium tungstate, that emits light when bombarded with x-rays. This light further exposes the x-ray film placed on it, making it possible to achieve a better x-ray picture while lowering the amount of radiation needed to produce it. *See* Image intensifier.

Intensity Modulation:

Process (or effect) of varying electron-beam current in a cathode-ray tube. Because the brightness of a particular spot on the tube becomes proportional to the magnitude of the signal, modulation allows a two-dimensional display to provide three simultaneous pieces of information: the x coordinate, the y coordinate, and brightness.

Intensive Care Unit (ICU):

Specialized hospital unit in which seriously ill patients are given continual nursing care (usually 1:1 or 1:2) aided by enhanced monitoring techniques. ICUs are often separated into surgical and medical divisions. The care in these units is always expensive, but its effectiveness is demonstrated when treating diseases that may be devastating but potentially reversible. *See* Figure.

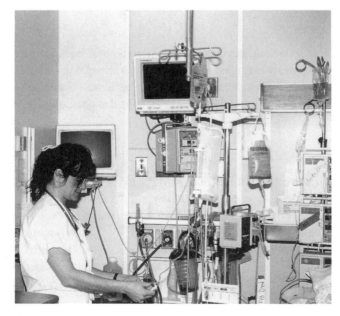

Intensive Care Unit: ICU Unit.

Intercostal Block:

Regional nerve block in which a local anesthetic is injected into the intercostal space(s). The block (1) provides pain relief after rib fractures or abdominal surgery, (2) facilitates deep breathing and coughing after surgery, and (3) is useful for superficial surgery of the chest, back, or abdominal wall. Production of a pneumothorax is the potential major complication of an intercostal block. *See* Figures.

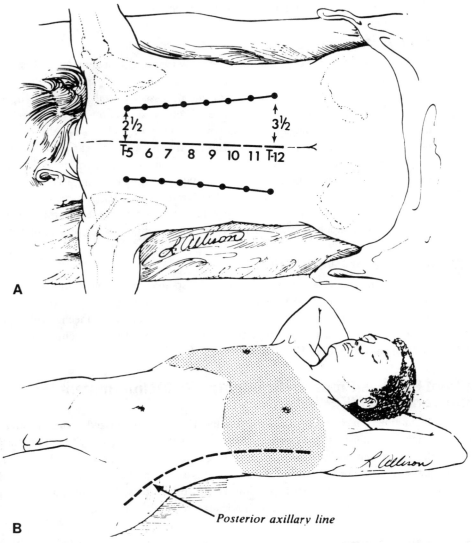

Intercostal Block: (A) Superficial landmarks for block of the intercostal nerves on the posterior aspect of the body. The needles are inserted 2½–3½ in. from the midline. The arms are drawn upward and outward to move the scapulae away from the field. (B) Position of the patient for block of the intercostal nerves along the posterior axillary line. The light shaded area shows the sensory distribution of the nerves more easily blocked in this position.

Interleukin-1 (IL-1):

See Endogenous pyrogen.

Intermittent Assisted Ventilation:

See Synchronized intermittent mandatory ventilation.

Intermittent Demand Ventilation:

See Synchronized intermittent mandatory ventilation.

Intermittent Flow Machine (Demand Flow Machine):

Type of anesthesia delivery system used mainly for outpatient dental anesthesia. There is a single control that continuously varies the percentages of O_2 and N_2O delivered by the machine. (The dentist is able to perform the necessary dental work while operating the simple control mechanism on the machine.) There is no gas flow out of the common outlet until a patient creates a negative pressure within the mask and the gas delivery hoses during inspiration. This negative pressure causes a valve to open and gas to be delivered in the proportion and pressure set by the adjustment controls. The intermittent flow system has some inherent disadvantages. Most commonly, the single mixture control can become blocked by dirt, rendering it inaccurate. The flow control is also subject to wide variation in calibration, so if a patient inspires deeply it is often impossible for the machine to produce enough flow to supply all the patient's required gas without being diluted by room air.

Intermittent Mandatory Ventilation (IMV):

Mode of mechanical ventilation where the spontaneously breathing patient triggers a ventilator that automatically interposes a mandatory mechanical inflation at a preset interval. IMV was initially used as a method to wean patients from mechanical ventilation. It since has been considered by some as a primary ventilatory technique. *See* Assisted mechanical ventilation; Ventilator; Weaning.

Intermittent Positive Pressure Breathing (IPPB); Intermittent Positive Pressure Ventilation (IPPV):

Technique of respiratory care by which the airway is pressurized during inspiration. Used extensively during the postoperative period to improve pulmonary function, it is based on the theory that positive pressure encourages the opening of closed, small airways. Airway pressure is allowed to fall to atmospheric pressure after inspiration, enabling the chest wall and lungs to recoil and permit expiration. (IPPB is also used to deliver aerosol drugs to the bronchopulmonary tree.) *See* Continuous positive airway pressure.

Internal Cardioversion:

See Cardioversion.

Internal Carotid Shunt:

See Stump pressure.

Internal Jugular Vein:

See Jugular veins.

International Anesthesia Research Society (IARS):

This organization was founded in 1922 and adopted its name in 1925 to "foster progress and research in all phases of anesthesia." The journal of the society, *Anesthesia and Analgesia,* has just entered its 70th year of publication and is the oldest journal in the specialty. The Society is based in Cleveland, Ohio.

International Classification of Diseases (ICD):

Coding system for human disease originally promulgated by the World Health Organization. This manual is now referred to as the International Classification of Diseases; 9th Revision Clinical Modification or ICDM-9-CM. The American edition is provided by the National Center for Health Statistics with input from such organizations as the American Hospital Association and the Council on Clinical Classifications. It is distributed by Healthcare Knowledge Systems in Ann Arbor, Michigan.

International System of Units (SI):

System of physical units in which fundamental qualities (length, time, mass, electrical current, temperature) correspond to the meter, second, kilogram, ampere and kelvin. SI with its official status, has been recommended for universal use by the General Conference on Weights and Measures. *See* SI unit.

Internodal Atrial Pathways:

See Heart, conduction system of.

Interposed Abdominal Compression:

Technique to enhance conventional cardiopulmonary resuscitation in which compression of the abdomen is applied during the relaxation phase of chest compression in an attempt to improve cardiac output. The technique appears to have promise but has not yet been accepted as standard practice.

Interscalene Block:

Alternative to the supraclavicular approach for blocking the brachial plexus. It has the advantage of giving good proximal shoulder anesthesia in combination with other local blocks. It requires the elicitation of paresthesias. The block is done in the interscalene grove. *See* Axillary nerve block; Brachial plexus block.

Interspinous Ligament:

See Lumbar puncture.

Interstitial Lung Edema:

Earliest form of pulmonary edema. It is characterized by engorgement of the peribronchial and perivascular spaces, which normally serve as conduits for fluids that might otherwise escape into the alveoli. Frank pulmonary edema occurs when the capacity of the lymphatics to drain these spaces is exceeded, forcing the fluid into the alveoli.

Intestinal Obstruction:

Blockage to the normal flow of solids and fluids in the intestine. It can be due to solid particles blocking the lumen, infection, inflammation, malignant tumor, extrinsic pressure, stricture, or twisted bowel. Any obstruction causes an increase in the anesthetic risk, as the elevated pressure proximal to the obstruction makes the patient more susceptible to esophageal reflux and possible aspiration. *See* Rapid sequence induction.

Intestinal Sterilization Syndrome:

Condition in which there is a marked decrease in the normal bacterial count in the intestine. It is seen in patients who have received large doses of antibiotics. Because bacteria produce most of the vitamin K normally available to the body, an effect on the prothrombin time may be evident within 7 days if vitamin K supplementation is not administered.

Intraaortic Balloon Pump (IABP):

Device used to assist or improve circulation in patients with inadequate cardiac output. The IABP may be used in patients (1) with ischemic heart disease due to cardiogenic shock, acute myocardial infarction, or refractory ventricular arrhythmias; (2) undergoing cardiac catheterization, cardiac surgery, or noncardiac surgery; or (3) with pediatric congenital heart disease. The IABP is inserted into the descending thoracic aorta; the tip of the balloon is inflated (with helium or CO_2) during diastole, thereby producing an increase in blood pressure and coronary blood flow. Ventricular afterload is decreased by balloon deflation just prior to systole. The actual inflation and deflation of the IABP is timed from the T wave (or dicrotic notch) and QRS complex of the electrocardiogram.

Intracardiac Electrocardiogram:

Graphic recording of electrical currents generated by the heart by means of an electrode introduced into the heart via an intravenous catheter. The technique requires precise placement of the catheter and monitoring of the movement of the catheter tip during introduction. Proper placement of the catheter is evidenced by an increasing amplitude of the P wave, which is upward deflecting as the catheter approaches the right atrium and downward deflecting as it traverses the right atrium and approaches the right ventricle.

Intracerebral Steal Syndrome:

Unpredictable shifts in the distribution of cerebral blood flow in damaged or diseased areas of the brain. One region may be hyperperfused while another may be ischemic due to the breakdown of normal autoregulatory control of cerebral blood flow. In the hypothetical Robin Hood syndrome, deliberate hypocapnia causes constriction of normal cerebral blood flow areas and redirects it to maximally dilated ischemic areas. In the hypothetical Sheriff of Nottingham syndrome, hypercapnia dilates normal areas, directing the blood flow away from ischemic areas that are already maximally dilated.

Intracranial Compliance:

Relation between the change in intracranial volume divided by the change in intracranial pressure or dV/dP. However, the relation between pressure and volume in the skull is more accurately called intracranial elastance which is change in pressure over change in volume (dP/dV). *See* Figures. *See* Intracranial hypertension.

Intracranial Elastance:

See Intracranial compliance.

Intracranial Hypertension:

Condition that exists when the measured intracranial pressure (ICP) is greater than 15 mm Hg (normal range is between 5–15 mm Hg). Elevated intracranial pressure, however, is not an absolute predictor of neurologic deficit. ICPs in the range of 80–100 mm Hg associated with low cerebral perfusion pressures have been demonstrated to exist in patients with little or no neurologic deficit, but, as a generality, neurologically significant intracranial hypertension is associated with rapid increases in the ICP. The relevance of ICP measurement to patient care is compromised in cases where there are bony defects due to traumatic, congenital, or surgical causes exist. *See* Table.

Intracranial Pressure Measurement:

Technique for determining the pressure within the cranium. Intracranial pressure (ICP) measurement is an invasive procedure and requires access through the skull. The measurement may be made via a fluid-filled catheter passing through the skull, brain, and into the cerebral ventricles, or it may be made via a small transducer resting on the dura or on the brain surface. The transducer technique, referred to as an intracranial screw or bolt, is less hazardous than the ventricular catheter but does not permit withdrawal of fluid. *See* Figure. *See* Subarachnoid screw.

Intragastric Pressure:

Pressure within the stomach that may vary with respiration. The pressure can increase dramatically during positive-pressure ventilation performed with an inadequate airway because gas is blown down the esophagus, inflating the stomach. It is believed that intragastric pressure rises significantly during the fasciculations induced by succinylcholine. *See* Sellick maneuver.

Intralipid:

See Lipid emulsion.

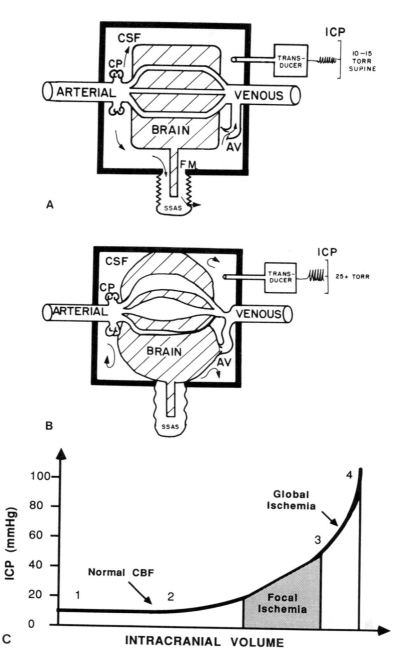

Intracranial Compliance: (A) Schematic representation of normal intracranial contents. Arrows indicate the direction of cerebrospinal fluid (CSF) flow and heavy lines represent the skull. (B) Schematic representation of intracranial contents during decompensated intracranial hypertension. Compressed as well as abnormally dilated cerebral vessels may coexist in different regions of the brain. Distortion of CSF circulatory pathways blocks CSF translocation-absorption processes, which tend to prevent intracranial hypertension. SSAS, spinal subarachnoid space; FM, foramen magnum; ICP, intracranial pressure; AV, arachnoid villi; CP, choroid plexus. (C) An idealized depiction of the intracranial volume-pressure relationship.

Intracranial Hypertension.

Etiology	Treatment
Intracranial mass	Surgical removal

Cerebral edema	Fluid restriction
	Diuretics
	  Osmotic
	  Tubular
	Steroids
	Hyperventilation
	Hypothermia
	Barbiturates
	Controlled hypotension
	Surgical decompression

Increased intravascular blood volume	Position Hyperventilation Blood pressure stability Muscle relaxants Barbiturates
CSF retention	Osmotic agents Reduction of CSF formation CSF shunting procedure

Intramedullary Anesthesia:

See Intraosseous anesthesia.

Intraocular Pressure (IOP):

Tension in the interior chamber of the eye produced mainly by the aqueous humor and, to a lesser extent, the vitreous humor. The aqueous humor is continually being formed and reabsorbed and the balance between the two processes regulates the total intraocular fluid volume and pressure. The normal IOP ranges from 10 to 30 mm Hg (average 15 mm Hg) and is measured clinically by tonometry or estimated by palpation of the eye. The IOP is elevated in patients with glaucoma. All anesthetic agents, with the exception of ketamine tend to decrease IOP, as do nondepolarizing muscle relaxants and intravenous barbiturates. Topical eye application of atropine, a mydriatic agent, increases IOP in eyes predisposed to closed-angle glaucoma. Succinylcholine can cause an elevated IOP, but this effect may be inhibited by prior administration of a nondepolarizing muscle relaxant. Succinylcholine must not be used in patients with penetrating eye wounds because even a transient increase in IOP would lead to the loss of vitreous humor. *See* Carbonic anhydrase; Glaucoma.

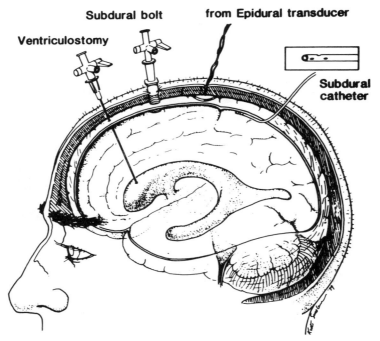

Ventriculostomy **Subdural bolt** **from Epidural transducer**

Subdural catheter

Intracranial Pressure Measurement: Commonly employed techniques and sites for ICP measurements.

Intraosseous Anesthesia:

Technique by which a local anesthetic solution is injected into the bone marrow of an extremity that is isolated from the systemic circulation by a tourniquet. Although similar in many respects to intravenous regional anesthesia, sterile technique is critical because of the possibility of directly introducing an infection into the bone. Intraosseous anesthesia may also be called intramedullary anesthesia. The latter term, however, is more frequently used to indicate spinal anesthesia.

Intraspinal:

Interchangeable with intrathecal. *See* Intrathecal.

Intrathecal:

Classically, "within a sheath," used in anesthesia as an *intrathecal injection;* injection below the dura into the cerebro-spinal fluid surrounding the spinal cord.

Intrathecal Injection:

Injection of a pharmacologic agent through the sheath (theca) of the spinal cord into the subarachnoid space. Spinal anesthesia is accomplished with an intrathecal injection. An alcohol or phenol intrathecal injection is given to alleviate intractable pain. Because both of these agents are neurolytic on direct contact with nerves, the technique requires great skill on the part of the operator.

Intrathecal Opioids:

Anesthetic technique using injection of narcotics into the subarachnoid space. A number of narcotics are used depending on the duration of pain relief required and the need to reduce side effects.

Intrauterine Pressure:

Pressure within the uterus measured near term by means of a catheter placed in the amniotic cavity. Normal baseline values are 8–20 mm Hg. Contractions occur between 25 and 75 mm Hg with peak values of 130 mm Hg occurring in conjunction with bearing down efforts. Uterine hypertonicity is a condition in which the baseline pressure is in excess of 20 mm Hg.

Intraval:

British trade name for thiopental sodium. *See* Barbiturate; Thiopental sodium.

Intravascular Electrocardiogram:

See Intracardiac electrocardiogram.

Intravenous Anesthesia:

Introduction of pharmacologic agents into a vein to create a general anesthetic state. Intravenous anesthesia is useful for surgical procedures of short duration or for induction purposes prior to inhalation anesthesia. It may also supplement regional anesthesia. Short-acting barbiturates such as thiopental and methohexital, are frequently used for intravenous anesthesia.

Intravenous Regional Anesthesia:

See Bier block.

Intravenous Solutions:

Any and all of the various sterile bagged or bottled liquids of wide composition that are used to maintain or replace blood loss or act as a vehicle for medications. Ever since the 1930s, it was recognized a patient who has been NPO for 6–8 hours prior to surgery arrives with a relative fluid deficit in the operating room. It gradually became the standard of care except for the most minor short procedures to "plug the patient in" to a running intravenous line in order to compensate for this relative lack of bodily fluid. *See* Tables. *See* Insensible loss and insensible water loss.

Intrinsically Safe Device:

Apparatus designed and built so that any internal spark that may occur or any point of high internal temperature cannot ignite an explosive mixture within or around the device. "Explosion-proof" indicates a device or apparatus enclosed in a case that is capable of withstanding an explosion without touching off surrounding explosive mixtures.

Intravenous Solutions: (A) Commonly used intravenous solutions.

SOLUTION	mEq/l	APPROX. pH	mOsm/l (calc)
5% dextrose in water	——	4.0	252
5% dextrose and 0.2% sodium chloride	Na 34 Cl 34	4.0	321
5% dextrose and 0.45% sodium chloride	Na 77 Cl 77	4.0	406
5% dextrose and 0.9% sodium chloride	Na 154 Cl 154	4.0	560
5% dextrose and Ringer's	Na 147.5 Ca 4.5 K 4 Cl 156	4.5	561
5% dextrose and lactated Ringer's	Na 130 K 4 Ca 3 Cl 109 Lactate 28	5.0	525
10% dextrose in water	——	4.0	505
0.45% sodium chloride	Na 77 Cl 77	5.0	154
0.9% sodium chloride	Na 154 Cl 154	5.0	308
Ringer's solution	Na 147.5 Ca 4.5 K 4 Cl 156	6.0	310
Lactated Ringer's solution	Na 130 K 4 Ca 3 Cl 109 Lactate 28	6.5	273

Intravenous Solutions: (B) Guidelines for routine fluids on the day of surgery.

Step 1
Replace insensible loss with maintenance-type solutions for interval since last oral intake.

Step 2
Change to replacement-type solution (such as LR, Normosol-R, or in some cases NaCl) for intraoperative insensible losses.

Step 3
Estimate surgical tissue trauma and add appropriate volume of replacement-type solution to that given in step 2:
Minimal trauma, add 4 ml/kg/hr
Moderate trauma, add 6 ml/kg/hr
Extreme trauma, add 8 ml/kg/hr

Step 4
Up to 15%–20% blood volume loss, replace with replacement solution three times the volume loss.
Over 15%–20% blood volume loss, replace additional blood loss with colloid solutions or blood products to maintain desired hematocrit.

Step 5
Monitor vital signs, urine output, and hematocrit to maintain urine output at about 1 ml/kg/hr.

Source: Glesecke AH, in *Anesthesia,* 2nd ed., perioperative fluid therapy-crystalloids, ed. Miller RD. Churchill Livingstone, New York, 1986.

Intrinsic Pathway:

Mechanism for activating blood coagulation by the formation of prothrombin activator. This pathway begins with trauma to the blood itself (or by contact with collagen in the vascular wall) that alters or damages factor XII and the platelets. The resulting activated factor XII and platelet factor III (platelet phospholipids) then activates factor XI, which in turn activates factor IX. Factor IX, with the aid of factor VIII and platelet factor III, then activates factor X. The last phase of the intrinsic pathway occurs when activated factor X combines with factor V and the platelet phospholipids to form the prothrombin activator complex which cleaves to form thrombin. Calcium ions are required for promotion of most of these reactions (except for the activation of factors XII and XI); clotting does not occur in the absence of calcium ions. Various substances (citrate ions or oxalate compounds) that decrease the concentration of calcium ions or deionize the calcium in the blood are used to prevent blood coagulation. The partial thromboplastin time (PTT) laboratory test is performed to evaluate the intrinsic pathway functions. *See* Blood coagulation; Extrinsic pathway.

Intrinsic PEEP:

See Pressure control inverse-ratio ventilation.

Intrinsic Sympathomimetic Activity (ISA):

Clinical effect of some beta antagonistic drugs when, at low doses, they have some sympathomimetic activity.

Intropin:

See Dopamine hydrochloride.

Intubation:

Process of passing a tube through the nose or the mouth so its tip rests below the vocal cords and above the division of the trachea into right and left main stem bronchi. This procedure ensures a patent airway if the tube remains mechanically intact. Intubation decreases the anatomic deadspace. Intubation is not a benign procedure because of the need for instrumentation and the introduction of a foreign body. It should be reserved for those patients who demonstrate difficulty in maintaining an airway or who require long-term respiratory support. *See* Double-lumen tube; Endobronchial intubation.

Intussusception:

Acute condition, most often seen in children, in which one part of the intestine becomes pushed into the lumen of an adjoining segment of the intestine.

Inulin:

Poorly metabolized polysaccharide (found in certain plants) used to measure the glomerular filtration rate to estimate kidney function. The test is known as inulin clearance. *See* Glomerular filtration rate.

Inverter:

Electronic or mechanical device that converts direct current (DC) into alternating current (AC). Inverters are often used in the operating room to provide standby AC service for emergency equipment. They allow a group of storage batteries with DC output to power AC equipment. An inverter also refers to an electronic device that inverts the polarity of a signal.

In vitro Study:

Test or observation made "within a glass," such as a test tube or Petri dish, or outside the intact organism (e.g., withdrawing an arterial blood sample for gas analysis in a blood gas machine).

In vivo Study:

Test or observation made within the intact organism (e.g., arterial pH measured by an appropriate electrode placed in an artery).

I/O:

See Input-output.

ION:

Atom or molecule that is either positively (cation) or negatively (anion) charged as a result of having lost or gained one or more electrons.

Ion Trapping:

Phenomenon of pharmacokinetics. It is based on the fact that the lipid-soluble, nonionized form of a drug can pass freely through lipid membranes leaving behind the non-lipid-soluble, ionized portion. For example, in the hypoxic fetus the more acidic fetal blood may accumulate or trap a local anesthetic, which is much more nonionized at the normal pH of the maternal blood than it is at the low pH of fetal blood.

Ionic Channel:

Concept that a specific enzyme or channel exists within a membrane otherwise highly resistant to ionic flow in one of many alternate configurations. This enzyme or channel vastly facilitates the passage of ions from one side of the membrane to the other. Modern theory postulates there are three basic states of the ion channel (particularly in reference to sodium channels) that play a major role in the mechanism of action of local anesthetics: (1) open, or conducting, where sodium ions flow through the channel; (2) resting, the normal state that can go to the open or conducting form; and (3) inactivated, in which the ion channel or gate cannot pass sodium ions without first reverting to the resting confirmation. Particularly in reference to the inhibition caused by local anesthetics to the movement of sodium ions through the sodium ion channels, current phraseology speaks of tonic inhibition and phasic inhibition (the word "block" and the word "inhibition" are here used interchangeably). Tonic inhibition is measured during infrequent stimulation (usually <2 Hz). Phasic block or inhibition (use-dependent block) is seen at higher rates of stimulation (>2 Hz) and is demonstrated when successive impulses show a smaller and smaller sodium ion flow. The explanation for this phenomenon is that local anesthetics bind preferentially to open gates; they do not attach to resting gates as avidly. As frequency of stimulation rises, more gates open and are then available to be blocked by local anesthetic molecules. Phasic inhibition was heretofore called "use-dependent" block.

Ionization:

Dissociation of compounds into their constituent ions. The process can occur spontaneously (in chemical reactions) or as the result of the deliberate bombardment of material with ionizing radiation. *See* Mass spectrometer.

Ionization Potential:

Minimum energy required to cause ionization of a particular atom or molecule.

Ionizing Radiation:

Any radiation of sufficient energy to cause ionization. Ionizing radiation can be either particulate (alpha and beta rays) or pure energy (gamma rays and x-rays).

IOP:

See Intraocular pressure.

IPPB:

See Intermittent positive pressure breathing.

IPSP:

See Inhibitory postsynaptic potential; Excitatory postsynaptic potential.

IR:

See Infrared radiation.

IRB:

See Institutional Review Board.

IRDS:

See Infant respiratory distress syndrome.

Iron Lung (Tank Ventilator; Cabinet Respirator):

Rigid tank encasing the entire body, it was the first successful long-term respirator for patients who were unable to ventilate themselves adequately. In current terminology it is classified as a negative-pressure ventilator. *See* Cuirass ventilator.

Irreversible Inhibition:

See Noncompetitive antagonism.

ISA:

See Intrinsic sympathomimetic activity.

Ismelin:

See Guanethidine.

Isobar:

One of two or more nuclides that have the same atomic weight but different atomic numbers.

Isoflurane (Forane):

Volatile anesthetic agent that is a stereoisomer of enflurane. Time periods for induction and recovery from anesthesia are somewhat shorter than with enflurane. Cardiovascular function is said to be less depressed with this agent than with earlier halogenated hydrocarbon anesthetics at comparable dosage levels. Isoflurane is metabolized only to a limited extent in the body. It has vaporization characteristics similar to those of halothane. *See* Enflurane. *See* Figure.

Isoflurane.

Isolated Forearm Technique:

Patient awareness assessment technique in which a pneumatic tourniquet is placed on the upper arm and inflated around the limb to a pressure that prevents entrance of the circulatory blood such that peripheral neuromuscular blockade cannot take place in this isolated appendage. This maneuver isolates the arm from a systemically administered muscle relaxant and allows the patient to respond to verbal command even though otherwise paralyzed. The technique may be used during general anesthesia with total paralysis. *See* Awareness.

Isolated Input:

See Isolated output.

Isolated Output:

Electronic design parameter in which the final (output) stage of a series of circuits has no direct connection with the previous circuits. Isolated input is an electronic design parameter in which the first of a series of circuits (input stage) has no direct connection with later circuits. Direct connection involves coupling the circuits by wiring or by bridging the two circuits with an active component, such as a capacitor. Isolation, on the other hand, is accomplished by interposing a transformer so a signal is transferred by interaction of electromagnetic fields or by optical isolation, in which the signal is transferred between circuits by a variable light beam. Modern electrocardiograph monitors have isolated inputs to protect them from a current surge caused by defibrillator discharge on top of an electrode. *See* Transformer.

Isolation Transformer:

Transformer used to separate a device from its power supply so that no direct connection between them can occur. Current from the power supply flows through the primary coil of the transformer, causing current to be induced in the secondary windings of the transformer. It is this current that powers the device. Modern operating rooms are powered through isolation transformers. *See* Ground.

Isomer:

Any compound that has the same molecular weight and chemical composition as another compound but that differs in some physical and chemical properties owing to varied structural arrangements of atoms within its molecules.

Isometric Change:

Change in a gas that occurs while the gas remains at a constant volume.

Isometric Contraction:

Muscle contraction with no change in muscle fiber lengths and associated with increased muscle tension. During the isometric contraction phase of the ventricle, the ventricular pressure rises but there is no change in the ventricular volume.

Isonatremic:

See Dehydration.

Isoprenaline:

See Isoproterenol.

Isopropyl Alcohol (Isopropanol):

Volatile, flammable alcohol (C_3H_8O) used as a topical bactericidal preparation in concentrations of 70–100%. (The 70% strength is known as rubbing alcohol.) The germicidal action is inconstant, however.

Isopropylnorepinephrine (Isopropylnoradrenalin):

See Isoproterenol.

Isoproterenol (Isuprel; Isoprenaline):

Synthetic drug closely related to the naturally occurring catecholamines, norepinephrine, epinephrine, and dopamine. (It is also known as isopropylnorepinephrine or isopropyl-noradrenalin.) Isoproterenol is a potent stimulator of beta receptors. It also has powerful positive inotropic and chronotropic effects on the heart and dilates bronchial smooth muscle and blood vessels. It is often used in aerosol form to treat bronchial asthma and related conditions. Overdosage of isoproterenol may cause tachycardia, angina, and headache. It increases cardiac O_2 consumption and stimulates cardiac output and, therefore it can increase the volume of infarcted tissue if administered during or immediately after a cardiac ischemic/infarct episode.

Isothermal Process:

Process that occurs at a constant temperature.

Isotonic Solution:

In biologic terms, a fluid having the same osmotic pressure as that of blood. Cells surrounded by an isotonic solution neither gain nor lose water.

Isotope:

Nuclide that has the same atomic number but a different atomic mass due to differences in the number of neutrons in the nucleus. Isotopes are nearly identical in chemical properties but vary in their physical properties. *See* Cesium 137; Gamma camera; Technetium 99; Xenon 133.

Isovolumic Contraction Time (ICT):

See Systolic time intervals.

IT:

See Implant tested; Z-79

J

Jackson, Charles:

See Morton, William T. G.

Jackson-Rees Apparatus:

Modification of the Ayre T-piece system for pediatric anesthesia. The basic change is that a double-ended bag is fitted to the expiratory limb of the T-piece. This bag allows breathing to be assisted or controlled. *See* Figure. *See* Bain circuit.

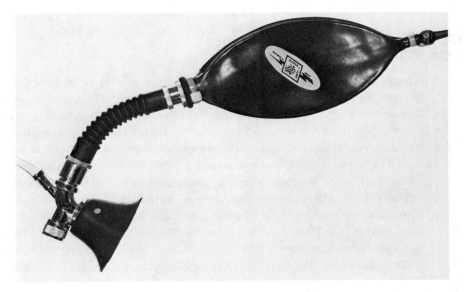

Jackson-Rees Apparatus: Jackson-Rees modification of an Ayre T-piece used for the administration of pediatric anesthesia.

JCAHO:

See Joint Commission on Accreditation of Health Care Organizations.

Jehovah's Witness:

International religious sect that originated in the United States at the end of the nineteenth century. Its members interpret the Old Testament literally. They believe that the soul resides in the blood and therefore consider transfusion with blood or blood derivatives to be a sacrilege. This presents a problem for major surgery as many hospitals require special permission forms for these individuals.

Jet Ventilation:

Various techniques that provide ventilation for a patient by means of a high pressure, high volume gas stream directed into the trachea. The key element in all jet ventilation is that the trachea is not occluded significantly so the high pressure jet stream does not literally burst the lungs. With all jet techniques, exhalation occurs when the jet is turned off and is caused by passive recoil of the chest wall. *See* High-frequency ventilation.

Jitter:

Short-term, often recurring instability during affecting either the phase or amplitude of a signal. This phenomenon is most often seen in a cathode-ray tube display.

JND:

See Just noticeable difference.

Joint Commission on Accreditation of Health Care Organizations (JCAHO):

Private, nonprofit organization. Originally founded in 1951 as the Joint Commission on Accreditation of Hospitals, the name was changed in 1987. JCAHO is governed by a 24-member Board of Commissioners representing the: American College of Physicians, American College of Surgeons, American Hospital Association, American Medical Association, American Dental Association, and three public members. The JCAHO currently accredits approximately 5400 hospitals and more than 3000 other related health care institutions such as community mental health centers and outpatient surgery centers. There are four categories of accreditation. Categories range from fully accredited to conditionally accredited to not accredited. The JCAHO stresses that its accreditation is voluntary by individual health care facilities. The accreditation is, in fact, mandatory in order for many institutions to receive funding from various public medical assistance programs. JCAHO headquarters is located in Oak Brook Terrace, Illinois.

Jones Solution:

See Howard Jones Solution.

Jorgensen Technique:

Method of sedation for dental procedures. Pentobarbital is injected slowly by the intravenous route until a predetermined point of patient relaxation is achieved. A fixed combination of meperidine and scopolamine is then injected slowly, followed by injections of appropriate intraoral anesthetic agents. Depending on the total dose of pentobarbital, the recovery can be prolonged.

Joule (J):

Standard international unit of measurement for all forms of energy. It is the energy equivalent to the work performed when a force of 1 newton moves a body a distance of 1 m. In electrical equivalence, 1 J = 1 watt-sec. In heat energy, 1 cal = 4.1868 J.

Joule Law:

Law stating that heat produced by an electrical current (I) flowing through a resistance (R) for a fixed time (t) is determined by I^2Rt. If the current is expressed in amperes, the resistance in ohms, and the time in seconds, the heat produced is expressed in joules.

Jugular Bulb:

Dilatation of the internal jugular vein just as it leaves the base of the skull. Blood removed from the jugular bulb is used to approximate mixed venous blood from the brain.

Jugular Veins:

Great veins of the neck composed of the external and internal jugular veins. The bilateral external jugular veins drain the blood from the parotid glands, facial muscles, and scalp into the subclavian veins. They run inferior and traverse the sternocleidomastoid muscle to a point opposite the middle of the clavicle, where they enter the subclavian veins. These veins are readily accessible in the patient who is in a Trendelenburg position (head down), but they are difficult to stabilize and therefore difficult to cannulate. This difficulty is due to several factors: the angle at which the external jugular veins enter the subclavian veins, the presence of valves in the external veins (impeding passage of the cannula), and the visibility of the external veins underneath the skin (which varies from individual to individual). The internal jugular veins begin in the base of the skull at the jugular fossae and are a continuation of the transverse sinuses of the brain. Coursing down through the neck, they accompany first the internal carotid arteries and then the common carotid artery. The internal jugular veins descend on either side of the neck and receive blood from the brain and superficial parts of the face and neck. They pass behind the clavicles and join with the right and left subclavian veins, forming the brachiocephalic veins and the superior vena cava. The internal jugular veins are fairly easily cannulated and are often used for central venous pressure monitoring or placement of a Swan-Ganz catheter. Right-sided cannulation is preferred because the right internal jugular vein leads directly into the superior vena cava. In addition, the apex of the right lung is lower than the left, thereby lessening the chances for inadvertent puncture of the lung. Furthermore, entry on the right side avoids possible injury to the thoracic duct, which is a left-sided structure. *See* Figures.

Jump Sign:

See Myofascial pain syndrome.

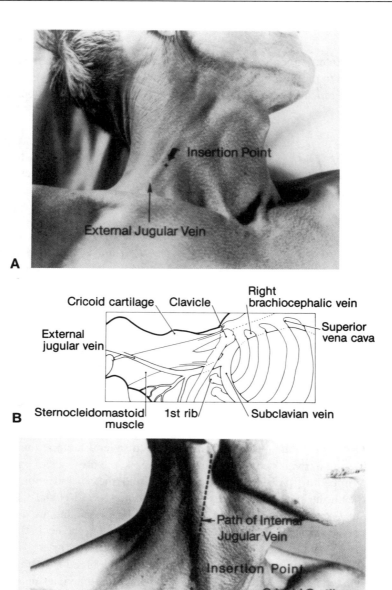

Jugular Vein: (A) External. Insertion point for external jugular venipuncture. (B) External. Anatomy of neck and upper thorax emphasizing relationships to the external jugular vein. (C) Internal. Insertion site for internal jugular venipuncture. SCM = sternocleidomastoid. (D) Internal. Anatomy of neck and upper thorax emphasizing relationships to internal jugular vein.

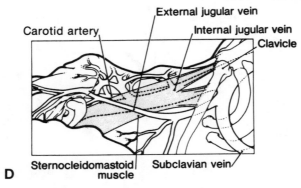

Jugular Vein *(continued)*

Just Noticeable Difference (JND):

Increase in the intensity of a painful stimulus that just barely causes an appreciable difference in the perception of pain. It has been shown that an average individual can distinguish approximately 22 JNDs measured from a level of no pain to a level of intense pain.

K

Kallidin:

See Kinins.

Kallikrein:

See Bradykinin.

Keeper:

Magnetic conductor placed over the ends of a magnet to prevent gradual loss of its magnetism.

Kelvin (K):

Standard international unit of temperature equal to 1/273.16 of the thermodynamic temperature of the triple point of water. On the K scale, 1 K = 1°C. Absolute zero on the K scale = –273°C, theoretically the lowest possible temperature. *See* Triple point of water.

Ketamine:

Nonbarbiturate intravenous general anesthetic. It is similar structurally to the veterinary anesthetic phencyclidine (Sernylan). Phencyclidine was abandoned for human use because of its propensity to cause severe and long-lasting hallucinations. Phencyclidine (angel dust) is popular for illicit drug use. Ketamine differs from the barbiturates because it tends to support, rather than depress, the cardiovascular system. With increased dosage, it causes epileptic-like electrical activity of the brain and, in general, enhances muscle tone. The anesthesia is of short duration and may increase the blood pressure and induce dreams, hallucinations, and psychological disturbances after recovery. The latter reactions are believed to occur less commonly in children. Ketamine produces "dissociative anesthesia"; i.e., the patient becomes unresponsive to pain and to the environment. *See* Dissociative anesthesia; neuroleptanesthesia.

Ketanserin:

Investigational drug that is an S_2-serotonergic receptor antagonist. The drug is being tested as an antihypertensive agent.

Ketone Body:

See Anion gap.

Keyed Filling Device:

See Agent-specific filling device.

Kidney:

Prime organ of the urinary system. The paired kidneys are located in the retroperitoneum, the right slightly lower than the left. The main function of the kidneys is regulation of the composition and volume of body fluids. They play a critical role in the maintenance of acid-base balance, excretion of unwanted metabolic end-products (e.g., urea, uric acid, and creatinine), and elimination of drugs. The kidneys also have an endocrine function in that they elaborate erythropoietin (erythropoietic stimulating factor) and renin (a proteolytic enzyme that activates the angiotensin-dependent vasoconstrictor mechanism). The kidneys produce erythropoietin when they are hypoxic and renin when they are ischemic and arterial pressure decreases. The functional unit in the kidney is the nephron; each kidney contains approximately one million nephrons. The loss or destruction of nephrons results in an increase in size of the remaining nephrons. Life may still be maintained with the loss of two-thirds of the nephrons. The components of the nephron include the glomerulus, proximal convoluted tubule, loop of Henle, and distal convoluted tubule. The distal convoluted tubule terminates by merging with the collecting duct. The circulation of the kidney is autoregulatory, i.e., the blood flow to the kidney remains constant within a range of mean arterial pressure of approximately 60–180 mm Hg. In general, inhalation anesthetics, such as ether, cyclopropane, isoflurane, enflurane, and methoxyflurane cause depression of renal blood flow and glomerular filtration rate; the degree of depression appears to be dose-related. A similar depression of renal blood flow is also seen with the use of the N_2O/O_2 muscle relaxant technique. Conversely, spinal anesthesia does not usually depress the glomerular filtration rate but may cause a decrease in the total renal blood flow. Epidural anesthesia appears to have little or no effect on renal blood flow. Of all the anesthetic agents, only methoxyflurane seems to be directly nephrotoxic, depending on dose and duration of administration. *See* Figure. *See* Glomerular filtration rate, Methoxyflurane.

Kilo- (k):

Prefix meaning 1000. In computer terminology it means 2^{10} (1024).

Kilogram (kg):

Standard international unit of mass (1 kg = 2.204 lb).

Kinesthesia:

Sensation mediated by end-organs in muscles, joints, and tendons. Movement is perceived by these end organs, enabling a person to estimate the relative position of the body parts.

Kinetic Energy:

Energy associated with motion. It is equal to the work that would be necessary to bring the system to rest. *See* Potential energy.

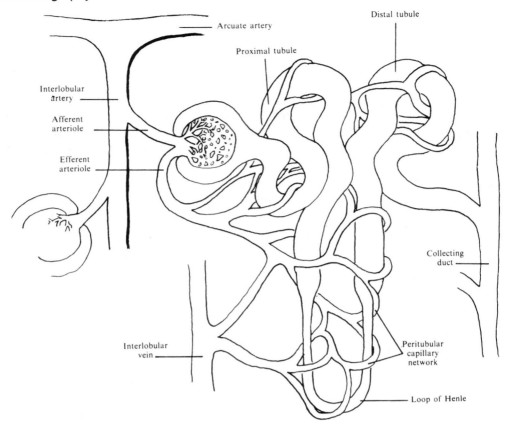

Kidney: Diagram of the nephron, the functional unit of the kidney.

Kinetocardiography:

See Apexcardiography.

Kinins:

Group of polypeptides that cause dilation of the blood vessels in kidneys, vascular smooth muscles, and some glands. Bradykinin, a plasma kinin, constricts the bronchial, uterine, and gastrointestinal smooth muscles. It also causes release of catecholamines (from the adrenal medulla), histamine (from mast cells), and prostaglandin (from the kidney). Kallidin, another plasma kinin, has pharmacologic properties similar to bradykinin. The kinins increase permeability in the microcirculation, thereby producing edema. They also evoke pain by stimulating nerve endings. Edema in conjunction with the nerve stimulation results in the "wheal and flare" reaction to intradermal injections. The kinins take part in inflammatory responses and allergic symptoms. *See* Allergic response; Bradykinin.

Korotkoff Sounds:

Sounds heard through the stethoscope during the auscultatory determination of arterial blood pressure. The blood pressure cuff is inflated to occlude the artery (usually brachial); then, as the pressure is slowly released, the blood can then flow through the partially collapsed artery. The resulting turbulence in the vessels is thought to produce the Korotkoff sounds. *See* Blood pressure.

Kupffer Cell:

See Macrophage.

Kussmaul Sign:

See Cardiac tamponade.

Kyphoscoliosis:

Lateral and backward curvature of the spinal column.

L

LA:

See Local anesthetic.

Labetalol (Normodyne):

Antihypertensive drug that blocks beta receptors. Used often for treatment of hypertension, its positive effects include a decreased or unchanged heart rate and decreased peripheral resistance. *See* Antihypertension drugs; Beta blocker.

Labor:

Process by which both fetus and placenta are expelled from the uterus through the vagina. Normal labor is divided into three stages. During stage 1, regular uterine contractions are accomplished by the complete dilation of the cervical os and effacement of the cervix. Stage 2, the stage of expulsion, begins when the os is fully dilated and ends with delivery of the fetus. Stage 3 involves expulsion of the placenta and membranes and ends with the final uterine contraction. False labor, common during late pregnancy, consists of brief, ineffective, irregular contractions not accompanied by cervical dilatation and effacement. *See* Figure.

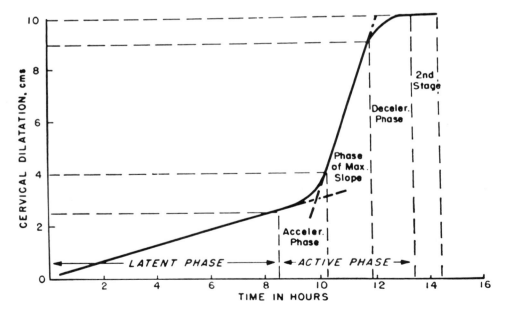

Labor: The mean labor curve (cervical dilation versus time) based on a graphicostatistical analysis of 500 primigravidas at term.

Lactate/Pyruvate Ratio:

Biochemical ratio measured in a blood sample that has been advocated as a possible indicator of tissue hypoxia. However, the lactate/pyruvate ratio has not been shown to add significantly to an understanding of patient status if other careful physiologic and metabolic monitoring has been performed.

Lactic Acid Acidemia:

Condition where lactic acid accumulates caused by improper utilization or transport of oxygen to the peripheral tissues.

Laerdal Valve:

See Nonrebreathing valve.

Laminar Flow:

Flow of an incompressible, viscous fluid in which the particles of the fluid move in distinct and separate layers (concentric laminae) parallel to each other and to the walls of a vessel or container. The velocity of the fluid particles is not uniform: there is little or no movement at the periphery of the flow and greatest movement in the center of the flow. It is different from turbulent flow, in which there is no order and all molecules tend to flow at approximately the same velocity. More energy is necessary to produce turbulent flow, and it often results in noise. *See* Figure. *See* Reynolds number; Turbulent flow.

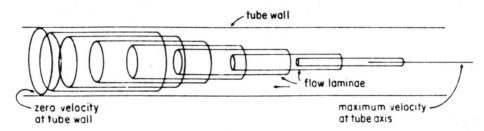

Laminar Flow: Laminar flow in a tube showing a few of the very large number of infinitely thin concentric flow laminae moving left to right. Each is at a different velocity, ranging from 0 at the tube wall to maximum at the tube center. The average velocity is half the maximum.

Laminar Flow Hood:

Enclosed work area (room, cabinet) that is protected from contamination by dust or microorganisms by HEPA filters. Air is continually moved in a single direction eliminating turbulence and backflow. Various units are available and are essential for use in laboratories for pharmaceutical research, tissue culture, and biomedical research and in hospital operating rooms. *See* HEPA filter.

Laparoscopy:

Method of visually examining the abdominal or pelvic organs by insertion of a specially equipped endoscope through a small incision in the abdominal wall. This method, also

357

known as peritoneoscopy, has both diagnostic and therapeutic value. Operative procedures, such as tubal ligation, ovarian or liver biopsy, gall bladder resection, and lysis of adhesions, may be performed through a laparoscope. *See* Insufflation; intraperitoneal.

Laplace Law:

Law of physics that has been applied to physiology. It defines the force that tends to stretch the muscle fibers in a vessel wall as proportional to the diameter (D) of the vessel × the pressure (P). The cardiac ventricular pressure depends on the tension produced by the contracting cardiac ventricular muscle and on the size and shape of the heart. This law helps explain the extra work load of the failing, dilated heart. As the diameter of the heart chamber is increased, more tension needs to develop in the myocardium to produce any given pressure, thereby increasing the work of the dilated heart in maintaining the same arterial pressure as in the healthy heart. In the lung, the radii of the curvature of the alveoli become smaller during expiration. The surface tension-lowering substance, surfactant, prevents the alveoli from collapsing. If the surface tension does not remain low, the alveoli would collapse according to the law of Laplace. In spherical structures such as alveoli, the distending pressure (P) equals two times the wall tension (T) divided by the radius (R): $P = 2T/R$. Therefore if T is not lowered as R is lowered, T overcomes P and collapse occurs. *See* Surfactant.

Large Samples:

Sample series large enough for the distribution of the individual observations to approach a normal distribution. *See* Normal distribution.

Larodopa:

See L-dopa; Levodopa.

Laryngeal Indices Caliper:

Device for determining relative laryngeal position as an aid to forecasting ease of intubation.

Laryngeal Mask Airway:

Airway consisting of a tube that at its distal end, has an elliptically shaped cuff resembling a miniature face mask. It is meant to be inserted blindly into the pharynx. The cuff then forms a low pressure seal around the upper larynx through which the patient can breathe spontaneously. *See* Figures.

Laryngitis:

Inflammation of the larynx often caused by a respiratory infection or irritant. It is characterized by dryness and soreness of the throat, hoarseness, cough, and loss of voice. It is a relatively common sequela of endotracheal intubation. It depends on cuff inflation pressure, tube position, duration of intubation, type of endotracheal tubing, and the technical competence of the anesthetist. *See* Endotracheal tube.

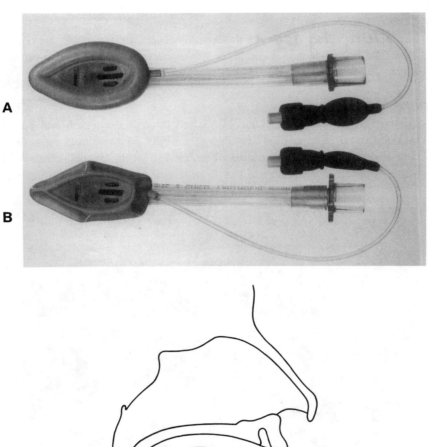

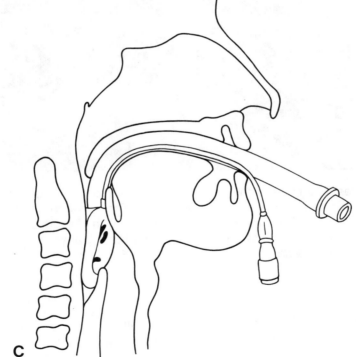

Laryngeal Mask Airway: (A) Cuff inflated. (B) Cuff deflated for insertion. (C) The laryngeal mask in position.

Laryngoscope:

Instrument for direct viewing of the larynx. Modern laryngoscopes are one- or two-piece units. The two piece unit is composed of a battery handle and an assortment of "blades" which are inserted through the mouth. *See* Laryngoscope blade.

Laryngoscope Blade:

The part of a laryngoscope that is inserted through the mouth and positioned in the hypopharynx in order to allow viewing of the larynx. Multiple and various modifications of the basic flat and curved blades have been made over the last half-century. The two basic blades currently in use are the Miller blade and the MacIntosh blades. *See* Figure.

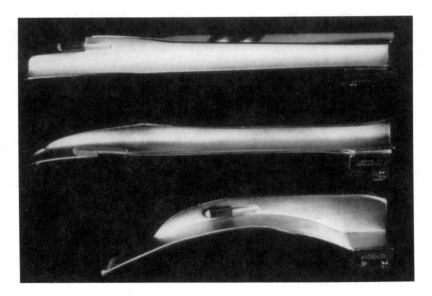

Laryngoscope Blades: Examples of the most frequently used detachable laryngoscope blades, which can be used interchangeably on the same handle. The uppermost blade is the straight or Jackson-Wisconsin design. The middle blade incorporates a curved distal tip (Miller). The lowermost blade is the curved or Macintosh blade. All three blades are available in lengths appropriate for neonates and adults.

Laryngoscopy:

Examination of the larynx either indirectly by means of a laryngeal mirror or directly by means of a lighted instrument, the laryngoscope.

Laryngospasm:

Sudden, forceful, and involuntary contraction (spasm) of the muscles of the larynx. Certain muscle groups normally act as sphincters to protect the airway, but during spasm they forcefully close, obscuring the true vocal cords and the glottis. Closure of these sphincters separates the larynx and trachea. These sphincters include the aryepiglottic folds, vestibular folds (false vocal cords), and true vocal cords. Laryngospasm can be a defensive reflex to prevent aspiration and is associated with a high-pitched squeak or whistle. (The complete absence of sound indicates that the vocal cords are in total opposition.) Laryngospasm can be a serious complication during induction of anesthesia caused by the seemingly innocuous manipulation of the upper airway. The administration of O_2 under pressure or injection of a fast-acting neuromuscular blocking agent, such as succinylcholine, may be useful in treating laryngospasm; however, the condition is easier to prevent than to treat. *See* Larynx.

Larynx (Voice Box):

Short passageway that connects the pharynx with the trachea. The walls of this musculocartilaginous structure are supported by nine pieces of cartilage. The larynx lies in the midline of the neck anterior to the fourth through the sixth cervical (C4-C6) vertebrae. It is lined with ciliated mucous membranes trapping particles not removed in the upper air passages. The vocal cords are usually thicker and longer in males and vibrate more slowly. *See* Figures.

Laser:

An acronym for "light amplification by stimulated emission of radiation." It refers to a device that transforms energy of various frequencies into a narrow, intense, nearly non-divergent beam of monochromatic (single-frequency) radiation in the optical, ultraviolet, and infrared regions. Lasers are capable of producing a great deal of heat and power; however, the conversion efficiency of the change from one form of energy to laser energy is inefficient. Laser techniques are being used with greater frequency in surgery for cutting and burning.

Lasix:

See Furosemide.

Latent Heat:

Amount of heat absorbed or released by a unit mass of a substance during isothermal changes of state (e.g., fusion, sublimation, or vaporization) at a constant pressure. For example, a gently heated mixture of ice and water remains at 0°C so long as there is any ice in the mixture. Latent heat becomes an important consideration in the vaporization of anesthetic liquids during anesthesia. For a liquid to vaporize at a constant rate, energy must be added to it to compensate for the heat loss and the resultant drop in temperature.

Lateral Femoral Cutaneous Neuralgia:

See Neuralgia paresthetica.

Latex Allergy:

Allergic response to natural latex rubber. It can manifest as a full-blown anaphylactic reaction when the mucus membranes of a patient come in contact with latex surgical gloves.

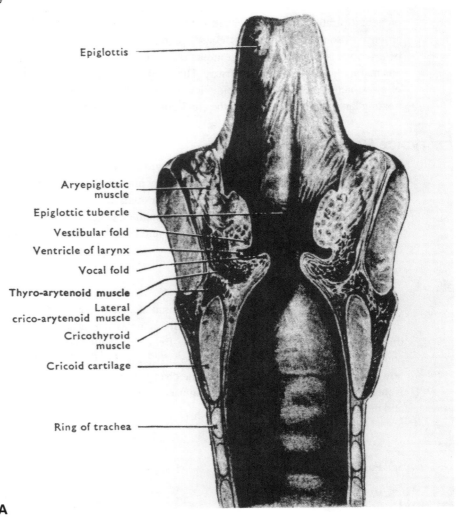

Epiglottis

Aryepiglottic muscle

Epiglottic tubercle

Vestibular fold

Ventricle of larynx

Vocal fold

Thyro-arytenoid muscle

Lateral crico-arytenoid muscle

Cricothyroid muscle

Cricoid cartilage

Ring of trachea

A

Larynx: (A) Coronal section of larynx to show situation of muscles. (B) Cartilages and ligaments of the larynx from the front. (C) Cartilages and ligaments of the larynx from behind.

Laudanosine:

Known convulsive agent. A minor metabolite of the muscle relaxant atracurium, it has no clinical significance in routine circumstances but may antagonize sedatives administered to treat the psychological effects of atracurium overdoses.

Laughing Gas:

See Nitrous oxide.

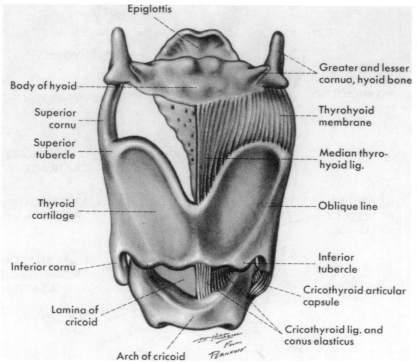

B

Epiglottis

Greater and lesser cornua, hyoid bone

Body of hyoid

Superior cornu

Thyrohyoid membrane

Superior tubercle

Median thyro-hyoid lig.

Thyroid cartilage

Oblique line

Inferior cornu

Inferior tubercle

Cricothyroid articular capsule

Lamina of cricoid

Cricothyroid lig. and conus elasticus

Arch of cricoid

C

Epiglottis

Triticeal cartilage in lat. thyrohyoid lig.

Greater cornu, hyoid bone

Thyrohyoid membrane

Sup. cornu, thyroid cart.

Corniculate cartilage

Vocal lig.

Arytenoid cartilage

Cricoarytenoid articular capsule

Muscular process

Post. cricoary-tenoid lig.

Inf. cornu, thyroid cart.

Cricothyroid articular capsule

Lamina of cricoid cartilage

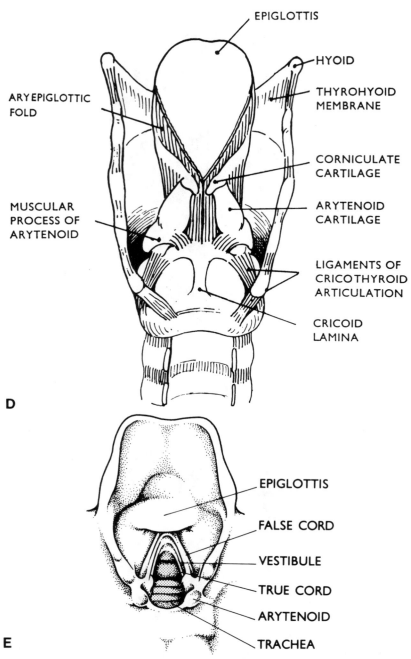

EPIGLOTTIS

HYOID

THYROHYOID
MEMBRANE

ARYEPIGLOTTIC
FOLD

CORNICULATE
CARTILAGE

ARYTENOID
CARTILAGE

MUSCULAR
PROCESS OF
ARYTENOID

LIGAMENTS OF
CRICOTHYROID
ARTICULATION

CRICOID
LAMINA

D

EPIGLOTTIS

FALSE CORD

VESTIBULE

TRUE CORD

ARYTENOID

TRACHEA

E

Larynx *(continued):* (D) The cartilages and ligaments of the larynx seen posteriorly. (E) View of the larynx at laryngoscopy.

Lavage:

Therapeutic washing out or irrigating of an organ, or cavity (i.e., peritoneal lavage) such as the lung, bowel, or stomach. *See* Pulmonary lavage.

Lay Standard Rule:

Legal principle that when obtaining informed consent the physician must disclose information that is material to the patient's decision. In general, this rule means that all information a "reasonable patient" would need to make a particular decision, should be disclosed. *See* Professional standard rule.

LCD:

See Liquid crystal display technology.

LD$_{50}$ (Lethal Dose 50%):

Dose of a pharmacologic substance that is fatal to 50% of test animals. As the difference between the LD$_{50}$ and the ED$_{50}$ (effective dose 50%) increases, so does the safety of the substance. *See* ED$_{50}$; Therapeutic index.

L-Dopa:

See Levodopa.

Lead (Lead Wire):

Conductor, such as an electrocardiograph lead, used to connect two points in a circuit. *See* Electrocardiogram.

Leading Edge Analysis (Spectral Edge Analysis):

Electroencephalograph (EEG) analysis technique. In this analysis EEG is displayed by compressed spectral array (CSA). The leading edge is the frequency below which a large percentage (90–98%) of the power in the EEG frequency band is contained. A shift in the leading edge from time interval to time interval on the CSA display is believed to indicate changes in depth of anesthesia. *See* Compressed spectral array; Fourier analysis.

Leakage:

Undesirable flow of electrical current in a path other than that intended, possibly due to imperfect insulation. *See* Fault current.

Least Squares, Method of:

Mathematical technique for finding the equation that best fits or describes the line or curve connecting points on a graph.

Leboyer Technique:

Named for a French obstetrician, the technique promotes "childbirth without violence." It is based on the belief that noise and bright lights can cause psychological trauma to the newborn.

Leclanche Cell:

Common dry cell, primary cell, or carbon-zinc battery in which the anode is made of carbon and the cathode is made of zinc. The least expensive of the common primary cells, it usually cannot be recharged. The voltage from a new cell is approximately 1.5 V, but it declines steadily with use. *See* Battery, electric.

Left Uterine Displacement (LUD):

Maneuver to prevent aortocaval compression by the gravid uterus. It can be accomplished either by manual displacement in which the uterus is lifted and pushed to the left or the patient can be positioned on her left side, or a mechanical arm (left uterus displacement device) can be used operating from the edge of the delivery table.

Left Ventricular Assist Device (LVAD):

Any and all devices designed to take over part or all of the pumping function of the left ventricle. Usually positioned downstream in the aorta, the device can have a number of configurations in practice or in research. It is usually paced by detection of electrical activity of the heart. *See* Intra-aortic balloon pump.

Left Ventricular Ejection Fraction:

See Muga scan.

Left Ventricular Ejection Time (LVET):

See Systolic time intervals.

Left Ventricular Stroke-Work Index (LVSWI):

Index of cardiac performance. It is the mean arterial pressure—the pulmonary capillary wedge pressure (PCWP) × the stroke volume index × a constant. *See* Pulmonary capillary wedge pressure.

Leritine:

See Anileridine; Narcotic.

LES:

See Lower esophageal sphincter.

Leu-Enkephalin:

See Enkephalins.

Leukotrienes:

See Eicosanoids.

Levallorphan (Lorfan):

Narcotic agonist/antagonist useful for treatment of significant narcotic-induced respiratory depression. It is ineffective for alleviating respiratory depression because of other causes and, if used, may actually potentiate the problem. The use of levallorphan has diminished with the introduction of the pure antagonist naloxone. *See* Naloxone.

Levarterenol:

See Norepinephrine.

Levodopa, L-dopa (Dopar; Larodopa):

Drug for treating Parkinson disease. Levodopa decarboxylates to dopamine, the neurotransmitter that is deficient in parkinsonian patients and must therefore be replenished. Relatively high doses of levodopa must be administered (orally) to produce the desired pharmacologic effects, e.g., reducing bradykinesia and rigidity. This treatment enables sufficient accumulation of the drug in the brain where the decarboxylation increases the dopamine concentration. (Dopamine itself does not readily penetrate the blood-brain barrier.) Side effects limit the usefulness of the drug, however.

Levophed:

See Norepinephrine.

Levorphanol Tartrate (Levo-Dromoran):

Synthetic molecule closely related to morphine. *See* Narcotic.

Lewis-Leigh Valve:

See Nonrebreathing valve.

L-Hyoscine:

See Scopolamine.

Libel:

Written, unjust statement that defames an individual's reputation. It is a possible basis for countersuit in malpractice actions.

Librium:

See Benzodiazepine.

Lidocaine (Xylocaine):

See Local anesthetic.

LIFO:

An acronym for "last in first out," referring to the ordering of machine tasks. The last task received is completed first.

Ligamentum Flavum:

See Lumbar puncture.

Light:

Electromagnetic radiation that is perceived by the eye. The visual spectrum is between wavelengths 390 and 770 nm. The photon is the unit of light energy. The velocity of light in free space, $2.997\ 925 \times 10^8$ m/second, is considered one of the prime constants in the universe.

Lignocaine:

British term for lidocaine.

Limbic System:

Portion of the brain composed of the limbic lobe (subcallosal, cingulate, and parahippocampal gyri), hippocampal formation, amygdaloid nucleus, hypothalamus, and anterior nucleus of the thalamus. The limbic system appears to be involved in emotional behavior, particularly fear, anger, and sexual behavior. The hippocampus appears to be concerned with recent memory.

Limits of Explosiveness:

See Detonability, limits of.

Limits of Flammability:

Upper and lower endpoints of the concentration range at which a fuel/oxidizer mix ignites. Generally, the upper and lower limits of flammability for a given fuel are much higher with O_2 than with air. *See* Cool flame.

Line Isolation Monitor:

Device that continually determines the electrical separation of the input and output sides of an isolated power supply. It measures the potential for current flow (electrical shock) if an individual simultaneously contacts a conductor located on the isolated side and a grounded conductor. *See* Ground; Ground fault circuit interrupter; Isolation transformer.

Lipid Emulsion (Intralipid):

Sterile mix of 10% soy bean oil, 1.2% egg phosphatide, and 2.25% glycerol. Used as the suspending medium for the intravenous anesthetic propofol.

Lipid Solubility Theory of Anesthesia (Meyer-Overton Theory):

Theory that correlates lipid solubility with the potency of an anesthetic agent. Anesthetics are lipophilic, and therefore the greater the solubility, the lower the concentration needed to be effective. In actuality, however, the theory does not explain anesthesia but only describes the actions of anesthetics in the lipid areas of body tissues.

Lipophilic:

Literally "fat loving," the tendencies of drugs to accumulate in fatty tissues. Usually drugs that are lipophilic are hydrophobic, which means they are not easily dissolved in water. The concept is used in anesthesia in epidural narcotics. A hydrophilic drug such as morphine administered by epidural, tends to accumulate in cerebrospinal fluid (CSF) and has a prolonged effect, as well as a great potential to produce respiratory depression. Drugs such as fentanyl and sufentanil, which are highly lipid-soluble, appear to have a low potential for producing depression of ventilation via epidural, which is probably due to their lower accumulation in the CSF.

Lipoxins:

See Eicosanoids.

Liquid Crystal Display (LCD) Technology:

Technique for displaying numbers or letters that employs the physical characteristics of liquid crystals. These semiamorphous materials reorient themselves internally when a voltage difference is placed across them. This internal reorientation changes the percentage of light reflected by the crystal. Such change in reflected light enables the liquid crystal element of the display to be seen. The LCDs have low power equirements and are not visible in darkness when no light exists for reflection. *See* Figures.

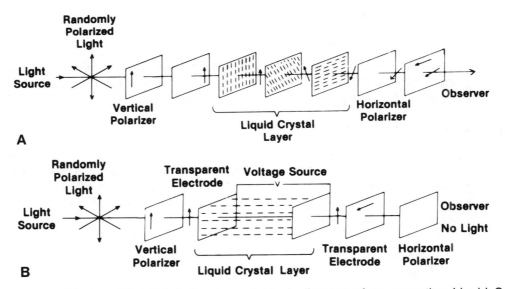

Liquid Crystal Display: (A) LCD Technology: A block diagram of an operating Liquid Crystal Display. (B) A diagram showing how an applied voltage changes the liquid crystal molecular shape, blocking light transmission.

Liquid Oxygen:

Oxygen cooled to $-183°C$ at 1 atmosphere pressure. It is the most convenient form for bulk movement of O_2. One cubic foot of liquid O_2 yields more than 24,000 L of gaseous O_2 at room temperature.

Liquid Ventilation:

Experimental technique in which gas exchange through the lungs is maintained by filling the lungs with a fluid. Liquid ventilation utilizes the properties of various silicone oils and fluorocarbons. Disadvantages of the technique include the viscosity of the fluid (which limits respiratory rate and tidal volume) and the long-term toxic effects on the cell linings of the alveoli. Theoretic advantages of the technique include the potential of delivering high O_2 concentrations while lowering O_2 toxicity and maintaining airway patency.

Lithium:

Metallic element of the alkali group with an atomic weight of approximately 7. The carbonate salt of lithium is widely used for treatment of the manic phase of manic-depressive psychiatric disease. Therapeutic doses of lithium carbonate have no discernible psychotropic effects in normal subjects. Its use is recommended only for medically healthy patients with acute mania or to prevent recurrences of manic-depressive states. Lithium toxicity is enhanced when sodium intake is lowered; this effect should be recognized if it is imperative to administer the drug to patients who are on intravenous therapy or have cardiac or renal disease. Toxic reactions and side effects include a benign, diffuse thyroid enlargement, vomiting, diarrhea, tremor, and polyuria.

Liver:

Large multilobulated organ in the upper right abdominal cavity. Responsible for multiple, profound chemical manipulations and metabolic processes that receives over 20% of resting cardiac output. *See* Liver function tests.

Liver Function Tests:

Series of blood tests that attempt to determine the functional integrity of the liver. Examples of such tests include prothrombin time, serum bilirubin, alkaline phosphatase, and serum glutamic oxaloacetic transaminase (SGOT). Because of the tremendous capacity of the liver to function despite injury, much of the liver has to be damaged before the tests show any deviations from normal.

LM:

See Lumen.

Lobar Atelectasis:

See Atelectasis.

Lobar Bronchi:

See Conducting airways.

Local Anesthetic (LA):

Agent that produces a transient/reversible loss of sensation in a circumscribed portion of the body. This primary effect of LAs is due to action on nerve fibers decreasing the permeability of the nerve membrane to sodium ions, thereby preventing an action potential. The nerve membrane remains in a polarized state, and the block produced by LAs is therefore known as a nondepolarizing nerve block. Modern LAs (all weak bases) are classified as either amides or esters depending on their chemical linkages. Most LAs are combined with an acid (usually hydrochloric) to form a salt that is stable and soluble in water. The specific method by which the amide or ester LA undergoes metabolic breakdown constitutes a major difference between the two classes. Esters such as procaine (Novocaine) and tetracaine (Pontocaine) are mainly hydrolyzed in the plasma by pseudocholinesterase, whereas amides, such as lidocaine (Xylocaine), dibucaine (Nupercaine), bupivacaine (Marcaine), and mepivacaine (Carbocaine), are metabolized in the liver. The toxicity of the LA depends on the plasma level of the drug, which in turn is influenced by the rate of absorption into the bloodstream, degree of plasma binding, rate of distribution to the tissues, and rate of removal via tissue metabolism or excretory pathways. Most LAs (except cocaine) have vasodilating properties, the clinical effects of which are to increase the rate of absorption of the drug in the blood, thereby increasing the anesthetic level in the blood and the potential for overdose. Absorption of the LA also depends on the injection site, the degree of vasodilation, the dose, and the presence of a vasoconstrictor in the solution. Vasoconstrictors, such as epinephrine, are frequently added to the LA solution (used for nerve block or infiltration) to prevent absorption of the drug, prolong its local pain control activity, and reduce systemic reactions. Once the LAs are absorbed from the injection site, they can affect the cardiovascular system and central nervous system (CNS) (paradoxical excitation and then CNS depression or linear cardiac depression with increasing dose). Side effects, such as anxiety, tachycardia, and hypertension, may be related to the added epinephrine. In general, toxic reactions are related to overdosage or, rarely, to allergic manifestations. Lidocaine is also used intravenously for its antiarrhythmic effect. *See* Table, Figure. *See* Dissociation constant; Ionic channel; Sodium channel.

Lockout Interval:

Parameter used for the programming of patient-controlled analgesia devices. It is the amount of time the operator mandates must be consumed before a new triggering of the infusion device is allowed. *See* Patient-controlled analgesia.

Lofentanil:

Probably the most potent synthetic opioid ever discovered. It is 10,000–13,000 times as potent as morphine. It has no practical use, as it appears to be nonreversible when administered to humans or animals. It may be the ultimate poison.

Logarithm:

System of notation in which every positive number is expressed as a power of 10. For example, 1000 can be expressed as 10^3 ($10 \times 10 \times 10$) or log 1000 = 3.

Long, Crawford:

See Morton, William T. G.

Local Anesthetic: Clinical profile of local anesthetic agents.

Agent	Concentration (%)	Clinical Use	Onset	Usual Duration (h)	Recommended Maximum Single Dose (mg)	Comments	pH of Anesthetic Solutions
Amides							
LIDOCAINE	0.5–1.0	Infiltration	Fast	1.0–2.0	300	Most versatile agent	6.5
	0.25–0.5	i.v. Regional			500 + epinephrine		
	1.0–1.5	Peripheral nerve blocks	Fast	1.0–3.0	500 + epinephrine	—	—
	1.5–2.0	Epidural	Fast	1.0–2.0	500 + epinephrine		
	4	Topical	Moderate	0.5–1.0	500 + epinephrine		
PRILOCAINE	5	Spinal	Fast	0.5–1.5	100	Least toxic amide agent	4.5
	0.5–1.0	Infiltration	Fast	1.0–2.0	600	Methemoglobnemia occurs usually above 600 mg	
	0.25–0.5	i.v. Regional			600		
	1.5–2.0	Peripheral nerve blocks	Fast	1.5–3.0	600		
MEPIVACAINE	2.0–3.0	Epidural	Fast	1.0–3.0	400	Duration of plain solutions longer than lidocaine without epinephrine. Useful when epinephrine is contraindicated	4.5
	0.5–1.0	Infiltration	Fast	1.5–3.0	500 + epinephrine		
	1.0–1.5	Peripheral nerve blocks	Fast	2.0–3.0			
	1.5–2.0	Epidural	Fast	1.5–3.0			
	4.0	Spinal	Fast	1.0–1.5	100		

Agent	Concentration (%)	Technique	Onset	Duration (h)	Maximum dose (mg)	Comments	pKa
BUPIVACAINE	0.25	Infiltration	Fast	2.0–4.0	175	Lower concentrations provide differential sensory/motor block. Ventricular arrhythmias and sudden cardiovascular collapse reported following rapid i.v. injection	4.5–6
	0.25–0.5	Peripheral nerve blocks	Slow	4.0–12.0	225 + epinephrine		
	0.25–0.5	Obstetrical epidural	Moderate	2.0–4.0	225 + epinephrine		
	0.5–0.75	Surgical epidural	Moderate	2.0–5.0	225 + epinephrine		
	0.5–0.75	Spinal	Fast	2.0–4.0	225 + epinephrine 20		
ETIDOCAINE	0.5	Infiltration	Fast	2.0–4.0	300	Profound motor block useful for surgical anesthesia but not for obstetrical analgesia	4.5
	0.5–1.0	Peripheral	Fast	3.06–12.0	400 + epinephrine		
	1.0–1.5	Surgical epidural	Fast	2.0–4.0	400 + epinephrine		
DIBUCAINE	0.25–0.5 hyperbaric	Spinal	Fast	2.0–4.0	400 + epinehprine 10	Recommended only for spinal and topical use	
	0.00067 hypobarbic	Spinal	Fast	2.0–4.0	10		
	1.0	Topical	Slow	30–60	50		
Esters **PROCAINE**	1.0	Infiltration	Fast	30–60	1000	Used mainly for infiltration and differential spinal blocks. Allergic potential after repeated use	5–6.5
	1.0–2.0	Peripheral nerve blocks	Slow	30–60	1000		
	2.0	Epidural	Slow	30–60	1000		
	10.0	Spinal	Moderate	30–60	200		

Local Anesthetic (continued)

AGENT	CONCENTRATION (%)	CLINICAL USE	ONSET	USUAL DURATION (h)	RECOMMENDED MAXIMUM SINGLE DOSE (mg)	COMMENTS	pH OF ANESTHETIC SOLUTIONS
CHLOROPROCAINE	1.0	Infiltration	Fast	30–60	800	Lowest systemic toxicity of all local anesthetics	2.7–4
	2.0	Peripheral nerve block	Fast	30–60	1000 + epinephrine	Intrathecal injection may be associated with sensory/motor deficits	
	2.0–3.0	Epidural	Fast	30–60	1000 + epinephrine		
					1000 + epinephrine		
TETRACAINE	0.5	Spinal	Fast	2.0–4.0	20	Use is primarily limited to spinal and topical anesthesia	4.5–6.5
	2.0	Topical	Slow	30–60	20		
COCAINE	40–10.0	Topical	Slow	30–60	150	Topical use only. Addictive. Causes vasoconstriction. CNS toxicity initially features marked excitation ("Fight or Flight" Response). May cause cardiac arrhythmias owing to sympathetic stimulation.	
—	—	—	—	—	—		
BENZOCAINE	Up to 20	Topical	Slow	30–60	200	Useful only for topical anesthesia	

*Note: Epinephrine-containing solutions have a pH 1 to 1.5 units lower than plain solutions.

Table 13–1. Clinical profile of local anesthetic agents. (Reprinted with permission from Covino BG. Clinical Pharmacology of Local Anesthetic Agents. In Cousins MJ, Bridenbaugh PO (eds). *Neural Blockade in Clinical Anesthesia and Management of Pain*. Philadelphia, JB Lippincott, 1988 pp 111–114.

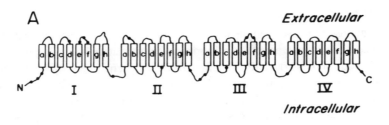

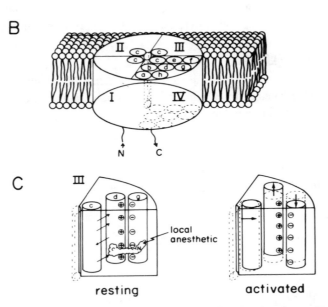

Local Anesthetic: A speculative model for the molecular mechanism of LA action. (A) The primary sequence of the large subunit of the Na^+ channel has four repeating domains (I–IV), each containing six to eight sequences of amino acids that probably form α-helical structures spanning the nerve membrane, denoted by the rectangles lettered a–h. (B) Montal et al. have postulated that these helices pack together in approximately fourfold symmetry with the polar edges of the four "c" helices forming the lining of the ion pore, projecting through the center of the complex. For simplicity, only the extracellular (top) and intracellular (bottom, dashed elipses) edges of the helices are shown in B. (C) A stripped-down view of quadrant III shows the postulated gating mechanism. Helix d is coupled to the pore-forming helix c and contains a series of basic amino acids that form a strip of positive charge. These charges are stabilized in the low dielectric milieu of the membrane interior by a strip of negative charges counterposed to them on helix g. membrane depolarization activates the channel by pulling the g helix in, pushing the d helix out, and thereby moving the c helix to open the channel pore. We speculate that a local anesthetic binds at a site near or on the gating helices, as drawn on the resting conformation, and prevents these conformational changes.

Long-Term Memory:

Construct used to describe human memory function. It has been compared to a library in that it contains large amounts of information appropriately indexed apparently indefinitely and without active effort. Information from long-term memory, to be useful, must be brought back to short-term memory. The long-term memory can be divided into declarative and nondeclarative memories. The declarative memory includes facts, for example, that can be explicitly retrieved. Nondeclarative memories are implicit, cannot be directly retrieved but can be demonstrated by performance. An example of nondeclarative memory is the ability to write or the ability to rollerskate. *See* Short-term memory.

Long-Term Potentiation (LTP):

Form of synaptic plasticity characterized by facilitation of synaptic transmission that is long-lasting and elicited by brief, high-frequency stimulation of certain presynaptic axons. It is believed to play a role in long-term memory.

Loop (Looping):

Closed series of computer instructions that are repeated continuously until a terminal condition is satisfied. The loop may start at any point, but it must return to that point for completion.

Lorazepam (Ativan):

See Benzodiazepine.

Lorfan:

See Levallorphan.

Lower Esophageal Sphincter (LES):

Junction between the lower esophagus and the cardia of the stomach. It must be active to prevent reflux. The usual pressure differential across the LES is on the order of 15–25 mm H_2O.

Low-Flow Anesthesia:

Concept of administration of inhalational anesthetics by which the continuous flow anesthesia machine is set to deliver a small fresh gas quantity per minute only replacing the amount of oxygen used by the patient as well as any anesthetic vapors lost through the skin or due to leaks. An elaborate way of administering anesthesia, certainly the most economical method for inhalational anesthesia, it is not generally used because of a small, but real chance that the patient may become hypoxic due to miscalculation of oxygen consumption. The use of pulse oximetry and end-tidal carbon dioxide measurement may make this technique popular once again. *See* Anesthesia system, closed.

Low-Flow Endobronchial Insufflation:

Technique for apneic oxygenation by which a continuous flow of compressed air is delivered by a specially designed tube with its forked ends resting in the main stem bronchi. *See* Apneic oxygenation.

L/S Ratio:

Ratio of lecithin to sphingomyelin usually determined by thin-layer chromatography done on amniotic fluid. A ratio higher than 1.0 to 3.5:1.0 seems to indicate a low risk for fetal development of infant respiratory distress syndrome (IRDS). *See* Foam test.

LTP:

See Long-term potentiation.

LUD:

See Left uterine displacement.

Ludwig Angina:

Diffuse suppurative infection of the connective tissues, muscles, and glands of the submaxillary area. This cellulitis may become so extensive as to cause respiratory embarrassment.

Lumbar Puncture:

Technique used to administer local anesthetics or to sample cerebrospinal fluid. A long spinal needle is inserted into the subarachnoid space, penetrating the supraspinous and interspinous ligaments, ligamentum flavum, and dura. See Figure. *See* Spinal anesthesia.

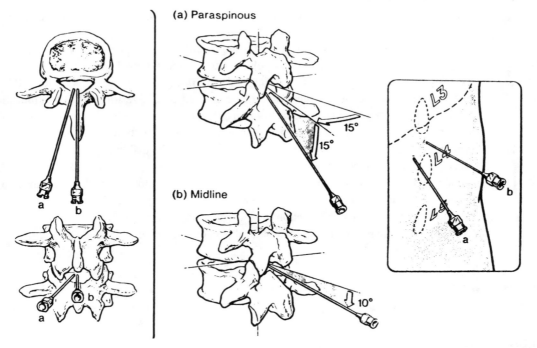

Lumbar Puncture: Two common techniques of lumbar puncture for spinal anesthesia. (a) Paraspinous, paramedian, or lateral approach. (b) Midline approach.

Lumen (LM):

Cavity of a tube or tubular organ. It is also the unit of measurement of light flux.

Luminal:

See Phenobarbital.

Luminescence:

Emission of electromagnetic radiation from a substance as the result of a nonthermal process. Luminescence also relates to visible radiation. If the luminescence terminates when the energy source is removed it is known as fluorescence, whereas if it persists it is phosphorescence. *See* Cathode-ray tube; Fluorescence; Phosphorescence.

Lung, Nongas Exchange Functions of:

Specific lung functions other than the oxygenation of blood. The lungs (1) act as a reservoir for blood and can increase their blood volume with only a slight increase in pulmonary and venous pressures; (2) act as a filter, removing thrombi and clots; (3) secrete the phospholipid dipalmitoyl lecithin, a major component of surfactant (necessary for lung expansion); (4) inactivate circulating serotonin, bradykinin, and some prostaglandins; and (5) primary site for conversion of angiotensin I to angiotensin II.

Lung Volumes and Capacities:

Nomenclature useful in respiratory physiology to describe the air in the lung at maximum inspiration, maximum expiration, and at agreed upon points in between. There are four primary volumes: (1) Tidal volume (TV) is the volume of air inspired or expired with each normal breath. (2) Inspiratory reserve volume (IRV) is the maximal amount of gas that may be inspired in excess of the normal tidal volume. (3) Expiratory reserve volume (ERV) is the maximal volume of gas that can still be expired by active forceful expiration after normal tidal expiration. (4) Residual volume (RV) is the gas remaining in the lungs after a maximal expiratory effect. Pulmonary capacities are combinations of two or more lung volumes. Total lung capacity (TV + IRV + ERV + RV) is the maximal volume to which the lungs may be expanded with maximum inspiration. Vital capacity (IRV + TV + ERV) is the greatest volume of air that can be expelled from the lungs following maximum inspiration. Functional residual capacity (ERV + RV) is the amount of air remaining in the lungs at the end of a normal tidal volume expiration (resting expiratory level). Inspiratory capacity (IRV + TV) is the maximum amount of air that can be inspired at the end of a normal tidal volume expiration. *See* Figure.

Lutz Needle:

See Epidural needle.

Luxury Perfusion:

Localized excessive cerebral blood flow in relation to metabolic requirements. *See* Intracranial hypertension.

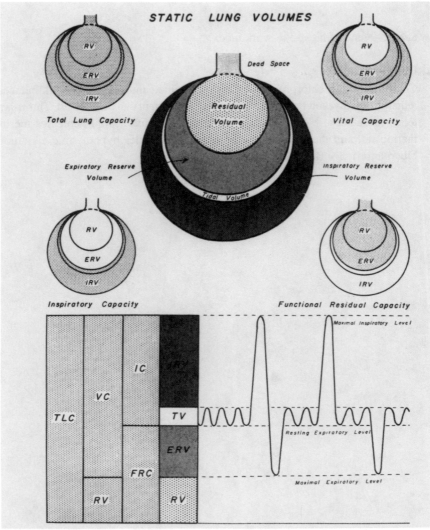

Lung Volumes and Capacities: Static lung volumes and their relationship to the capacities of the lung.

LVAD:

See Left ventricular assist device.

LVEF:

See Muga scan.

LVET:

See Left ventricular ejection time.

LVSWI:

See Left ventricular stroke-work index.

Lytic Cocktail:

Combination of chlorpromazine, promethazine, and meperidine. It induces a state of lethargy, apathy, and tranquility from which a patient can be aroused. This mixture of drugs tends to decrease blood pressure as well. The lytic cocktail depresses the hypothalamic thermostat, and the patient may be maintained under hypothermic conditions (artificial hibernation). *See* Brompton mixture.

M

MAC:

See Minimum alveolar concentration.

MAC Awake:

Minimum alveolar concentration of an inhalation anesthetic at which 50% of a patient population responds to simple direct verbal commands.

Macroglossia:

Enlargement of the tongue frequently seen in congenital disorders such as Down syndrome. Airway maintenance is a potential problem with this disorder. In patients with macroglossia, abnormal positioning of the head during general anesthesia may occlude venous outflow of the tongue, making it even larger.

Macrophage (Histiocyte):

Large phagocytic cell of the reticuloendothelial system. These cells are found in the loose connective tissue and are capable of engulfing bacteria and cellular debris, thereby providing a defense mechanism against foreign matter. Tissue macrophages include the Kupffer cells in the liver and alveolar macrophages (dust cells) in the lung. *See* Alveolar cell types.

Macroshock:

Electrical current passing through the body that is strong enough to produce a physically perceptible response. This response can take the form of sensory stimulation, muscular contraction, or burns. The threshold of perception for 60-cycle alternating current is approximately 1 mA. *See* Microshock.

Magill System:

Modification of the basic Ayre T-piece for pediatric anesthesia purposes. It is useful with spontaneous, assisted, or controlled ventilation. In the Mapleson classification of breathing systems, the Magill system is known as the A system, based on the relative positions of the fresh gas flow, expiratory valve, and reservoir bag. *See* Ayre T-piece.

Magnesium (Mg):

Silvery, metallic element with atomic number 12 and atomic weight 24.3. Its salts are essential in nutrition. Magnesium is necessary as a catalyst for many intracellular enzymatic reactions, especially those pertaining to carbohydrate, lipid, and protein metabolism. Normal extracellular Mg concentration is approximately 1.8–2.5 mEq/L. Hypomagnesemia

(<1 mEq/L), seen in alcoholic cirrhosis, chronic nephritis, prolonged parenteral fluid therapy (without Mg supplementation), and some cancers, is characterized by neuromuscular and central nervous system (CNS) hyperirritability, cardiac arrhythmia, convulsions, depression, and psychotic behavior. Hypermagnesemia (>3 mEq/L), associated with chronic renal disease and magnesium sulfate enemas, is characterized by drowsiness, CNS depression, and decreased skeletal muscle contraction (similar to hyperkalemia). The body's normal Mg content is approximately 25 g, half of which is in the bone. *See* Eclampsia; Ion.

Magnesium Hydroxide (Milk of Magnesia):

Useful antacid and cathartic.

Magnesium Sulfate (Epsom Salt):

Magnesium salt useful as a cathartic and antacid. It is also used to treat seizures associated with acute nephritis and eclampsia. Magnesium sulfate may accentuate the action of muscle relaxants. *See* Eclampsia.

Magnetic Resonance Imaging (MRI):

Expensive hi-tech technology for two-dimensional imaging of planes internal to the body. Capable of resolution and exactness heretofore impossible to achieve by x-ray technology or computerized axial tomography (CAT scanning), the technique involves placing the body (in whole or in part) in an intense electromagnetic field, which causes shifting of electrons, particularly in water molecules. When the field is turned off, these molecules release energy that can be detected and interpreted as variable densities. If anesthesia or sedation is required for patients undergoing this technique, it is imperative that nonmagnetic materials be used as magnetic materials move violently in the magnetic field.

Mainstream Sampling:

Type of gas sampling usually associated with capnography in which the entire gas sample is passed through a detection chamber, for example, when a photocell is placed on the expiratory limb of the anesthesia circuit. Sidestream sampling occurs when a small stream of gas is pulled off from the anesthesia circuit and taken to an appropriate test chamber.

Malignant Hyperpyrexia:

See Malignant hyperthermia.

Malignant Hypertension:

Progressive elevation of blood pressure that ultimately produces degenerative changes in the walls of blood vessels; papilledema; retinal, cerebral, and renal hemorrhages; and left ventricular hypertrophy. A persistent diastolic blood pressure of 120 mm Hg associated with these clinical features is indicative of malignant hypertension. Approximately 1% of patients with essential hypertension develop malignant hypertension. Untreated patients usually live less than 1 year and typically die of uremia, heart failure, or stroke. Diet and drug therapy are implemented to reduce the hypertension, and many of these patients may survive for several years without renal disease. *See* Hypertension.

Malignant Hyperthermia (MH; Malignant Hyperpyrexia):

Genetically determined (autosomal dominant) syndrome that manifests following an abnormal reaction to various anesthetic agents. Although any potent inhalation anesthetic agent or skeletal muscle relaxant may precipitate an acute crisis of MH in susceptible individuals, the most frequently implicated are halothane and succinylcholine. Malignant hyperthermia can also occur following the use of a monoamine oxidase inhibitor or psychotropic agent. Malignant hyperthermia is characterized by a markedly elevated body temperature, tachycardia, unstable blood pressure, arrhythmias, cyanosis, skin mottling, and profuse diaphoresis. Muscle rigidity may or may not be present. (Temperatures as high as 44°C have been recorded.) Laboratory findings include respiratory and metabolic acidosis; hyperkalemia; hypercalcemia; and elevated levels of serum creatine phosphokinase (CPK), lactic dehydrogenase, and myoglobin. The overall incidence of MH during anesthetic administrations is approximately 1/15,000 in children and 1/50,000 in adults. Mortality rate is approximately 60% if treated late or inadequately. The ability to determine susceptibility to MH preoperatively would aid in decreasing this rate. Evaluation of patients should include a complete medical history and physical examination to detect subclinical muscle weakness or abnormality. Specific information about anesthetic exposures in family members should be obtained as well. Measurement of CPK levels, although not completely reliable, may be used as a screening test. Muscle biopsies may be taken for halothane-caffeine contraction tests and for light and electron microscopic studies to determine certain myopathies in patients susceptible to MH. Awareness of MH susceptibility should alert the anesthetist to use neuroleptanesthesia (fentanyl and droperidol), pancuronium, or a barbiturate/N_2O/narcotic combination and to avoid succinylcholine and other depolarizing relaxants, local anesthetics of the amide type, and halogenated anesthetic agents. The classic presentation of MH (in a previously unsuspected case) is muscle rigidity (frequently jaw muscles) following intravenous succinylcholine administration. Anesthesia should be terminated immediately, and if the surgery is of an emergency nature, neuroleptanesthesia should be administered. Dantrolene, a muscle relaxant which acts directly on skeletal muscle, should be given intravenously as soon as MH is recognized. It decreases the amount of calcium released from the sarcoplasmic reticulum, thereby reversing the probable defect found in MH, i.e., an inability to control calcium levels within the muscle fibers that leads to an elevated intracellular calcium concentration. *See* Caffeine test; Creatine phosphokinase; Dantrolene.

Malignant Hyperthermia Association of the United States (MHAUS):

Organization that is primarily educational. It was founded in 1981 and has its headquarters in Westport, Connecticut. MHAUS actively assembles and disseminates information to medical professionals and individuals who are susceptible to malignant hyperthermia. *See* Malignant hyperthermia.

Malignant Hyperthermia Group:

Organization set up in 1987 by representatives of each Malignant Hyperthermia Diagnostic Center across North America. The group met to standardize the caffeine and halothane contracture test (CHCT). The criteria included reliance on two diagnostic tests, one utilizing halothane and the other incremental caffeine and requiring a minimum of three fresh muscle strips for each test.

Malpractice:

Treatment rendered by a health practitioner that is improper, unskillful, and possibly injurious to the patient. An acceptable level of professional skill, "the standard of care," is not rendered. This "standard" varies with the amount and type of training the individual practitioner possesses and is determined by expert testimony.

Mandatory Minute Volume (MMV):

Technique of ventilatory support in which the overall minute volume is maintained at a preset level. The patient's responses regulate the volume supplied by spontaneous respiration, and the remainder is supplied by intermittent positive-pressure breathing.

Mandible:

Lower jaw. It is the largest and strongest facial bone and the only movable bone in the skull. It consists of the body, ramus, angle, coronoid process, and condylar process. (The condylar process forms part of the articulation of the temporomandibular joint.) The mental nerve and vessels pass through the mental foramen, and the inferior alveolar nerve and vessels pass through the mandibular foramen. These sites are frequently used for dental local anesthetic injections. *See* Figure.

Mannitol:

Naturally occurring sugar alcohol that is useful as a diuretic when administered intravenously. It rapidly decreases brain mass and cerebrospinal fluid pressure by an osmotic gradient created in plasma prior to neurosurgery and intraocular tension during an acute attack of congestive glaucoma or prior to ophthalmic surgery. Mannitol is known as an osmotic diuretic because it filters at the glomerulus, is not reabsorbed by the tubules, and is resistant to metabolic changes. In large amounts it adds to the osmolality of the plasma, the glomerular filtrate, and the tubular fluid. The extracellular fluid volume increases after administration of mannitol.

Manometer:

Instrument for measuring the pressure of liquids and gases. A sphygmomanometer, for example, measures blood pressure.

MAO:

See Monoamine oxidase inhibitor.

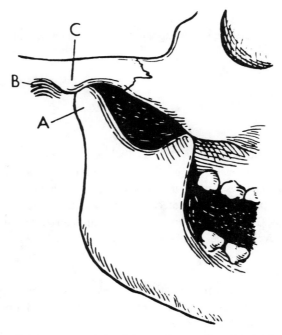

Mandible: Dislocated mandible, a potential mishap of anesthesia which can occur with muscle paralysis and manipulation of the mandible. The condyle (A) is out of the fossa (B) in the base of the skull and has jumped anterior to the articular eminence (C). Direct movement posteriorly is impossible. The condyle must descend before it can move posteriorly to regain normal position.

MAP:

See Mean arterial pressure; Muscle action potential.

Mapleson System:

See Ayer's T-piece.

Marcaine (Bupivacaine):

See Local anesthetic.

Marfan's Syndrome:

Autosomal dominant defect that is the result of abnormal synthesis and consequent accumulation of defective collagen. The clinical manifestations of this syndrome include aortic regurgitation and weak arterial walls. These complications eventually lead to the death of the patient before age 30.

Marijuana:

See Cannabis.

Mask, Anesthesia:

Device for delivering gas and vapor to the nose and mouth simultaneously while sealing out atmospheric air.

Mass Number:

See Nucleus, atomic.

Mass Reflex:

Automatic response exhibited by an area innervated by a segment of the spinal cord distal to a cord disruption. It may be evident in paraplegic individuals. A mild stimulus to the denervated area causes uncontrolled massive sympathetic discharge, resulting in sweating, pallor, blood pressure shifts, defecation, and urination. There may be a withdrawal response in the limbs. The fluctuation in blood pressure can be harmful to the patient, as it may potentially overload the circulatory system.

Mass Spectrometer:

Analytic instrument which identifies a substance by separating and quantifying its ions according to their mass. A mass spectrometer may be used for rapid analysis of respiratory gases accurate to a few parts per million. *See* Figure.

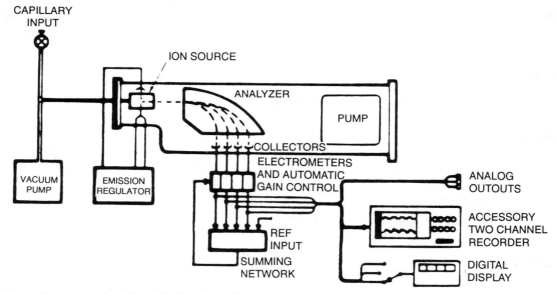

Mass Spectrometer: Simplified schematic.

MAST:

See Military antishock trouser.

Mast Cell:

See Alveolar cell types.

Material Risk:

In law, it is the principle of quantifiable risk, which a reasonable person would want to know before deciding on having or foregoing a proposed therapy. *See* Informed consent.

Maxilla:

Paired bones that form the upper jaw. It articulates with every facial bone except the mandible and forms the floor of the nasal cavities and part of the floor of the orbit and palate. The infraorbital nerve and artery pass through the infraorbital foramen, an opening in the maxilla inferior to the orbit. The incisive foramen and greater and lesser palatine foramens are other canals through which nerves and vessels travel. These are common sites for dental local anesthetic injections.

Maximal Surgical Blood Order Schedule (MSBOS):

Method for minimizing blood utilization while appropriately maximizing blood bank facilities. Based on the blood transfusion experience for a particular group of surgical cases, the MSBOS is a predetermination of the maximum number of units of blood that a blood bank routinely crossmatches for a given procedure. The schedule tends to restrain excessive crossmatching. *See* Blood types.

Maximum Breathing Capacity (MBC):

See Maximum voluntary ventilation.

Maximum Voluntary Ventilation (MVV):

Volume of air that can be breathed per minute by the greatest voluntary effort. To test the MVV, a patient is asked to breathe as deeply and rapidly as possible for 15 seconds. The MVV is reduced in patients with such conditions as airway obstruction and emphysema. MVV is also known as maximum breathing capacity (MBC). *See* Pulmonary function tests.

MBC:

See Maximum voluntary ventilation.

Mcginnis Balloon System:

Endotracheal tube mechanism in which both the endotracheal cuff and the pilot balloon are inflated in parallel. When a fixed pressure in the system is reached, the pilot balloon fills preferentially. It is designed to keep lateral tracheal wall pressure at a minimum.

MDDRG:

See Physician Diagnostic Related Groups.

Mean Arterial Pressure (MAP):

Average blood pressure throughout the cardiac cycle. There is a formula used to approximate this pressure: MAP = diastolic pressure + one third pulse pressure (systolic pressure – diastolic pressure). *See* Arterial blood pressure.

Measured Flow Vaporizer:

See Vaporizer.

Mechanical Nebulizer:

See Nebulizer.

Mechanical Ventilation:

See Ventilator.

Meconium:

Intestinal contents (usually dark green) of the newborn child.

Meconium Aspiration Pneumonitis:

Leading cause of respiratory death in the term newborn. The presence of thick, particulate meconium in the amniotic fluid requires immediate suctioning of the infant mouth and nose. Immediate endotracheal intubation should be considered.

Median:

Middle number of a set of numbers arranged in order of magnitude. For example, the median of the set of serum sodium values 135, 138, 139, 140, 142, 142, and 145 is 140. Note that it is not the same as the arithmetic mean.

Median Power Frequency (MPF):

Means of analysis of an electroencephalograph (EEG) signal along with the peak power frequency (PPF). The MPF and PPF are determined after the EEG signal is analyzed by Fourier computations. Shifts in the MPF and PPF have been used to monitor changes in depth of anesthesia. The MPF is the median frequency of the set of frequencies determined by the Fourier equation. The PPF is the component frequency with the highest amplitude in the same set. *See* Fourier analysis; Leading edge analysis.

Mediastinal Flap:

Movement of the heart and great vessels in the mediastinum toward the unaffected lung during ventilation when one lung has collapsed. It may be a dangerous occurrence, because the entire weight of the mediastinal contents compresses the normal lung.

Mediastinal Shift:

Abnormal position of the mediastinum, which can be visualized by roentgenography. It occurs in patients with significant lung atelectasis.

Mediastinoscopy:

Examination of the mediastinum using a lighted endoscope inserted through a cervical incision at the suprasternal notch. The instrument is passed along the anterior surface of the trachea to the bifurcation of the trachea. Direct visualization allows the surgeon to perform a biopsy of a suspicious area, e.g., lymph nodes or bronchi. This procedure, which requires general anesthesia, is used to evaluate hilar adenopathy and metastatic bronchogenic cancer. It is a potentially hazardous procedure, however, because of the possibility of injury to the great vessels present in the area due to improper scope manipulation.

Mediastinum:

Tissues and organs between the pleura of the lungs that extend from the sternum to the vertebral column. It is subdivided into the superior mediastinum (containing many large vessels), anterior mediastinum (containing the thymus gland), middle mediastinum (containing the pericardium and heart), and posterior mediastinum (containing the esophagus, trachea, and many large lymphatic and blood vessels).

Medical Group Management Association (MGMA):

Founded in 1926, MGMA is an organization for professionals in medical management. The organization is headquartered in Englewood, Colorado.

Medlars:

Acronym for MEDical Literature Analysis and Retrieval System. It is a computerized service of the National Library of Medicine (available to most medical and dental school libraries) that organizes published material into key words and topics to aid a complete literature search.

Mega-:

See SI unit.

Membrane Oxygenator:

Method to facilitate gas exchange in the extracorporeal circulation. The blood and the gases are separated by a membrane which allows diffusion of O_2 and CO_2. It attempts to simulate the physiologic state (no gas-blood contact). This type of oxygenator is expensive and difficult to use, however, and its capacity is limited. *See* Cardiopulmonary bypass; Extracorporeal membrane oxygenation.

Membrane Stabilizing Activity (MSA):

Effect seen with some beta-blockers that have local anesthetic-like activity, usually at high doses, in which they stabilize the cell membrane, causing a slowing of conduction.

Memory, Computer:

Mechanism used for the storage of information within a designated system. Many categories of memory exist: (1) volatile, a temporary type in which power loss causes a loss of the information; (2) nonvolatile, a permanent type whereby loss of electrical power leaves the information intact; (3) random access memory (RAM) in which all stored information is available in the same amount of time; (4) read-only memory (ROM) which is information that can only be read out and not added to by the user; and (5) programmable read-only memory (PROM) which is where ROM can be changed or added to in toto. Reprogramming this type deletes all earlier information. (In the changing world of microelectronics, these definitions are subject to alteration at least every 18 months.)

Mendelson Syndrome:

See Aspiration.

Meperidine (Demerol):

Synthetic opioid analgesic drug that is useful as a supplement to N_2O/O_2 anesthesia. Meperidine is the ancestor of the fentanyl class of synthetic narcotics. In overdose, it can cause EEG activation. *See* Narcotic.

Mephentermine (Wyamine):

Drug related to ephedrine that has both direct and indirect vasoactive properties. It causes the release of endogenous norepinephrine and has a positive inotropic effect on the heart.

Mepivacaine (Carbocaine):

See Local anesthetic.

Meprobamate (Equanil; Miltown):

Drug with mild sedative and tranquilizing properties. Side effects tend to be dose-related; high doses cause drowsiness and may induce allergic reactions (skin rash and itching). Meprobamate has an additive effect with alcohol and other central nervous system depressants.

Mercury Switch:

Device whereby electrical contact can be established between a pair of electrodes by a drop of mercury enclosed in a glass cylinder. Depending on the tilt of the cylinder, the mercury moves either toward or away from the contacts to make or break a circuit.

Mesh:

Network or screen composed of small openings that allow various sized particles to pass through or be retained. Mesh size is designated according to the number of openings per linear inch and is used to grade soda lime granules. *See* Carbon dioxide absorption.

Mestinon:

See Pyridostigmine.

Metabolic Acidosis:

Condition in which there is a decrease in the pH of the body fluids not caused by an excess of CO_2. Metabolic acidosis may result from severe diarrhea (which would eliminate excessive amounts of sodium bicarbonate), kidney malfunction (which would interfere with normal excretion of metabolic acids), excessive amounts of metabolic acids in the body (from exogenous or endogenous sources), or a loss of alkali from body fluids. It depresses the central nervous system to such a level that it may lead to coma. The acidic pH also leads to an increased rate and depth of respiration (compensatory respiratory alkalosis). *See* Anion gap.

Metabolic Alkalosis:

Condition in which there is an increase in the pH of the body fluids not caused by reduction in CO_2. It may result from excess ingestion of alkaline substances, excessive vomiting of gastric contents (and a subsequent decrease in acid content), or excessive secretion of aldosterone by the adrenal gland. Metabolic alkalosis tends to overexcite the nervous system and leads to tetany.

Metabolic Compensation:

See Acid-base compensation.

Metabolite:

Substance produced by metabolism. Metabolites are classified pharmacologically as active or inactive. Active metabolites can produce further changes in physiologic function; inactive metabolites are breakdown products that cause little or no change in physiologic function. Halothane is a general anesthetic with active metabolites from undergoing metabolic breakdown in the body. Up to 30% of inhaled halothane is transformed to nonvolatile metabolites. It is now postulated that bromine (a known sedative), which is a metabolite of the halothane molecule, may account for prolonged awakening after a long halothane anesthetic.

Metaclopromide (Reglan):

A dopamine antagonist, which promotes gastric emptying and increases muscle tone of the lower esophageal sphincter.

Metaraminol (Aramine):

Antihypotensive drug that causes profound peripheral vasoconstriction by acting directly on alpha receptors. *See* Receptor/receptor site.

Metarteriole:

See Microcirculation.

Met-enkephalin:

See Enkephalins.

Meter (m):

Standard international unit of length (approximately equal to 39.37 inches), which is defined in terms of the wavelength of the orange light emitted during electrical excitation of krypton.

Methadone (Amidone; Dolophine):

Synthetic narcotic related to meperidine. Although it has an analgesic potency approximately equal to that of morphine, it has a much longer duration of action. It produces respiratory depression but causes less sedation, nausea, and constipation than morphine. Oral methadone is useful for treatment of narcotic addiction. Subsequent withdrawal symptoms are less severe but may be more prolonged. *See* Narcotic.

Methamphetamine:

See Amphetamine.

Methemoglobin:

See Hemoglobin.

Methohexital (Brevital):

See Barbiturate.

Methoxamine (Vasoxyl):

Sympathomimetic drug that acts directly on alpha receptors. It tends to increase blood pressure by causing vasoconstriction and is therefore used primarily to treat hypotensive states. It has no significant stimulant effect on the heart. *See* Receptor/receptor site.

Methoxyflurane (Penthrane; 2,2-dichloro-1,1-difluoroethyl methyl ether):

Halogenated hydrocarbon that is liquid. It is used as a general anesthetic. It is lipid-soluble and has a low vapor pressure at room temperature. It produces analgesia and relaxation of skeletal muscles. Its use is limited to short-term intermittent administration to lessen the accumulation of the agent in the body. (It may be used during the first stage of labor for its analgesic properties.) Methoxyflurane is nephrotoxic as the drug is metabolized to free fluoride ions and other toxic derivatives that may cause permanent renal damage and high output renal failure. *See* Figure.

Methoxyflurane.

Methylcholine:

Parasympathetic agonist that is a derivative of acetylcholine. Methylcholine along with two other choline esters, bethanechol and carbachol, has a marked decrease in susceptibility to hydrolysis by serum cholinesterase. They effectively, for a short time, mimic the muscarinic activities of acetylcholine. They decrease heart rate, conduction and contractility; increase bronchial smooth muscle contraction; increase bladder motility and bladder sphincter relaxation; and increase sweating and salivation. *See* Acetylcholine.

Methyldopa (Aldomet):

Antihypertensive agent that decreases both blood pressure and total peripheral resistance. It has been reported to both maintain cardiac output and decrease cardiac output. Its precise mechanism of action is unknown, but it is currently believed to act primarily on the central nervous system. Methyldopa, given orally or parenterally, tends to produce sedation and some depression. This drug and its metabolites interfere with laboratory tests for catecholamines, and their presence in blood and urine produces false-positive results for pheochromocytoma.

Methylene Blue:

Dark green crystalline powder that produces a distinct blue color in solution, which is a useful histologic-biologic stain. Because it can be reduced to a colorless form and oxidized to its blue form, methylene blue may be used as an indicator in reversible oxidation-reduction reactions. The dye has weak bactericidal properties but is no longer used for this purpose. Currently, methylene blue in low doses is relied on as a treatment for methemoglobinemia. It hastens the conversion of methemoglobin to hemoglobin. Conversely, high concentrations of methylene blue oxidize the ferrous ion of reduced hemoglobin to the ferric form, thereby inducing methemoglobinemia.

Methyl Methacrylate:

Volatile flammable liquid that is easily polymerized. It is useful as a monomer for resins and as a bone cement. To form the cement, a powder (polymer that contains short chains of methyl methacrylate) and a liquid (monomer that contains single molecules) are rapidly mixed to form a semiviscous mass that hardens as molecular chains lengthen and cross-link (polymerization). There is controversy as to what effect this semisolid material has on the circulation when placed onto raw bone surfaces; i.e., both hypertension and hypotension are seen.

Methylmorphine (Codeine):

See Narcotic.

Methylparaben:

See Preservative.

Metoprolol:

Drug that is a relatively selective β_1 blocking drug that has β_2 blocking effects in higher doses. It has neither intrinsic sympathomimetic activity nor membrane stabilizing effects.

393

Metrazol:

See Pentylenetetrazol.

Metubine:

See Dimethyl tubocurarine iodide; Neuromuscular blocking agent; Tubocurarine chloride.

Metycaine:

Also called monocaine, piperocaine and neothesin. It was the first local anesthetic introduced into clinical practice after the discovery and use of procaine. The use of this agent has recently been confined to dentistry. *See* Local anesthetic.

Meyer-Overton Theory:

See Lipid solubility theory of anesthesia.

Mg:

See Magnesium.

MG:

See Myasthenia gravis.

MGMA:

See Medical Group Management Association.

MH:

See Malignant hyperthermia (malignant hyperpyrexia).

MHAUS:

See Malignant Hyperthermia Association of the United States.

MI:

See Myocardial infarction.

Microbicide:

Agent that kills all organisms.

Microcirculation:

Part of the vascular network comprising the arterioles, capillaries, and venules, and their smaller branches. The arterioles divide into metarterioles (precapillaries), which are lined with discontinuous muscle cells. Blood flows from the metarterioles into the venules via a capillary thoroughfare vessel. True capillaries are connecting side branches of this thoroughfare vessel or channel and are lined with a single layer of endothelial cells. The openings of the true capillaries are surrounded by smooth muscle precapillary sphincters, which regulate the surface area of the capillary-venule network. Venules merge to form collecting venules, which drain the entire microcirculatory unit. Arteriovenous anastomoses provide extensive collateral circulation. (Many capillaries originate from single metarterioles, and branch and anastomose repeatedly to provide increased surface area, which effectively lowers the velocity of blood flow.) Sympathetic blockade causes the musculature of the metarterioles and precapillary sphincters to relax, making the entire capillary bed available for blood passage. If it occurs over a large enough portion of the microcirculatory bed, it can cause a profound drop in blood pressure as the resultant intravascular volume is suddenly three to four times that of circulating blood. Sympathetic blockade does not cause a maximal increase in intravascular volume because the capillary beds have an intrinsic vasomotor tone affected by the sympathetic nervous system. This vasomotor tone can be disturbed by histamine or local acid-base derangements. *See* Acid-base balance; Histamine; Microsphere, biologic.

Microfuel Cell:

See Oxygen analyzer.

Micrognathia:

Congenital or acquired condition in which the jaws are abnormally small. This disorder is significant in anesthesia because a satisfactory fit of the mask is difficult to achieve, and maintenance of the airway is therefore not optimal. *See* Pierre Robin syndrome.

Microhematocrit:

Rapid determination of erythrocyte volume in a small quantity of blood. The measurement is accomplished using a capillary tube of blood in a high-speed centrifuge.

Microshock:

Electric shock of small magnitude that is hazardous to patients with pacemakers, cardiac catheters, or other low-resistance current paths to the heart. Currents smaller than 2 μA appear to be safe irrespective of route. *See* Macroshock.

Microsphere, Biologic:

Minutely sized sphere (5–50 μm) composed of an inert material (cannot be broken down in the circulation) or albumin (can be broken down). Microspheres are used to determine the extent and size of the microcirculation in an organ or part of an organ. They can be prepared so they contain at least eight different radioisotopes. The spheres function by flowing distally with the blood and then lodging, according to size, in the capillaries. They can be identified microscopically (tissue sections) or radiographically (if they are tagged with a radiotracer).

Microwave:

Electromagnetic wave of high frequency (1–300 GHz) and short wavelength (0.1–100 cm) that is not sharply distinguishable from either infrared or radio waves. Microwaves are used for radar surveillance and cooking.

Midazolam:

Water-soluble benzodiazepine derivative that is virtually painless on injection and lessens the incidence of venous thrombosis. It is apparently three to four times as potent as diazepam, has a much shorter half-life, and finds significant use for conscious sedation. *See* Antianxiety; Benzodiazepine; Flumazenil.

Military Antishock Trouser (MAST):

Method of augmenting venous return to the thorax by inflating air sacks encased in a specially designed trouser worn around the lower limbs. It has been used intraoperatively to prevent venous air embolism during sitting craniotomies. *See* Air embolus.

Milliequivalent:

See Equivalent system of measurement.

Millihenry:

See Henry.

Millimeters of Mercury (mm Hg):

Unit of pressure measured by the height (in millimeters) of a column of mercury at standard gravity. One standard atmosphere equals 760 mm Hg.

Milliosmole:

See Osmole.

Mill Wheel Murmur:

Aberrant cardiac sound associated with venous air embolism. It is a relatively insensitive indicator of this condition and is often misinterpreted. [Having listened to a mill wheel on many occasions, I do not find it similar to the murmur of venous air embolism. The mill wheel was courtesy of the Mt. Vernon Historical Society, Alexandria, Virginia.] *See* Embolism.

Miltown:

See Meprobamate.

Mimosa Z:

Indicating agent for absorbents. When fresh, it is red; when exhausted, it is white. *See* Indicator dye.

Mini Mental State Test (MMS):

This test tries, in a brief period of time, to access cognitive functioning. It consists of 11 sections, such as short-term recall, language ability, and orientation to time and to place.

Minimum Alveolar Concentration (MAC):

Anesthetic concentration at 1 atmosphere (after the alveolar gas has equilibrated with the inhaled gas mixture) that is necessary to produce a lack of response to a standard skin incision in 50% of subjects tested. MAC is the best available method for comparing the potencies of inhaled anesthetics. *See* MAC awake.

Minimum Blocking Concentration (C_m):

The lowest level of local anesthetic that blocks nerve impulse conduction. Each anesthetic has its own C_m; and the smaller the C_m, the more effective is the agent. The thicker nerve fibers require a higher concentration of local anesthetic. *See* Duality of pain transmission; Nerve fiber, anatomy and physiology of.

Minute Volume:

Total volume of air leaving the lung each minute, calculated by multiplying the tidal volume by the respiratory rate. The volume of air that enters the lung is slightly greater than the volume of air that leaves the lung because more O_2 is inhaled than CO_2 is exhaled. *See* Lung volumes and capacities.

Miosis:

Contraction of the pupil of the eye.

Miotic:

Agent that produces miosis.

Mitral Regurgitation (Mitral Insufficiency):

Condition in which the mitral (bicuspid, left atrioventricular) valve fails to close completely, thereby allowing reflux from the left ventricle into the left atrium. Chronic mitral regurgitation is usually the result of rheumatic heart disease and can remain stable for many years. Acute mitral regurgitation can occur owing to papillary muscle dysfunction or rupture of the chorda tendineae cordis. (The cusps of the mitral valve are attached by means of the chorda tendineae cordis to papillary muscles which are located on the inner surface of the ventricles. Functioning chorda tendineae cordis and the papillary muscles keep the valve flaps pointing in the direction of the blood flow. Contraction of these muscles prevents the valve from swinging upward into the atrium.) Acute mitral regurgitation is poorly tolerated and may result in death. As the left atrium becomes a low-pressure shunt for left ventricular ejection, the total stroke volume of the left ventricle consists of backflow into the atrium and forward flow into the aorta, which causes left atrial hypertrophy. Symptoms of mitral insufficiency include easy fatigability, exertional and nocturnal dyspnea, and ultimately congestive heart failure. Deliberate peripheral vascular dilatation (with nitroprusside) significantly decreases backflow into the atrium and enhances forward flow.

Mitral Stenosis:

Narrowing of the orifice of the mitral valve that causes obstruction of blood flow from the left atrium to the left ventricle. It is the most common form of rheumatic valvular heart disease in adults. The normal area of the adult mitral valve is 4–6 cm. When progressive narrowing of the valve reduces this area to 1 cm^2 or less, a mean left atrial pressure (LAP) of 25 mm Hg (normal LAP is 8–12 mm Hg) is required to maintain minimally adequate left ventricular filling and cardiac output. This elevated LAP eventually causes an increase in pulmonary arterial and right ventricular pressures, which produces symptoms such as dyspnea on exertion and paroxysmal nocturnal dyspnea. As the disease progresses, orthopnea and fatigue become prominent and acute pulmonary edema may occur. Adequate control of the cardiac rate is an anesthetic consideration for a patient with this condition. Drugs that may induce tachycardia should be avoided. Mitral valve prostheses are employed to replace the diseased valve surgically.

Mitral Valve Prolapse (Click Murmur Syndrome, Barlow Syndrome):

Anatomic abnormality of the mitral valve support structure that results in prolapse of the mitral valve into the left atrium when the left ventricle contracts. This finding is present in approximately 5–10% of the adult population.

Mivacurium (Mivacron):

A new short-acting nondepolarizing neuromuscular blocking agent with minimum cardiovascular effect, hydrolyzed by plasma cholinesterase. *See* Neuromuscular blockade, assessment of.

MMS:

See Mitral valve prolapse.

MMV:

See Mandatory minute volume.

Mode:

Value that occurs most frequently in a set of variables.

Modem:

Acronym for *mod*ulator/*dem*odulator. It is a device that transforms or converts signals from one type of equipment into a form for use in another type. It is typically used to modulate and demodulate signals transmitted over communication networks.

Modulation:

Controlled variation of frequency, phase, or amplitude of a wave to transmit a message.

Mogadon (Nitrazepam):

See Benzodiazepine.

Moisture Exchanger (Artificial Nose):

Device, composed of a condenser or filter, that allows efficient humidification for a patient who is breathing through a tracheostomy or endotracheal tube. Because the temperature of the exchanger is lower than that of the body, some water vapor from expiration condenses on its inner surface and is thereby able to humidify the inspired air. This apparatus lessens fluid loss seen when the upper airways are bypassed. It also helps prevent excessive drying of the lower air passageways.

Molal Solution:

Solution that contains 1 mol solute dissolved in 1 kg solvent.

Molar Pregnancy (Hydatidiform Mole):

Abnormal pregnancy resulting from a pathologic ovum. The chorionic villi become hydropic and trophoblastic tissue proliferates. This condition is more common in older women. Most hydatidiform moles are benign. Urinary human chorionic gonadotropin (hCG) hormone levels are markedly elevated.

Molar Solution:

Solution in which each liter contains 1 gram-molecule of the dissolved substance.

Mole (mol):

See Gram-molecular weight.

Molecule:

Smallest quantity into which a substance may be divided while still retaining all its chemical properties.

Monitor:

Instrument used to measure, display, and record (continuously or intermittently) certain physiologic variables, such as pulse, blood pressure, and respiration.

Monoamine Oxidase (MAO) inhibitor:

Drug that blocks MAO, an enzyme important in catecholamine degradation. When this enzyme is inhibited, an increase in the concentration of norepinephrine, dopamine, and serotonin results, producing side effects such as orthostatic hypotension, nervousness, and insomnia. Severe adverse reactions (hypertension, headache, heart palpitations) occur in patients who have ingested tyramine-rich foods and beverages (e.g., aged cheese, Chianti wine) or certain drugs (e.g., meperidine, barbiturates, sympathomimetic amines). MAO inhibitors were originally introduced to treat depression, Because the pronounced side effects they can produce, however, their use has decreased. Newer MAO inhibitors are becoming available with fewer side effects.

Montage:

Term for the layout of multiple sampling electrodes, particularly in electroencephalography.

Montando Tube:

U-shaped endotracheal tube used to deliver anesthetic gases through a tracheostomy.

Montevideo Unit:

System for determining the relative force of uterine contractions using intrauterine pressure (in mm Hg) × the frequency of contractions during a 10-minute period.

Morbidity:

Condition of being ill. In common usage, morbidity describes the possibility and type of untoward effects following a specific procedure. For example, morbidity associated with endotracheal anesthesia includes sore throat or damaged teeth. In statistics, morbidity indicates the relative incidence of disease.

Morbid Obesity:

A condition which is present when the body weight is more than twice normal. *See* Broca index.

Morphine:

Naturally occurring narcotic analgesic obtained from opium. It is the standard of comparison of potency for all narcotics. *See* Figure. *See* Narcotic.

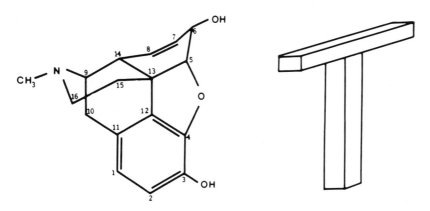

Morphine: The T-shaped molecule of morphine.

Mortality:

Condition of being subject to dying. In common usage, mortality describes the possibility of dying from a given procedure or technique. In statistics, mortality rate indicates the proportion of deaths in a population.

Morton, William T. G.:

Dentist and medical student who gave the first successful demonstration of general anesthesia, employing diethyl ether, at the Massachusetts General Hospital on October 16, 1846. (The operating room, known as the Etherdome, still exists as a memorial.) Diethyl ether was brought to the attention of Morton by Charles Jackson, his chemistry professor. Crawford Long, a Georgia surgeon, used diethyl ether as a general anesthetic on his own patients at least 4 years earlier (but without publishing). Gardner Quincy Colton demonstrated the use of N_2O as an anesthetic in Connecticut in 1844. Horace Wells, a dentist in the audience, was so impressed with the agent that he offered to test it on himself. Wells demonstrated N_2O the next year at Harvard, but the results were unfavorable and the technique was thought to be useless. Controversy developed as to who should receive recognition for inventing anesthesia. No one profited from the discovery and most of those involved spent the rest of their lives in litigation.

Mouth-to-Mouth Resuscitation:

Method of artificial ventilation in which the rescuer's mouth is placed over the victim's mouth (mouth and nose in an infant) and air is blown forcefully into the lungs at a rate of 12 times/minute in an adult or 30 times/minutes in an infant. It provides adequate O_2 for life support even though exhaled breath contains only 14–18% O_2. This technique is combined with external cardiac massage in cardiopulmonary resuscitation (CPR) to resuscitate patients with cardiac arrest. *See* Cardiopulmonary resuscitation.

MPF:

See Median power frequency.

MRI:

See Magnetic resonance imaging.

MSA:

See Membrane stabilizing activity.

MSBOS:

See Maximal surgical blood order schedule.

Mucociliary Transport:

Cleansing action of the cilia in the trachea and respiratory passageways. Cilia are fine, hair-like structures, approximately 7.0 µm long and 0.3 µm thick, projecting from specialized columnar cells of the mucous membrane. Ciliary movement occurs at a rate of 10–15 times/second to move mucus and trapped foreign material upward toward the hypopharynx for swallowing. Ciliary activity is optimal at 28–33°C, stops at 7–10°C, and decreases at about 35°C. In actuality, however, ciliary activity is directly influenced by the quantity of mucus secreted rather than by temperature changes. Low concentrations of volatile general anesthetics stimulate ciliary activity, whereas high concentrations depress it. (N_2O has no effect on ciliary transport.) Nonhumidified gases dry the mucous membranes and hinder ciliary movement. This effect is even more pronounced following concomitant use of atropine as a premedicant.

Mucolytic Agent:

See Respiratory care.

Mucomyst:

See Respiratory care.

Mucus:

Viscous fluid suspension secreted by the mucous membranes and composed of mucin (a complex polysaccharide), water, desquamated cells, leukocytes, and inorganic salts. Mucus moistens and protects the respiratory tract and is essential for ciliary activity. *See* Mucociliary transport.

Muga Scan (Multiple Uptake Gated Acquisition Scan):

A test of cardiac function using radionuclide cineangiography. The test measures the left ventricular ejection fraction (LVEF), which is the change in blood volume in the left ventricle between diastole and systole divided by the volume of blood in the left ventricle during diastole. The scan outlines the wall of the heart and therefore can detect abnormal wall movements. LVEF has been proposed as a good predictor of perioperative cardiac complications, particularly for large vascular procedures.

Multibreath Test:

Test used to determine the rate of washout of pulmonary N_2 when 100% O_2 is administered starting at the end of a normal expiration. The N_2 concentration, continuously measured at expiration by an N_2 analyzer, is nearly linear (on semilogarithmic paper) when plotted against the number of breaths in normal patients, which is explained by the fact that the remaining N_2 in the lung is successfully diluted by each breath of pure O_2, thereby causing an exponential decay in N_2 concentration. When ventilation is uneven, as in a diseased lung, the line becomes successively curved because different regions of the lung eliminate N_2 at different rates. At the end of the test, only the N_2 left in the least ventilated spaces is being washed out. The test can be modified to determine the functional residual capacity (FRC). FRC = volume of N_2 washed out × 100/78 (since 78% of the gas in the lungs is N_2). *See* Infrared analyzer; Single-breath test.

Multiple Sclerosis:

Acquired (immunologic?) disease of the central nervous system whose symptoms usually appear in patients between the ages of 15 and 40. Characterized by demyelination of neurons in the brain and spinal cord along cerebrospinal fluid pathways, the specific symptoms depends on the site of demyelination, and they can wax and wane for years.

Multiplex:

Simultaneous transmission of two or more signals via a common carrier wave by means of time, frequency, or phase divisions. *See* Modulation.

Muscarine:

Naturally occurring alkaloid that acts like acetylcholine on receptors of smooth muscles and glandular cells. These receptors are blocked by atropine. Muscarine is not used clinically at the present time. *See* Neuromuscular blocking agent; Pilocarpine.

Muscarinic Drug:

Drug that produces effects similar to those of muscarine. Such effects include marked diaphoresis, salivation, noticeable drop in blood pressure, and temporary slowing or cessation of the heart rate. Examples of muscarinic agents are acetylcholine, methacholine, bethanechol, and carbachol.

Muscle Action Potential (MAP):

See Neuromuscular blocking agent.

Muscle Contraction/Relaxation:

See Actomyosin.

Muscle Relaxant:

See Neuromuscular blocking agent.

Muscle Twitch:

Sudden solitary muscle contraction of extremely short duration (approximately 7.5–100.0 ms). The twitch can be elicited by exciting the motor nerve or by passing an electrical current through the muscle itself.

Muscular Dystrophy:

Group of hereditary diseases characterized by progressive atrophy of the muscles and by the absence of central nervous system (CNS) involvement. Many types of muscular dystrophy have been described. Duchenne, the most common type, is sex-linked and is therefore confined to young boys. Serum enzyme studies reveal markedly elevated levels of creatine phosphokinase (CPK). Female carriers may be identified with moderate increases in the serum CPK levels. Pseudohypertrophy of the calf muscles, due to replacement of muscle cells by fatty and fibrous tissues, is evident. Cardiac abnormalities occur in many of these patients. Most Duchenne patients die within a decade from respiratory infection or cardiac failure. With other forms of muscular dystrophy, symptoms tend to appear later in life, and localized areas of the body become affected.

Mushroom Valve:

Type of valve made up of a balloon that when inflated occludes a passageway.

Mutagenicity:

Ability of a substance (mutagen) to produce a permanent alteration in the genetic material. Mutagens include radioactive substances and some chemotherapeutic agents.

MVV:

See Maximum voluntary ventilation.

Myasthenia Gravis (MG):

Chronic disease characterized by muscle weakness and easy fatigability. Typically, there are alternating periods of remission and exacerbation of symptoms. Ptosis and diplopia are common early signs. Myasthenia gravis appears to be caused by an abnormality at the neuromuscular junction that prevents the muscle from contracting normally in response to nerve impulses. Functionally, it appears that either (1) the neurons fail to release enough acetylcholine; or (2) excessive cholinesterase present in the neuromuscular junction destroys acetylcholine (ACh); or (3) there is a decrease in acetylcholine receptors. (Motor neurons stimulate contraction of muscle fibers by releasing ACh.) Although the exact etiology of MG is unknown, it is thought to be an autoimmune disorder based on the following: (1) Evidence exists that thymectomy may produce clinical improvement.

(Organ-specific autoimmunity has been established to have a pathogenic role.) (2) Autoantibodies to ACh receptors have been demonstrated in the sera of MG patients. MG results from this autoimmune damage to the ACh receptors, which in turn results in failure of neuromuscular transmission. (3) Malignant thymomas may occur in patients with MG. Confirmation of an MG diagnosis may be accomplished by the "edrophonium test." An intravenous injection of edrophonium chloride, a short-acting anticholinesterase agent, produces a brief increase in muscle strength in the extremities. A nondepolarizing muscle relaxant may also be administered for diagnostic purposes; however, adequate means for patient resuscitation must be available. Patients with MG are sensitive to drugs that produce respiratory depression (sedative-hypnotics and opiates) and to drugs that produce muscle weakness, e.g., neuromuscular blocking agents. These effects are potentiated with certain antibiotics (kanamycin, streptomycin, and neomycin) and some general anesthetics (ether, halothane, methoxyflurane, and cyclopropane). *See* Neuromuscular blocking agent.

Myasthenic Syndrome:

Weakness of the peripheral musculature usually seen in association with bronchial carcinoma. Patients with myasthenic syndrome are highly sensitive to muscle relaxant agents. It differs from myasthenia gravis (MG) in that it first attacks limb muscles rather than ocular muscles and has a poor response to anticholinesterases. *See* Myasthenia gravis.

Mycifradin:

See Neomycin.

Mydriasis:

Excessive or extreme dilatation of the pupil. Unless induced by drugs or trauma, pupil dilatation is considered to be a sign of significant central nervous system damage. *See* Miosis.

Myelin Sheath:

Lipid-ladened material that surrounds the axon of large nerve fibers. Its presence is critical for the rapid conduction of nerve impulses. It acts as an electrical insulator by preventing the flow of ions between the axon and the extracellular fluid and as a pharmacologic insulator by protecting a nerve fiber from the actions of local anesthetics. It is possible for a local anesthetic to reach the nerve membrane only at the nodes of Ranvier, where the myelin thins out or is absent. Furthermore, these nodes act as shortcuts for electrical impulses, i.e., impulses can actually jump from node to node faster than they can travel down the nerve membrane. This jumpwise conduction is called saltatory conduction. As a consequence of *saltatory conduction,* local anesthetics must cover a distance of at least two or three nodes (which in practical terms is a span of approximately 8–10 mm) to block myelinated fibers. *See* Figure. *See* Nerve fiber, anatomy and physiology of.

Myelography:

Roentgenographic visualization of the spinal subarachnoid space following a lumbar or cisternal puncture and injection of air or an opaque medium.

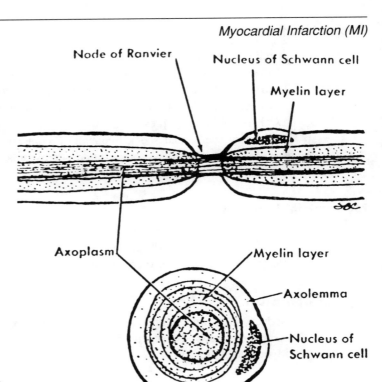

Myelin Sheath: Structure of a myelinated nerve fiber.

Myelomeningocele:

Congenital defect of the spinal canal through which the cord and its meninges protrude. Myelomeningoceles most frequently occur in the lumbosacral region. The abnormality is either exposed or covered by atrophic skin and infection is therefore a frequent complication. Paraplegia, absence of bowel and bladder control, and sensory disturbances below the level of the lesion are common. Surgical repair is aimed at preventing infection and correction of spinal abnormalities.

Mylaxen:

See Hexafluorenium.

Myocardial Hibernation:

Persistently impaired myocardial function caused by reduced coronary blood flow. The function can be restored, partially or completely, by improving blood flow or reducing oxygen demand. *See* Myocardial stun.

Myocardial Infarction (MI):

Syndrome resulting from sudden and persistent curtailment of myocardial blood supply due to a thrombus, embolus, or spasm (?) in a coronary artery. It is characterized by severe and prolonged chest pain (described as crushing or compressing) and electrocardiographic (ECG) and laboratory evidence of myocardial necrosis. There is a rise in non-cardiac-specific serum glutamic-oxaloacetic transaminase (SGOT) and in the serum levels of cardiac-specific isoenzymes of creatinine phosphokinase (CK) and lactic dehydrogenase (LDH). SGOT and CK rise and fall rapidly. Although LDH rises slowly, the rise is sustained. The size of the infarct can be correlated with the amount of enzyme released. The ECG irregularities, if present, are usually abnormal Q waves and ST segment changes. Pulmonary edema and shock frequently accompany MI, and pulmonary embolism and cardiac arrest are common complications. Paroxysmal atrial or ventricular arrhythmias may occur after MI. *See* QRS complex.

Myocardial Irritability:

Tendency of the myocardium toward arrhythmia. Irritability is enhanced by circulating catecholamines, lowered body temperature, myocardial ischemia, acid-base imbalance, electrolyte abnormalities (particularly potassium), and certain drugs, e.g., halothane.

Myocardial Stun:

Reduced myocardial function due to inadequate coronary blood flow that is not partially or completely restored when oxygen demand is decreased or blood flow is restored. *See* Myocardial hibernation.

Myocardium:

Specialized muscle tissue of the heart. Cardiac muscle fibers are involuntary and striated, and are responsible for the contraction of the heart. The myocardial tissue layer lies between the epicardial and endocardial layers. Cardiac muscle tissue contracts rhythmically about 70–80 times/minute. Specialized conducting tissue of the heart transmits electrical impulses that stimulate cardiac contraction. Two networks of cardiac muscle fibers exist: the muscle walls and the septum of the ventricles. Each fiber is separated from the next by an intercalated disk. When a single fiber is stimulated, all the fibers in that network become progressively stimulated. Each network therefore contracts as a functional unit. *See* Heart, conduction system of.

Myoclonic Seizure:

Type of seizure often associated with degenerative or metabolic brain disease. It manifests as isolated clonic jerks, usually in response to a sensory stimulus. *See* Epilepsy.

Myofascial Pain Syndrome (Myofascial Syndrome, Myofascitis):

Chronic pain syndrome that depends on an aberrant feedback cycle to the central nervous system from myofascial "trigger points." A trigger point is a localized area of tenderness and sensitivity in skeletal muscle. They can be identified by a positive "jump sign." The jump sign is a visible shortening of that part of the muscle that contains the myofascial band when it is stimulated by direct contact. These trigger points appear to have distinct histologic changes of degeneration and destruction of muscle fibers with fatty infiltration. The entire syndrome of myofascial pain syndrome can be ameliorated by direct injection of local anesthetic, at times with added steroids.

Myoglobin:

O$_2$ transport and storage protein complex found in muscle fibers.

Myoneural Junction:

See Neuromuscular blocking agent.

Myotonia:

Increased irritability and contractility of a muscle or group of muscles. It is temporary when brought about by excessive exercise. Myotonia is identical with tonic muscle spasm and is seen in various disease states.

Myotonia Atrophica (Myotonic Dystrophy; Steinert Disease):

Rare, hereditary (autosomal dominant) disease characterized by a degenerative myotonia and subsequent atrophy of the muscles (especially of the face and neck). Ptosis, cataracts, testicular atrophy, endocrine dysfunction, and mental retardation are associated with this disorder. Some patients develop diabetes mellitus. Cardiac musculature is frequently affected. The patients are particularly prone to cardiorespiratory abnormalities and therefore pose problems for anesthetic management. When continued muscle contraction occurs in this disease, neuromuscular blocking agents do not relax the affected muscles because the motor nerves are uninvolved.

Myotonia Congenita (Thomsen Disease):

Rare, inherited (autosomal dominant) disease characterized by rigidity and the tonic spasm of muscles upon movement after a period of rest. (The stiffness disappears after continual use of the muscles.) The disease is manifested clinically in the entire somatic and branchiomeric muscular system. Patients complain of difficulty chewing, swallowing, talking, and walking and show evidence of muscle cell hypertrophy. Although myotonia congenita is not often debilitating, patients with the disease present anesthetic problems similar to those of patients with muscular dystrophy. *See* Muscular dystrophy.

Myotonic Dystrophy:

See Myotonia atrophica.

Mytolon:

See Benzoquinonium.

N

n-Butyl p-aminobenzoate (BAB):

Molecule that is a highly lipid-soluble congener of benzocaine. Used at one time as a local anesthetic, it may have neurotoxic and neurolytic effects.

N$_2$:

See Nitrogen.

N$_2$O:

See Nitrous oxide.

NACS:

See Neurologic and adaptive capacity score.

Nadolol:

Noncardioselective beta-blocking agent with no intrinsic sympathomimetic activity or membrane stabilizing activity. It is approximately equal in potency to propranolol.

Nalbuphine (Nubain):

Partial agonist/antagonist opioid that has a ceiling effect for both pain relief and respiratory depression. *See* Ceiling effect.

Naloxone (Narcan):

Derivative of oxymorphone (Numorphan), it is a popular narcotic antagonist that is neither analgesic nor addicting. It reverses the respiratory depressant action of drugs such as morphine, meperidine, and methadone. Naloxone administered alone does not cause respiratory depression, pupillary constriction, sedation, or analgesia. *See* Figure.

Naltrexone:

Long-acting narcotic antagonist that can be administered orally. It is used both for the treatment of opioid addiction and to decrease the incidence of side effects of epidural opioids.

Nano-:

See SI unit.

Naloxone.

Nanoequivalents:

System of units used as an alternate to quantitating hydrogen ion concentration. *See* pH.

Narcan:

See Naloxone.

Narcotic:

A term referring to any group of drugs that cause narcosis. The elements of narcosis are pain relief, insensibility, and stupor (a sleep-like state). A particular drug may have highly variable amounts of each element. Addiction potential is also considered a characteristic of narcotics. Morphine (a product of the poppy plant), was the original narcotic. Although used for at least a thousand years, it was first isolated chemically during the nineteenth century. Since that time, hundreds, if not thousands of derivatives, which are partially or wholly synthetic, have been made. In potency, they range from codeine, which is approximately 25–50 times less potent than morphine, to the illegal lofentanil, which is about 13,000 times as potent as morphine. *See* Table. *See* Lofentenil; Morphine.

Narkotest Meter:

Device for indicating the percentage of halogenated hydrocarbon anesthetics in the gas mixture of an anesthetic circuit. Values are registered by changes in the length of Silastic bands attached to a lever that moves in proportion to the concentration of anesthetic absorbed. The Narkotest meter is not accurate, requires a large gas sample, is affected by water vapor, and has a slow response time. *See* Halothane analyzer.

Nasal Catheter (Nasal Cannula):

Device that is inserted into the nose to supply O_2 enrichment to the inspired breath or to maintain an airway. Nosebleed is a fairly common consequence of its use. Nasal cannulas augment inspired O_2 only up to a limit of approximately 50%; the high volumes of fresh gas flow required for this level of augmentation dry out the nasal mucosa, causing the patient discomfort.

Narcotics: A comparison of opioid analgesics with respect to dosage, duration of action, withdrawal symptoms, and distinguishing features.

NONPROPRIETARY NAME	TRADE NAME	DOSE * (*mg*)	DURATION OF ACTION * (*hours*)	WITHDRAWAL SYMPTOMS	DISTIN-GUISHING FEATURES ▲
Morphine		10	4–5	*see* text	*see* text
Heroin (diacetyl-morphine)		4 (2–8)	3–4	like morphine	2
Hydromorphone (dihydromorphinone)	DILAUDID	1.5	4–5	like morphine	
Oxymorphone (dihydro-hydroxymorphinone)	NUMORPHAN	1.0–1.5	4–5	like morphine	
Metopon (methyldihydro-morphinone)		3.5	4–5	like morphine	3
Codeine		120 (10–20)	(4–6)	*see* text	*see* text
Hydrocodone (dihydro-codeinone)	HYCODAN †	(5–10)	(4–8)	between morphine and codeine	4,8
Drocode (dihydrocodeine)	SYNALGOS-DC †	60	4–5	between morphine and codeine	
Oxycodone (dihydro-hydroxycodeinone)		10–15 (3–5)	4–5 (4–5)	close to morphine	8
Pholcodine (β-morph-olinylethylmorphine)		(5–15)	(4–5)	much less than codeine	3,4,5
Levorphanol	LEVO-DROMORAN	2	4–5	like morphine	6,8
Methadone	DOLOPHINE	8–10	3–5	*see* text	6,8
Dextromoramide	PALFIUM	5–7.5	4–5	like methadone	3,6,8
Dipipanone		20–25	4–5	like methadone	3,6,8,9
Phenadoxone		10–20	1–3	less than morphine	3,9
Meperidine	DEMEROL, *etc.*	75–100	2–4	*see* text	1,7
Alphaprodine	NISENTIL	40	1–2	like meperidine	1,7

* *Dose* shown is the amount given *subcutaneously* that produces approximately the same analgesic effects as 10 mg of morphine administered subcutaneously. The figures in *parentheses* are the *doses* and the *duration of action* for *oral, antitussive* doses; they are not necessarily equieffective doses. *Duration of action* shown is for analgesic effects after *subcutaneous* administration; after *intravenous* administration, peak effects are somewhat more pronounced but overall effects are of shorter duration. The doses and durations shown in this table are based primarily on papers reviewed by Eddy and coworkers (1957), Reynolds and Randall (1957), and Lasagna (1964), and are augmented by more recent studies of newer drugs.

▲ 1 = causes little or no constipation; 2 = manufacture or importation into the United States illegal; 3 = not available in the United States; 4 = by tradition used mainly as an antitussive; 5 = little or no analgesic or euphorigenic activity; 6 = may exhibit cumulative effects on repeated dosage; 7 = retains 25 to 40% of efficacy when given orally; 8 = retains 50% or more of its analgesic efficacy when given orally; 9 = marked irritation at injection sites.

† These opioids are marketed in the United States only in combination with additional ingredients.

Nasotracheal Tube (Nasoendotracheal Tube):

Endotracheal tube that is introduced into the trachea via the nose. It has a smaller diameter than an orotracheal tube and less curvature, so it passes easily along the posterior pharyngeal wall. Nasotracheal intubation is usually used for oral and maxillofacial operations and in patients with jaw fractures or trismus. *See* Endotracheal tube.

National Fire Protection Association (NFPA):

Voluntary nonprofit organization that writes codes and standards for fire prevention and safety for both the public and private sectors. It was founded in 1896, and its headquarters are in Boston. The NFPA has developed and continues to update approximately 240 codes and standards, which cover such diverse areas as smoke detectors, firefighter clothing, stairway fire door standards, transportation of hazardous materials, electric wiring, and qualifications to be a firefighter. The single most popular code is the National Electric Code (NEC). *See* Central gas supply.

Nausea:

Distinctly unpleasant sensation in the epigastrium or abdomen described as "bloating," "fullness," or "need to vomit."

NBAS:

See Neonatal behavioral assessment scale.

Near-Field Potential:

A change in electrical potential (signal), particularly during evoked potential recording that is detected by an electrode close to the neurogenerator that initiates the signal. Signal strength fades as the distance from the neurogenerator to the recording site increases. Therefore the amplitude of near-field sensory evoked potentials is larger than far-field potentials by approximately an order of magnitude. *See* Far-field potential.

Nebulizer:

Device that disperses water into a fine droplet spray. It is used to humidify the respiratory airways. Two types exist: the high-pressure gas nebulizer and the ultrasonic nebulizer. The high-pressure gas type produces droplets of large diameter (5–20 µm). The ultrasonic type produces droplets approximately 1 µm in diameter, which easily penetrate to the terminal bronchioles.

Needle Valve:

See Flow control valve.

Negative Water Balance:

Condition in which total water loss (sweat, urine, feces, lungs) exceeds water intake. Positive water balance exists when water loss is less than water intake. Negative water balance leads to dehydration; positive water balance leads to overhydration and water intoxication. *See* Water balance.

Negligence:

Legal term for failure to administer ordinary care (standard of care) to an individual resulting in harm to that person.

Negligence, Gross:

Legal term indicating willful behavior compounding neglect. It may be grounds for punitive damages as well as malpractice.

Nembutal:

See Barbiturate; Pentobarbital.

Neomycin (Mycifradin):

Broad-spectrum antibiotic of the aminoglycoside series. It is used topically against infections from burns, wounds, or ulcers and orally to reduce the microbial content in the intestines prior to bowel surgery. Intestinal malabsorption syndrome and yeast infection may result, however. Toxic effects such as renal damage and nerve deafness may occur with parenteral use. *See* Antibiotic.

Neonatal Behavioral Assessment Scale (NBAS):

See Brazelton score.

Neoprene:

See Elastomer.

Neostigmine (Prostigmin):

Reversible anticholinesterase drug used to improve neuromuscular transmission in patients with diseases such as myasthenia gravis (alleviating muscle fatigue) and to reverse non-depolarizing muscle relaxants. It is also used to treat glaucoma and urinary retention, and to enhance gastrointestinal smooth muscle tone. Intramuscular injections of neostigmine produce elevation of skin temperature, diaphoresis, salivation, constriction of the intestines, bradycardia, and fasciculations. Atropine antagonizes the muscarinic effects of neostigmine but does not antagonize the general fasciculations.

Neo-Synephrine:

See Phenylephrine.

Nerve Action Potential (NAP):

See Action potential; Depolarization.

Nerve Conduction:

See Action potential, Depolarization.

Nerve Conduction Velocity:

See Nerve fiber, anatomy and physiology of.

Nerve Fiber, Anatomy and Physiology of:

Long pathways of electrically conducting tissue constituting a peripheral nerve and composed of both motor and sensory fibers. These fibers vary in size and are myelinated or unmyelinated. (Generally, large diameter fibers are myelinated, and small ones are unmyelinated.) These nerve fibers are classified as either A, B, or C based on anatomic and functional differences. The A and B fibers are both myelinated, whereas the C fibers are not. The A fibers are divided into alpha, beta, gamma, and delta types. The A-alpha fibers, which range in size from 6 to 22 μm, are concerned with proprioception, motor function, and reflex activity. The A-beta fibers, 5–22 μm in size, are responsible for touch and pressure sensations. The A-gamma fibers are 2–8 μm in diameter and serve muscle tone. The A-delta fibers, only 1–5 μm in diameter, are concerned with pain, temperature, and touch. The B fibers are preganglionic sympathetic (autonomic) fibers less than 3 μm in diameter. The C fibers (postganglionic sympathetic fibers) measure only 0.1–1.3 μm in diameter and are important in temperature, pain, and reflex responses. The diameter of a nerve fiber is important for determining its ability to carry impulses and its sensitivity to local anesthetics. The larger (myelinated) nerve fibers can conduct impulses at an approximate rate of 100 m/second, whereas the smaller (unmyelinated) fibers conduct impulses at an approximate rate of 0.1 m/second. Nerve fiber susceptibility to local anesthetics depends on the circumstances of the investigation being done. For example, the large A fiber has been shown to be blocked both faster and slower than the small diameter C fibers! The classic description of peripheral nerve blockade onset was loss of sympathetic function, then loss of pinprick sensation, then loss of touch and temperature sensation, and then loss of motor function. At a nerve trunk, the local anesthetic effect progresses from the outer layer of fibers (mantle fibers) toward the inner layer of fibers (core fibers) and spreads in a proximal to distal direction. As the anesthesia wears off, this direction of diffusion reverses, so that sensation is restored first to the proximal and then to the distal areas. With intravenous regional anesthesia (Bier block), the anesthetic effect is reversed and progresses from the core fibers to the mantle fibers. *See* Duality of pain transmission; Local anesthetic; Minimum blocking concentration; Myelin sheath. *See* Table.

Nerve Fiber, Anatomy and Physiology of: Classification of Nerve Fibers.

CONDUCTION/ BIOPHYSICAL CLASSIFICATION	ANATOMIC LOCATION	MYELIN	DIAMETER (μ)	RATE (m·s⁻¹)	FUNCTION
A-FIBERS A-alpha A-beta	Afferent to and efferent from muscles and joints	Yes	6–22	30–85	Motor and Proprioception
A-gamma	Efferent to muscle spindles	Yes	3–6	15–35	Muscle Tone
A-delta	Sensory roots and afferent peripheral nerves	Yes	1–4	5–25	Pain Temperature Touch
B-FIBERS	Preganglionic sympathetic	Yes	<3	3–15	Vasomotor Visceromotor Sudomotor Pilomotor
C-FIBERS sC	Postganglionic sympathetic	No	0.3–1.3	0.7–1.3	Vasomotor Visceromotor Sudomotor Pilomotor
drC	Sensory roots and afferent peripheral nerves	No	0.4–1.2	0.1–2.0	Pain Temperature Touch

Nerve Gas:

Organophosphorus compounds that have been used as war agents. They interfere with nerve transmission and cause profound cardiac and respiratory interference. They are classed pharmacologically as permanent anticholinesterase inhibitors. First invented in Germany during World War II, there are now at least four major types. The "V" agents can be absorbed through the skin and can persist in the environment for hours or days once sprayed in the atmosphere. *See* Organophosphorus compounds; Pralidoxime.

Nerve Membrane:

See Action potential; Myelin sheath; Nerve fiber, anatomy and physiology of.

Nerve Palsy:

Paralysis of a peripheral nerve. Inadvertent compression or stretching of the nerve or poor positioning of the limbs during operations may lead to nerve palsy. Injection of an irritating solution into or near the nerve trunk may produce the same effect. Post-operative assessment of nerve damage is possible if knowledge of the preoperative condition exists. Diseased nerves are more susceptible to trauma, and certain illnesses such as diabetes mellitus, periarteritis nodosa, and alcoholism predispose the nerves to injury.

Nerve Stimulator:

See Peripheral nerve stimulator.

Nesacaine (Chloroprocaine):

See Local anesthetic.

Neuralgia:

Acute paroxysmal pain radiating along peripheral nerves.

Neuralgia Paresthetica:

Neuralgia characterized by numbness, burning pain and tingling in the anterior lateral aspect of the thigh. It is frequently associated with obesity and prolonged pressure from belts. Although it may be due to nerve entrapment, it is not easy to identify a cause. Injection of a local anesthetic into the lateral femoral cutaneous nerve near the superior iliac spine can provide both diagnosis and pain relief. *See* Causalgia.

Neuritis:

Inflammation of a nerve or group of nerves that causes pain, sensory disturbances, or impaired reflexes. *See* Neuropathy.

Neuritis, Alcohol:

See Alcohol neuritis.

Neuroleptanalgesia:

See Neuroleptanesthesia.

Neuroleptanesthesia (Neuroleptanalgesia):

State of altered awareness, restfulness, and unconsciousness produced by the combined administration of (usually) intravenous Innovar (droperidol plus fentanyl, a butyrophenone and opioid, respectively) with N_2O/O_2. The use of Innovar alone causes neuroleptanalgesia during which the patient remains conscious and minor surgical procedures such as bronchoscopy and cystoscopy may be performed. Neuroleptic agents have antipsychotic activity and typically belong to either the butyrophenone or phenothiazine group. *See* Fentanyl; Innovar; Ketamine.

Neurologic and Adaptive Capacity Score (NACS):

For newborns, the test combines elements of the Amiel-Tison neurologic examination and other procedures. This test is specifically designed to detect central nervous system depression caused by drugs, distinguishing it from depression caused by perinatal deprivation of oxygen or trauma. *See* Brazelton score.

Neurolysis:

Destruction of nerve fibers. Substances that can cause this destruction are called neurolytic agents and include solutions of alcohol or phenol. They are used to treat intractable pain. *See* Neurotoxin.

Neurometrics:

Three-dimensional display technique for electroencephalographic data. It shows the variables of time, frequency, and amplitude.

Neuromuscular Blockade, Assessment of:

Technique by which the adequacy of muscular relaxation is determined. (1) *Twitch response:* After a single electrical shock to a large motor nerve, the strength of the subsequent contraction of the muscles the nerve supplies is evaluated. When the twitch response is nearly gone, the neuromuscular blockade is suitable for even the most severe retraction during surgery. (When curare is used, at least 75% of the receptors must be blocked in order to obtain a significant decrease in twitch response.) (2) *Tetanic response:* Normally follows administration of rapid, repeated shocks to a large motor nerve: No relaxation occurs between shocks, with continuous contraction being seen. Frequent shocks deplete acetylcholine levels in the nerve endings and, when this effect is combined with endplate blockade, the tetanic response fades with continued stimulation. Commonly used frequencies to demonstrate tetany are 30, 50, 100, and 200 Hz. The higher the frequency of the stimulus, the more is the demand put on the neuromuscular junction. The rate of fade is related to the profoundness of the neuromuscular blockade. (3) *Train-of-Four:* Four supramaximal shocks (above the current required to obtain a maximal response) are given a half-second apart, and the ratio of the height of the fourth twitch to that of the first twitch is used to determine the degree of block. (4) *Physical diagnosis:* Such tests include hand squeeze on command, ability to raise the head from a pillow and hold for 5 seconds on command, and respiratory measurements, such as vital capacity and inspiratory and expiratory force. *See* Figure. *See* Blockade monitor; Double-burst stimulation.

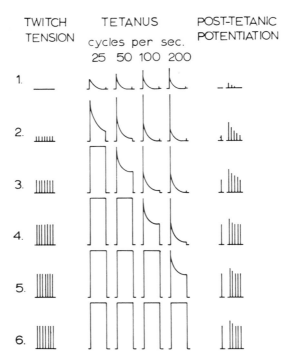

| | TWITCH TENSION | TETANUS cycles per sec. 25 50 100 200 | POST-TETANIC POTENTIATION |

Neuromuscular Blockade: Neurally evoked muscle tension. Idealized diagram of twitch, tetanus at 25, 50, 100 and 200 Hz, and posttetanic potentiation following neuromuscular block. Row 6 indicates normal response without neuromuscular block.

Neuromuscular Blocking Agent:

Drug that produces skeletal muscle relaxation by altering the ability of the neurotransmitter acetylcholine (ACh) to activate the postsynaptic cholinergic receptor of the muscle fiber. Neuromuscular blocking agents are classified as nondepolarizing (competitive) or depolarizing (noncompetitive). Nondepolarizing drugs compete with ACh for the cholinergic receptor sites. If enough nondepolarizer is present, it prevents ACh from interacting with these receptors. Therefore depolarization and contraction of the muscle cannot occur. (This sequence is called competitive inhibition.) These effects may be reversed if a cholinesterase inhibitor (e.g., neostigmine) is administered, which increases available ACh. Examples of nondepolarizers are tubocurarine chloride (Tubarine), gallamine (Flaxedil), dimethyl tubocurarine iodide (Metubine), and pancuronium (Pavulon). Depolarizing drugs, such as succinylcholine, structurally resemble ACh and have a shorter duration of action than nondepolarizing agents. They cause an initial depolarization and muscle contraction (fasciculation) followed by a block. Serum enzyme pseudocholinesterase quickly inactivates the succinylcholine. Depolarizing blockers are noncompetitive, i.e., they are not displaced from the cholinergic receptor by any increase in ACh. Currently, there is no reliable antagonist to depolarizing agents. Their action is terminated by diffusion away from their site of action and metabolism. All neuromuscular blocking agents impair respiration and can produce apnea. Ventilation must therefore be controlled until spontaneous respiration occurs. Neuromuscular blocking agents are useful during general anesthesia to aid in muscle relaxation and endotracheal intubation. Because patient response to neuromuscular blockers differs, it is recommended that a monitoring device, e.g., peripheral nerve stimulator, be used to determine the effectiveness of the drug. *See* Action potential; Neuromuscular blockade, assessment of; Succinylcholine.

Neuromuscular Junction:

Specialized synapse between a nerve fiber and a muscle membrane. *See* Figure. *See* Neuromuscular blocking agent.

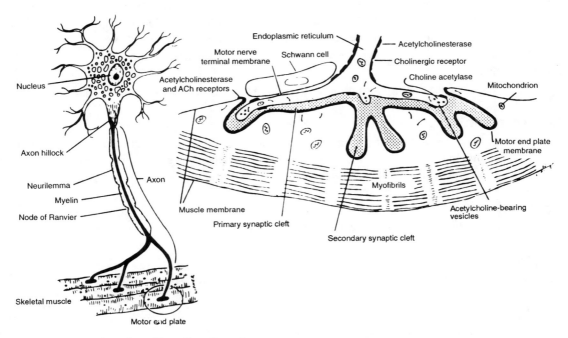

Neuromuscular Junction: Functional anatomy.

Neuromuscular Relaxant:

See Neuromuscular blocking agent.

Neuromuscular Transmitter, Quantal Release of:

Unit of release of acetylcholine from the presynaptic membrane of a nerve terminal. Acetylcholine is stored in the nerve terminal as separate "quanta." A nerve action potential appears to release many quanta. In the absence of an action potential, intermittent spontaneous release of single quanta occurs from the presynaptic membrane. The release of quanta increases exponentially with each stepwise increase in depolarization caused by the action potential. For every 15-mV difference during depolarization there is a 10-fold increase in quanta release. *See* Acetylcholine; Neuromuscular blockade, assessment of.

Neuropathy:

Functional or pathologic disturbance caused by degeneration affecting the peripheral nerves. Neuropathy refers to noninflammatory lesions of the peripheral nervous system, whereas neuritis refers to inflammatory lesions. Possible causes of neuropathy include diabetes, alcoholism, trauma, nutritional deficiencies, and, indirectly, cancer. Less commonly, there are a few inherited neuropathies. Occasionally, no specific etiology is discovered. One nerve, several nerves, or bilaterally symmetric nerves may be affected.

Neuropeptide Y (NPY):

A 36-amino acid peptide that is found in blood vessels having sympathetic innervation; it appears to be stored along with the classic neurotransmitter norepinephrine. It seems to modulate norepinephrine action and induce contractions of vascular walls.

Neurotoxin:

Substance that is injurious or destructive to nerve tissue. *See* Intrathecal injection.

Neurotransmitter:

Any of a number of pharmacologically active small molecules that act as synaptic transmission elements in both the central and peripheral nervous systems. *See* Table. *See* Acetylcholine; Norepinephrine; Receptor/receptor site.

Neutron:

Uncharged elementary particle found in all known atomic nuclei except hydrogen.

Newton:

Force that gives a mass of 1 kg an acceleration of 1 m/second.

NFPA:

See National Fire Protection Association.

Nicotine:

Natural poisonous, colorless, soluble, liquid alkaloid obtained from the tobacco leaf. It is used as an agricultural insecticide and veterinary external parasiticide. In humans, nicotine in small doses causes ganglionic stimulation and peripheral constriction. With larger doses, stimulation is quickly followed by neuromuscular blockade, decreased blood pressure, and diminished peripheral resistance. Nicotine also causes the release of catecholamines in some organs. It stimulates the central nervous system, producing tremors, and with large doses, convulsions. Toxic effects of nicotine are observed in children who ingest tobacco products. Nicotine poisoning may also result from the ingestion of insecticide-laden substances. Symptoms of acute nicotine poisoning include nausea, salivation, abdominal pain,

Neurotransmitter: Some Known and Possible Neurotransmitters and Neuromodulators.

Substance	Site of action	Type of action	Status*
Acetylcholine	Vertebrate skeletal muscle; neuromuscular junction	Excitatory	Est.
	Autonomic nervous system:		
	preganglionic sympathetic	Excitatory	Est.
	pre- and postganglionic parasympathetic	Excitatory or inhibitory	Est.
	Vertebrate CNS	Excitatory	Est.
	Various invertebrates	Various	Est.
Norepinephrine	Most postganglionic sympathetic, CNS	Excitatory or inhibitory	Est.
Glutamic acid	CNS	Excitatory	Poss.
	Crustacea, CNS and PNS	Excitatory	Est.
Aspartic acid	Vertebrate retina	—	Poss.
γ-Aminobutyric acid (GABA)	CNS	Inhibitory	Est.
	Crustacea, CNS and PNS	Inhibitory	Est.
Serotonin (5-hydroxytryptamine)	Vertebrate and invertebrate CNS	—	Est.
Dopamine	CNS	—	Est.
Octopamine	Insect CNS	Excitatory modulation	Est.
Substance P	CNS	Inhibitory modulation	Est.
Various peptides	Vertebrate and invertebrate CNS; gut	Various	Est.

*Est. = established transmitter; Poss. = possible transmitter.

vomiting, diarrhea, cold sweat, headache, dizziness, mental confusion, and weakness. A decrease in blood pressure, dyspnea, and a weak, rapid, irregular pulse follow. Death due to respiratory failure may result. Chronic nicotine abuse (smoking) is now thought of by many (except smokers!) as a true addiction.

Nifedipine:

Calcium channel blocking drug used for the prevention of coronary ischemia, treatment of chronic stable angina, and control of hypertension. *See* Calcium channel blocker.

Nipride:

See Sodium nitroprusside.

Nisentil:

See Alphaprodine; Narcotic.

Nitrazepam (Mogadon):

See Benzodiazepine.

Nitric Oxide:

Naturally found oxide of nitrogen. Toxic in all but tiny quantities, it appears to have profound pharmacologic effects mostly unexplored. It is also probably a limited neuro-transmitter.

Nitrogen (N_2):

Gaseous, soluble element that is colorless, odorless, and tasteless. Its atomic number is 7, and atomic weight is 14. It constitutes 78% of the atmosphere by volume and is a constituent of all proteins. At pressures over 5 atmospheres, N_2 may be a general anesthetic agent (in combination with O_2). This anesthetic ability of N_2 parallels its lipid solubility. Liquid N_2 (at $-196°C$) is useful as a coolant in the laboratory. *See* Nitrogen narcosis; Nitrous oxide.

Nitrogen Analyzer:

See Infrared analyzer.

Nitrogen Dioxide (NO_2):

A reddish brown, poisonous, irritant gas prepared from nitric oxide and air. Under pressure, it becomes nitrogen tetroxide (N_2O_4). NO_2 is an intermediate in the production of nitric and sulfuric acids. Inhalation of NO_2 at concentrations of more than 100 ppm leads to pulmonary edema and possible death. It was a significant contaminant in early nitrous oxide production.

Nitrogen Narcosis:

Condition caused by excessive exposure to high N_2 pressure (e.g., hyperbaric chamber, deep-sea diving) and characterized by stupor and central nervous system depression. These symptoms usually begin with pressures higher than 5 atmospheres for at least 1 hour. *See* Caisson disease.

Nitrogen Tetroxide:

See Nitrogen dioxide.

Nitroglycerin (Nitrol; Nitrostat):

Yellowish, volatile liquid, also known as glyceryl trinitrate, formed by the action of nitric and sulfuric acids on glycerin. It is useful as a vasodilator for the management of angina pectoris. Nitroglycerin administered sublingually produces almost immediate pain relief from an acute anginal attack. (Given prior to exercise or stressful situations, nitroglycerin may be used to reduce the patient's susceptibility to an attack.) The mechanism of action appears to be reduction of the work load of the cardiac muscles by decreasing after-load, production of coronary artery vasodilation and a decrease in the venous return to the heart. Nitroglycerin may also be administered topically, as it is absorbed by the skin. This latter method has a much slower onset of action, although its effectiveness is longer lasting.

Nitroprusside:

See Sodium nitroprusside.

Nitrous Oxide (N_2O; Laughing Gas):

Colorless gas with a slight sweetish odor and taste. It is used as an inhalation anesthetic and analgesic. It is the only inorganic gas useful as a general anesthetic agent. Although N_2O is neither flammable nor explosive, it supports combustion. It is both rapidly absorbed and eliminated from the body. The maximum concentration of N_2O that can be given safely is approximately 75%; over prolonged periods it must be administered with at least 25% O_2 to prevent hypoxia. To provide complete anesthesia, supplementation with a barbiturate (e.g., thiopental sodium) or narcotic, and a neuromuscular blocking agent is advocated. When 70% N_2O in O_2 is used in conjunction with a halogenated hydrocarbon anesthetic, lower levels of the hydrocarbon may be used and a reduction in respiratory and circulatory depression occurs. In hyperbaric chambers, N_2O becomes a total general anesthetic, i.e., supplementation is no longer required. In concentrations below 50%, N_2O is often used as an analgesic during dental procedures. Chronic exposure to N_2O has been implicated in occupational disease among anesthesia and operating room personnel. *See* Figure.

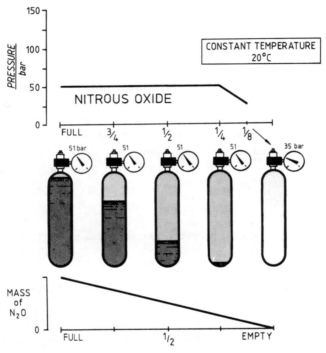

Nitrous Oxide: Relationship between the pressure in a cylinder and the amount of nitrous oxide in it at constant temperature.

Nitrous Oxide Analyzer:
See Infrared analyzer.

NMR (Nuclear Magnetic Resonance):
See Magnetic resonance imaging.

Nociceptive-Specific Neurons:
See Wide dynamic range neurons.

Nociceptor: Properties and Presumed Physiological Role of Nociceptive Afferents Sensitive to Mechanical and Heat Stimuli.

Property	CMHs*	Type I AMHs†	Type II AMHs
Receptive field area (mm²)	19 ± 3‡	37 ± 4¶	1–4††
Skin type	Glabrous and hairy	Glabrous and hairy	Hairy only
Heat threshold (°C)	43.6 ± 0.6‡	>49¶	43††
Receptor utilization time (to heat) (ms)	>50§	Long (>600)**	Short (<200)**
Heat response characteristic	Slowly or quickly adapting§	slowly adapting¶	quickly adapting**
Mechanical threshold (bars)	6.0 ± 0.6‡	3.5 ± 0.3¶	1.7 (0.4 gm)††
Conduction velocity (m/s)	0.8 ± 0.1‡	31.1 ± 1.5¶	15.2 ± 9.9††
Presumed physiological role	Burning pain (second pain) Hyperalgesia in hairy skin	Primary hyperalgesia after injury to glabrous and possibly hairy skin	Pricking pain (first pain) ?Role in hyperalgesia

* CMHs = C-fiber mechano-heat afferents.
† AMHs = A-fiber mechano-heat afferents.
‡ From reference 124.
§ From reference 161.

¶ From reference 31.
** From reference 30.
†† From reference 56.

Nociceptor:

Nerve receptor that perceives pain. Nociceptors are end-organs for A-delta fibers and C fibers. They have a high threshold to their specific stimulus but once activated do not show adaptation (rising threshold in response to a constant stimulus). In fact, reverse adaptation can take place when the threshold is lowered after prolonged stimulation. Subclasses exist that are determined by the initial stimulus causing the response. Such stimuli include temperature extremes, mechanical deformation, and locally released chemicals, such as histamine and acetylcholine. *See* Table.

Noise:

Extraneous, unwanted disturbance in a communications or electronic system.

Nomogram:

Graphic representation of interrelated variables. The Radford nomogram, for example, was designed to show the relation between body weight in pounds, respiratory rate, and basal tidal volume. When the first two are known, the third can be determined from the nomogram. Corrections for fever, altitude, and so on must always be taken into consideration. *See* Figure.

Noncompetitive Antagonism (Irreversible Inhibition):

Pharmacologic phenomenon seen when an agonist is prevented from acting at a specific receptor site by an antagonist, irrespective of the concentration of either. *See* Competitive antagonism; Receptor/receptor site.

Nondeclarative Memory:

See Long-term memory.

Nondestructive Monitor:

See Noninvasive monitor.

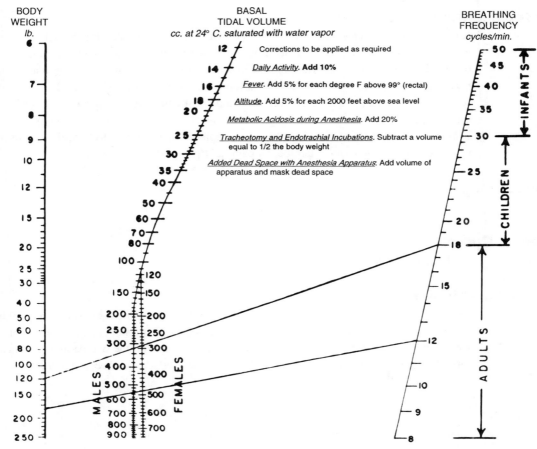

BODY
WEIGHT
lb.

BASAL
TIDAL VOLUME
cc. at 24° C. saturated with water vapor

Corrections to be applied as required

Daily Activity. **Add 10%**

Fever. Add 5% for each degree F above 99° (rectal)

Altitude. Add 5% for each 2000 feet above sea level

Metabolic Acidosis during Anesthesia. Add 20%

Tracheotomy and Endotrachial Incubations. Subtract a volume equal to 1/2 the body weight

Added Dead Space with Anesthesia Apparatus. Add volume of apparatus and mask dead space

BREATHING
FREQUENCY
cycles/min.

INFANTS

CHILDREN

ADULTS

MALES

FEMALES

Nomogram: Radford nomogram.

Nonfade:

See Oscilloscope; Shift register.

Noninvasive Monitor:

Instrument used to observe physiologic functions that does not invade or puncture tissues. It is also called a nondestructive, indirect, external, or transcutaneous monitor. Conversely, invasive monitoring techniques enter, puncture, or penetrate intact tissues.

Nonrebreathing Valve:

Type of valve found in a respiratory apparatus that directs fresh gas to the patient and allows the release of exhaled gas into the atmosphere. These valves are useful in pediatric anesthesia and in portable resuscitators. There are three functional types of nonrebreathing valves: (1) spontaneous ventilation (Stephen-Slater valve); (2) controlled ventilation (Ambu valve); and (3) spontaneous and controlled ventilation (Ambu E, Ambu Hesse, Ambu E2, Fink, Frumin, Laerdal, Lewis-Leigh, and Ruben valves).

423

Norepinephrine (Levophed):

Naturally occurring catecholamine produced by the adrenal medulla. It acts mainly on the alpha receptors and is a potent vasoconstrictor. Norepinephrine (also known as levarterenol or noradrenaline) increases systolic and diastolic pressures, mean arterial pressure, and peripheral resistance. Adverse effects of norepinephrine associated with high doses include severe hypertension, diaphoresis, vomiting, and chest pain. Arrhythmias may occur if the drug is given with some general anesthetic agents. The sympathetic nervous system stimulates production of norepinephrine and epinephrine during physiologic "flight-or-fight" responses. *See* Catecholamine; Dopamine; Epinephrine.

Norcuron:

See Muscle relaxants; Vecuronium.

Normal Curve:

See Frequency curve.

Normal Distribution:

Display of many data points that are symmetric to either side of the mean (the center of the distribution). The standard deviation (SD) measures the variation of each measurement. A normal curve, which displays a normal distribution, depends on the two parameters, mean and SD, and is illustrated by a symmetric, bell-shaped curve. *See* Frequency curve; Standard deviation.

Normality:

Number of gram-equivalent weights of a solute per liter of solution.

Normocapnia:

Normal concentration of CO_2 in the arterial blood in young healthy individuals ($PaCO_2$ = 36–44 mm Hg).

Normothermia:

Oral temperature of 37°C (98.6°F).

Normoxia:

Normal concentration of O_2 in the arterial blood of young, healthy individuals (PaO_2 = 96–104 mm Hg).

North American Drager:

World leader in manufacturing sophisticated anesthesia workstations (i.e., Narkomed 4). They are headquartered in Telford, Pennsylvania.

Novocaine:

See Local anesthetic; Procaine hydrochloride.

Noxious:

Substance that is harmful and destructive.

NPY:

See Neuropeptide Y.

Nucleus, Atomic:

Central, positively charged, dense portion of an atom. Constituting nearly the entire mass of the atom, the nucleus is composed of protons and neutrons (nucleons). The atomic number (Z) is equal to the number (constant) of protons in each element, whereas the mass number (A) is equal to the number of neutrons. The mass number may vary depending on the various isotopes of each element. Most naturally occurring atoms have stable nuclei, whereas naturally occurring radioactive atoms do not. This instability gives rise to nuclear transmutations involving atomic and chemical alterations. Artificial nuclei are produced by bombarding a stable nucleus with charged particles of high energy. This bombardment leads to the creation of a new nucleus and the possible ejection of one or more particles. *See* Alpha particle.

Nucleus, Cell:

Membrane-bound organelle that controls cellular structure and activity. The nucleus contains the genetic (chromatin) material deoxyribonucleic acid (DNA). (A mature red blood cell does not contain a nucleus and is therefore unable to reproduce.) The nucleolus, a protein structure containing ribonucleic acid (RNA), is present within the nucleus. Multiple nucleoli may be present. The nucleolus is important in protein synthesis and becomes enlarged when active (during growth, repair, tumor formation). Microscopic abnormalities in the size and characteristics of the nucleus and nucleolus are evident in malignant cells.

Null Hypothesis:

Statistical theory to be tested and accepted or rejected in favor of an alternative. A null hypothesis is used to aid in the design of appropriate experiments that prove or disprove a set of related statements. Any hypothesis that differs from a null hypothesis is known as an alternate hypothesis. *See* Type I error; Type II error.

Nupercaine:

See Local anesthetic.

Nuromax:

See Doxacurium chloride.

Nutritional Assessment:

A series of anthropometric variables such as weight, height, tricep skinfold thickness, etc. Used to assess the presence of malnutrition and progress in its treatment. Often hastily performed on self to justify early lunch break.

O₂:

See Oxygen.

Obesity:

Condition characterized by excessive accumulation of body fat. Obesity may be due to exogenous (overeating) or endogenous (endocrine, metabolic, or hypothalamic abnormality) causes. *See* Morbid obesity; Pickwickian syndrome.

Obesity Hypoventilation Syndrome (OHS):

See Pickwickian syndrome.

Obstruction:

Blockage of vessels, ducts, or organs. For example, respiratory obstruction may occur if the upper airways are blocked by foreign material, tissue swelling, or the tongue falling backward in the unconscious patient.

Obstructive Pulmonary Disease:

See Chronic obstructive pulmonary disease.

Occlusion Pressure:

Amount of pressure required in an external circumferential cuff to prevent inflow of arterial blood to a limb. Usually believed to be 100 mm Hg above systolic blood pressure.

Occupational Exposure:

Unavoidable contact with a potentially harmful substance due to its presence in the work environment. Individuals working in operating rooms have an inevitable exposure to N_2O and other gaseous agents. Studies have shown that, at least at high concentrations, chronic exposure to N_2O is deleterious to health. The Occupational Safety and Health Administration (OSHA) determines the maximum safety levels for various toxic agents.

OCR:

See Optical character reader.

Octanol:Buffer Partition Coefficient:

Ratio at equilibrium of the neutral and charged components of a particular drug at a particular pH in an octanol:buffer solution, which represents an organic solvent in contact with an aqueous solution. The coefficient is related to the potency of an anesthetic.

Ohm:

Unit of electrical resistance in the meter-kilogram-second (MKS) system of measurement equal to the resistance of a circuit in which a potential difference of 1 V produces a current of 1 ampere.

Ohm Law:

Expression of the relation between the current, potential difference (voltage), and resistance. The current in a conductor is proportional to the potential difference between its ends. A voltage (E) across a direct current circuit is the current (I) in amperes × resistance (R) of the circuit (E = IR). *See* Impedance.

OHS:

See Obesity hypoventilation syndrome.

Omphalocele:

Congenital condition characterized by protrusion of part of the intestine through a defect in the abdominal wall at the umbilicus. It results from failure of the intestine to return to the abdominal cavity during fetal development. A translucent amniotic sac covers the exposed intestine. The umbilical cord is generally located at the apex of the sac. If the amniotic sac ruptures in utero, chronic peritonitis results. If it ruptures at birth, emergency treatment to cover the viscera is necessary. Silastic sheets may be used to cover an intact omphalocele after birth, which allows for a slow, progressive reduction of the intestine into the growing abdominal cavity. Total parenteral feeding is necessary to provide adequate nutrition for the infant, who at this stage is unable to tolerate oral feedings. *See* Gastroschisis.

OMV Inhaler (Oxford Miniature Vaporizer):

Device developed during the early 1960s to deliver halothane in precise concentrations for use in medically unsophisticated areas. It is fairly light and relatively easy to use. *See* EMO inhaler.

Oncotic Pressure:

Osmotic pressure at the capillary membrane caused by the plasma colloids. Normal oncotic pressure is approximately 28 mm Hg. *See* Osmotic pressure.

OND:

See Ondansetron.

Ondansetron (OND):

Antiemetic for use during the postoperative period.

One Day Stay Procedure:

Operative procedure limited as to complexity such that the patient need only stay overnight after the procedure to be street ready. *See* Outpatient anesthesia.

One-Lung Anesthesia:

See Bronchial blocker; Double-lumen tube; Pulmonary alveolar proteinosis.

One-Tailed Test:

See Two-tailed test.

On-Line:

Term describing a device or process that is directly connected to or controlled by a central processing unit or computer.

Open Chest Massage:

See Cardiac massage.

Open Circuit, Anesthesia:

See Anesthesia system, open; Nonrebreathing valve.

Open Circuit, Electrical:

Circuit in which either the input side or the output side (source-load-source connection) is cut (opened), stopping current flow.

Open Drop Technique:

Method for administering inhaled anesthetics introduced in 1847 for use with chloroform. The technique involved dropping a volatile liquid anesthetic onto a gauze-covered mask frame made of wire mesh. When used with diethyl ether, the mask temperature could reach 0°C. Aside from use in emergencies or adverse field conditions, the technique is rarely employed today.

Operating Room Air Circulation Systems (Air Handlers):

There are two basic types of air circulation system in operating rooms: nonrecirculating and partial recirculating. The nonrecirculating, or one-path, system takes in fresh air, heats or cools it as appropriate, filters it, then circulates it through the operating room, and exhausts it outside the building. The partial recirculating, or two-path, system does not vent all air to the outside but filters and places back in the room some previously circulated air. The former is costly, as each new batch of air must be modified to bring it to temperature and humidity standards. The latter system, on the other hand, although less expensive to operate, only slowly reduces room concentrations of anesthetics. Two methods of air handling are turbulent and laminar. Turbulent flow systems put in high velocity air through a small grill, whereas laminar systems put in low velocity air via a large grill, which can typically comprise an entire wall or most of the ceiling (Allander air curtain). National Fire Protection Association codes require at least five complete air changes per hour in operating rooms; partial recirculating systems, which balance expense versus dilution of contaminants, have five to six complete changes per hour with 80% recirculation, meaning that air is completely filtered at least 25 times/hour. (It is to be remembered that with modern air conditioning systems the older consideration that anesthetics were heavier than air and could therefore be safely assumed to settle to the floor is no longer operative.) The modern systems, to a large but variable degree, stir waste anesthetics throughout the entire room. *See* Allander air curtain; HEPA filter.

Operating Room Electrical Concepts:

See Grounding; Isolation transformer.

Operating Room Utilization:

Nebulous term, usually hospital specific, meaning in general the hours of time patients are in a particular operating room versus the total number of hours available. *See* Turnover time.

Operational Amplifier:

Type of amplifier that uses voltage feedback between output and input. Operational amplifiers are used to perform functions such as integrating, adding, and differentiating. Combinations of operational amplifiers can carry out complex mathematic manipulations on a signal. *See* Amplifier.

Opiate:

One of a group of chemical compounds extracted or derived from the opium poppy (Papaver somniferum). Opiates are used mainly for relief of moderate to severe pain. They depress respiration and may produce bronchoconstriction. Opiates induce a feeling of euphoria and tranquillity in combination with analgesia. Adverse effects include nausea, vomiting, orthostatic hypotension, constipation, and urinary retention. Opiates have significant abuse potential. Overdose or opiate poisoning renders the patient comatose and cyanotic; pinpoint pupils are common; respiratory failure is a prime cause of death. *See* Figure. *See* Narcotic.

Opioid Receptor:

Those cellular receptors, particularly in the central nervous system that act as binding sites for the large pharmaceutical class known as the opioids. It appears that these binding sites are the natural active binding points for the neurotransmitters of the endorphin class. Opioid receptors are known to have at least six subclassifications, with each subclass responsible for a different effect when stimulated. Synthetic opioid molecules are now being tailored for each receptor subset. *See* Table. *See* Morphine; Receptor/receptor site; various individual opioids such as Fentanyl, Sufentanil.

Opium:

See Opiate.

Opiate: Phenylpiperidine skeleton structure and synthetic phenylpiperidine opioids, meperidine and fentanyl.

Opioid Receptor: Characteristics of Opioid Receptors.

Receptor	Tissue Bioassay	Agonists	Major Actions
Mu			
Mu$_1$	Guinea pig ileum	Morphine Meptazinol Phenylpiperidines	Analgesia Bradycardia Sedation
Mu$_2$	Guinea pig ileum	Morphine Phenylpiperidines	Respiratory depression Euphoria Physical dependence
Delta	Mouse vas deferens	*d*-Ala-*d*-Leu Enkephalin	Analgesia (weak) Respiratory depression
Kappa	Rabbit vas deferens	Ketocyclazocine Dynorphin Nalbuphine Butorphanol	Analgesia (weak) Respiratory depression Sedation
Sigma		SKF 10,047 Pentazocine	Dysphoria-delirium, mydriasis Hallucinations Tachycardia Hypertension
Epsilon	Rat vas deferens	β-Endorphin	Stress response Acupuncture

Optical Character Reader (OCR):

Light-sensitive photoelectric device used for data processing. It scans printed material and produces digital signals corresponding to the characters it views. Optical scanners are simpler devices that produce signals proportional to the shades of light and dark that the scanner views.

Optical Density:

Determination of the degree of opacity of a translucent medium. It is calculated as the log of the intensity of the ray of light incident to the medium divided by the log of the intensity of the transmitted light.

Optical Isolation:

See Isolated output.

Optical Scanner:

See Optical character reader (OCR).

Optic Nerve:

See Cranial nerves.

Oral Transmucosal Fentanyl Citrate (OTFC):

Technique for administering premedication, particularly the opioid fentanyl to children. It involves putting a fixed dose of fentanyl in a candy base on a stick. It is controversial in that this technique may be considered too casual, giving the wrong impression about powerful medicants.

Organophosphorus Compounds:

Highly toxic alkyl phosphate compounds that irreversibly bind with, and inactivate, cholinesterase. They were developed as chemical warfare agents and are now modified as insecticides (Malathion; Diazinon). Poisoning by these agents may result in paralysis and respiratory depression leading to death. Pralidoxime may be administered intravenously to counteract these anticholinesterase effects. Topical organophosphorus compounds may be used to treat glaucoma. *See* Nerve gas; Pralidoxime.

Orinase:

See Tolbutamide.

Orthostatic Hypotension:

Drop in blood pressure that is evident after changing from a supine or prone position to a standing or sitting position. The transient decrease in venous return and cardiac output causes a reduction of the blood pressure. Orthostatic hypotension may be due to drugs that impair autonomic reflexes, hypovolemia or excessive doses of antihypertensive agents.

Oscillation:

Periodic variation between minimal and maximal values or a single swing of an object or current between the two extremes of its arc or travel.

431

Oscillator:

Electronic device that converts energy from a direct current source to a periodically varying electrical output. An oscillator is also a mechanical or electrical device that, in the absence of external forces, regularly and repeatedly changes position, e.g., a pendulum.

Oscillometry Method of Taking Blood Pressure:

See Arterial blood pressure.

Oscilloscope:

Instrument that displays the instantaneous values and waveforms of electrical currents on the fluorescent screen of a cathode-ray tube. Most commonly, electrocardiographic recordings are visualized on an oscilloscope. The bouncing ball and nonfade display techniques are two common methods used to display this information. The bouncing ball display shows a bright spot that moves along the screen from left to right. The light is nonpersistent and disappears within seconds. In contrast, the nonfade display remains on the screen until a blanking area clears the screen. Combinations of these two methods are possible; parts of the screen may use different methods. *See* Cathode-ray tube; Phosphorescence.

Oscillotonometer:

Instrument used for indirect measurement of blood pressure. It is most accurate during hypotensive states. *See* Figure. *See* Arterial blood pressure.

Osm:

See Osmole.

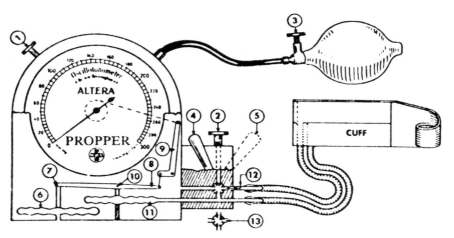

Oscillotonometer: Working elements. 1. Zero adjust. 2. Bleed valve adjustment screw. 3. Bulb pressure release valve. 4. Control valve lever: normal position, read pressure. 5. Control valve lever: position to bleed, observe oscillometry. 6. Pressure wafer. 7., 10., 8. Pivot points on internal lever. 9. Bell crank. 11. Sensitive oscillometric wafer. 12. Connection port to valve rotor shown in pressure or normal position (control lever in position 4). 13. Position of valve rotor to bleed, observe oscillometry. From Instruction Pamphlet of Oscillotonometer[®].

Osmolarity:

Osmotic concentration of a solution expressed as the number of osmoles of the dissolved substance per liter of solution.

Osmole (osm):

Unit of measurement of osmotic activity based on the actual number of particles in solution, regardless of their charge. In physiologic practice, it is usually designated in milliosmoles (mOsm). One osmole is the number of particles in 1 gram-molecular weight of an undissolved solute; however, if that solute dissociates into two ions, 1 gram-molecular weight equals 2 Osm.

Osmometer:

Instrument that measures osmotic pressure.

Osmosis:

Movement of fluid across a semipermeable membrane in response to solute concentrations.

Osmotic Pressure:

Amount of force necessary to prevent osmosis across a semipermeable membrane. The actual osmotic pressure is dependent on the number of particles in solution per unit volume of solution. Serum osmotic pressure is the osmotic pressure exerted by the serum and is primarily the result of concentrations of sodium, chloride, and bicarbonate, although sodium plays the dominant role. Serum protein and metabolites play a lesser role, although high levels of urea or glucose can increase the serum osmotic pressure. Urea can penetrate membranes and therefore does not produce long-term marked osmotic shifts. In contrast, glucose does not equilibrate well without sufficient insulin and can be responsible for maintaining osmotic differences across membranes. Normal serum osmotic pressure is 290 ± 5 milliosmoles. The body, exquisitely sensitive to changes in serum osmolarity, expends great effort to maintain serum osmolarity in a narrow normal range. *See* Osmole.

Ostwald Solubility Coefficient (Lambda):

Means for describing the equilibrium distribution between a gas and a solvent. The Ostwald solubility coefficient equals the volume of gas absorbed per unit volume of the solvent when the partial pressure of the gas is 760 mm Hg. This coefficient is numerically equivalent to the partition coefficient. The Bunsen solubility coefficient (alpha) is the Ostwald solubility corrected to standard temperature (273° absolute). *See* Partition coefficient.

OTFC:

See Oral transmucosal fentanyl citrate.

Ouabain:

Most rapid and shortest acting of all the cardiac glycosides. *See* Digitalis.

Outpatient Anesthesia:

Multiple techniques by which anesthesia is administered to individuals undergoing surgery who plan to leave the hospital, clinic, or office the same day. These patients are expected to be street ready hours after surgery. *See* Street ready.

Output:

Electronics term relating to the current, power, voltage, driving force, or information that a device or circuit delivers. It is also an automatic data-processing term indicating the data that have been processed.

Output Impedance:

See Impedance.

Output Transformer:

Coupling transformer between an output (e.g., amplifier) circuit and a load. *See* Transformer.

Overcurrent Protection Device:

Instrument that prevents excessive electrical current flow. Two types exist: (1) a fuse that melts if too much current passes through it, thereby opening the circuit, and (2) a circuit breaker that uses the excessive current to create a magnetic field of sufficient strength to open a movable contact, thereby breaking the circuit.

Overhydration:

See Dehydration; Water balance.

Overspill Valve:

See Pop-off valve.

Overwedging:

Unfortunate problem that occurs when the balloon of a Swan-Ganz catheter is overinflated and starts to occlude the opening of the distal tip of the catheter. The result mimics an elevated pressure. *See* Swan-Ganz catheter.

Oxalosis (Primary Hyperoxaluria):

Pathologic accumulation of calcium oxalate crystals, usually occurring in the kidneys, although it may also occur in the bones, arteries, or heart. The inhalation anesthetic methoxyflurane is metabolized, in part, to oxalate. Oxalosis is considered one of the possible causes of the nephrotoxicity of methoxyflurane. *See* Methoxyflurane.

Oxazepam (Serax):

Antianxiety drug of the benzodiazepine class. It is recommended for elderly patients or those with impaired liver function. *See* Benzodiazepine.

Oxidative Phosphorylation:

Process of obtaining adenosine triphosphate (ATP) from adenosine diphosphate (ADP) and phosphate by utilizing the energy produced when hydrogen molecules are oxidized to water. This process is performed by a complicated system of enzymes known as the cytochrome chain. *See* Figure. *See* Adenosine triphosphate; Cytochrome P-450 system.

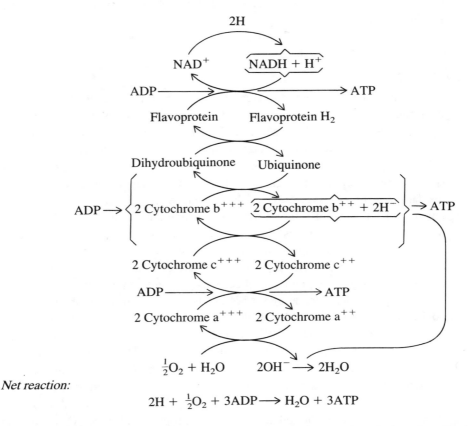

Net reaction:

$$2H + \tfrac{1}{2}O_2 + 3ADP \longrightarrow H_2O + 3ATP$$

Oxidative Phosphorylation: Chemical processes of oxidative phosphorylation showing the ionization of H_2O and adenosine triphosphate.

Oximeter:

Photoelectric instrument designed to measure the amount of O_2 in whole blood. The instrument operates on the principle that the optical density of hemoglobin at specific red and infrared wavelengths is linearly related to the percentage of O_2 saturation. *See* Optical density; Pulse oximeter.

Oxygen (O₂):

Element that is present freely in the atmosphere as a colorless, odorless, tasteless gas (comprising approximately 21% of air volume.) It is frequently found in combination with

435

many solids, liquids, and gases. It has an atomic number of 8 and an atomic weight of 16. Oxygen has a critical temperature of $-183°C$ below which it becomes a liquid. It is often supplied commercially in bulk in the liquid state and stored in vacuum containers to remain cold. Smaller supplies of O_2 are delivered in standard colored cylinders (American color for O_2 is green; international color is white). Oxygen is an essential component for cellular respiration and combustion processes. *See* Atmosphere; Cylinder, gas; Liquid oxygen; Paramagnetism.

Oxygen Analyzer:

Device that measures the percentage of O_2 in a mixture of gases. Two basic modes of operation exist: the discrete sampler and the continuous sampler. The discrete samplers (Pauling, Paramagnetic Analyzer) have been in use since the early 1940s. They operate on the principle that O_2 molecules, unlike all other commonly encountered gases, exhibit magnetic properties. Samples of unknown gas are drawn into a test chamber spanned by a permanent magnetic field. The O_2 molecules migrate to one side and displace any other gas present. This imbalance in the magnetic field changes the position of a mirror reflecting a light beam along a calibrated scale dependent on the percentage of O_2. Continuous O_2 analyzers place a sensor in the gas volume to be tested and a reading is constantly displayed (except for a lag in time as the sensor responds to changes in O_2 content). Two types of sensor are commonly in use today: the galvanic cell (often wrongly called microfuel cell) and the polarographic cell. The galvanic cell is made up of a lead anode and a gold cathode sealed in a membrane (filled with a potassium hydroxide electrolyte bath) which allows for easy diffusion of gases but not of large molecules (proteins). When O_2 crosses the membrane and comes in contact with the gold, it is reduced to hydroxide ions (OH^-). These ions migrate to the lead anode and form lead oxide, releasing electrons which flow from the anode back to the cathode through a resistor that is external to the sensor. A sensitive meter measures the voltage across the external resistor and registers on a scale calibrated in O_2 concentrations. The cell life of the galvanic sensor is proportional to the O_2 concentration to which it is exposed because the electrodes are consumed in the process. The galvanic sensor is slow to respond and is expensive owing to its gold content. However, it is rugged, easy to use, and requires no power input to the sensor. The galvanic sensor is rated in percent hours: 100% O_2 lasts x hours, 50% O_2 lasts x/2 hours. The polarographic O_2 sensor is a two-electrode system: a silver anode and a gold or platinum cathode, which are surrounded by an electrolyte solution of potassium chloride. The cathode is insulated from the electrolyte solution (except at its tip, which is covered by a membrane through which gas can permeate) and is kept negative in respect to the anode by an external battery. Oxygen crosses the membrane, is broken down at the cathode, and alters the conductivity of the electrolyte solution. Current flow between the electrodes is proportional to the O_2 concentration. Polarographic sensors are less expensive than galvanic sensors but require frequent electrolyte changes and careful maintenance. They respond faster than galvanic sensors but require an external power source. *See* Figures.

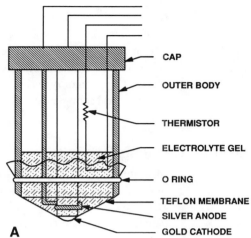

CAP

OUTER BODY

THERMISTOR

ELECTROLYTE GEL

O RING

TEFLON MEMBRANE

SILVER ANODE

GOLD CATHODE

A

Oxygen Analyzer: (A) Schematic diagram of a Plarographic Sensor. (B) Schematic diagram of a Galvanic (Micro-Fuel) Cell. (C) Configuration of a paramagnetic oxygen analyzer.

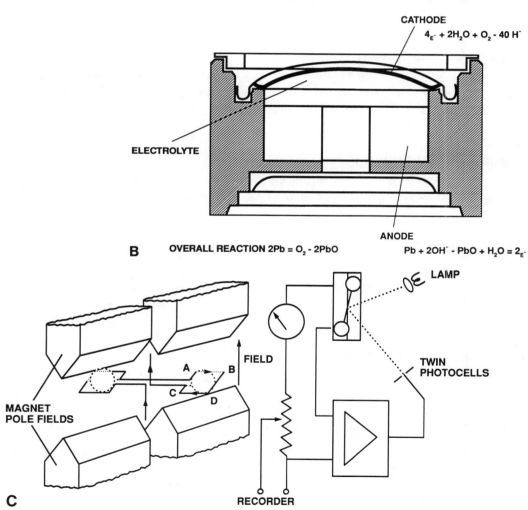

CATHODE

$4_{e^-} + 2H_2O + O_2 - 40 H^-$

ELECTROLYTE

ANODE

B OVERALL REACTION $2Pb = O_2 - 2PbO$

$Pb + 2OH^- - PbO + H_2O = 2_{e^-}$

LAMP

FIELD

TWIN PHOTOCELLS

MAGNET POLE FIELDS

A B
C
D

RECORDER

C

Oxygenator:

Mechanical device that oxygenates venous blood extracorporeally. In combination with one or more pumps, an oxygenator can maintain circulation during open heart surgery. (CO_2 is passively eliminated by diffusing from venous blood into the O_2 in contact with the blood.) Oxygenator types include bubble, membrane, rotating disk, and screen. *See* Bubble oxygenator; Membrane oxygenator; Rotating disk oxygenator; Screen oxygenator.

Oxygen Carrying Capacity:

Maximum amount of O_2 that can be combined with hemoglobin (Hb) when the blood is fully saturated with 100% O_2 at a PO_2 of 760 mm Hg. One gram of Hb can bind with 1.34–1.39 ml O_2; the O_2 capacity of normal blood is therefore approximately 21 ml O_2/dl blood. (Normal blood contains 15 g Hb/dl.) At PO_2 760 mm Hg, the amount of dissolved O_2 is 0.3 ml/dl blood. *See* Oxygen content.

Oxygen Consumption:

Amount of oxygen utilized in the body for metabolism per minute. For the mythical 70-kg adult at normal body temperature, oxygen consumption is approximately 250 ml/minute. Oxygen consumption rises dramatically during exercise or fever.

Oxygen Consumption Index:

Oxygen consumption per minute divided by the calculated surface area of the patient. Relates oxygen consumption in a crude way to body size and mass.

Oxygen Content:

Amount of O_2 that can be extracted from 100 ml blood. It includes both the amount that is physically dissolved in plasma plus the amount bound to hemoglobin. The O_2 content of partially desaturated blood is below the theoretic maximum. *See* Oxygen carrying capacity.

Oxygen Dissociation Curve:

See Oxygen-hemoglobin dissociation curve.

Oxygen Electrode (Clark Electrode):

One of three standard electrodes that make up a blood-gas analyzer. It is a device for determining PO_2 in solution. Oxygen molecules cross a plastic membrane and are ionized by a platinum cathode, which is kept negative with respect to a silver/silver chloride anode. By various corrections the ionic current of O_2 between cathode and anode is converted to a reading of PO_2. *See* Figure.

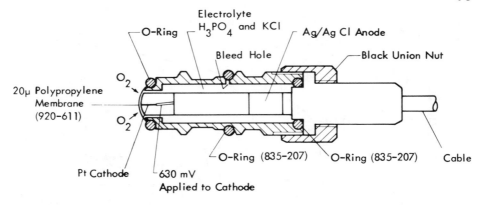

E5049 Po$_2$ Electrode

Oxygen Electrode: Standard O$_2$ electrode. From ABL2 Users' Handbook.

Oxygen Flush Valve:

Valve that directs high-flow O$_2$ (at least 35–75 L/minute) through an anesthesia machine outlet. Standards require that the O$_2$ flush valve be spring-loaded so that when pressure on the valve button or handle is removed the flow shuts off. On some machines activation of the O$_2$ flush valve eliminates all O$_2$ flow through integral vaporizers. This flow must be restored manually when O$_2$ flushing ceases. Modifications of O$_2$ flush valves exist that vary the effect on other gases that may be flowing when the valve is activated, i.e., the flow may stop or be vented into the atmosphere. *See* Continuous flow anesthesia machine.

Oxygen-Hemoglobin Dissociation Curve:

Graphic representation of the relation of hemoglobin-oxygen saturation related to PaO$_2$. Three major conditions affect the curve: pH, temperature, and concentration of 2,3-diphosphoglycerate (2,3-DPG) in the red blood cell. A decrease in temperature or 2,3-DPG or an increase in pH (i.e., decreased CO$_2$) of the blood shifts the curve to the left. Conversely, an increase in temperature or 2,3-DPG or a decrease in pH (i.e., increased CO$_2$), of the blood shifts the curve to the right. (The concentration of 2,3-DPG is elevated in chronic hypoxia and at high altitudes.) P$_{50}$ indicates the PO$_2$ at which hemoglobin is half-saturated with O$_2$. The decrease in the affinity of hemoglobin for O$_2$ when the pH of blood falls is known as the Bohr effect. *See* Figure.

Oxygen Hood:

See Oxygen tent.

Oxygen Point:

Temperature at which gaseous and liquid O$_2$ are in equilibrium at 1 standard atmosphere (–183°C).

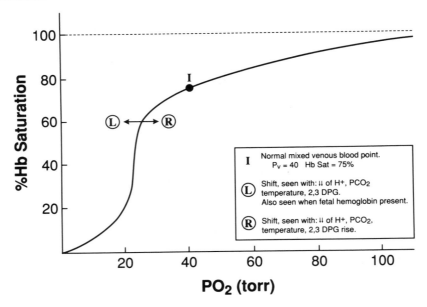

Oxygen-Hemoglobin Dissociation Curve: Oxygen-Hemoglobin Dissociation Curve and the parameters which determine left or right shift of the curve. a = Point indicating normal mixed venous blood that has P_vO_2 40 torr and Hb 75 percent saturated; b = Cyanosis not normally apparent until PaO_2 drops to approximately 50 torr (80 percent saturation) or less. Also, below this level a drop in PO_2 is related to a large drop in percent Hb saturation (the neonate with fetal Hb will have a much lower than 50 torr PaO_2 level at 80 percent saturation); c = Right shift of curve with increased H^+, PCO_2, temperature and 2,3 DPG; d = Left shift of curve with decreased H^+, PCO_2, temperature and 2,3 DPG; also, left shift with HbF. (HbF, therefore, holds onto O_2 "tighter" and gives up O_2 at tissue level less readily.)

Oxygen Saturation:

Ratio of oxyhemoglobin to total hemoglobin in a given blood sample, expressed as a percentage. Normally, blood leaving the lungs via the pulmonary vein is approximately 97% saturated. *See* Oxygen capacity; Oxygen content; Oxygen-hemoglobin dissociation curve.

Oxygen Tent (Oxygen Hood):

Light, portable, transparent, tent-like structure that is placed around a patient's head (hood) or bed (tent) and used for administration of O_2. The O_2 concentration within the tent may be increased by higher flow rates, elimination of leaks, or use of a smaller tent. This concentration rarely exceeds 50% and may be as low as 25%. In contrast, the O_2 concentration of a head hood may reach 90–100%. The low O_2 concentration of the tent and the restricted patient accessibility of the hood limit the usefulness of this method for O_2 administration.

Oxygen Therapy:

Treatment that involves administration of O_2 by means of inhalation via an O_2 tent or hood, nasal cannula, or face mask. Such therapy is employed to treat hypoxia.

Oxygen Toxicity:

Injurious prolonged exposure to excessive concentrations of inhaled O_2. Rapid O_2 toxicity occurs only under hyperbaric conditions. Chronic O_2 toxicity, occurring when O_2 concentrations over 70% are inhaled at atmospheric pressure for a long period of time, may be due to the deactivation of surfactant and damage to the alveolar epithelium. (Clinically, exposure to 100% O_2 for 24 hours may be considered injurious, to some extent, to all patients whereas it may take more than a week for 70% O_2 to cause damage.) During the first stage of toxicity (exudative) the lungs become edematous and there is evidence of hemorrhage and capillary damage. During the second stage (proliferative), there is marked scarring and fibrosis. Some degree of tolerance to high concentrations of O_2 occurs in some patients. No patient, however, should be denied high O_2 concentrations because of a potential for O_2 toxicity if it is the only means to prevent hypoxia. Premature infants are susceptible to eye manifestations of O_2 toxicity. *See* Retrolental fibroplasia.

Oxymorphone (Numorphan):

See Naloxone; Narcotic.

Oxytocin:

Hormone formed in the hypothalamus and stored in the posterior lobe of the pituitary gland (neurohypophysis). It has weak but noticeable contractile effects on smooth muscle, a characteristic it shares with vasopressin (antidiuretic hormone, ADH), the other major hormone released by the posterior pituitary. Oxytocin's primary use is to increase the strength of uterine contractions. *See* Antidiuretic hormone; Hormone.

P

PABA:

See Para-aminobenzoic acid.

Pacemaker:

Implantable device used for long-term management of patients with cardiac rhythm abnormalities, particularly symptomatic bradycardia due to sinus node dysfunction or heart block. It is also used to manage some tachydysrhythmias. A specialty variant is called an automatic implantable cardioverter defibrillator (AICD). This device is battery powered and senses cardiac electrical activity by means of sensing leads attached to the heart. When it senses a life-threatening dysrhythmia, it fires a defibrillating shock. The Inter Society Commission for Heart Disease uses a five digit pacemaker identification code to form the basis for pacemaker identification. For example, with a AOO, DOO, or a VOO, one or both chambers of the heart are paced without regard to spontaneous electrical activity. This technique is called A-synchronous pacing. AAI or VVI pacemakers operate on demand: They are inhibited if they sense atrial or ventricular electrical activity. *See* Figures, Table.

Pacemaker-Mediated Tachycardia (PMT):

Also called endless loop tachycardia, it is a phenomenon that can occur with atrial activity scensing pacemakers in patients who have ventricle to atria retrograde conduction capability. What occurs is that a ventricular premature beat is conducted back to the atria, triggering a paced ventricular beat. The paced ventricular beat is also conducted back to the atria and the process repeats itself. PMT can be terminated by converting the pacemaker to A-synchronous operation. *See* Pacemaker.

Pain:

Unpleasant sensation, either conscious or unconscious, that signals the body that some tissue damage is occurring. In one system, pain sensation is classified into three major types: pricking, burning, and aching. Pricking pain and burning pain are felt at the skin surface, whereas aching pain is felt below the surface. In a second system, pain is described in terms of (1) onset; (2) severity; (3) quality; (4) duration; and (5) etiology. In a third system, pain is classified according to origin: (1) peripheral; (2) cerebral; or (3) psychogenic. *See* Nerve fiber, anatomy and physiology of; Nociceptor.

Pacemaker: Glossary of Pacemaker Terminology.

Pacemaker	The complete unit, consisting of computer governor (electronic hardware), generator, lead, and electrode.
Generator	The portion of the pacemaker that contains the energy storage device (eg, nickel-lithium battery; in older models, plutonium), produces the electrical current, and detects intrinsic myocardial electrical activity.
Electrode	The portion of the pacemaker that is in physical contact with the atrium or ventricle.
Lead	The entire length of insulated wire that leads from the generator to the electrode.
Current threshold	The number of milliamperes that is just able to stimulate myocardial contraction.
Voltage threshold	The number of volts that is just able to stimulate myocardial contraction
Pulse duration	The breadth of each pulse; the usual duration is between 0.5 and 1.0 milliseconds.
Bipolar	The circuit created (both positive and negative leads) lies within the heart. Two leads emanate from the generator. When an AICD has been implanted, a bipolar pacemaker is used.
Unipolar	The circuit created has its negative (or stimulating) electrode within the heart, and the positive (or ground) electrode is within the generator. A single lead emanates from the generator.
Pulse interval (automatic interval)	The amount of time in milliseconds between consecutive pacing impulses.
Escape interval	The amount of time in milliseconds between the patient's R wave and the following paced beat.
Hysteresis	The difference in the duration of the pacemaker escape interval, depending on whether it is started by a sensed or paced event.
R-wave sensitivity	The number of millivolts required to inhibit the generator from firing.
Ventricular triggered	Triggered when the R wave causes the pacemaker to fire during the refractory period of the myocardium.
Ventricular Inhibited	Inhibited when the R wave causes the pacemaker not to fire an impulse.
Overdrive pacing	Pacing at a more rapid rate than an underlying tachycardia in order to interrupt and terminate a reentrant arrhythmia.
Asynchronous	The pacemaker is insensitive to incoming signals from the chamber being paced. NB: The antonym of *asynchronous* in pacing terminology is not synchronous; it is responsive.
Synchronous	The pacemaker generates a response to a sensed event after an appropriate delay.

Pacemaker: Traditional Five-Letter Code for Pacemaker Systems.

1st Letter Chamber Paced	2nd Letter Chamber Sensed	3rd Letter Mode of Response	4th Letter (if Used) Programmable Features	5th Letter (if Used) Arrhythmia Treatment
A = atrium V = ventricle D = double	A = atrium V = ventricle D = double O = none	T = triggered I = inhibited D = double O = not applicable	P = programmable M = multiprogrammable O = not programmable	B = burst N = normal S = scanning E = external

443

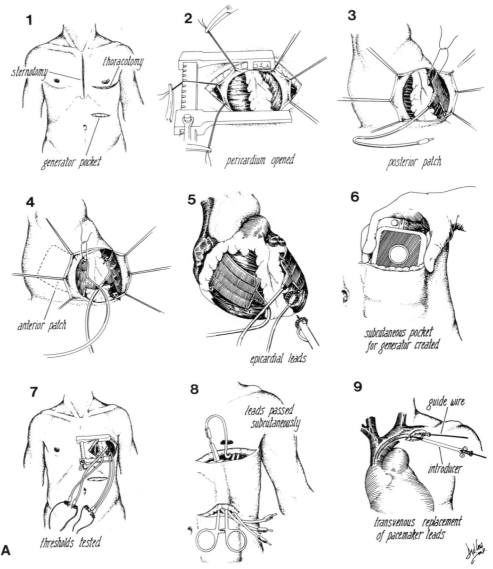

Pacemaker: (A) Automatic internal cardiac defibrillator. (B) Transvenous pacemaker.

Pain, Gate Theory of:

See Gate theory of pain.

Pain, Local Mechanism of:

See Pain signal transmission.

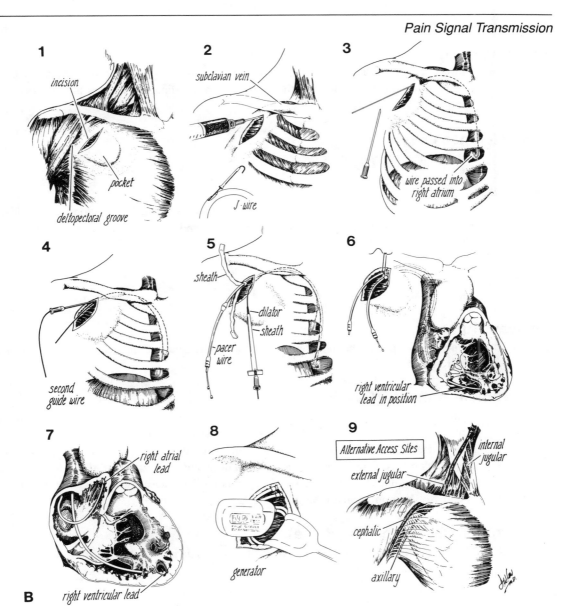

1 incision
pocket
deltopectoral groove

2 subclavian vein
J-wire

3 wire passed into right atrium

4 second guide wire

5 sheath
dilator
sheath
pacer wire

6 right ventricular lead in position

7 right atrial lead
B right ventricular lead

8 generator

9 Alternative Access Sites
internal jugular
external jugular
cephalic
axillary

Pacemaker *(continued)*.

Pain Signal Transmission:

Sensation of two types of pain because of the presence of two pain pathways (slow and fast). The first half of the double sensation is a pricking pain sensation which is carried rapidly by the small A-delta fibers at velocities of approximately 5–25 m/second. The second part of the sensation is a burning sensation that is transmitted more slowly by type C fibers at velocities of 0.1–2.0m/second. *See* Gate theory of pain; Nerve fiber, anatomy and physiology of.

Pain Threshold:

Lowest intensity of a pain stimulus that elicits the sensation of pain. Implicit in the concept of pain threshold is the idea that the more intense the stimulus, the less time it has to be applied before it elicits a response.

Pain Tolerance Level:

Greatest intensity of pain a subject can tolerate, usually as part of an experiment.

Palladium:

Rare metal often found in conjunction with platinum. It is used in electrical components because of its resistance to oxidation and corrosion and in jewelry because of its beautiful silver color.

Palsy:

See Paralysis.

Pancoast Tumor:

Tumor of the apex of the lung that may spread to the adjacent brachial plexus. *See* Horner syndrome.

Pancuronium Bromide (Pavulon):

Competitive neuromuscular blocking agent that is approximately five times as potent as d-tubocurarine. Because it does not appear to cause ganglionic blockage or histamine release, Pavulon does not (especially upon rapid intravenous injection) precipitate a rapid drop in blood pressure. Rather, depending on dose and administration, it is more likely to cause tachycardia (by some degree of vagus nerve blockage) and an increase in cardiac output. *See* Neuromuscular blockade, assessment of.

Papaveretum (Omnopon; Opoidine):

Mixture of all the water-soluble alkaloids of opium in their natural proportions (available in Great Britain).

Papaverine:

Naturally occurring alkaloid of opium. It is neither a narcotic nor an analgesic, and it is nonaddictive. Its major effect is smooth muscle relaxation. It has been used to treat peripheral vascular disease and has been advocated on occasion as a treatment for the inadvertent intraarterial injection of irritants such as thiopental and diazepam.

PAR:

See Postanesthetic recovery room.

Para-Aminobenzoic Acid (PABA):

Acid associated with the vitamin B complex. Often used in topical preparations as a sunscreen, it has been reported to have some cross-sensitivity with the ester group of local anesthetics. PABA is a breakdown product of procaine and a potent inhibitor of the bacteriostatic effects of the sulfonamides. *See* Procaine hydrochloride.

Paraben Preservatives:

See Preservative.

Paracervical Block (Uterosacral Block):

Anesthetic nerve block of the inferior hypogastric plexus. The block interrupts uterine and cervical sensation and is therefore performed to ease pain during labor. The procedure has fallen into disfavor because of the possible inadvertent injection of local anesthetic into the placental circulation, which delivers a high concentration of local anesthetic to the fetus, causing bradycardia. *See* Figure.

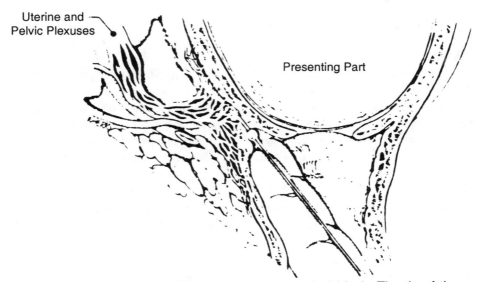

Paracervical Block: Schematic representation of paracervical block. The tip of the needle just penetrates the mucosa and points away from the myometrium and the fetal presenting part.

Paradoxical Air Embolus:

Condition that occurs when air or other foreign material crosses the septum between the right and the left atria and appears in the systemic circulation rather than going directly to the lungs. Potentially seen in patients with patent foramina ovale. It is highly dangerous. *See* Venous air embolus.

Paradoxical Oxygen Death:

Clinical circumstance that occurs when the respiratory center adapts and no longer responds normally by increasing ventilation in response to elevated $PaCO_2$ but is, in fact, being driven by the carotid bodies responding to low O_2. Arterial CO_2 rises so high that it acts as a depressant. The administration of high O_2 concentrations to the patient is detected first by the carotid bodies. They cease stimulating the respiratory center, which shuts down completely, and the patient dies paradoxically from hypoxia and hypercapnia in the presence of adequate O_2. Paradoxical O_2 death is seen in respiratory cripples, e.g., those with end-stage emphysema. Avoiding this iatrogenic catastrophe requires controlled administration of mildly elevated O_2 concentrations to correct hypoxia and mechanical ventilation with adjustment of acid-base balance as necessary. *See* Carotid body.

Paradoxical Respiration:

Phenomenon seen after a crush injury to the chest wall (flail chest) or surgical removal of part of the rib cage. On normal inspiration, the chest rises up and out. With paradoxical respiration, the normal side behaves as noted, but the damaged side is sucked inward. Similarly, on expiration, the unaffected side falls inward, and the affected side balloons outward. This reversal of normal movement of the chest wall is deleterious to normal respiratory function. *See* Flail chest.

Paraldehyde:

Cyclic ether that is an effective hypnotic. It was formerly administered to treat delirium tremens, psychiatric disorders characterized by excitement, or convulsions due to tetanus or eclampsia; and it has been given for basal and obstetric anesthesia. Paraldehyde has been implicated in both chronic intoxication (despite its unpleasant odor and taste) and fatal toxic reactions. It is damaging to tissues at the site of injection and has been replaced by other sedatives that do not have the offensive taste and odor and are not irritating on injection.

Parallel Circuit:

Circuit with elements that connect across the same pair of terminals, ensuring that the voltage is constant across each element. *See* Figure.

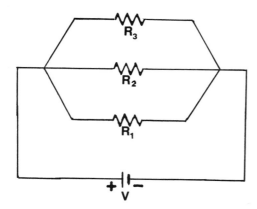

Parallel Circuit: Simple parallel circuit made up of three resistors connected across the same voltage source.

Paralysis (Palsy):

Loss of motor function. Paralysis has also been used to mean loss of any organic function.

Paramagnetism:

Physical property of certain substances, such as O_2, in which the molecules behave as if they carry a magnetic charge.

Paramedian Approach:

Spinal anesthetic technique in which the needle is placed offset from the midline below and to the side of the interspace and aimed cephalad. This technique is used when the usual midline perpendicular approach is not easily accomplished. *See* Spinal anesthesia.

Paraplegia:

Paralysis of the lower part of the body and of both legs.

Parasympathetic Division (Craniosacral Division):

Craniosacral portion of the autonomic nervous system. There are two divisions of this system: the cranial outflow and the sacral outflow. The cranial outflow supplies the visceral structures of the head, thorax, and upper abdomen via the oculomotor, facial, glossopharyngeal, and vagus nerves. The sacral portion varies with each individual but most frequently consists of the second, third, and fourth sacral segments. Parasympathetic preganglionic fibers go to discrete ganglia nearest the organ they innervate. The parasympathetic ganglia include the ciliary, pterygopalatine, submandibular, and otic ganglia. Within the chest and abdomen, parasympathetic ganglia are diffuse and are therefore referred to as plexuses. They include the superficial cardiac, deep cardiac, pulmonary, myenteric, and mucosal. The afferent fibers of the parasympathetic system travel from the area they are monitoring to their cell bodies. The cell bodies of the cranial portion are in the sensory ganglia of the cranial nerves; the cell bodies of the sacral portion are in the posterior root ganglia of the spinal nerves. The major difference between the sympathetic and parasympathetic systems (aside from their antagonistic effects on various organs) is that the sympathetic system has a wide, diffuse effect owing to its remote ganglia and multiple, branching postganglionic fibers, whereas the parasympathetic system, owing to its few ganglia located near the organ affected and its short postganglionic fibers, has a more local, discrete effect. *See* Autonomic nervous system; Cranial nerves.

Parasympathetic Nervous System:

See Autonomic nervous system.

Parasympathetic Tone:

See Sympathetic tone.

Parasympatholytics:

Agents that abolish the action of the parasympathetic nervous system. Atropine is the prototypical parasympatholytic.

Paravertebral Block:

Introduction of a local anesthetic alongside the vertebrae with the purpose of blocking the injected level of the sympathetic chain. *See* Paravertebral lumbar sympathetic block.

Paravertebral Lumbar Sympathetic Block:

Injection of a local anesthetic into the area of the first or second lumbar vertebra (unilateral or bilateral) to block the sympathetic chain. This technique provides excellent analgesia for the first stage of labor but is inadequate for delivery. (Local anesthetics cross the placental barrier, and high blood levels may cause circulatory and central nervous system depression in the fetus.) The paravertebral lumbar block is also useful for treating vascular disorders in the lower limbs. It relieves vascular spasms and dilates blood vessels.

Parenteral Fluids:

Solutions composed of various proteins, calories, and essential minerals, and designed to be administered by direct intravenous injection usually on a continuous basis, with the prime purpose of restoring and maintaining circulating volume. *See* Transfusion therapy.

Paresthesia:

Inappropriate sensation in a body part or over a portion of the body surface, usually described as burning, stinging, or tingling. It can be a symptom of neurologic disease. With regional anesthesia, "eliciting paresthesia" by probing for a nerve trunk with a needle prior to injection is a technique for determining proper deposition of a local anesthetic solution.

Pargyline (Eutonyl):

Monoamine oxidase inhibitor that is useful as an antihypertensive agent. Administration of pargyline is contraindicated in patients taking antidepressants or indirect sympathomimetics, or after ingestion of tyramine-containing foods.

Parotitis:

Infection of the parotid gland characterized by swelling and reduced salivary flow. Treatment includes systemic antibiotic therapy and, if necessary, surgical intervention.

Partial Pressure:

Contribution to the total pressure made by each gas in a mixture of gases. In a fixed volume, each gas exerts the pressure it would exert if it were alone. *See* Charles law; Vapor pressure.

Partial Pressure Crossover Point:

See Respiratory failure.

Partial Thromboplastin Time (PTT):

Test of the clotting mechanism that determines the relative intactness of the intrinsic clotting system. The measurement is of the time necessary for recalcified citrated plasma to clot in the presence of a standardized platelet substitute (cephalin) and standardized activating surface (provided by kaolin). *See* Prothrombin time, one-stage prothrombin time.

Partition Coefficient:

Ratio of the concentrations in each phase of a substance in equilibrium between two phases. For example, the drug methoxyflurane has a fat/blood partition coefficient of 49; i.e., at equilibrium there are 49 times the number of molecules of methoxyflurane in fat versus the number of molecules of methoxyflurane in the blood flowing through the fat. Because a partition coefficient can be determined for any two phases in contact with one another, one can determine the blood/gas partition coefficient, the tissue/blood partition coefficient, or the oil/gas partition coefficient. Any determination of the partition coefficient assumes that equilibration of partial pressures of the gas in question has occurred in the two phases. *See* Ostwald solubility coefficient.

Pascal:

Either a procedure-oriented computer programming language or a unit of pressure symbolized as Pa, which is equal to the force 1 newton acting uniformly over an area of 1 square meter. *See* Pressure.

Password:

Unique set of characters or digits used to identify a particular individual or user of a computer facility. It can be used to restrict an individual to only certain parts of a computer facility or parts of a computer memory. It is usually used to upgrade the security of a computer facility.

Patch Clamp:

Direct method for observing ion channel activity in which a tiny patch of membrane is clamped to electrochemical values chosen by an investigator. The technique requires the heat-polished tip of a glass micropipette gently touching the surface of a cell membrane. Suction is applied to the micropipette interior so the membrane patch covered by the tip is pulled up into the aperture. The receptors in the "trapped" patch of membrane can then be examined under controlled conditions.

Patchy Atelectasis:

See Atelectasis.

Patent Ductus Arteriosus (PDA):

Abnormal persistence in the newborn of a channel in the ductus arteriosus connecting the pulmonary artery with the thoracic aorta. This condition, common in premature infants, can be life-threatening, as it can act as a left-to-right shunt (to a variable degree) causing severe cardiac decompensation and increased pulmonary blood flow. In normal infants, the ductus closes shortly after birth, probably due to local prostaglandin activity. *See* Figure. *See* Fetal circulation; Prostaglandin.

Pathway:

Route that a nerve impulse takes from the periphery to the spinal cord and upward into the brain or reverse. Depending on the type of signal and the requirements for the body to respond to it, the pathway can be made up of a single long nerve fiber or tract or numerous short fibers that communicate between multiple junctions (synapses).

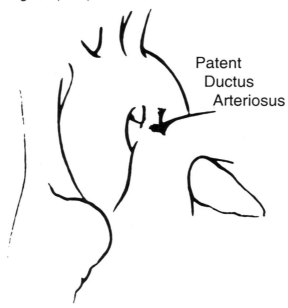

Patent Ductus Arteriosus: Patent ductus arteriosus connecting the thoracic aorta with the pulmonary artery.

Patient-Controlled Analgesia (PCA):

Modern technique of pain control based on systemic drugs being administered parenterally by a patient's controlling an intravenous infusion pump. The pump is directed by a sophisticated microprocessor, which can be preset as to dose, interval, and continuous or intermittent automatic augmentation. *See* Figure. *See* Bolus; Epidural narcotics; Lockout interval; Transcutaneous electrical nerve stimulation.

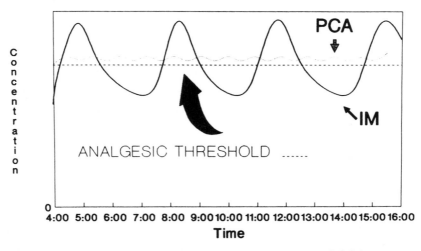

Patient-Controlled Analgesia: Narcotic plasma concentration: IM vs. PCA (computer simulated).

Patient-Controlled Epidural Analgesia (PCEA):

Technique for providing continuous pain control for a patient using an epidural catheter connected to a programmable infusion pump containing several possible drugs or drug combinations, including local anesthetics and opioids. The patient self-administers pain relief by activating the pump; the program of the pump prevents overdosage by lockout intervals and size of bolus. *See* Epidural narcotics; Lockout interval; Patient-controlled analgesia.

Patient Positioning (Posture):

Position in which the patient is placed during anesthesia. In order to meet the requirements for access for a particular surgical procedure, modern operating room tables can fold the human body into a number of positions. In most regions of the United States, it has been determined that the anesthesia personnel are legally responsible for properly positioning the patients. Reported complications of incorrect patient positioning include nerve palsies, pressure atrophy of the skin, bone breaking, (i.e., limbs caught between folding table parts), and special conditions (e.g., electrosurgical burns and direct damage caused by the weight and position of such items as endotracheal tube connectors, hoses, and head straps). Position is usually noted by a stick figure drawn on the anesthesia record. *See* Figures, Table.

Patient-Triggered Mechanical Positive Pressure Ventilation:

See Assisted mechanical ventilation.

Pattern Recognition:

Ability to identify one symbol or object among many symbols or objects. Pattern recognition appears to be one of the basic functions of intelligence. *See* Optical character reader.

Pauling Analyzer:

See Oxygen analyzer.

Pavulon:

See Pancuronium bromide.

PCA:

See Patient-controlled analgesia.

PCEA:

See Patient-controlled epidural analgesia.

PCP:

See Phencyclidine.

PCRIV:

See Pressure control inverse-ratio ventilation.

PCWP

See Pulmonary capillary transit time.

Patient Positioning: Some of the affected nerves and the sites of lesions caused by poor patient positioning.

Nerve	Site of lesion	Cause
Supraorbital	Orbital ridge	Pressure of a face mask; pressing on nerve to provide a painful stimulus for assessment of coma.
Brachial plexus	Stretching over head of humerus	Shoulder rests placed in root of neck. Over 90° abduction of the supinated arm. Hyperextension of head.
Radial	Radial groove in humerus	Arm falling down during surgery. Badly applied tourniquet.
Radial	At wrist	Placing patient's hands under buttocks.
Ulnar	Epicondylar groove	Resting arm on unpadded arm board.
Sciatic	Posterior roots	Failing to flex both legs together when adopting lithotomy position.
Lateral popliteal	Head of fibula	The unpadded knee in the lateral position: pressure from lithotomy poles on unprotected knee.
Lingual	Tip of tongue	Biting of tongue following laryngeal spasm.
Cervical cord	C3-4	Extension of head in the presence of subluxation of cervical vertebrae (e. g., injury or rheumatoid arthritis)

Supine
Arms at side, face up

Supine
Arms out, face up

Sitting
Arms on chest

Trendelenburg
In Operating Room Parlance,
head down, body straight.
True Trendelenburg, patient supine
on a surface at a 45° angle, head at
lower end, knees flexed over upper end.

Reverse Trendelenburg
In Operating Room Parlance, head
up, body straight. True Reverse
Trendelenburg, patient supine on
surface at 45° angle, head at highest end.

Lithotomy
Patient supine with hips
and knees flexed, thighs
abducted and externally
rotated.

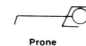

Prone
Face down

A

Patient Positioning: (A) Stick drawings of the various positions of the patient on the operating table.

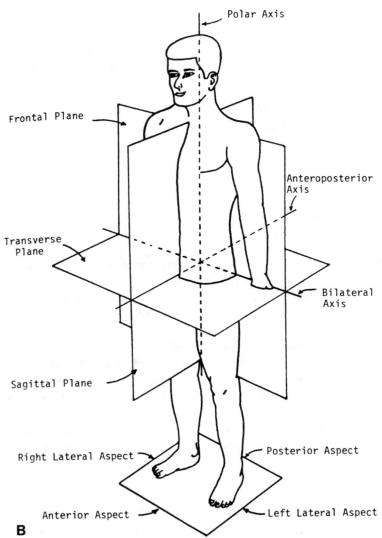

B

Patient Positioning *(continued):* (B) Cardinal planes and axes of the human body.

PDA:

See Patent ductus arteriosus.

"P" Depletion Test:

Test of cognitive ability used to determine recovery of individuals from outpatient anesthesia. It requires the recovering patient to cross out all examples of the letter "P" found in a complicated series of letters. The test is scored quantitatively. *See* Street ready; Trieger dot test.

455

PDPH   Postdural puncture headache. *See* Spinal headache.

Peak Flowmeter:

Device for measuring (in liters per minute) the rate at which a patient can exhale during forced expiration.

Peak Power Frequency (PPF):

See Median power frequency.

PEEP:

See Positive end-expiratory pressure.

Peltier Effect:

See Thermocouple.

Pemphigus:

Disease of the skin in which vesicles and blisters may involve extensive areas including the mucous membranes. Denuding of the skin and blister formation can result in significant fluid and protein loss. Gentle handling of the skin and the prevention of secondary infections is important during administration of anesthesia for these patients.

Penaz Continuous Blood Pressure Method:

Technique for continuous blood pressure determination by means of a small cuff wrapped around a finger and inflated. The operating point pressure in the external cuff is the mean arterial pressure. The pressure in the external cuff is constantly changing, as a computer adjusts the pressure based on readings of a light source and light sensor attached to the cuff detecting volume changes in the finger and modifying the pressure accordingly, such that the pressure in the cuff is linear with the systolic to diastolic change in the digital arteries. *See* Finipres.

Pendelluft:

Pendulum-like movement of the lungs seen when the patient is breathing spontaneously in the presence of an open pneumothorax. On inspiration, the normal side fills partially from the trachea and partially from the lung on the injured side. On expiration, air returns up the trachea and into the partially deflated lung on the injured side. *See* Pneumothorax.

Penicillin:

First available effective biologic antibiotic, discovered by Alexander Fleming in 1928. Its use has been limited in recent years because of the proliferation of resistant strains of microorganisms. Multiple derivatives of the drug have the potential for causing allergic reactions in susceptible individuals. Various preparations can carry a significant ionic load (sodium, potassium) upon massive injection. *See* Table. *See* Antibiotic.

Pentamorphone:

Designed drug modifying the basic structure of morphine to enhance analgesia without increasing respiratory depression. Pentamorphone is approximately 1.5–8.0 times more potent than fentanyl and 300–2500 times more potent than morphine. Its course of action is roughly equivalent to that of fentanyl.

Penicillin: Penicillin and Penicillin Derivatives.

Generic Name (Representative Trade Name*)	Spectrum	Penicillinase-Resistant	Acid-Stable	Route	Comments
Penicillin G (Pentids) Potassium Sodium	G⁺, some G⁻ (Escherichia coli, <u>Proteus mirabilis</u>, <u>Hemophilus influenzae</u>, Salmonella, Shigella, and strains of Enterobacter aerogenes), Leptospira, and Treponema.	No	No	PO	Penicillin and its derivatives are bactericidal in action. The penicillins can cause various side effects, including anaphylaxis, skin rash, Coombs-positive hemolytic anemia, fever, interstitial nephritis, angioedema, and serum sickness.
Benzathene (Bicillin)				IM	
Procaine (Wycillin)				IM	
Penicillin V (Pen-Vee K)	Same as penicillin G	No	Yes	PO	Penicillin V is well-absorbed orally.
Ampicillin (Omnipen)	Broad spectrum, especially against G⁻ rods.	No	Yes	PO IM IV	Ampicillin is well-absorbed orally. Side effects include GI upset, anaphylaxis, increased SGOT, and skin rash.
Hetacillin (Versapen)	Same as ampicillin	No	Yes	PO	Hetacillin is metabolized to ampicillin in the body.
Cyclacillin (Cyclapen)	Similar to ampicillin though less broad.	No	Yes	PO	Cyclacillin may show less incidence of GI upset and skin rash than ampicillin.
Amoxicillin (Amoxil)	Broad spectrum	No	Yes	PO	Amoxicillin is absorbed better orally than ampicillin. It is reported to show higher blood levels, and less incidence of diarrhea than ampicillin.
Carbenicillin (Pyopen)	Broad spectrum with a high activity against Proteus and Pseudomonas and occasional strains of G⁻ rods such as <u>Bacillus fragilis</u>	No	Yes	IM IV	Carbenicillin's side effects are similar to other penicillins but also include possible abnormalities in coagulation tests. It is very useful for severe urinary tract infections. Nephrotoxicity may be seen in large doses.

Penicillin (*continued*)

Generic Name (Representative Trade Name*)	Spectrum	Penicillinase-Resistant	Acid-Stable	Route	Comments
Ticarcillin (Ticar)	Similar to carbenicillin including G⁻, especially Pseudomonas	No	No	IM IV	
Methicillin (Celbenin)	G⁺, including penicillinase-resistant Staphylococci	Yes	No	IM IV	One of the first penicillinase-resistant penicillins.
Bacillin (Bactocill)	Same as methicillin	Yes	Yes	PO IM IV	Side effects include GI upset, fever, skin rash, decreased hemoglobin, neutropenia, increased SGOT, and transient hematuria in infants.
Cloxacillin (Tegopen)	Same as methicillin	Yes	Yes	PO	Cloxacillin and dicloxacillin do not show complete cross-sensitivity with penicillin G.
Dicloxacillin (Dynapen)	Same as methicillin	Yes	Yes	PO IM	Dicloxacillin is the best orally absorbed penicillinase-resistant penicillin.
Nafcillin (Nafcil)	Same as methicillin	Yes	Variable	PO IM	Nafcillin is not particularly well-absorbed orally. Its side effects are similar to those of oxacillin.

* Particularly for the older preparations many trade names exist for the same product. At times the trade name covers all forms of administration, other times it does not.

Pentazocine (Talwin):

Synthetic analgesic with moderate potency and short duration. Originally believed to be completely nonaddictive, it has been shown to have a low addiction capability. It is available for use as subcutaneous, intravenous, and intramuscular injection. The drug is only one-third as effective in oral tablet form as when given parenterally. Pentazocine has been used as a premedicant and for pain relief in the recovery room. It may cause discomforting hallucinogenic activity. *See* Narcotic.

Penthrane:

See Methoxyflurane.

Penthrane Analgizer:

Simple lightweight disposable device that can deliver a range of approximately 0.3% to 0.9% of methoxyflurane. Used as a self-administered analgesic for obstetric patients, its function is similar to that of the Cyprane or Duke inhaler.

Pentobarbital (Nembutal):

Popular barbiturate for preanesthetic medication. *See* Barbiturate.

Pentolinium (Drug C-5):

Ganglionic blocking agent no longer available clinically.

Pentothal:

See Thiopental sodium.

Pentylenetetrazol (Metrazol):

Central nervous system stimulant that is useful as a diagnostic aid in epilepsy. A patient's response to the drug is monitored with electroencephalography to evaluate the cerebral disorder.

Penumbra:

In cerebral physiology, that area of the brain that lies between infarcted tissue and normal tissue. It is thought that approximately half the neurons in this zone are still alive. Most efforts for cerebral resuscitation are aimed to benefit this area.

PEP:

See Preejection period.

Percutaneous Infusion System:

System that is capable of delivering a small, continuous stream of a drug or medication into a patient through a catheter that traverses the skin. It is used most often to supply terminally ill cancer patients with low doses of morphine for analgesic purposes. *See* Subdermal pump.

Percutaneous Transtracheal Jet Ventilation (PTJV):

Technique for emergency ventilation in which a large-bore intravenous catheter is inserted into the cricothyroid membrane aimed downstream and an interruptible high pressure source of oxygen is used to ventilate the patient. *See* Jet ventilation.

Perfusion:

Passage of a fluid through a vessel, tissue, or specific organ of the body. The fluid usually perfusing the body tissue is blood, but techniques have been developed in which an organ or limb is isolated as to its arterial inflow and venous return and is then perfused with various solutions or drugs, such as chemotherapeutic agents. The definition of perfusion has been extended to include cardiopulmonary bypass. (The technician operating the cardiopulmonary bypass pump and oxygenator apparatus is known as a perfusionist.)

Perfusion Abnormality:

See Ventilation/perfusion abnormality.

Perfusionist:

See Cardiopulmonary bypass; Perfusion.

Perfusion Limitation:

See Diffusion limitation.

Perfusion, Pulmonary:

See Pulmonary perfusion, zones of.

Peridural Anesthesia:

See Epidural anesthesia.

Period (T):

Duration of a single repetition of a cyclic phenomenon or the time occupied in one complete to-and-fro movement of a given oscillation or vibration.

Periodic Breathing:

Period of apnea followed by a gradual crescendo and then decrescendo of respiratory volume, terminating again in apnea. In healthy individuals, periodic breathing can be demonstrated after a period of deliberate hyperventilation. The hyperventilation causes hypocapnia, and this lack of CO_2 causes apnea. During this apneic period, arterial O_2 tension falls off. There then arises a situation of relative hypoxia, which drives respiration to begin again. The hypoxic drive is satisfied by a few good respirations; however, the CO_2 has not built up yet due to tissue metabolism and respiration therefore ceases. This cycle continues until CO_2 is built up to a normal range again, whereupon it resumes control of respiration.

Periodic Table:

Table of the elements displayed in sequence according to atomic number and atomic weight and arranged in horizontal rows (periods) and vertical columns (groups). *See* Table.

Peripheral Chemoreceptors:

Small mass of cells (carotid and aortic bodies) that respond to changes in PCO_2, PO_2, and the pH of blood. They appear to be most sensitive to the PO_2. A fall in O_2 tension causes a rise in ventilation. *See* Carotid body.

Peripheral Nerve Stimulator:

Device that can deliver precise amounts of electrical current to excite a peripheral nerve. The stimulators may be used to evaluate neuromuscular blockade and to prevent overdose with blocking agents. A supramaximal stimulus is applied to the skin electrodes (previously needle electrodes) and the movements of the tested areas (e.g., fingers) are observed. The output voltage under no-load conditions of a typical device can be in excess of 250 V. The output current is usually adjustable between 0 and 50 mA. *See* Figure. *See* Blockade monitor; Neuromuscular blockade, assessment of.

Peripheral Nervous System (PNS):

Part of the nervous system exclusive of the brain and spinal cord. *See* Autonomic nervous system.

Peripheral Vascular Resistance:

See Total peripheral resistance.

Peritoneal Dialysis:

Procedure, useful in patients with acute or chronic renal failure, that aids in the removal of toxic waste material from the blood and maintenance of fluid, electrolyte, and acid-base balance. It is accomplished by means of selective exchange or diffusion across the peritoneal surface (a semipermeable membrane). Peritoneal dialysis involves passing a large volume of dialyzing fluid (dialysate) through the abdominal wall, waiting while exchange takes place, then removing the introduced fluid. Although peritoneal dialysis is easier than hemodialysis, it is a more time-consuming procedure. *See* Hemodialysis.

Peritoneal Insufflation:

See Insufflation, intraperitoneal.

Peritoneoscopy:

See Laparoscopy.

Permanent Gas:

Gas that can be liquefied only by the combination of extreme pressure and cooling.

Periodic Table: Periodic table of the elements.

Horizontal Period	IA	IIA		IIIB	IVB	VB	VIB	VIIB		VIIIB		IB	IIB	IIIA	IVA	VA	VIA	VIIA	O
1	1 **H** 1.0079																		2 **He** 4.0026
2	3 **Li** 6.941	4 **Be** 9.012												5 **B** 10.81	6 **C** 12.011	7 **N** 14.007	8 **O** 15.9994	9 **F** 18.9984	10 **Ne** 20.179
3	11 **Na** 22.990	12 **Mg** 24.31												13 **Al** 26.98	14 **Si** 28.09	15 **P** 30.974	16 **S** 32.064	17 **Cl** 35.453	18 **Ar** 39.948
4	19 **K** 39.102	20 **Ca** 40.08		21 **Sc** 44.96	22 **Ti** 47.90	23 **V** 50.94	24 **Cr** 52.00	25 **Mn** 54.94	26 **Fe** 55.85	27 **Co** 58.93	28 **Ni** 58.71	29 **Cu** 63.546	30 **Zn** 65.38	31 **Ga** 69.72	32 **Ge** 72.59	33 **As** 74.92	34 **Se** 78.96	35 **Br** 79.904	36 **Kr** 83.80
5	37 **Rb** 85.47	38 **Sr** 87.62		39 **Y** 88.91	40 **Zr** 91.22	41 **Nb** 92.91	42 **Mo** 95.94	43 **Tc** 98.91	44 **Ru** 101.07	45 **Rh** 102.91	46 **Pd** 106.4	47 **Ag** 107.868	48 **Cd** 112.4	49 **In** 114.82	50 **Sn** 118.69	51 **Sb** 121.75	52 **Te** 127.60	53 **I** 126.90	54 **Xe** 131.30
6	55 **Cs** 132.91	56 **Ba** 137.34		57 **La*** 138.91	72 **Hf** 178.49	73 **Ta** 180.95	74 **W** 183.85	75 **Re** 186.2	76 **Os** 190.2	77 **Ir** 192.2	78 **Pt** 195.09	79 **Au** 196.97	80 **Hg** 200.59	81 **Tl** 204.37	82 **Pb** 207.20	83 **Bi** 208.98	84 **Po** (209)	85 **At** (210)	86 **Rn** (222)
7	87 **Fr** (223)	88 **Ra** 226.0		89 **Ac†** (227)	104 **Rf**	105 **Ha**	106												

Transition elements

KEY
Electron Configuration
Atomic number
Symbol
Atomic mass

*lanthanide elements

| 58 **Ce** 140.12 | 59 **Pr** 140.9 | 60 **Nd** 144.24 | 61 **Pm** (145) | 62 **Sm** 150.4 | 63 **Eu** 151.96 | 64 **Gd** 157.25 | 65 **Tb** 158.93 | 66 **Dy** 162.50 | 67 **Ho** 164.93 | 68 **Er** 167.26 | 69 **Tm** 168.93 | 70 **Yb** 173.04 | 71 **Lu** 174.97 |

†actinide elements

| 90 **Th** 232.04 | 91 **Pa** 231.04 | 92 **U** 238.03 | 93 **Np** 237.05 | 94 **Pu** (244) | 95 **Am** (243) | 96 **Cm** (247) | 97 **Bk** (247) | 98 **Cf** (251) | 99 **Es** (254) | 100 **Fm** (257) | 101 **Md** (258) | 102 **No** (255) | 103 **Lr** (260) |

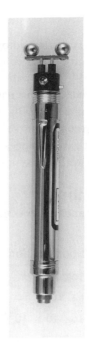

Peripheral Nerve Stimulator: Typical bipolar peripheral nerve stimulator used for assessing neuromuscular blockade.

Permeability Theory of Anesthesia:

Theory proposing that anesthetics reduce permeability to ions that affect synaptic transmission of the central nervous system. In experimental systems, some anesthetics can change membrane permeability. Other drugs, however, which are not anesthetics are able to affect this alteration as well. Therefore this theory does not fully explain the anesthetic state. *See* Lipid solubility theory of anesthesia.

Pethidine:

British term for meperidine (Demerol).

Petite Mal Seizure:

Seizure disorder characterized by brief loss of awareness; it may appear to occur without loss of consciousness and may manifest only as staring, blinking, or rolling of the eyes. This type of seizure usually lasts less than 30 seconds and is rarely associated with postural muscle tone loss. *See* Epilepsy.

Petrolatum (Petroleum Jelly):

Hydrocarbon obtained during the fractional distillation of petroleum. It is used as an emollient, lubricant, and ointment base.

PFT:

See Pulmonary function tests.

pH:

Symbol for hydrogen ion concentration. It is the negative logarithm to the base 10 of the hydrogen ion concentration and is used in measuring acidity and alkalinity on a scale of 0–14 with 7 indicating neutrality. The system serves the useful purpose of restating small values within a narrow range of larger numbers. For example, the hydrogen ion concentration of extracellular fluid is normally 4×10^{-8} Eq/L. The pH is inversely proportional to the hydrogen ion concentration; i.e., as pH increases, the hydrogen ion concentration decreases. A suggestion has been made that hydrogen ion concentration be reported directly in the linear system of nanoequivalents. *See* Table. *See* Acid-base balance.

Phantom Limb:

Phenomenon occurring in recent amputees in which the patient claims that he or she

pH: (A) Normal blood pH derivative. (B) Hydrogen ion nEq/L related to pH.

$$pH = - \log H^+$$
Normal $H^+ = 40 \times 10^{-9}$ Eq. L (40 nEq. L)
$$pH = - \log 40 \times 10^{-9}$$
$$= - (\log 40 + \log 10^{-9})$$
$$= - (\log 4.0 + \log 10^{-8})$$
$$= - (0.59 - 8)$$

A $= - (-7.4) = 7.4$

$[H^+]$ (nEq. L)	pH
125	6.8
100	7.0
40	7.4
25	7.8
15	8.0

B

can still feel, locate in space, and experience pain in the missing limb. It is sometimes reported by patients who have had adequate regional anesthetics. The "phantom" position most often reported is the limb position at the onset of motor blockade. Phantom limb pain is a particularly perplexing problem because regional block done in amputees often does not alleviate the pain and actually makes it worse. *See* Central pain.

Pharmacodynamics:

Measurement of what a drug does in the body, specifically its therapeutic, toxic, and pharmacologic effects. It includes analysis of the mechanism of drug action and measurement of response versus dose or plasma concentration.

Pharmacokinetics:

Study of the relation between time and serum concentration of a drug and its metabolites. It is usually broken down into subcategories of absorption, distribution, and elimination. The latter is a combination of metabolism and excretion. *See* Table.

Pharmacokinetics: Volatile agents.

A₁ Coefficients × 1000

Compartment	Desflurane	Sevoflurane	Isoflurane	Halothane
Lungs	875 ± 64	861 ± 66	779 ± 71[a]	664 ± 95[a]
Vessel-rich group	118 ± 29	107 ± 29	165 ± 38[a]	208 ± 57[a]
Muscle group	39.8 ± 7.5	48.0 ± 17.3	60.3 ± 11.0	108 ± 20[a]
Fourth compartment	4.60 ± 0.87[a]	8.20 ± 0.74[a]	11.5 ± 2.3[a]	20.9 ± 2.8[a]
Fat group	0.349 ± 0.175	0.661 ± 0.372	1.05 ± 0.49[b]	2.29 ± 0.96[a]

Values are mean ± SD.
[a]Significantly different from the other anesthetics ($P < 0.05$).
[b]Significant versus desflurane ($P < 0.05$).

Pharyngolaryngoscope:

Device used for viewing both the pharynx and larynx, particularly when edema has distorted the upper airways. It consists of a tubular blade on a specially constructed handle that gives an unobstructed view by pushing edematous tissue aside. *See* Figure.

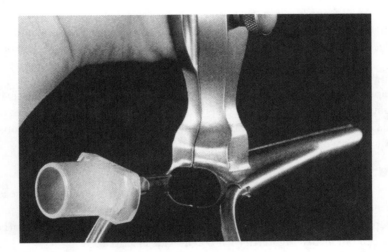

Pharyngolaryngoscope: In vitro recreation of the intraluminal insertion of an endotracheal tube through the tubular laryngoscope blades and into the trachea with bright illumination provided by dual fiberoptic light sources in each blade.

Pharynx:

Mucous membrane-covered muscular sac that is the communication between the nares and mouth superiorly and the esophagus and larynx inferiorly. Specifically, the nasopharynx is the part of the pharynx above the level of the soft palate that is continuous with the nasal passages and contains the opening for the eustachian tubes to the inner ear. The lower part of the pharynx from the soft palate to the upper edge of the epiglottis forming the rear of the mouth is called the oropharynx. The laryngopharynx (hypopharynx) is that part of the pharynx contained between the upper edge of the epiglottis continuous with the larynx and the esophagus.

465

Phasic Block (Inhibition):

See Ionic channel.

Phase I Block:

Normal neuromuscular blocking effect of depolarizing muscle relaxants on the motor endplate area. Agents such as succinylcholine react with the receptors of the motor endplate and depolarize the endplate membrane. The depolarization of the endplate region persists until succinylcholine is metabolized. This continuous action eventually leads to inexcitability in the muscle membrane adjacent to the endplate and to neuromuscular blockade. With phase I block, there is prolonged response to a single twitch, sustained tetanus, no posttetanic facilitation, and train-of-four, each of which is equally depressed. Initial onset of a phase I block causes muscle twitching (fasciculation). *See* Neuromuscular blockade, assessment of.

Phase II Block (Desensitization Block, Dual Block):

Poorly understood phenomenon that occurs after prolonged depolarizing neuromuscular blockade. With this block the muscle membrane becomes at least partially repolarized but does not normally respond to acetylcholine by depolarizing. A phase II block resembles a nondepolarizing block in that tetanus is poorly sustained, posttetanic facilitation is present, and a train-of-four ratio of less than 50% has been observed. Response to anticholinesterase reversal is variable, however. *See* Neuromuscular blockade, assessment of.

Phasic Component of Pain:

Rapid onset of pain sensations felt immediately after injury. The phasic component is in contradistinction to the tonic component which is the longer lasting persistent phase. It is this latter that is believed to enforce rest, care, and protection so as to promote healing. *See* Gate theory of pain; Pain signal transmission.

pH Electrode:

Device that determines the hydrogen ion concentration in a solution as the ions cross a glass membrane to reach an electrode, thereby causing or forming an ion current. This current is proportional to the pH of the solution. The current is read out in units of pH or hydrogen ion concentration. *See* Figure. *See* Carbon dioxide electrode.

Phenacetin:

Analgesic and antipyretic agent often used in conjunction with salicylates. It is an aniline (coaltar) derivative in which the active metabolite is acetaminophen. These agents offer only weak antiinflammatory activity. Overdosage with phenacetin may lead to methemo-globinemia, cyanosis, respiratory depression, and cardiac arrest. *See* Acetaminophen.

Phencyclidine (Sernylan, "Angel Dust," PCP):

Nonbarbiturate compound originally proposed as a human anesthetic but not used clinically because of the high incidence of hallucinations. (It is, however, used as a veterinary anesthetic.) It is chemically related to ketamine. A widely abused drug that can be easily manufactured, it can cause severe toxic psychosis, convulsions, and death. Some anecdotal evidence exists that it can cause permanent personality changes after single- or short-term use, an attribute that would make it a unique pharmacologic entity. *See* Figure.

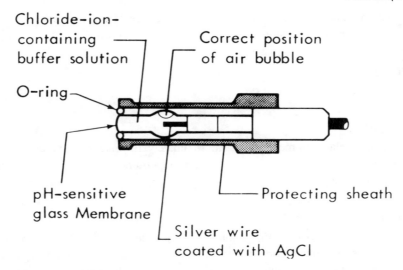

pH Electrode.

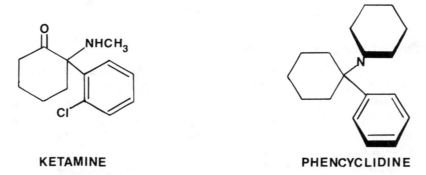

KETAMINE   **PHENCYCLIDINE**

Phencyclidine: Molecular diagrams of ketamine and phencyclidine showing the similarity.

Phenergan:

See Phenothiazine; Promethazine hydrochloride.

Phenobarbital (Luminal, Phenobarb):

Barbiturate used as a sedative, hypnotic, and anticonvulsant. It is more potent as an anticonvulsant than as a sedative. After even short-term use, phenobarbital stimulates liver enzyme systems that metabolize many similar drugs. It can therefore, theoretically at least, shorten the action of those agents that depend on metabolism to terminate their actions. *See* Barbiturate; Cytochrome P-450 system.

Phenol (Carbolic Acid):

First widely used antiseptic. Many dilute phenol derivatives are employed to disinfect equipment and furniture surfaces that do not come in contact with patients. Phenol is highly toxic and may cause convulsions and renal damage. It may be used clinically for neurolytic injection in the treatment of intractable pain. *See* Neurolysis.

Phenolphthalein:

See Indicator dye.

Phenoperidine:

Narcotic related to meperidine. Approximately 10 times more potent than morphine, it is available in England under the trade name Operidine. The drug is a long-acting respiratory depressant. *See* Narcotic.

Phenothiazine:

Widely used group of drugs that are employed primarily for treatment of psychiatric disorders and are important also as antiemetic and antihistaminic agents. Although not addictive, they can produce some degree of physical dependence. The phenothiazines are weak α-adrenergic blocking agents and can therefore enhance hypotension seen during anesthesia. They can produce acute parkinsonian-like rigidity that can lead to respiratory embarrassment. *See* Antipsychotic agent; Lytic cocktail.

Phenoxybenzamine (Dibenzyline):

α-Adrenergic blocking agent closely related to the nitrogen mustards, that effectively prevents responses mediated by alpha receptors, producing a "chemical sympathectomy." Phenoxybenzamine lowers blood pressure and may produce orthostatic hypotension. It is used for presurgical treatment of pheochromocytoma. In this role it controls the episodic hypertension and sweating that characterize this disease. It has also been used to alleviate vasospastic peripheral vascular disease. Adverse side effects of phenoxybenzamine include tachycardia, miosis, and orthostatic hypotension. *See* Phentolamine.

Phentolamine (Regitine):

Imidazoline with a wide range of pharmacologic actions, the most important of which is its alpha receptor blockade. It is used to prevent or control the hypertensive episodes of a patient with pheochromocytoma. It is also used in the Regitine test to assist in the diagnosis of pheochromocytoma. An intravenous injection of phentolamine produces a rapid fall in blood pressure in a patient with the adrenal tumor. An alternate use of the drug is in the treatment of dermal necrosis caused by extravasation of norepinephrine from an intravenous site. Adverse side effects include tachycardia, cardiac arrhythmia, angina, abdominal pain, nausea, vomiting, diarrhea, and exacerbation of peptic ulcer. *See* Phenoxybenzamine.

Phenylephrine (Neo-Synephrine):

Potent pressor agent (raises blood pressure) and a powerful alpha receptor stimulant with little effect on beta receptors. It produces a marked reflex bradycardia, increases peripheral resistance, and slightly decreases cardiac output. Because of its potency, it is administered in highly dilute form in an intravenous bolus or drip; because of its rapid onset, it requires careful management. It is also used topically as a nasal decongestant and as a mydriatic agent.

Pheochromocytoma:

Tumor arising from the chromaffin cells in sympathetic ganglia. It is capable of secreting vasoactive substances, particularly epinephrine and norepinephrine, and may be found anywhere in the body where sympathetic nervous tissue is found, most typically in the adrenal medulla. This type of tumor is particularly significant to anesthesia; premedication with alpha-blocking agents, e.g., phenoxybenzamine, to block the action of the agents secreted by the tumor is absolutely essential. At times, even in the face of adequate long-term blockade, the anesthetic course is uneven with wild shifts in blood pressure and cardiac output as the tumor is manipulated. Pheochromocytoma tends to be familial and is often associated with medullary carcinoma of the thyroid gland. *See* Table. *See* Phenoxybenzamine; Phentolamine.

Pheochromocytoma: Symptoms and signs.

Hypertension	Psychosis
Palpitations	Syncope
Sweating	Convulsions
Pallor	Tinnitus
Flushing	Blurred vision
Angina	Weight loss
Dyspnea	Anorexia
Headache	Nausea
Nervousness	Epigastric pain
Weakness	Back pain
Dizziness	Neck pain
Tremors	Flank pain

pHisoHex:

See Hexachlorophene.

Phosgene (Carbonyl Chloride):

Highly toxic, colorless gas ($CoCl_2$) that condenses at 0°C to a fuming liquid. It is a breakdown product of trichloroethylene (an obsolete anesthetic). Phosgene was used as a poisonous gas during World War I and is now used in the manufacture of organic compounds. *See* Trichloroethylene.

Phospholine:

See Echothiophate iodide.

Phosphor:

Substance capable of emitting light when excited by radiant energy. *See* Cathode-ray tube.

Phosphorescence:

Luminescence seen after bombardment with electromagnetic energy and visible for a time after the excitement has ceased. *See* Luminescence. *See* Cathode-ray tube.

Photocell (Photoelectric Cell):

Solid-state photosensitive electronic device. Its resistance to electric current flow is a function of incident radiation. It is also known as an electric eye, because of its use as a sensor in burglar alarm systems. *See* Photoconductivity.

Photoconductivity:

Subclass of the photoelectric effect that describes the ability of specific elements or compounds to change (usually by lowering) their electrical resistance when illuminated by a light frequency specific to the compound. It is the basic process that makes photocells possible.

Photoelectric Determination of Blood Pressure:

Technique for determining blood pressure using a light source, a photocell, and a blood pressure cuff. A light source is aimed at a particular area of tissue. The amount of light reflected or transmitted through the tissue changes with each pulse, and the amount of light received by a photoconductive cell fluctuates. Because the resistance of the cell changes with light striking it, current flowing through it pulsates with tissue blood flow. Quantitating pressure changes requires slow deflation of a proximal blood pressure cuff while watching for a pulse indication from the photocell. *See* Arterial blood pressure.

Photoelectric Effect:

Physical property that allows certain substances to use energy contained in incident electromagnetic radiation (particularly light) to raise the energy level of electrons in the substance. This phenomenon underlies photoconductivity and photoelectric emission.

Photoelectric Emission (Photoemission):

Physical property of certain substances that causes electrons to be randomly emitted when the substance is struck in a vacuum by electromagnetic energy such as light. Elements that exhibit this property include barium, cesium, and lithium. *See* Photovoltaic effect.

Photomultiplier:

Device that detects light by converting light energy to an electric current and then amplifying the current. For example, with liquid scintillation counters light flashes strike a photocathode, which exhibits the photoelectric effect (photons of light energy are converted to free-moving electrons). These electrons are then accelerated by a magnetic field and are used to strike subsequent cathodes, liberating more electrons. The strength of the ultimate electron cascade is the function of the strength of the magnetic field used to guide it and the number of cathodes.

Photon:

A discrete unit of electromagnetic radiation that has no rest mass and travels at the speed of light. Its energy is the product of its frequency, in cycles per second, times the Planck constant, i.e., $E = hf$.

Photovoltaic Effect:

Production of an electrical field or voltage in a substance by absorption of the energy contained in the light striking the substance. As a subclass of the photoelectric effect, it is the phenomenon underlying solar cells. The efficiency of the process of converting one form of energy to another is at best 20–25%. *See* Photocell.

Phrenic Nerve:

Paired main motor nerves that arise from the cervical plexus at levels C3–C5 and innervate the diaphragm. Paralysis of the phrenic nerve(s) may result from neck fracture or inadvertently from brachial plexus block, high epidural, or high spinal anesthesia. Deliberate phrenic nerve block was an old method of treating intractable hiccup. *See* Electrophrenic respiration.

pH Stat Management (Strategy):

Technique for managing hypothermic cardiac pulmonary bypass. It maintains $PaCO_2$ at 40 mm Hg and pH at 7.50 after correction for body temperature. *See* Alpha stat management.

Physical Status Classifications, ASA:

Evaluation of the patient's overall health as it would influence the conduct and outcome of anesthesia or surgery. Physical status can be defined within one of five assigned classes. (1) Class 1 patients have no organic, physiologic, biochemical, metabolic, or psychiatric disturbance. The operation to be performed is for a local pathologic process and has no systemic effect. An example of a class 1 patient is an athlete who requires repair of an inguinal hernia. (2) Class 2 patients have a systemic disturbance that may be of a mild to moderate degree but that is either controlled or has not changed in its severity for some time. Examples are patients with controlled diabetes, controlled hypertension, or mild nonlimiting organic heart disease. Often anesthetists consider healthy individuals at the extremes of age (neonate or octogenarian) to be class 2 patients. (3) Class 3 patients suffer from significant systemic disturbance, although the degree to which it limits the patient's functioning or causes disability may not be quantifiable. Examples include severe organic heart disease, severe diabetes with vascular or kidney involvement, pulmonary insufficiency, angina pectoris, or an old myocardial infarction. (4) Class 4 patients have severe systemic diseases that are already life-threatening and may or may not be correctable by surgery. An example is a patient with initial signs of cardiac failure, advanced liver or renal disease, or intractable angina. (5) Class 5 patients are considered to have little or no chance of survival in the short term (< 24 hours) and are submitted to operation in desperation. An example of a class 5 patient is an individual with a massive pulmonary embolus, major cerebral trauma, or severe and progressive compromised respiratory gas exchange. As a further subclassification of physical states, any patient falling naturally into one of the five classes who comes to an operation as an emergency has the letter E placed after the classification number. For example, the patient scheduled for emergency nephrectomy due to rejection of a transplanted kidney would be classified 4E.

Physician Diagnostic Related Groups (MDDRG):

Financial reimbursement scheme that would pay physicians based on the patient's diagnosis rather than the time or effort spent with a particular patient. It is considered to be unfavorable to anesthesiologists who work in academic situations, where surgical procedures tend to take longer.

Physician-Patient Relationship:

The contract for services between patient and physician that contains the following legal considerations: (1) The physician must personally render the care agreed on; the patient suffers injury in a legal sense if another physician is substituted without permission of the patient. (2) The physician has the responsibility of working to the standard set by similarly trained physicians with similar experience in similar communities. (3) The physician has a duty or obligation not to cease rendering care without the permission of the patient. (4) The physician must maintain the trust of the patient and not reveal publicly details of the patient's care that are of a confidential nature. When a contract for service has been established with a physician, the patient has the following obligations and duties: (1) The patient is required to follow the instructions, prescriptions, and advice of the physician. (2) The patient is obligated to pay for the services he or she receives. If any of the above duties are not carried out, one or the other of the parties to the agreement may have legal recourse. *See* Informed consent.

Physiologic Dead Space:

Portion of a tidal volume that is not available for gas exchange. It includes the anatomic deadspace and those alveoli that, although ventilated, are not perfused. *See* Alveolar deadspace, Anatomic deadspace.

Physostigmine; Eserine (Antilirium):

Anticholinesterase agent useful for treatment of glaucoma. It is capable of penetrating the blood-brain barrier. It has been used to reverse the cardiovascular and central nervous system (CNS) effects of acute atropine and scopolamine overdose. It has also been reported to be an effective antidote to a variety of CNS depressants; however, it can cause profound bradycardia.

Pickup:

Device that converts a sound or other form of mechanical vibration into an electrical signal. Such devices include microphones and phonograph cartridges.

Pickwickian Syndrome:

Condition involving morbid obesity with various associated problems such as somnolence, cyanosis, intermittent respiration, secondary polycythemia, and right-sided cardiac failure.

Total lung capacity, vital capacity, and respiratory reserve volume are all decreased. The work of breathing is increased as the amount of energy required to move the chest mass is elevated. *See* Morbid obesity.

Pico-:

Prefix meaning 10^{12}. (This term replaces micromicro-.) *See* SI unit.

Picrotoxin:

Convulsant that acts as a γ-aminobutyric acid (GABA, a neuroinhibitory transmitter) antagonist. It functions by binding directly to GABA receptors. This action prevents the normal inhibitory influence of GABA and results in seizure activity.

Pierre Robin Syndrome:

Congenital syndrome that combines micrognathia with cleft palate and glossoptosis. Glossoptosis, displacement or retraction of the tongue into the hypopharynx, may produce intermittent airway obstruction.

Piezoelectric Effect:

Property of certain crystals to produce an electrical signal (oscillate) when subjected to mechanical stress (pressure, expansion, twisting). The electrical charges are proportional to the tension applied. Depending on size, shape, and composition (quartz, barium tartrate), the frequency at which a crystal oscillates is controllable and exact. Crystals are therefore used for precision clocks or timing circuits.

Pilocarpine:

Naturally occurring alkaloid that mimics the effects of acetylcholine in the heart, salivary glands, and sweat glands. It is most commonly used as a topical miotic agent.

Pindolol:

Drug that is a nonselective beta-blocker. It has both membrane-stabilizing activity and intrinsic sympathomimetic activity. It is anywhere between 10 and 40 times as potent as propranolol.

Pin-Index Safety System:

Safety system that prevents the wrong gas cylinder from being placed in a yoke. The pin-index safety system is used with small cylinders (size E or less) and consists of two pins on the yoke that fit into two corresponding holes in the cylinder valve. If the pins and holes cannot be aligned, the cylinder port will not fit against the washer of the yoke. The system uses various combinations of six locations of holes and pins. Anesthetic disasters have occurred when the pin-index system was deliberately defeated by extracting the pins or using double washers as a temporary convenience. *See* Diameter index safety system.

Pin Valve:

See Flow control valve.

Pipecuronium (Arduan):

Nondepolarizing neuromuscular blocking agent structurally similar to pancuronium and vecuronium. The drug appears to be somewhat more potent than pancuronium. It may also preserve cardiovascular stability.

Piperocaine (Metycaine):

Local anesthetic agent with properties similar to those of procaine. *See* Local anesthetic.

pKa:

See Dissociation constant.

Placental Drug Transfer:

Concept that drugs administered to the pregnant patient cross the placenta and reach the fetus. Placenta transfer of particular drugs is determined by their maternal plasma binding, maternal pH, drug solubility, and drug molecular size. *See* Ion trapping.

Planck Constant (h):

Universal constant that relates the frequency of radiation to its quanta of energy; it has a value of 6.25×10^{-27} erg second.

Planck Law:

Basis of quantum theory used to describe the behavior of electromagnetic radiation. It states that the energy of electromagnetic radiation is in the form of small individual packets called photons. *See* Photon.

Plasma:

Clear straw-colored liquid portion of the blood in which the formed elements, (cells) float and proteins and other molecules are dissolved. *See* Serum, blood.

Plasma Expander:

Solution used to replace critical loss of blood plasma. Plasma expanders may be non-blood-derived starch solutions such as dextran or hetastarch or blood-derived such as Albumin, and are administered intravenously. *See* Albumin; Dextran; Hetastarch.

Plasma Half-Life:

The time it takes for a drug detected in plasma to be half eliminated by metabolism, excretion, or redistribution.

Plasma Kinin:

See Bradykinin.

Plasmapheresis:

Removal of plasma from drawn blood and retransfusion of the formed elements of that blood back to the donor. Most often used pre- or perioperatively. (If done, for example, prior to extracorporeal circulation, it is referred to as acute plasmapheresis. The technique tries to minimize the use of homologous blood and blood products and improves coagulation in cardiac surgery. The plasma may be reinfused to compensate for acute blood loss.

Platelet (Thrombocyte):

Anucleate, disk-shaped cell 2–4 μm in diameter that is a constituent of mammalian blood and important in coagulation. Normal levels range from 150,000 to 400,000 platelets/mm^3 blood. Platelets can change shape and accumulate at the site of vascular injury (platelet aggregation). Platelet aggregation and adhesion occur in response to the contact of platelets with a nonvascular surface. These two processes cause many products to be released from cytoplasmic granules in the platelets, the most important being adenosine diphosphate (ADP). (Other substances released include serotonin, epinephrine, calcium, and clotting factors.) ADP is a potent agent for causing further platelet aggregation. Aggregation, adhesion, and release are collectively called platelet activation and, once having reached a threshold, it is a self-sustaining process. *See* Blood coagulation.

Platelet Concentrate:

Pooling of platelet-rich plasma produced by the differential centrifugation of several units of whole blood. Stored at room temperature, the concentrate contains a significant number of viable platelets for 72 hours. Platelets stored at 4°C retain viability for only 24 hours. The concentrate, used for platelet transfusion, temporarily prevents or reduces bleeding associated with platelet-deficient diseases, such as acute leukemia, thrombocytopenia, and aplastic anemia.

Platinum:

Grayish white metallic element that, because of its malleability and high electrical and corrosive resistance, is used in alloys, jewelry, and electrical and electronic equipment. It acts as a catalyst for many chemical reactions. *See* Oxygen analyzer.

Plethysmograph:

See Blood flow, methods for measuring; Body plethysmograph.

Pleura:

Collective name for the two layers of serous membrane that enclose and protect the lungs. The parietal pleura, the outer layer, is attached to the walls of the pleural cavity; the visceral pleura, the inner layer, lines the lungs. The potential space between the two layers of the pleura is called the pleural cavity and contains a lubricating fluid secreted by the membranes.

Plexus:

See Ganglion.

Ploss Valve:

See Stethoscope.

PMN:

See Polymodal nociceptors.

PMT:

See Pacemaker-mediated tachycardia.

PNCG:

See Pneumocardiography.

Pneumatics:

Branch of physics that deals with the mechanical properties of gas.

Pneumocardiography (PNCG); thoracic air plethysmography:

Recording variations in heart functions by monitoring the respiration. The pneumocardio-graph senses changes in thoracic cavity dimensions and changes in bronchial pressure with each heartbeat. This procedure is most conveniently done in the apneic patient.

Pneumocephalus:

Condition that can occur as a result of neurosurgery when the skull is opened. When cerebrolspinal fluid (CSF) is drained for access purposes, space is made available within the skull that allows air to become trapped. This accumulation of air may cause untoward pressure on brain tissue when repairs are complete. Also: an early technique of radiologic imaging that replaces CSF with air through a spinal tap. *See* Nitrous oxide.

Pneumocyte:

See Alveolar cell types.

Pneumotachograph (Fleisch Pneumotachograph):

Device for measuring gas flow. It operates by placing a mesh screen in the path of a moving gas. The resistance of the mesh screen causes a pressure drop across its surface, and the magnitude of this decrease in pressure is related to the volume of gas passing the screen. By measuring the pressure difference, the volume of gas that has passed the screen per unit of time can be approximated. The device tends to become inaccurate at low flows or if the screen becomes obstructed. *See* Anemometer, hot wire.

Pneumothorax:

Presence of free air in the pleural cavity. It may occur traumatically after puncture or penetration of the chest wall or pleura, or it may appear spontaneously after blowout of a bleb on the surface of the lung. An open pneumothorax occurs when a wound of external entry remains exposed. The air space then enlarges with each inspiration as the negative pressure in the chest sucks air simultaneously down the trachea and through the hole in the chest wall. A closed pneumothorax is the aforementioned air space with no communication with either the external chest wall or the air passageways of the lung. The closed pneumo-thorax may become a tension pneumothorax if the pressure of the air in the pleural cavity rises above that in the lung. The best explanation of the mechanism of tension pneumotho-rax is to consider the communication with the pleura as a ball valve that enlarges the pneumothorax space at peak inspiratory pressure but closes when expiratory pressure would push air out of the cavity. The trapped air compresses the affected lung. Tension pneumothorax can be exacerbated by the use of N_2O during anesthesia. Nitrous oxide, because it diffuses across membranes so rapidly (faster than the N_2 it replaces), diffuses into the closed air space, continually pressurizing and expanding it. It progressively encroaches on the lung volume and may lead to severe respiratory embarrassment. Signs and symptoms of pneumothorax include pain, dyspnea, effusion (hydropneumothorax), and absence of breath sounds. *See* Figure.

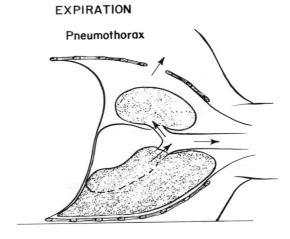

EXPIRATION

Pneumothorax

INSPIRATION

Pneumothorax

Pneumothorax: Pneumothorax and paradoxic respiration during spontaneous breathing. Note collapse of lung during inspiration, and expansion during expiration.

Pneumotaxic Center:

See Respiratory centers.

PNS:

See Peripheral nervous system.

Podophyllum:

Natural resin mixture obtained from the various parts of the May apple. It has been a popular remedy for constipation and has been used for topical treatment of various wart-like conditions. It can be toxic after both oral ingestion and topical application.

Poiseuille Law:

Physical principle determining flow of fluid in a tube or vessel. Flow rate is directly proportional to (1) the pressure drop along the length and (2) the fourth power of the tube radius. Flow is inversely proportional to tube length and fluid viscosity. In practical terms, doubling the height of an intravenous bottle roughly doubles flow; doubling the radius of an intravenous cannula increases flow 16 times.

Polarization:

State of matter in which two surfaces have opposite, and often equal, electrical charges. For example, in a polarized membrane of a nerve cell the outside surface is positive and the inside surface negative. Differences in electrical potential are normally measured in volts. Generally, when a skin electrode is polarized, a difference measurable in volts (millivolts) exists between the electrodes and the skin.

Polarography:

Electrochemical technique of analysis in which changes in the chemical or physical composition of a solution create changes in its electrical conductivity, thereby effecting a change in any electrical current passing through the solution. Thus in accordance with the Ohm law, changes in the voltage difference across the solution can be measured and reflect the changing conditions in the solution. Polarography is most immediately applicable to O_2 analysis where the presence or absence of O_2 changes the electrical conductivity of an ionic solution and this change is used to measure O_2 concentration. *See* Oxygen analyzer.

Polio Blade:

Adaptation of the Macintosh laryngoscope blade, which sits at an obtuse angle on the handle to allow intubation of a patient in an iron lung. *See* Laryngoscope.

Polymerization:

Process of forming a polymer by bonding monomers of repeating structural units. Polymers may be naturally occurring (e.g., rubber, proteins, starches) or man-made (e.g., nylon, Teflon, polyvinyl chloride).

Polymodal Nociceptors (PMN):

See Somatic pain.

Polymyxin B (Aerosporin):

Potent peptide antibiotic of the polymyxin group produced from a strain of soil bacillus (*Bacillus polymyxa*). It is active against gram-negative bacteria. Polymyxin B is administered parenterally [intravenously (IV), intramuscularly (IM), intrathecally], topically (usually in combination with bacitracin as an ointment), or orally. Untoward side effects include pain (after IM injection), renal toxicity, nausea, vomiting, diarrhea, headache, meningeal irritation (after intrathecal injection), diplopia, ptosis, and generalized areflexia. Polymyxin E, commonly known as colistin (Coly-Mycin), is another member of this antibiotic group. *See* Table. *See* Antibiotics.

Polymyxin B: Polymyxins.

Generic Name (Trade Name)	Spectrum of Activity	Comments

Polymyxin B (Aerosporin)
  Topical
  IM
  PO
  Otic Solution
	G^- bacilli, including Pseudomonas, Escherichia, Enterobacter, Klebsiella, Hemophilus, Salmonella and Shigella. Proteus is resistant.	Polymyxin B, like the other polymyxins, is bactericidal and is associated with certain side effects, including nephrotoxicity and neurologic disturbances such as vertigo, paresthesias, and neuromuscular blockade. It is not absorbed orally but is used orally for the treatment of GI infections.

Colistin (Coly-Mycin S)
  PO
  Otic Solution
	Similar to polymyxin B.	Colistin is used in treating diarrhea caused by *E. coli* and Shigella in children with enteritis. Side effects include superinfection within the GI tract, especially by Proteus.

Colistimethate (Coly-Mycin M)
  IM
  IV
	Similar to polymyxin B.	Colistimethate can cause nephrotoxicity, neuromuscular blockade, and transient neurologic disturbances. Its therapeutic uses are essentially the same as polymyxin B.

Polypeptide:

Peptide composed of three or more amino acids joined by peptide bonds, i.e., a carbon atom linked to a nitrogen atom in an alternating chain. The size of the polypeptide depends on the number of amino acids in the chain.

POMS:

See Profile of mood states.

Ponderal Index:

Calculation in which the patient's height is divided by the cube root of the patient's weight. It is used as one of the indices of morbid obesity. *See* Morbid obesity.

Pontocaine:

See Local anesthetic; Tetracaine hydrochloride.

Pop-Off Valve (Expiratory Valve; High-Pressure Relief Valve):

Valve downstream from the patient in a gas delivery system, that relieves the excess volume that continuously builds up when the fresh gas flow into the system exceeds the O_2 uptake of the patient. *See* Figure.

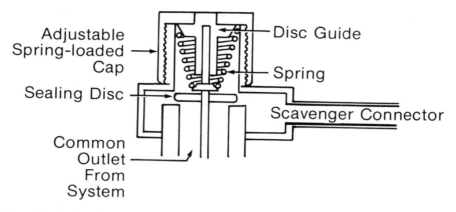

Pop-Off Valve: Typical spring-loaded pop-off valve showing the various internal parts.

Porphyria:

Hereditary disease that involves errors in the formation or excretion of porphyrins. Porphyrins are molecular components of hemoglobin, myoglobin, various enzymes concerned with oxidation reactions such as the cytochromes, and other proteins concerned with oxidation and electron transport. They are chemically related to plant chlorophyll. There are two basic types of porphyria: (1) erythropoietic, in which the metabolic disturbance is in the bone marrow; and (2) hepatic, in which the metabolic disturbance is in the liver. Hepatic porphyrias—of clinical interest to the practice of anesthesia—are divided into three types: acute intermittent porphyria, variegate porphyria, and hereditary coproporphyria. The latter is a rare type that clinically mimics either of the first two. Acute intermittent porphyria is characterized by attacks that are irregular and unpredictable. The attacks can consist of abdominal pain, various moderate to severe neurologic abnormalities involving both central and peripheral nervous systems, motor disturbances, seizure activities, psychiatric aberrations, and cardiovascular involvement. The patients ultimately die from the additive effect of multiple central nervous system lesions. Anesthetic interest lies in the fact that intravenous barbiturates in the dose used for anesthesia induction allegedly can trigger an attack of acute intermittent porphyria, which can lead to cardiovascular collapse.

Positive End-Expiratory Pressure (PEEP):

Modality for the treatment of patients who require ventilatory support. When PEEP is employed, the airway pressure is never allowed to return to "zero" (atmospheric). At the end of expiration, when airway pressure would normally be at its lowest point, it is artificially held at positive pressure by the PEEP apparatus. It can be held there simply by using a water trap into which the exhalation hose is dipped. The amount of pressure placed on the gas in the hose is directly readable as the number of centimeters the hose dips below the surface of the water. The prime purpose of PEEP is to keep the small airways open and stabilize the structural integrity of the lung. The positive pressure "splints" open airways that would otherwise close (due to loss of support) and thereby trap air. Side effects of peep include decreased venous return and increased risk of pneumothorax. High PEEP levels are associated with more risk. *See* Pneumothorax.

Positive-Pressure Respiration, Positive-Pressure Ventilation:

Technique of providing ventilation for a patient by means of positively pressurizing gas so it enters the lungs. Normal respiration depends on a negative pressure being created in the chest with the drop of the diaphragm and the lifting up of the rib cage, sucking air into the lungs.

Positive Water Balance:

See Negative water balance.

Positron:

Elementary particle with an identical mass and positive charge equal in strength to the negative charge of an electron.

Postanesthetic Recovery Room (PAR):

See Recovery/recovery room.

Postdural Puncture Headache (PDPH):

See Spinal headache.

Postherpetic Neuralgia:

See Herpetic neuralgia.

Postoperative Visit:

Bedside visit by the anesthetist to the postoperative patient with the purpose of evaluating the outcome of anesthesia and recording appropriate remarks on the patient's chart. A postoperative visit is a requirement for hospital accreditation, particularly for those patients who are in the hospital for at least 24 hours postoperatively.

Poststimulus Latencies:

Amount of time (usually measured in milliseconds) between stimulation while testing for evoked potentials and dominant components in the elicited waveforms. Poststimulus latencies are usually described as long, intermediate, or short. Short latencies are usually less than 20 ms and occur when the electrical signal arises near the site of sensory stimulation. Intermediate latencies occur between 20 and 120 ms after stimulation. Electrical signals that arise more than 120 ms after the stimulation are called long latency events. *See* Far-field potential.

Postsynaptic Membrane:

See Neuromuscular blockade, assessment of.

Postsynaptic Potential:

See Neuromuscular blockade, assessment of.

Posttetanic Count (PTC)::

Method of monitoring neuromuscular transmission during periods of intense neuromuscular blockade. Although the technique is not yet standardized, in general, it uses a tetanic stimulation such as 50 Hz for 5 seconds after train-of-four or single twitch in sequence for 4–6 minutes. *See* Neuromuscular blockade; assessment of.

Posttetanic Facilitation:

See Neuromuscular blockade, assessment of.

Postural Drainage:

Technique of respiratory therapy that uses gravity to mobilize excess lung secretions. The patient is positioned so the affected area of the lung is superior to the trachea. Postural drainage is often used with chest percussion to "shake" secretions loose.

Potassium (K):

Element that occurs abundantly in nature; it is the principal cation of intracellular fluids. Its atomic number is 19 and its atomic weight 39. The potassium balance of the body is important to both the integrity of cellular function and, more specifically, the maintenance of normal cardiac rhythmicity. The normal 70-kg man has a total body content of exchangeable potassium of approximately 3200 mEq; about two-thirds of this amount is intracellular. The concentration in intracellular water is approximately 160 mEq/L. Extracellularly, the serum potassium normally ranges from 3.5 to 5.5 mEq/L. Under normal circumstances with normally functioning kidneys, the minimum daily requirement approaches 30 mEq. Problems arise with potassium control that do not exist with the control of sodium concentration because the kidney is not as well equipped to conserve potassium when potassium is depleted in the body. Manditory loss is in the range of 20 mEq/24 hours. Particularly in those instances where a normal adult continues to receive sodium but whose potassium intake is restricted for as little as 7 days, significant potassium depletion can occur. Potassium and hydrogen ions compete for exchange with sodium ions in renal tubules; and when sodium is provided, adrenal steroids increase renal potassium loss. When the patient is stressed and has normal kidneys, excretion may reach levels in excess of 100 mEq/24 hours. Of particular interest to individuals managing patients with acid-base imbalances is the fact that plasma potassium increases approximately 0.6 mEq/L for each 0.1-unit fall in blood pH. Conversely, plasma potassium decreases about 0.6 mEq/L for each 0.1-unit rise in blood pH. It is difficult to raise serum potassium levels in alkalotic patients. Because of the interchangeability, so far as the body is concerned, of potassium and hydrogen. *See* Table. *See* Cardiac glycosides; Electrocardiogram.

Potassium Channel (Potassium Tunnel):

Name given to the opening in the membrane of a nerve that allows passage of the potassium ion outward into the extracellular fluid during depolarization. The potassium channel is a theoretic entity. Unlike the sodium pore, which appears to occur in areas of the membrane that are thin, the potassium pore (channel) occurs in areas of the membrane that are of normal thickness. The nature of the gate in the potassium tunnel is not well defined. *See* Ionic channel; Sodium channel.

Potassium: Clinical entities associated with serum potassium changes.

Causes of Potassium Elevation	Causes of Potassium Depletion
Excess oral or parenteral intake	Dietary insufficiency
Use of potassium-sparing diuretics, i.e., aldactone, dyrenium	Diarrhea
	Alkalosis
Acidosis	Potassium-losing renal disease
Acute hemolysis of red cells	Aldosteronism
Muscle necrosis	Nasogastric suction
Renal insufficiency	Therapy with diuretics
Addison disease	Secondary to glucose and insulin administration
Hypoaldosteronism associated with diabetes	Villous adenoma of the intestine

Potency:

Relative strength of a drug determined by the dose (measured by weight) that produces pharmacologic effects (especially intensity and duration of action) equal to those of a reference compound. For example, milligram for milligram, tetracaine has been determined to be approximately 10 times more potent than procaine.

Potential Energy:

Energy a body or system has by virtue of its position. It is equal to the work that was done in bringing that system to its current position.

Potentiation:

Increase in the power of an activity, e.g., the greater force of contraction of the heart on administration of a positive inotropic drug. It is used frequently but less correctly as a synonym for synergism in reference to drug interaction. *See* Synergism.

Potentiometer:

Variable resistor in electronic circuits with resistance changes from zero up to its rated resistance in ohms, depending on the position of a moving contact. It is also an instrument for measuring voltage.

Potts Shunt:

Side-to-side anastomosis of the descending thoracic aorta and the left pulmonary artery. It is performed as a palliative surgical procedure to help patients with reduced pulmonary blood flow, e.g., congenital pulmonary artery stenosis. It has been largely replaced by the Blalock-Taussig shunt because of the difficulty of controlling blood flow through the anastomosis.

Poynting Effect:

Ability of N_2O and O_2 in a premixed cylinder to exist as a single-phase gas at a pressure below 2000 1b/in at room temperature. This effect is due to the solvent action of O_2.

PPF:

See Peak power frequency; median power frequency.

Practolol (Eraldin):

ß-Adrenergic blocking agent said to have a predilection for beta sites in the myocardium. It has been used to treat hypertension but produces toxic side effects after long-term use. It is not available for use in the United States.

Pralidoxime (Protopam; 2-PAM):

Specific drug used to treat organophosphate poisoning. It reactivates cholinesterase by causing its release from the organophosphate to which it has been bound. Without 2-PAM, nonspecific cholinesterase is regenerated by the liver in about 2 weeks, whereas acetylcholinesterase may take up to 3 months to be regenerated. *See* Organophosphorus compounds.

Prazocin (Minipress):

Drug used to treat both hypertension and ischemic cardiomyopathy, causing venodilation and arterial dilation. It is an α_1-adrenergic receptor blocker. It has anticholinergic effects and has been associated with palpitations, dizziness, vertigo, depression, and muscle weakness.

Preamplifier:

Amplifier used to provide moderate amplification of an incoming signal before it reaches the main amplifier. Using one amplifier to power another allows for a better signal-to-noise ratio; by placing the preamplifier close to the signal source, the initial signal is amplified before noise from transmission lines can occur.

Preanesthetic Visit (Preoperative Evaluation):

Introduction of the anesthetist to the patient prior to surgery. Aside from any social purpose the preoperative visit may accomplish, it allows the patient to see and identify the individual who will have a profound effect upon his or her immediate future. This visit alone often allays patient anxiety. The preoperative visit also allows the anesthetist to evaluate the patient's medical history and review pertinent operative and hospital records. A physical examination can be done as required; and subtle clues, such as respiratory rate, skin color, motor coordination, and emotional level, can be ascertained. The preoperative visit is always a good idea and is the only way the anesthetist can obtain informed, intelligent consent to anesthetic procedures. *See* Informed consent.

Precision:

Term used to classify error. It is an index of the repeatability of a measurement. It quantifies the random error associated with multiple determinations. *See* Accuracy.

Precision Vaporizer:

See Vaporizer.

Prednisolone (Delta-Cortef; Meticortelone):

Glucocorticoid with a higher antiinflammatory potency than cortisol. Prednisolone has a slightly lower tendency than cortisol to cause sodium retention. *See* Corticosteroid.

Prednisone (Meticorten; Deltasone):

Glucocorticoid with a higher antiinflammatory potency than cortisol. It also has less tendency than cortisol to cause sodium retention. *See* Corticosteroid.

Preeclampsia:

Toxemia of unknown etiology that occurs during late pregnancy. It is characterized by generalized hypertension, edema, and the appearance of albumin in the urine. When these phenomena are accompanied by seizure activity, the patient is considered to be eclamptic. Preeclampsia and eclampsia are obstetric emergencies; patients manifesting these symptoms are considered increased anesthetic risks. *See* Eclampsia; Magnesium.

Preejection Period (PEP):

Time interval between the onset of ventricular depolarization and the onset of left ventricular ejection time (LVET) on the electrocardiogram. The PEP is used as a qualitative estimate of left ventricular performance. *See* Systolic time intervals.

Pregnancy Risks:

Categorization of drugs that may affect the fetus in utero if taken by the pregnant mother. There are four categories—A through D—with category B subdivided into three sub units. *Category A* comprises drugs that are used by a large number of pregnant women and are not associated with any disturbances in the reproductive process. *Category B* comprises drugs that have not been associated with harmful effects but have been used by only a limited number of patients. *Group B1* comprises those drugs for which reproduction studies in animals have not indicated a harmful effect. *Group B2* comprises drugs for whom reproduction and toxicology studies are incomplete. *Group B3* drugs are those for which reproduction or toxicology studies have shown an increased incidence of reproductive or fetal damage. *Category C* comrises drugs that have been shown to cause or are suspected of causing disturbances in the reproductive process without being related to teratogenicity in the fetus. *Category D* comprises drugs that have been known to cause fetal malformation.

Preload Recruitable Stroke Work (PRSW):

Index of myocardial contractility that requires implantation of miniature ultrasonic length transducers in the myocardium. It is a reliable and relatively afterload insensitive measure of intrinsic inotropic state. It demonstrates a relation between regional stroke work and end-diastolic length.

Premedication:

Concept that appropriate administration of drugs facilitates anesthetic induction. In many ways it is an idea that grew up with and was made mandatory by the use of diethyl ether as an anesthetic, as one of the outstanding characteristics of diethyl ether is irritation to the respiratory tree on inhalation. The initial purpose of premedication was to prevent outpouring of secretions in the respiratory tree that could precipitate respiratory obstruction. Therefore atropine and scopolamine, which decrease salivation and other secretions, were important in early premedicant regimens. In addition, because of the irritation, diethyl ether anesthetic inductions were often stormy. This reaction led to the use of sedative drugs to allay anxiety and make the perioperative experience smoother. With the use of intravenous induction agents and the more modern, less irritating halogenated hydrocarbon general anesthetics, the absolute requirement for premedication (in particular the antisecretory drugs) has diminished, but ritualistic dousing of patients with premedication has continued to be a part of anesthetic practice and appears to have a firm hold on the future. *See* Atropine; Basal anesthesia; Preanesthetic visit.

Preoperative Evaluation:

See Preanesthetic visit.

Preoxygenation:

See Denitrogenation.

Preservative:

Chemical additive that prevents decomposition as well as growth and multiplication of microorganisms. Benzoic acid (0.1%) is a common pharmacologic preservative, as are its parahydroxy variations, such as methylparaben, ethylparaben, propylparaben, and butylparaben (all used in concentrations of 0.1–0.3%). All preservatives are justifiably considered to have low systemic toxicity, but allergies to preservatives are encountered in medical practice. Preparations without preservatives are available, although they have a short shelf-life once exposed to room air. They are used in circumstances in which any irritation or toxicity must be avoided, such as spinal anesthesia or intravenous therapy for cardiac arrhythmias.

Pressoreceptor:

See Baroreceptor.

Pressure (P):

Force exerted per unit area in any direction from any point. In a liquid the pressure varies with the depth. The standard international (SI) unit of pressure is the pascal, but pressure can also be measured in millibars, millimeters of mercury (mm Hg), atmospheres, centimeters of water (cm H_2O), or pounds per square inch (psi or lb/in^2).

Pressure Control Inverse-Ratio Ventilation (PCRIV):

Type of ventilation in which exhalation times are short compared with times needed for complete exhalation; and in fact, exhalation may be shorter than inspiration. With this technique, intrathoracic pressure at the end of passive expiration does not reach zero; it is called intrinsic PEEP. *See* Mechanical ventilation; PEEP.

Pressure Effect:

See Pumping effect, pressure effect.

Pressure-Equalizing Valve:

Combination valve that can be set to act either as a low-pressure relief valve or as a safety feature to prevent a pressure buildup in a gas system. This function depends on the position of the toggle handle, which controls an internal valve disk in the valve body.

Pressure Head:

Height of a column of liquid necessary to exert a specific pressure.

Pressure-Limited Ventilator:

See Ventilator.

Pressure Rate Quotient (PRQ):

Hemodynamic indices that are derived by dividing the mean arterial pressure by the heart rate.

Pressure-Reducing Valve; Pressure Regulator:

Device that converts the high, variable pressure within a gas cylinder to a lower, more constant gas pressure. For example, a standard O_2 regulator reduces the input pressure of a full tank of O_2 at 2200 $1b/in^2$ to an output pressure of approximately 50 $1b/in^2$.

Pressure Reversal of Anesthesia:

See Anesthesia, pressure reversal of.

Pressure Support Ventilation:

Newer mode of mechanical ventilation. It is designed to overcome the inspiratory resistance of endotracheal tubes and ventilator hose circuitry, thereby reducing patient work of breathing. When the ventilator detects a drop in pressure, caused by the initiation of a spontaneous inspiratory effort, the ventilator triggers a high gas flow, raising the inspiratory pressure to a preselected maximum. The pressure is maintained until the patient's total flow falls to 25% of initial peak flow. At this point, the ventilator cycles off. Pressure support ventilation can be used in conjunction with positive-end expiratory pressure (PEEP) and continuous positive airway pressure (CPAP) and is a more sophisticated version of the earlier demand "ventilation" as used on early ventilators. *See* IMV; PEEP; Ventilators.

Prilocaine (Citanest):

Amide-type local anesthetic that undergoes rapid biotransformation in the liver and kidney. *See* Local anesthetic.

Primary Atelectasis:

See Atelectasis.

Primary Fibrinolysis:

Rare disorder in which the fibrinolytic system is inappropriately activated without prior existence of large-scale clotting. The clinical picture resembles disseminated intravascular coagulation (DIC). The differential diagnosis is often made by a platelet count, with a normal count ruling out DIC. The clinical course is complicated by the fact that severe primary fibrinolysis can drop the platelet count as fibrin degradation products tend to clump platelets. Secondary fibrinolysis is an appropriate response to DIC, as it is an attempt by the body to compensate for inappropriate clotting. ε-Aminocaproic acid (EACA) blocks the fibrinolytic system and is a specific treatment for primary fibrinolysis, but it can cause a disaster in secondary fibrinolysis because the clotting mechanism of the underlying DIC is unchecked. Because primary fibrinolysis usually does not cause massive bleeding and is rare, EACA should not be empirically administered for emergency treatment of hemorrhage. *See* Blood coagulation; Disseminated intravascular coagulation.

Primary Winding:

See Transformer.

Priming Principle:

Concept of administering slow-onset, nondepolarizing muscle relaxants by first administering approximately one-tenth of the calculated total dose required by the patient, waiting either a fixed time interval or until the patient reports weakness, followed then by the calculated intubating dose of the drug. A fixed time interval such as 90 seconds is allowed to pass, or a rough estimate of muscle relaxation is made on clinical grounds, whereupon the trachea is intubated. It is a controversial technique not yet generally accepted. *See* Muscle relaxant; Timing principle.

Primum Non Nocere:

Considered by many to be the fundamental goal of medicine. In translation, this expression means: "In the first place, do no harm." It has been reinterpreted to the more useful: "Help, but at least do no harm."

Printer:

Device using characters that produces copy interpretable by a human user. Subcategories are determined by the manner in which the printer converts encoded signals into characters, e.g., electrostatic, type face, heat.

Priscoline:

See Tolazoline hydrochloride.

Privileged Communication:

Right of the patient, in a medicolegal context, to expect that the physician will not divulge any personal information concerning the patient to the public. It forms part of the physician-patient relationship. The extent to which the doctrine of privileged communication applies depends on state law. *See* Physician-patient relationship.

Probability:

Likelihood that a stated result will occur. Probability is expressed as a number between 0 and 1. If the result cannot occur, its probability is 0. If it must occur, it is a certainty and its probability is 1.

Procainamide (Pronestyl):

Effective, quinidine-like antiarrhythmic agent that is pharmacologically similar to procaine. The drug decreases cardiac automaticity. It retards electric conduction in the atrium and ventricle and enhances atrioventricular block. Effective against a wide range of arrhythmias, procainamide can cause, on rapid intravenous injection, a precipitous drop in blood pressure. The drug can be administered intravenously, intramuscularly, or orally.

Procaine Hydrochloride (Novocain):

First successful local anesthetic to be synthesized (by Einhorn in 1905). An ester-type drug, it is the standard measure of relative potency for other local anesthetic agents. *See* Local anesthetic.

Professional Standard Rule:

Legal principle applied to a concept of informed consent that held that a physician needs to explain the consequences of a procedure only as much as would another reasonable practitioner. *See* Lay standard rule.

Profile of Mood States (POMS):

Rating scale technique that is useful for accessing acute changes in mood states during situations that are stress-producing.

Progesterone:

Ovarian steroid hormone, the effects of which include glandular development of the breasts and cyclic glandular development of the endometrium of the uterus. It increases body temperature and has effects on carbohydrate, protein, and lipid metabolism.

Program, Computer:

Sequence of instructions by which a computer manipulates data; performing various tasks and solving problems using the computer central processing unit (CPU). Programs can range from simple and direct, e.g., hand-held calculators, to thoroughly complex so it is necessary to use a small computer to program a larger computer. *See* CPU.

Progress of Labor:

Orderly procedure of normal childbirth with increasing cervical dilatation and effacement with a continuous descent into the pelvis of the presenting fetal part over a period of time. *See* Labor.

Prolactin:

Single-chain protein originating in the anterior pituitary that stimulates breast development and milk production. Controlled via a feedback loop with the hypothalamus, prolactin is the primary hormone responsible for lactation.

Prolapse:

Falling down or sinking of a part or an organ. For example, in the multiparous patient weakening of the pelvic floor can lead to uterine prolapse, a condition in which the uterus appears outside the lower abdominal cavity.

Promethazine Hydrochloride (Phenergan):

Phenothiazine derivative that, in addition to being a potent antihistamine and sedative, can be used as a mild tranquilizer, hypnotic, and antiemetic. Although its mechanism of action is unknown, promethazine clearly enhances the actions of drugs that depress the central nervous system. *See* Antipsychotic agent.

Pronestyl:

See Procainamide.

Propanidid (Epontol):

Eugenol (oil of cloves) derivative used in Europe as an intravenous anesthetic, it is not available in the United States. As fast-acting as thiopental, electroencephalographic changes seen with its use are similar to those of barbiturates. Excitatory muscle movements in patients receiving propanidid appear to be dose-related. Hypersensitivity reactions to the drug have been reported. Propanidid increases apnea caused by succinylcholine, transiently decreasing serum pseudocholinesterase levels.

Propofol (Diprivan):

Hypnotic drug used for induction; it causes unconsciousness within one arm-to-brain circulation time. A unique characteristic of the drug is rapid awakening upon stopping of infusions due to the drug having little accumulation at usual doses. *See* Intralipid.

Propoxyphene (Darvon):

Close chemical derivative of the narcotic methadone. Although no longer considered as potent as codeine, it is known to be an abused drug. Overdose resembles narcotic poisoning and is treated with narcotic antagonists. Abrupt termination of drug administration (following chronic ingestion of high doses) may produce withdrawal symptoms.

Propranolol (Inderal):

Competitive antagonist of catecholamines at beta receptors throughout the body. It precipitates bronchoconstriction, can have a negative chronotropic effect, and can decrease the strength of cardiac contractions. Currently, it is used to treat arrhythmias, hypertension, angina, thyrotoxicosis, pheochromocytoma, and some intrinsic cardiac diseases. In high concentrations, it attenuates the fight-or-flight reaction. It was originally believed to be dangerous to anesthetize patients taking propranolol. More recently, however, it has been shown that, at least in cases in which it is given for hypertensive disease or angina, withdrawal of the drug can precipitate a crisis of hypertension or angina. *See* Beta-blocker.

Proprietary Pharmaceutical:

Drug or chemical that is exclusively or privately owned, usually by patent.

Propylene Glycol:

Simple molecule used as antifreeze for automobiles or as a solvent for some anesthetic intravenous agents.

Propylparaben:

See Preservative.

Prostacyclin (PGI₂):

Prostaglandin with a half-life of approximately 3 minutes. A major source for this most potent of the vasodilators is vascular endothelium. Prostacyclin has been used to treat pulmonary artery hypertension seen during adult respiratory distress syndrome and has been implicated in the hypotension seen upon administration of d-tubocurarine.

Prostaglandin:

Originally named because of its initial isolation from human prostate. It is now recognized as a widely distributed family of oxygenated, cyclized, 20-carbon fatty acids that are structurally similar but with strikingly independent biologic properties. They are not stored within cells but are manufactured from precursors in response to various stimuli. Prostaglandins are rapidly degraded within the systemic circulation. They function as local hormones or autacoids. At least nine prostaglandin groups have been recognized (PGA through PGI); all share the 20-carbon molecular skeleton. Appropriate prostaglandins can be used to close a patent ductus arteriosus. *See* Figure.

Prosthetic Heart Valve:

Device that can be surgically implanted to replace a diseased heart valve, particularly an aortic or mitral valve. These valves are available in various designs or by harvest from pigs, and with continued refinement have become functionally more efficient as replacements for stenosed (narrowed) or regurgitant (permitting backflow) valves. *See* Figure.

Prostigmin:

See Neostigmine.

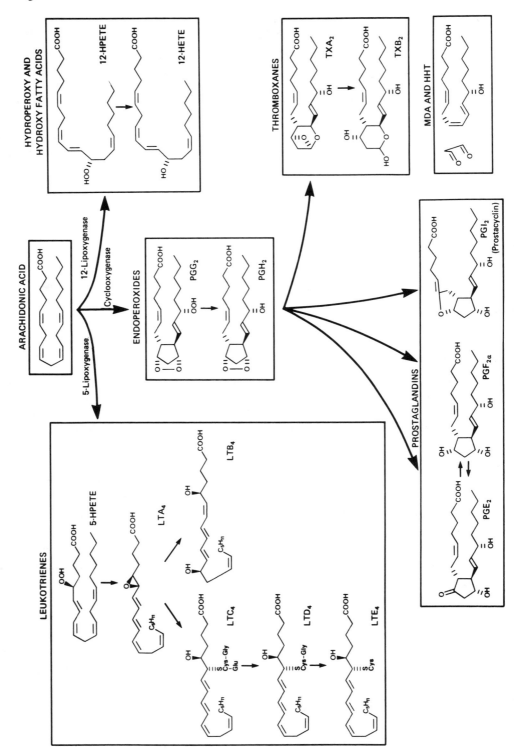

Prostaglandin: Major enzymatically derived products of arachidonic acid metabolism.

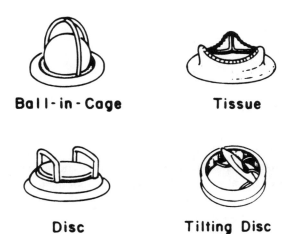

Ball-in-Cage   Tissue

Disc   Tilting Disc

Prosthetic Heart Valves: Common types of valve prostheses.

Protamine Sulfate:

Naturally occurring (found in certain fish sperm) low molecular weight protein used to block and reverse the anticoagulant action of heparin. Protamine is used clinically to antagonize heparin after extracorporeal circulation. Rapid intravenous injection may cause direct peripheral dilatation, cardiac depression, and severe hypotension. *See* Anticoagulant; Heparin; Heparinoids.

Protein Hydrolysate:

See Amigen.

Prothrombin Time, One-Stage Prothrombin Time (PT):

Test of the clotting mechanism that determines the relative intactness of the extrinsic clotting system. The time necessary for recalcified citrated plasma to clot in the presence of tissue thromboplastin is measured. *See* Blood coagulation; Extrinsic pathway; Intrinsic pathway; Partial thromboplastin time.

Proton:

Positively charged elementary particle that is a constituent of all nuclei. It forms the nucleus of the hydrogen atom. It is approximately 1836 times heavier than the electron.

Protopam:

See Pralidoxime.

Proximate Cause:

Action that immediately precedes and gives rise to an effect. For example, in the case of a patient death due to drug allergy, the injection, rather than the preparation of the injection, would be the proximate cause of death.

PRQ:

See Pressure rate quotient.

PRSW:

See Preload recruitable stroke work.

Prune-Belly Syndrome:

Congenital syndrome characterized by a protruding abdomen with wrinkled, thin skin. This appearance is due to absence of the lower portion of the rectus abdominis and the medial parts of the oblique muscles. Usually, along with this defect the bladder and ureters are dilated, and the kidneys are small, dysplastic, and hydronephrotic. In males, the testes are undescended. *See* Gastroschisis.

Pseudocholinesterase:

See Acetylcholinesterase; Dibucaine number; Succinylcholine.

Pseudohypoxemia:

Condition that results in inaccurate in vitro measurement of blood gas tension in patients with leukemia and thrombocytosis. Often undetected, pseudohypoxemia involves the rapid decline of oxygenation in a blood sample as a result of rapid cell metabolism of oxygen in the sampling tube.

Psoas Compartment Nerve Block:

Nerve block done in such a manner as to deposit local anesthetic's solution into the psoas compartment between the two muscle masses of the psoas major anteriorly and the quadratus lumborum posteriorly, so the solution is distributed around the lumbar plexus. The compartment is approached either posteriorly or perivascularly.

Psychogenic:

Having an origin in the mind. *See* Psychogenic pain.

Psychogenic Pain:

Circumstance that occurs when patients use the language and behavior normally describing tissue damage to describe anxiety and depression. It is as if the central nervous system augments what would otherwise be a trivial injury into significant distress. The Anesthesia Boards cause psychogenic pain.

Psychometric Testing:

Measures for testing mental functioning, mental efficiency, and various aspects of mental acuity. *See* Controlled oral word association test; Finger oscillation test; Wechsler Memory Scale-revised.

Psychomotor Seizure:

Type of seizure characterized by impaired consciousness, inappropriate but purposeful motor acts, and at times hallucinations, illusions, amnesia, and sudden feelings of fear. This type of seizure is often proceeded by an aura. *See* Epilepsy.

Psychotropic (Psychoactive) Drug:

Pharmacologic agent used to treat psychiatric disorders. Examples of psychotropic drugs are antipsychotics (phenothiazines, thioxanthenes, butyrophenones), antidepressants, anti-anxiety-sedatives (benzodiazepines), and mood stabilizers. *See* Antipsychotic agents; Benzodiazepine.

PT:

See Prothrombin time, one-stage prothrombin time.

PTC:

See Posttetanic count.

PTJV:

See Percutaneous transtracheal jet ventilation.

PTT:

See Partial thromboplastin time.

Pulmonary Alveolar Proteinosis:

Chronic lung disease of unknown etiology. Clinical manifestations of the disease range from asymptomatic involvement to total disability or death due to respiratory insufficiency, secondary infection (e.g., Nocardia), or cor pulmonale. Pulmonary alveolar proteinosis is characterized pathologically by alveoli filled with periodic acid-Schiff (PAS)-positive dense granular material (a lipoprotein). Bronchopulmonary lavage is an effective treatment for patients with significant symptoms. *See* Double-lumen tube; Pulmonary lavage.

Pulmonary Artery Banding:

Operation performed to correct excessive pulmonary blood flow, as in the congenital disorder of common ventricle. A band is tightened around the external circumference of the pulmonary artery, thereby increasing pulmonary outflow resistance.

Pulmonary Artery Catheter:

See Figure. *See* Swan-Ganz catheter.

Pulmonary Blood Vessels:

Vessels (i.e., arteries, arterioles, capillaries, venules, and veins) that transport blood through the pulmonary circulation, starting at the pulmonary artery outflow and returning via the pulmonary veins to the left atrium.

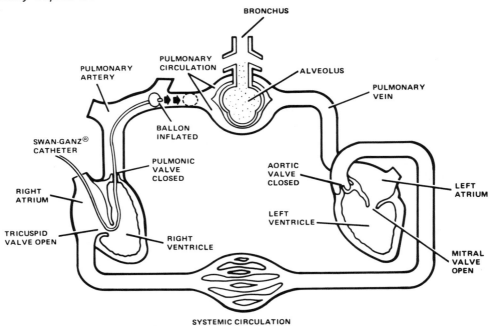

Pulmonary Artery Catheter: Heart in Diastole (Ventricles Relaxed).

Pulmonary Capillaries:

Minute blood vessels connecting the pulmonary metarterioles and venules. The pulmonary capillaries form a continuous network of blood (flowing sheet) in the alveolar wall. This network constitutes an effective arrangement for pulmonary gas exchange.

Pulmonary Capillary Transit Time:

Length of time it takes (usually less than 1 second with normal cardiac output) for blood to traverse the pulmonary capillaries. A single red blood cell traverses two or three alveoli during this time period. Oxygen equilibration is essentially complete within approximately 0.3 second. Carbon dioxide equilibrium is attained even faster.

Pulmonary Capillary Wedge Pressure (PCWP):

Pressure distal to the inflated balloon tip of a well positioned Swan-Ganz catheter. This reading approximates the left atrial pressure. *See* Swan-Ganz catheter.

Pulmonary Edema (PE):

Presence of excessive amounts of fluid in the interstitial spaces of the lung or in the alveoli. PE is usually the result of left-sided heart failure, which tends to increase pulmonary capillary pressure to such a degree that the interstitial spaces are overloaded. Pulmonary edema may also be due to destruction of the capillary membranes by noxious vapors or can be caused by aspiration pneumonitis. Severe pulmonary edema involving the alveoli often leads to death by suffocation. *See* Congestive heart failure.

Pulmonary Function Tests (PFT):

Combination of clinical and laboratory tests designed to assess the patient's ability to perform the functions of ventilation, i.e., increase PaO_2 decrease $PaCO_2$ to normal levels in venous blood returned to the lungs. PFTs also establish the norms of the various lung volumes for a particular patient and his or her ability to move air at maximal rates. In their simplest form, PFTs consist of the measurement of vital capacity and arterial blood gases. At a more sophisticated level, the next test usually performed is measurement of forced expiratory volume (FEV) in 0.5 second ($FEV_{0.5}$) or 1 second (FEV_1). The results from a particular patient can be compared with standards for age, sex, and body size. It must be kept in mind, however, that normal problems with the apparatus, such as maintenance of an airtight seal at the machine-patient interface, and patient motivation, are critical factors in obtaining an accurate, repeatable result. *See* Forced expiratory volume; Maximum voluntary ventilation; Vital capacity.

Pulmonary Hypertension:

Morbid condition said to be present when the systolic pressure in the pulmonary artery consistently rises above 30 mm Hg. This rise may be due to an increase in pulmonary-vascular resistance or to blood backup behind a failing left side of the heart.

Pulmonary Lavage:

Therapeutic "washing out" or irrigating of the air passages of a lung performed with general anesthesia via a double-lumen tube. A hazardous procedure usually employed as a specific treatment for pulmonary alveolar proteinosis, it is performed on one lung at a time with a recovery period between procedures. Recovery is complicated by the fact that surfactant is also "washed out," making reinflation of the washed lung difficult. *See* Double-lumen tube; Pulmonary alveolar proteinosis.

Pulmonary Perfusion, Zones of:

Model for the way in which blood flow from the right side of the heart perfuses the lung. In this model, the lung is divided into three zones. *Zone 1*, the superior zone, is that area in which alveolar gas pressure is higher than pulmonary artery pressure (due to gravitational forces). In this abnormal state the alveolar capillaries are so constricted that blood flow is prevented, which gives rise, therefore, to a portion of the lung that is ventilated but not perfused (alveolar deadspace). In *zone 2,* further down in the lung, pulmonary arterial pressure rises and exceeds alveolar pressure. In this zone, flow is determined by the difference between arterial and alveolar pressures rather than arterial and venous pressures. Flow occurs when arterial pressure becomes higher than alveolar pressure for part of the cardiac cycle and ceases as systolic pressure wanes toward diastolic pressure. The effect seen in *zone 2* is called a Starling resistor, "sluice," or waterfall effect. In *zone 3,* still further down the lung, not only is pulmonary arterial pressure higher than alveolar pressure, but venous pressure is now high enough for flow to be determined in the normal manner, i.e., the difference between arterial and venous pressures. There are no sharp distinctions between zones; they are dependent on the patient's body position. *See* Figure. *See* Ventilation/perfusion abnormality.

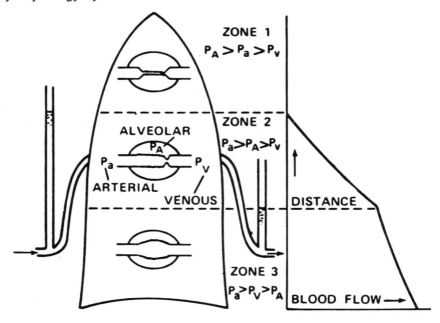

Pulmonary Perfusion, Zones of: Supposed behavior of the small vessels in various parts of the lung which cause regional differences in the blood flow. The lung is shown in a vertical position.

Pulmonary Physiology Symbols:

See Table.

Pulmonary Stenosis:

Narrowing in the pulmonary vasculature that causes elevated right ventricular pressure.

Pulmonary Vascular Resistance (PVR):

Resistance to blood flow out of the right ventricle. It can be calculated given the fact that the pulmonary vasculature carries the same volume of blood as the systemic vasculature over time (conveniently calculated at 1 minute). Under normal circumstances the pulmonary pressure drop from the pulmonary artery to the left atrium is only one-eighth to one-tenth that of the pressure drop in the systemic circulation. Pulmonary vascular resistance is therefore, one-eighth to one-tenth the systemic vascular resistance. It can also be calculated as the pulmonary artery pressure minus the pulmonary capillary wedge pressure divided by the cardiac output. *See* Swan-Ganz catheter.

Pulmonary Vascular Resistance Index:

Derived value equal to the pulmonary artery pressure minus the pulmonary capillary wedge pressure divided by the cardiac index. *See* Cardiac index; Pulmonary capillary wedge pressure.

Periodic Table: Periodic table of the elements.

SPECIAL SYMBOLS

— Dash above any symbol indicates a *mean* value.
. Dot above any symbol indicates *a time derivative.*

FOR GASES

PRIMARY SYMBOLS (Large Capital Letters)

Symbol	Definition	EXAMPLES
V	= gas volume	V_A = volume of alveolar gas
$\dot{V}$	= gas volume/unit time	$\dot{V}_{O_2}$ = O_2 consumption/min
P	= gas pressure	$P_{A_{O_2}}$ = alveolar O_2 pressure
$\bar{P}$	= mean gas pressure	$\bar{P}_{C_{O_2}}$ = mean capillary O_2 pressure
F	= fractional concentration in dry gas phase	$F_{I_{O_2}}$ = fractional concentration of O_2 in inspired gas
f	= respiratory frequency (breaths/unit time)	
D	= diffusing capacity	D_{O_2} = diffusing capacity for O_2 (ml O_2/min/mm Hg)
R	= respiratory exchange ratio	R = $\dot{V}_{CO_2}/\dot{V}_{O_2}$

SECONDARY SYMBOLS (SMALL CAPITAL LETTERS)

EXAMPLES

Symbol	Definition	Example
I	= inspired gas	$F_{I_{CO_2}}$ = fractional concentration of CO_2 in inspired gas
E	= expired gas	V_E = volume of expired gas
A	= alveolar gas	$\dot{V}_A$ = alveolar ventilation/min
T	= tidal gas	V_T = tidal volume
D	= dead space gas	V_D = volume of dead space gas
B	= barometric	P_B = barometric pressure

STPD = 0°C, 760 mm Hg, dry
BTPS = body temperature and pressure saturated with water vapor
ATPS = ambient temperature and pressure saturated with water vapor

FOR BLOOD

PRIMARY SYMBOLS (Large Capital Letters)

EXAMPLES

Symbol	Definition	Example
Q	= volume of blood	Q_c = volume of blood in pulmonary capillaries
$\dot{Q}$	= volume flow of blood/unit time	$\dot{Q}_c$ = blood flow through pulmonary capillaries/min
C	= concentration of gas in blood phase	$C_{a_{O_2}}$ = ml O_2 in 100 ml arterial blood
S	= % saturation of Hb with O_2 or CO	$S\bar{v}_{O_2}$ = saturation of Hb with O_2 in mixed venous blood

SECONDARY SYMBOLS (small letters)

EXAMPLES

Symbol	Definition	Example
a	= arterial blood	$P_{a_{CO_2}}$ = partial pressure of CO_2 in arterial blood
v	= venous blood	$P\bar{v}_{O_2}$ = partial pressure of O_2 in mixed venous blood
c	= capillary blood	$P_{c_{CO}}$ = partial pressure of CO in pulmonary capillary blood

FOR LUNG VOLUMES

VC	= Vital Capacity	= maximal volume that can be expired after maximal inspiration
IC	= Inspiratory Capacity	= maximal volume that can be inspired from resting expiratory level
IRV	= Inspiratory Reserve Volume	= maximal volume that can be inspired from end-tidal inspiration
ERV	= Expiratory Reserve Volume	= maximal volume that can be expired from resting expiratory level
FRC	= Functional Residual Capacity	= volume of gas in lungs at resting expiratory level
RV	= Residual Volume	= volume of gas in lungs at end of maximal expiration
TLC	= Total Lung Capacity	= volume of gas in lungs at end of maximal inspiration

Pulse:

Physical manifestation of the blood pressure as it waxes and wanes in a palpable artery. The pulse can be counted to determine the number of heartbeats per minute. In electronics, a pulse is considered to be a discrete, transient phenomenon of short duration.

Pulse Contour:

Computer-derived approximation of cardiac output obtained by measuring the area under the curve of the peripheral vascular trace acquired through use of an indwelling arterial cannula, usually calibrated against a thermodilution cardiac output determination. *See* Area under the curve; Thermodilution cardiac output.

Pulse Oximeter:

Monitoring device for on-line continuous evaluation of oxygen delivery to tissue. A significant element in increased patient safety during anesthesia. *See* Oximeter.

Pulse Pressure:

Difference between diastolic and systolic pressure extremes in the arterial circulation. If the blood pressure is recorded as 120/80 mm Hg, the pulse pressure would be 40 mm Hg.

Pulse Pressure Tracing:

Oscillographic or paper representation of the pulse pressure contours as recorded with the y-axis representing pressure and the x-axis representing time. The shape of the generated tracing changes with the location at which it is transduced (aortic arch, peripheral artery), the force of cardiac contraction, and the peripheral vascular resistance. A qualitative interference of myocardial function can be derived from the changing shape of this tracing.

Pulsus Alternans (Alternating Pulse):

Pulse in which a weak beat alternates with a strong beat. It is most often found in conjunction with left ventricular failure. A failing ventricle changes its strength of contraction with minor changes in left ventricular muscle fiber length.

Pumping Effect, Pressure Effect:

Two effects reported with the variable bypass vaporizer (precision vaporizers, agent-specific vaporizers) in which back pressure to the vaporizer changes the anesthetic output delivered. The pumping effect is seen when the vaporizer output is increased, whereas the pressure effect is seen when the vaporizer output is decreased. Three factors influence the effect that predominates: the magnitude of the back pressure fluctuations, the amount of flow through the vaporizer, and the vaporizer dial setting. Design changes in vaporizers produced during the late 1980s to early 1990s eliminated, or significantly attenuated, these variations in vaporizer output. The simplest modification for preventing the pressure and pumping effects is to place a backflow check device between the vaporizer and the patient circuit. *See* Figures.

500

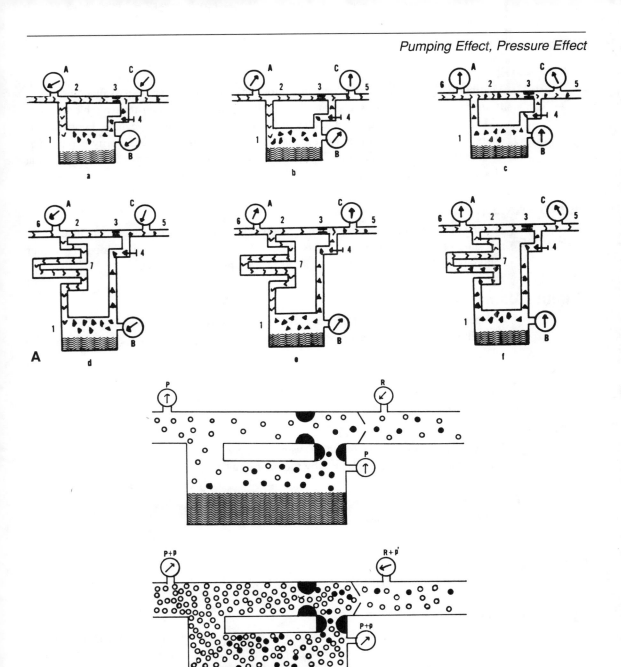

Pumping Effect; Pressure Effect: (A) The pumping effect in a variable bypass vaporizer. a, b, and c, during exhalation gas containing anesthetic vapor flows into the bypass, increasing the vaporizer output. d, e, and f, the long spiral tube prevents vapor-laden gas from reaching the bypass. (B) The pressurizing effect. An increase in pressure (p') causes an increase in pressure (p) inside the vaporizer. The vapor pressure of the volatile anesthetic is unaffected by changes in the total pressure of the gas mixture above it. As a result, the concentration is reduced.

501

Pump Lung:

Ventilatory dysfunction seen in patients following cardiopulmonary bypass machine usage. It appears to be caused by a group of unrelated factors, including massive blood transfusion, concomitant infection, and altered hemodynamics following bypass. Pump lung is characterized by diffuse pneumonitis, pulmonary edema, or both. Its severity is related to the following factors: total time the patient remains on extracorporeal circulation, total blood loss, and total blood replacement. *See* Cardiopulmonary bypass.

Pump Prime:

Volume of fluid initially within the oxygenator and fluid circuits of a heart-lung machine at the start of cardiopulmonary bypass. Pump primes are often whole blood, but other solutions are becoming popular as well. *See* Cardiopulmonary bypass.

Punitive Damages:

Compensation awarded to an injured party in order to punish the individual judged to have committed the injury. Compensatory damages recompense for the injury itself. *See* Damages.

Pure Cut:

See Cutting current.

Purging:

Deliberate high flow of gas through a system particularly when it is new or reconfigured so as to reduce leftover contamination by room air or a test gas.

Purkinje Fibers:

See Heart, conduction system of.

PVR:

See Pulmonary vascular resistance.

Pyloric Stenosis:

Severe congenital anomaly that occurs once in every 300–900 live births; there is a 4:1 male predominance. The pathophysiology of the disease is that the pylorus (outlet of the stomach) becomes progressively more hypertrophic and obstructive. The condition appears to be self-limiting, and if nutritional support can be maintained long enough it disappears without surgical intervention. If nutritional support cannot be maintained, however, the operation of choice is called a pyloromyotomy. An anesthetic consideration for this procedure is patient dehydration due to the prolonged vomiting. Also, full stomach precautions are necessary.

Pyrexia:

See Hyperpyrexia.

Pyridostigmine (Mestinon):

Anticholinesterase agent closely related to neostigmine but with fewer side effects. It is used for the treatment of myasthenia gravis and as a reversal agent for neuromuscular blockade. *See* Neuromuscular blockade, assessment of.

Pyrometer:

Instrument for measuring high temperatures.

Q

QRS Complex:

Electrocardiographic representation of the electrical impulses through the ventricles. Q wave is the first negative (downward) deflection; R wave is the first upward deflection regardless of whether it is preceded by a Q wave; and the S wave is a negative deflection following an R wave. *See* Electrocardiogram.

Quaternary Ammonium Compound:

Molecule containing a nitrogen atom bonded to four other atoms. With this charged quaternary binding, the nitrogen atom is relatively deficient in electrons and therefore behaves as if it is positively charged. These compounds are relatively incapable of passing through biologic membranes that reject charged molecules. For example, neostigmine is a quaternary ammonium compound that does not readily cross the blood-brain barrier. *See* Physostigmine.

Queckenstedt Sign:

Test for intact cerebrospinal fluid (CSF) pathways in the central nervous system. It is based on the fact that unilateral or bilateral compression of the internal jugular vein(s) in the neck causes a rise in cerebral venous pressure and an increase in cerebral blood volume. This leads to a rise in intracranial and CSF pressures. This elevation of pressure decreases on release of the compression on the neck. No CSF pressure rise measured by spinal tap indicates a blockage of the path of egress of the CSF (the Queckenstedt sign is positive). This blockage may be due to tumor, blood clot, or cord transection. The test is dangerous in cases of elevated intracranial pressure, as it can precipitate cerebral herniation. *See* Cerebrospinal fluid.

Quick Connector:

Device that allows a rapid, often one-handed connection between a gas line and a wall receptacle.

Quinidine:

Isomer of quinine used for its antifibrillatory and antiarrhythmic effects on cardiac musculature. It decreases automaticity and conduction velocity in the heart. Quinidine depresses all muscle tissue. If administered to a patient with myasthenia gravis, it produces marked weakness. It is given either orally or intramuscularly. As with many antiarrhythmic drugs, toxic effects include arrhythmias; these effects may be additive to other antiarrhythmic drugs being given. *See* Procainamide.

R

Rad:

Acronym for radiation absorbed dose. It is the unit of absorbed dose of ionizing radiation. One rad is equal in energy to 100 ergs/g of irradiated material and is approximately equal to the energy absorbed by soft tissue when it is exposed to 1 R (roentgen) of medium voltage x-rays. Total body irradiation with as little as 50–100 rad can cause severe injury. *See* Roentgen-equivalent-man.

Radford Nomogram:

See Nomogram.

Radioactivity:

Spontaneous change in the nucleus of certain atoms resulting in the formation of an element with different chemical properties. This change also results in a change of the element's atomic number when accompanied by emission of either alpha or beta particles. The atomic number does not change when only a gamma ray is emitted, but the nucleus drops to a lower energy state. For any given number of molecules of a radioactive element, half of these molecules decay within a period of time that is constant and characteristic of that element (half-life), ranging from millionths of a second to thousands of years.

Radiofrequency (RF) Choke:

Small electrical component consisting of a tuned coil that offers high resistance to frequencies in the radio band of the electromagnetic spectrum. In medical equipment the purpose of the RF choke is to prevent RF energy from following pathways that can lead to patient injury. RF chokes are often used in the inputs of electrocardiograph (ECG) machines to prevent electrosurgical instruments from establishing an energy return path using the ECG leads.

Radionuclide Angiography:

Technique that uses a gamma camera placed over an appropriate portion of the body to scan for the flow of a radioactive "dye." It is performed most commonly to determine flow through the heart. The radionuclide used is technetium 99m (^{99m}Tc). *See* Technetium-99m.

Radiosensitivity:

Relative destructibility of a tissue exposed to ionizing radiation. A concept used both to treat neoplastic disease and to calculate the exposure limits of those individuals who must work around sources of radiation.

Radiotherapy:

Utilization of ionizing radiation, including gamma rays, electron beams, and x-rays to treat disease.

Raman Technique:

Technique for gas analysis in which the sample gas is passed into a chamber and exposed to the monochromatic light generated by a laser. The gas molecules in the mix scatter the incident light, and the amount of scatter is specific to the type of molecule doing the scattering. It is used to monitor gas mixture. *See* Mass spectrometer.

Random Access:

Specific type of memory device that allows immediate access to a piece of information without having to review all the data contained in the memory. Each piece of information has a particular address or physical location in the memory. *See* Memory, computer.

Random Numbers:

List of numbers in which one particular number has no discernible relation to any other number in the list. The concept of random numbers has its greatest usefulness in statistics.

Range, Statistical:

Difference between the largest and smallest numbers in a set. With these serum potassium values—3.5, 4.0, 4.5, 5.0, 5.5, 6.0—the range is 2.5.

Rapid Eye Movement (REM):

See REM.

Rapid Sequence Induction:

See Induction; Sellick maneuver.

Rapid Twitch Muscle:

See Type II muscle fiber.

Rare Gases:

Collective name given to five elements: helium, neon, argon, krypton, and xenon. These gases are rare because they have low partial pressures at ordinary temperatures and are found in minute quantities in the atmosphere. Under normal circumstances the gases are not bound chemically to any other element. They are also referred to as inert gases. *See* Air.

Rate-Pressure Product (RPP):

Index of cardiac O_2 consumption. It is obtained by multiplying the systolic blood pressure by the heart rate. A product of more than 12,000 is considered a sign of possible ischemia in patients with coronary artery disease.

Rauwolfia Alkaloid:

Generalized name for preparations, (e.g., reserpine) obtained from a climbing shrub indigenous to India. *See* Reserpine.

Ray:

Moving photon or particle of ionizing radiation.

RBRVS:

See Resource-based relative value scale.

RDS:

See Respiratory distress syndrome.

Reactive Hyperemia:

See Tourniquet.

Readily Releasable versus Depot Acetylcholine:

Two forms in which acetylcholine is believed to exist in a nerve terminal. The readily releasable fraction is immediately available for use as a transmitter, whereas the large depot store serves to replenish the readily releasable stock as required. The readily releasable portion appears to be contained in vesicles close to or attached to the portion of the nerve terminal membrane that borders the synaptic cleft. The depot store would be contained in vesicles further back. There appears to be some delay in the conversion of depot acetylcholine to readily releasable acetylcholine. The readily releasable fraction then becomes partially exhausted by frequently repeated action potentials, as seen with tetanic nerve stimulation. This partial exhaustion appears to be responsible for the fade seen during tetanic stimulation when a nondepolarizing block exists. *See* Neuromuscular blockade, assessment of; Neuromuscular transmitter, quantal release of.

Read Only Memory (ROM):

See Memory, computer.

Real-Time Analysis:

Examination that takes place concurrently with the process being analyzed. The implication is that real-time analysis can be used to guide the process. For example, arterial CO_2 analysis using the Van Slyke-Cullen method takes many hours and is of no use for regulating respiration by ventilator. However, continuous end tidal sampling via a mass spectrometer gives values second by second in real time.

Rebreathing Bag:

See Breathing bag.

Receptor Occlusion:

Concept that during neuromuscular blockade a percentage of neuromuscular receptors must be unblocked in order for normal responses to be elicited by testing. This percentage is usually derived by determining the amount of depolarization seen with a fixed dose of succinylcholine in the presence or absence of block by a known quantity of a nondepolarizing muscle relaxant. The fraction of receptors that remain unblocked by the nondepolarizing relaxant can be estimated from the dose ratio between the succinylcholine and the nondepolarizing agent. It comes as somewhat of a surprise that a significant number of receptors can still be blocked, and yet normal responses are elicited by neuromuscular block testing techniques. *See* Neuromuscular blockade, assessment of; Tetanic stimulation; Train-of-four.

Receptor/Receptor Site:

Cellular phenomenon that allows a small quantity of drug or hormone to produce large changes in a tissue or organ. A receptor site is a specialized area on a cell's surface having a three-dimensional configuration or electrical charge capable of interacting with specific substances to cause a change in the entire cell. Receptor sites allow for economy and efficiency by acting as tiny switches that control the function of the cell as a whole. An example of a receptor site is the specialized portion of a motor endplate that interacts with acetylcholine to trigger an action potential. Acetylcholine acts only at this special area and does not affect the remainder of the cell. Receptors for the neurotransmitters released by the adrenergic (norepinephrine-releasing) fibers of the sympathetic nervous system have been extensively classified. Alpha receptors divided into alpha1 and alpha2 subtypes mediate vasoconstriction, mydriasis, and intestinal relaxation. Beta1 receptors are responsible for cardiac stimulation and also lipolysis. Beta2 receptors are involved with adrenergic bronchodilatation and vasorelaxation. Dopaminergic receptors seem to be present in only certain vascular networks. Dopamine produces vasoconstriction in the intracerebral, renal mesenteric, and coronary arteries. Cholinergic (acetylcholine-releasing) fibers interact with specific receptors to mediate the function of the parasympathetic nervous system. Neurons of the central nervous system (CNS) have receptors for the enkephalins and endorphins and are stimulated by narcotics. Many hormones achieve their results by mating with a cell receptor. The combination of hormone and receptor causes the intracellular formation of a "second messenger" which then alters cytoplasmic function. Identified second messengers are cyclic 3,′5′–adenosine monophosphate (cAMP) and cyclic 3,′5′-guanosine monophosphate (cGMP). Within the context of the nervous system, a receptor is the specialized ending of a sensory nerve fiber that converts a stimulus into a nerve impulse. An example of this type of receptor is the stretch receptor or muscle spindle, which responds to elongation of the muscle and informs the CNS continuously of the muscle's degree of contraction. Specific receptors also exist for such entities as pain and temperature sensation. *See* Figure, Tables.

Receptor Reserve:

Concept of agonist/receptor interaction in which a high efficiency agonist requires a smaller number of receptor sites to generate a given endpoint. For example, sufentanil, a highly potent narcotic, requires occupancy on fewer cellular receptor sites than morphine to effect a given amount of pain relief, which means that sufentanil has a higher receptive reserve than morphine. The efficacy of the agonist is defined by the fraction of the total specific receptor population that must be occupied to produce the given effect. It is called fractional receptor occupancy (FRO). *See* Agonist; Antagonist; Receptor/receptor site.

Receptor/Receptor Site: Characteristic interactions of agonists and antagonists at the adrenergic receptors.

Receptor	Agonist Potency*	Antagonist Potency	Agonist Effect on Adenylate Cyclase Activity
Alpha$_1$	Same for a_1 and a_2.	Prazosin > phentolamine > yohimbine.	None
Alpha$_2$	Epinephrine slightly > norepinephrine >> isoproterenol.	Phentolamine slightly > yohimbine >> prazosin.	Decrease
Beta$_1$	Isoproterenol > epinephrine $\cong$ norepinephrine.	Metoprolol > butoxamine.	Increase
Beta$_2$	Isoproterenol > epinephrine >> norepinephrine.	Butoxamine > metoprolol.	Increase

*These potencies are defined by studies of binding competition and pharmacologic response.

Recirculation Curve:

See Cardiac output.

Record:

Documentation of an event or process on paper, tape, or film. For example, in operating room practice the anesthesia record is the real-time recording and, in fact, often the only evidence of the conduct of an anesthetic.

Recovery/Recovery Room:

Time period between emergence from anesthesia and stabilization of the patient's vital signs and state of consciousness. The patient typically spends this time in the postanesthetic recovery room (PAR), a way station between the intense monitoring of the anesthetic period and the more casual monitoring of the patient's ward. The PAR was not typical of operating technique until the 1940s. Prior to that time, the patient would have been transported directly from the operating room to the ward bed. Because recovery rooms are now the standard of practice, emergence from anesthesia blends into the recovery period, and postoperative patient safety is much improved.

Receptor/Receptor Site: Adrenergic responses of selected tissues

Organ or Tissue	Receptor	Effect
Heart (myocardium)	β_1	Increased force of contraction Increased rate of contraction
Blood vessels	a	Vasoconstriction
	β_2	Vasodilatation
Kidney	β	Increased renin release
Gut	a, β	Decreased motility and increased sphincter tone
Pancreas	a	Decreased insulin release Decreased glucagon release
	β	Increased insulin release Increased glucagon release
Liver	a, β	Increased glycogenolysis
Adipose tissue	β	Increased lipolysis
Most tissues	β	Increased calorigenesis
Skin (apocrine glands on hands, axillae, etc)	a	Increased sweating
Bronchioles	β_2	Dilatation
Uterus	a	Contraction
	β_2	Relaxation

Chloride channel

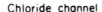

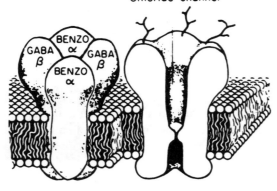

Receptor/Receptor Site: Model of the GABA$_A$-BZ-chloride ionophore receptor complex.

Rectal Anesthesia:

Method of inducing anesthesia via the rectum. Dosage of the anesthetic agent is calculated according to the patient's weight. Rectal anesthesia is believed to provide a smoother, less psychologically traumatizing method of induction, particularly for children. However, speed of onset and total absorption are unpredictable. The method has become less popular since the introduction of the nonirritating inhalation anesthetics. Bromethol (Avertin, Tribromoethanol) was a popular agent for this technique but became obsolete because of its tendency to produce liver and kidney damage.

Rectal Temperature Measurement:

Means of temperature measurement that is advantageous because the monitoring site (rectum) is usually undisturbed during surgery. A disadvantage of this method is that it is slow to reflect the actual core temperature.

Rectifier:

Device found in electrical circuitry that permits current to flow in only one direction. It can thus change alternating current (AC) into direct current (DC) because it suppresses or attenuates alternate half-cycles of the current waveform. In order to generate a steady direct current, rectifiers must contain mirror image components, each of which operates on only half of the current cycle.

Redundancy:

Part of the total amount of information that can be eliminated without destroying the essential message. In a broader sense, it refers to the number and effectiveness of backup systems of a particular process.

Reference Electrode:

Electrode with an electrical potential difference from a second electrode. This difference is constant owing to the chemical makeup of the reference electrode.

Reference, External or Internal:

Known or given value or quantity that is used to determine the accuracy of a particular piece of equipment. For example, during the calibration of a blood-gas analyzer, an external reference would be a fluid of known gas values fed into the machine to check the machine's performance. An internal reference is a known constant already "on board." Most modern scintillation counters contain a precisely known quantity of radioactive material that can be used to check the accuracy of the instrument at any time.

Referred Pain:

Pain characterized by the central nervous system (CNS) reporting injury at one location whereas the injury is occurring at another. For example, it is not unusual for decay in one tooth to be referred to opposing undamaged teeth . Although referred pain rarely jumps the midline, it can in specific cases. The explanation for referred pain relies on common use pain pathways in the CNS causing confusion to higher center information processing. It is probably not that simple. *See* Somatic pain; Visceral pain.

Reflection Coefficient:

See Staverman reflection coefficient.

Reflux:

See Esophageal reflux.

Refractory:

Term meaning highly resistant to therapy. Refractory also means the ability to withstand high temperatures (at least 1580°C) without physical change. The most common and oldest refractory material is clay. Refractory residents require more heating.

Refractory Period:

Time period when a membrane is relatively incapable of depolarization. During the shorter absolute refractory period no amount of stimulation depolarizes the membrane.

Refrigerant:

Gas or liquid with an extremely low boiling point that is used to absorb heat in refrigerating machines. The most common refrigerants used today are from the group of fluorinated hydrocarbons called Freons. *See* Fluorocarbon; Freon.

Regenerative Depolarization:

Description of the effect of sodium pores on nerve action potential. The sodium pores amplify or regenerate the action potential that would be attenuated because of continuous diffusion of ions away from the nerve through the conducting fluid that surrounds the nerve membrane. Sodium pores, however, increase the ionic current as the action potential passes them. Two other physiologic entities allow the action potential to travel a greater distance before requiring amplification. One is an increase in the diameter of the axon, which reduces the internal resistance to current flow; and the other is the myelin sheath, which surrounds and insulates the axon, thereby reducing the loss of current through direct and capacitive leakage. *See* Action potential; Depolarization; Sodium channel.

Regional Wall Motion Abnormalities:

One finding from radionuclide angiography of the heart. Wall motion may be normal or can be rated as diakinetic, akinetic, or unsynchronized in various degrees. *See* Radionuclide angiography; TEE.

Register:

High-speed but usually temporary storage device where an intermediate value can be stored until called for by the program of a computer. *See* Shift register.

Regitine:

See Phentolamine.

Regulator:

See Pressure-reducing valve.

Regurgitation:

See Esophageal reflux.

Relative Value Guide (RVG):

Reimbursement plan for physicians most extensively used by anesthesiologists that relates reimbursement in "units" for particular surgically named procedures. The reimbursement for each procedure is made up of "base units," which is a measure of the difficulty of the procedure, and in time units, which are usually calculated in 15-minute increments. *See* Usual, customary, and reasonable charges.

Relaxant:

See Neuromuscular blocking agent.

Relay:

Electrical device in which one current controls the switching on or off of an independent current. Relays, for example, isolate strong power currents from weak control currents.

Reliability:

Estimate of the trustworthiness of the output of a device. In reference to medical equipment, such as patient-monitoring instruments, reliability implies both repeatability under similar circumstances and the capability to tolerate gross malmanipulation by the maladroit.

REM:

Acronym for rapid eye movement. It is used to describe a stage of sleep during which dreaming is associated with muscle jerks and rapid eye movements.

Remak Fiber:

See Nerve fiber, anatomy and physiology of.

Remote Access:

Ability to receive or handle information at a distance from the place where it is generated or stored. A computer terminal on the ward that communicates with the main hospital computer that stores laboratory values is an example of remote access.

Renal Toxicity, Anesthesia:

Deleterious effects of anesthesia on the kidney. With the exception of methoxyflurane (Penthrane), anesthetics in general do not damage the kidney. Decreased renal blood flow usually accompanies the anesthetic state, however, and it can exacerbate preexisting renal disease. *See* Methoxyflurane.

Rendell-Baker Soucek Mask:

Type of mask used in pediatric anesthesia and characterized by low deadspace between the surface of the mask and the patient's face. *See* Figure. *See* Face mask.

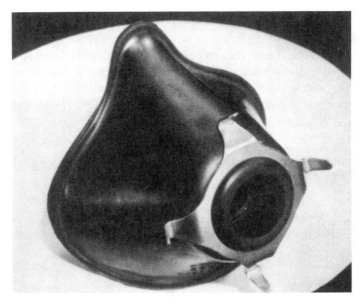

Rendell-Baker Soucek Mask: Face mask.

Renin:

Proteolytic enzyme with a molecular weight of approximately 40,000 daltons. Produced by the juxtaglomerular cells in the kidney, renin acts on a circulating substrate called angiotensinogen to form angiotensin I. This molecule is nonactive pharmacologically; it is, however, converted to angiotensinogen II by the action of Converting Enzyme. Angiotensin II has a half-life of less than 1 minute. *See* Angiotensin.

Reproducibility:

Ability of a piece of equipment to reliably reach the same determination when presented with the same specimen on numerous occasions. Reproducibility does not imply accuracy, as a piece of equipment can make the same mistake again and again if, for example, it is improperly calibrated. *See* Reliability.

Reserpine (Serpasil):

Naturally occurring plant product of the climbing shrub *Rauwolfia serpentina* (hence the name rauwolfia alkaloid) used for thousands of years in Hindu medicine. Introduced to modern clinical medicine for its antipsychotic properties, it is currently used only as an antihypertensive agent. When reserpine is combined with a hypotensive anesthetic agent such as halothane, cardiovascular failure is a distinct possibility. Its greatest common drawback, however, appears to be related to its central nervous system actions, causing depression, drowsiness, and lethargy.

Reservoir Bag:

See Breathing bag.

Residual Volume (RV):

Amount of gas remaining in the lung after maximal expiration. *See* Lung volumes and capacities.

Resin:

Group of substances originally obtained from tree gum. Resins have been used from earliest times for such things as pharmaceuticals, lacquers, varnishes, adhesives, inks, and building materials. Synthetic resins are a huge class of similar, usually polymerized, chemicals such as polyvinyl, polyethylene, polystyrene, and polyester that can be either thermoplastic or thermosetting.

Res Ipsa Loquitur Doctrine:

A legal doctrine, first delineated over a hundred years ago in England, stating "the thing speaks for itself." In malpractice cases it means that the negative outcome of a particular doctor-patient relationship was so obviously caused by negligent behavior (as understood by the average individual) that no proof of negligence is required. An obvious case in which the doctrine of *res ipsa loquitur* could be applied is when forceps are left in a patient after surgery.

Resistance, Airway:

Measurement of the pressure differential necessary to move air from the nose and mouth to the alveoli. It is expressed in centimeters of water per liter per second. Airway resistance rises with obstruction. Measured by body plethysmograph, airway resistance is 0.05–1.5 cm H_2O/L/second in normal adults. An indirect clinical evaluation of airway resistance is measurement of the timed vital capacity. *See* Airway obstruction; Pulmonary function tests; Pulmonary physiology symbols.

Resistance, Electrical:

Ratio of the potential difference (voltage) across a conductor to the current flowing through the conductor. Resistance is measured in ohms. *See* Impedance; Ohm law.

Resistance to Air in Lung:

See Lung volumes and capacities.

Resistance Vessels:

Vessels mainly comprising the arterioles that, by means of sympathetic stimulation, can change their lumen size and thereby alter the resistance offered to blood flow. In contrast to the resistance vessels are the capacitance vessels, which are composed of the medium and large veins and can, by means of sympathetic stimulation, change their cross-sectional dimensions to act as reservoirs for part of the circulating volume. They can therefore actively alter the blood volume returned to the heart. *See* Central venous pressure.

515

Resistance Wire:

Wire that deliberately heats when an electric current is passed through it. Usually these wires are made of nickel and chromium and are not oxidized at high temperatures.

Resource-Based Relative Value Scale (RBRVS):

Scheme for reimbursement of physician services based on resource cost rather than historic charges. It is designed to compensate specialists on the basis of their work, the cost of their practices, and the duration of their training. *See* Relative value guide.

Respiration:

Chemical and physical process by which either a single cell or an entire organism utilizes O_2 and disposes of CO_2. The terms *respiration* and *respirators* are often used interchangeably with the terms *ventilation* and *ventilators*. Strictly speaking, ventilation refers to the movement of gas in and out of the lungs. Therefore, it is appropriate to speak of cellular respiration but not of cellular ventilation.

Respiratory Acidosis:

Rise of $PaCO_2$ above the normal range of 36–44 mm Hg which does not occur in order to compensate for metabolic alkalemia. Respiratory acidosis augments neuromuscular block by d-tubocurarine and limits and opposes reversal of the block by neostigmine.

Respiratory Alkalosis:

Fall in $PaCO_2$ below the normal range of 36–44 mm Hg, which does not occur in order to compensate for metabolic acidemia.

Respiratory Care:

Activities that, taken as a whole, aid in patient respiration, including such modalities as intermittent positive-pressure breathing, humidification of inspired gases, and chest physiotherapy. Other techniques in respiratory care include incentive spirometry, in which the patient breathes from or into a device designed to demonstrate and encourage maximal effort. Respiratory care can also involve the administration of drugs by inhalation therapy, such as mucolytic agents, which are designed to increase fluidity and decrease the viscosity of secretions. Examples of mucolytic agents include acetylcysteine (Mucomyst) and the pancreatic enzyme dornase (Dornavac). *See* Postural drainage.

Respiratory Centers (Regulation of Respiration):

The seat of breathing in the brain, the respiratory center, is composed of several widely dispersed neuronal groups located bilaterally in the medulla oblongata and the pons. Respiratory function is initiated by the inspiratory center, which is also referred to as the dorsal respiratory group of neurons. Stimulation of these neurons always causes inspiration. This group generates the basic rhythm of respiration by emitting repetitive bursts of inspiratory action potentials. The pneumotaxic center, located in the upper pons, has the primary effect of switching off the inspiratory signal of the inspiratory center. There appears to be an expiratory center as well, called the ventral respiratory group of neurons.

It does not appear to function unless an overdrive mechanism is necessary to increase ventilation. A poorly understood area is the apneustic center, which appears to send signals that prevent switching off the inspiratory movements. The function of this center in health is poorly understood. All of the aforementioned centers are influenced by higher central nervous system centers, which in turn respond to and are modified by central sensors for of $PaCO_2$ and pH. *See* Figure.

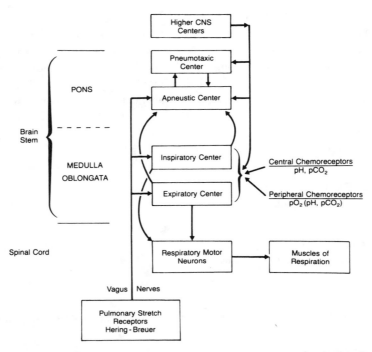

Respiratory Centers (Regulation of Respiration): Schematic diagram of classic CNS respiratory centers. Diagram illustrates major respiratory centers, neurofeedback circuits, primary neuro-humoral sensory inputs, and mechanical outputs.

Respiratory Distress Syndrome (RDS):

See Adult respiratory distress syndrome; Infant respiratory distress syndrome.

Respiratory Effort:

See Work of breathing.

Respiratory Exchange Ratio; Respiratory Quotient (RQ):

Ratio of the minute production of CO_2 to the minute consumption of O_2. Both are determined by tissue metabolism and are normally measured in a steady state. In the 70-kg man at rest, 200 ml CO_2 is exhaled/minute while 250 ml O_2 is consumed, for an RQ of 0.8.

Respiratory Failure:

Inability of a patient to maintain appropriate lung ventilation to prevent hypoxia or hypercapnia without mechanical assistance. For practical purposes, in acute situations active, forceful intervention to assist respiration is done when the $PaCO_2$ rises above 50 mm Hg and arterial oxygenation falls below 50 mm Hg. This point is called the *partial pressure crossover point*.

Respiratory Gas Exchange, Altitude Effects on:

Consequences of altitude changes on oxygenation. The barometric pressure of air decreases as the distance from the earth's surface increases. At 18,000 feet, the barometric pressure is approximately one-half the normal 760 mm Hg. Among the body processes that adapt to high altitudes are (1) hyperventilation based on hypoxic stimulation of the peripheral chemoreceptors; (2) polycythemia, in which the hemoglobin concentration is increased by 3–5 g/dl; (3) a shift to the right of the O_2-hemoglobin dissociation curve; and (4) an increase in maximum breathing capacity when the air is less dense. *See* Oxygen-hemoglobin dissociation curve.

Respiratory Lobule:

See Secondary lobule.

Respiratory Quotient:

See Respiratory exchange ratio.

Respiratory Rate:

Number of complete respirations (inspirations and expirations) per minute.

Respiratory Resistance:

See Forced expiratory volume.

Respiratory Sparing Effect:

See Tubocurarine chloride.

Respiratory Therapy:

Application of various physical and physiologic techniques, including chest palpation and percussion and aerosol therapy to optimize lung function. Most efficacious in those cases where liquids or solids have obstructed the air passageways.

Respiratory Tree:

See Conducting airways.

Respiratory Zone:

Area of the lung beyond the connecting pathways that contain alveoli for gas exchange.

Respirometer:

See Spirometer.

Respirometer, Hot Wire:

See Anemometer, hot wire.

Resting Membrane Potential:

See Action potential.

Resuscitation:

See Cardiopulmonary resuscitation.

Retrieval, Data:

Ability to call back data by search, retransmission, or in some cases recreation from a file, data bank, or other storage unit.

Retrobulbar Block:

Local anesthetic block where solution is deposited behind the globe of the eye. It is a good anesthetic for procedures on the anterior chamber. The block is usually performed by the ophthalmologic surgeon rather than the anesthesiologist and is popular for cataract surgery in the elderly. *See* Figure.

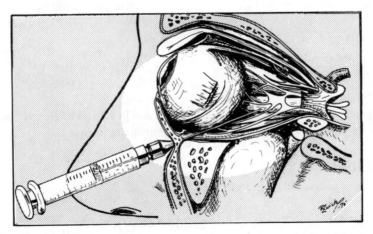

Retrobulbar Block: Direction of the needle in the orbit during retrobulbar block.

Retrofit:

Ability to add new capabilities or modes of action to an already existing piece of equipment, usually implying that no major function is lost in the process. A digital display added to an electrocardiograph (ECG) machine so it can simultaneously display pulse rates and the ECG is an example of retrofit.

Retrograde Amnesia:

Loss of memory material that had been intact up to a particular event, such as a blow to the head. Retrograde amnesia is specifically not caused by the benzodiazepine class of drugs. In fact, these drugs may demonstrate retrograde facilitation in that they appear at times to improve the retention of material learned before they are administered. *See* Anterograde amnesia.

Retrograde Facilitation:

See Retrograde amnesia.

Retrolental Fibroplasia (RLF):

Formation of a fibrovascular membrane behind the lens of the eye, leading to blindness. Almost exclusively confined to premature infants who have been exposed to high concentrations of O_2, it is one of the most feared outcomes of supportive O_2 therapy for these infants.

Return to Flow Method:

Technique for determining the accuracy of blood pressure recorded from an arterial line. The technique involves inflating a blood pressure cuff above the point of entry of the arterial line until the trace is abolished, then slowly deflating the cuff until the beginning of the trace is just detected. This point is the systolic pressure, and the cuff pressure can now be read to determine the calibration and accuracy of the arterial tracing.

Revell Circulation:

See Circulator, Revell.

Reverberation:

Persistence of sound (after its source has ceased) in a series of closely spaced echoes so the listener perceives a continuous sound of diminishing intensity.

Reversible Inhibition:

See Competitive antagonism.

Reye Syndrome (Acute Toxic Encephalopathy):

Disease that occurs in small numbers of pediatric patients following an otherwise uneventful respiratory or varicella (chickenpox) infection. The mortality rate associated with Reye syndrome is at least 15–20%. The disease is characterized by recurrent vomiting, stupor, and coma, with continually deepening depression terminating in death. The key to treatment of Reye syndrome appears to be monitoring for an acute elevation in intracranial pressure and then taking appropriate measures to reduce it. A link is suspected between aspirin usage during a viral syndrome and subsequent development of Reye syndrome. Aspirin is usually avoided in individuals under 21 years of age. *See* Table. *See* Cerebral blood flow.

Reye Syndrome: Signs, symptoms, and stages of severity of Reye syndrome.

Stage 1:	1) vomiting, lethargy**, sleepiness
	2) liver dysfunction
	3) type I EEG
Stage 2:	1) disorientation**
	2) delirium, combativeness
	3) hyperventilation
	4) hyperactive DTR's
	5) type II EEG
Stage 3:	1) obtunded, coma**
	2) decorticate rigidity**
Stage 4:	1) decerebrate rigidity**
	2) loss of oculocephalic reflexes
	3) large, fixed pupils
	4) type III or IV EEG
Stage 5:	1) seizures, loss of DTR's
	2) respiratory arrest**
	3) flaccidity**
	4) type IV or V EEG
	5) hepatic function often normal

* Lovejoy, 1974
** Best clinical signposts delineating stage of encephalopathy.

Reynolds Number:

Measurement of the tendency for turbulence to occur in a vessel or container. The Reynolds number relates the change in fluid flow pattern from laminar to turbulent. This change is related to velocity, viscosity, and length and diameter of the conducting tube or vessel. *See* Critical velocity; Laminar flow; Poiseuille law; Turbulent flow.

RF:

See Radiofrequency choke.

Rh Factor:

See Blood types.

Rheology:

Branch of science that studies the deformation and flow of matter.

Rheomacrodex:

See Dextran.

Rheostat:

Type of potentiometer used for large electric currents.

Rhizotomy:

Technique of sectioning nerve roots for the treatment of intractable pain. *See* Chondrotomy.

Right, Legal:

Legally enforceable expectation on the part of an individual owed a duty that the duty will be carried out. For example, if a patient enters into a contract with a physician for an operative procedure, the physician has a duty to perform the operation and the patient has a right to expect the physician to do so. *See* Duty.

Ritodrine:

See Tocolytic.

RLF:

See Retrolental fibroplasia.

RMS Value:

See Root mean square.

Ro 15-1788:

See Flumazenil.

Robert Shaw Tube:

See Double-lumen tube.

Robin Hood Syndrome:

See Intracerebral steal syndrome.

Robinul:

See Glycopyrrolate.

Rocking Boat Movement:

Paradoxical depression of the chest wall during inspiration coupled with flaring of the lower chest margins and bulging of the abdomen. This movement is seen when diaphragmatic action is unopposed by normal intercostal contraction. It can occur with upper airway obstruction, partial muscle paralysis, or deep general anesthesia.

Roentgen:

International unit of x-radiation/gamma radiation. It is quantity of radiation that, when absorbed completely, produces in 1 cc dry air at 0°C and standard pressure, ions carrying 2.58×10^{-4} coulomb of electric charge of either sign. *See* Rad; Roentgen-equivalent-man.

Roentgen-Equivalent-Man (rem):

Unit of exposure to ionizing radiation that has the same biologic effectiveness as 1 rad of x-rays. *See* Rad.

ROM:

See Read only memory; Memory, computer.

Root Mean Square (RMS Value; Effective Value):

Effective current or voltage is a function of the peak current or voltage divided by the square root of 2 in any situation where current or voltage alternates in magnitude. By convention, the root mean square value is used when speaking about supplied current or voltage. Therefore when one speaks of a wall supply being 115 V, one is actually speaking of a wall voltage that peaks at approximately 145 V.

Ropivacaine:

Amide local anesthetic structurally similar to bupivacaine with approximately the same or somewhat shorter time course of action, but definitely appearing less cardiotoxic.

Rotameter:

Common float used in flowmeter tubes that resembles a skirted, upside-down cone. The grooves cut in the skirt cause the rotameter to turn when it is freely suspended in the gas stream of a flowmeter tube. If the rotameter is suspended in the gas stream but not turning, it is an indication that it may be jammed in the flowmeter tube. The rotameter is read at the rim. *See* Flowmeter.

Rotating Disk Oxygenator:

Device for gas exchange used during the early years of extracorporeal circulation. Such a device consisted of a row of metal disks threaded on a common shaft that rotated in a cylinder half-filled with the patient's venous blood. The gas over the blood was O_2. Gas exchange occurred on the thin blood film on the upper half of the disks. This technique was relatively atraumatic to blood, but it did require gas and metal contact with the blood. *See* Extracorporeal circulation.

Rouleau Formation:

Arrangement of red blood cells piled one on top of another like a stack of coins. If present to any great extent in the circulation, it causes clogging and cessation of flow in the microcirculation. The red blood cells of patients with sickle cell disease are particularly prone to rouleau formation.

Routine (Subroutine):

Circumscribed set of instructions that allows a machine to carry out a well-defined function. For example, when determining patient charges, a hospital computer in a cashier's office might have a routine or subroutine as part of its master program that would query the hospital's laboratory computer for laboratory charges to the particular account in question.

RPP:

See Rate-pressure product.

RQ:

See Respiratory exchange ratio, respiratory quotient.

Rubber/Gas Coefficient:

Concentration of a gaseous agent, particularly an anesthetic agent, in contact with rubber materials at equilibrium. Rubber/gas coefficients range from 1.2 for N_2O to 120 for halothane, and to over 600 for methoxyflurane. Therefore these rubber items are a significant source of gas cross contamination when they are used for more than one patient. *See* Partition coefficient.

Ruben Valve:

See Nonrebreathing valve.

Rule of Nines:

Method of rapidly estimating the extent of body burns. According to this rule, the head and each arm are figured to have 9% of the body surface area. Each leg has 18%, as does the front and the back of the torso, respectively. The perineal area is credited with the remaining 1%.

Rumpel-Leede Phenomenon (Sign, Test):

Test for coagulopathy disorders, particularly platelet deficiencies in which the formation of petechiae below an occlusive band circumferentially applied to a limb are counted.

RV:

See Residual volume.

RVG:

See Relative value guide.

S

SAAC:
See Society of Academic Anesthesia Chairmen.

Sacral-Epidural Anesthesia:
See Caudal anesthesia.

Safety Release Device:
The part of a gas cylinder valve designed to release the contents of the tank to the atmosphere when internal pressure conditions rise to explosive levels. The device consists of three operating segments: (1) frangible disk assembly (frangible disk and safety caps), which blocks the path to the outside atmosphere and bursts whenever a minimum pressure behind it is exceeded; (2) fusible plug, a low melting point alloy that occludes a discharge channel and melts at a predetermined temperature, and (3) safety relief valve, which contains a spring that holds the valve against a seat until the pressure within the tank exceeds that for which the spring is set. The valve then opens, and gas escapes through the safety valve vents until the pressure is lowered, causing the valve to close again. These three devices are often used in combination.

Salicylate:
See Acetylsalicylic acid.

Saltatory Conduction:
See Myelin sheath.

Salting Out Effect:
Observation that increased electrolytes in the blood decrease the aqueous solubility of an anesthetic agent. This effect is normally outweighed by the increased solubility associated with elevation in protein and lipid components of the blood.

SAMBA:
See Society of Ambulatory Anesthesia.

Same Day Surgery:
See Outpatient anesthesia.

Sanders Jet (Jet Anesthesia):

Device used to ventilate patients during bronchoscopy. A jet injector is attached to the bronchoscope, and a thin stream of high-pressure O_2 is delivered down the trachea alongside the bronchoscope. This high-pressure jet draws air down the trachea or through the lumen of the bronchoscope by the principle of entrainment. The jet is pulsed to initiate inspiration and then stopped so passive expiration can take place. *See* Figure. *See* High-frequency ventilation.

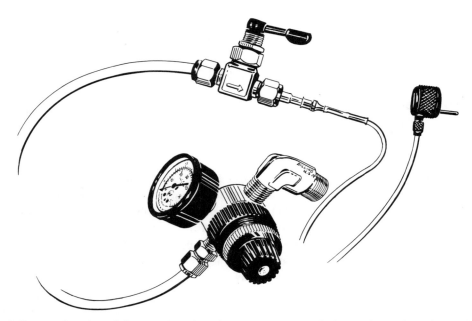

Sanders Injector: Sanders injector showing the pressure regulating valve, triggering valve, and the gas jet which is aimed down the trachea.

SA Node:

See Heart, conduction system of; Sinoatrial node.

Sarcomere:

See Actomyosin.

Saturated Vapor:

See Vapor, saturated.

Scaler:

Circuit that produces an output pulse when a specified number of input pulses have been received.

Scanner:

See Optical Character Reader.

Scanning:

Process by which a particular area is searched or explored in a methodic manner to peruse or examine displayed or stored information. There are two general types of scanning. In the first, a beam from a sensor, which could be made up of particles such as electrons or waves from the electromagnetic spectrum, sweeps across the area to be scanned. The other method of scanning has a receiver tracking across a field or body in a preconceived pattern sensitive, for example, to radiation emitted from various parts of the body. This technique is utilized in medicine for liver, spleen, and lung scans. Radioisotopes are administered to the patient, and the detector then searches for alterations in density and concentration of the radioisotope.

Scattering:

Random deflection of electromagnetic energy. For example, an x-ray beam is both absorbed and deflected (scattered) by shielding.

Scavenger System:

Device used to remove waste anesthetic gases from the immediate operative environment. (Before the advent of scavengers, excess gases were freely released into the operating room). Waste gas is collected into a reservoir bag or tube and continuously exhausted into the centralized suction system of the hospital. Paradoxically, this improvement in the operating room atmosphere has led to a deterioration of the atmosphere in and around the central suction pumps. *See* Figure.

Schimmelbusch Mask:

Classic, much feared mask for open drop ether induction of anesthesia. This mask is an open framework of wire or brass over which a gauze sponge has been fitted. The anesthetic agent is dripped on to the gauze after the mask has been placed on the patient's face. As the changeover from flammable to nonflammable agents has occurred in the United States, these masks are an increasingly popular item on the antique market. *See* Face mask.

Sciatic Nerve Block:

Injection of a local anesthetic solution around the sciatic nerve for relief of chronic pain or as part of a series of nerve blocks prior to surgery on the leg.

Sciatic Nerve Palsy:

Neuropathy of the sciatic nerve resulting from trauma due to improper injection technique. It may be seen as an iatrogenic injury. *See* Nerve palsy.

Scientific Notation:

Shorthand expression of quantities denoted as a value times 10 to the nth power. It is particularly useful for extremely large or extremely small numbers. For example, the number 0.005678 is 5.678×10^{-3} in scientific notation.

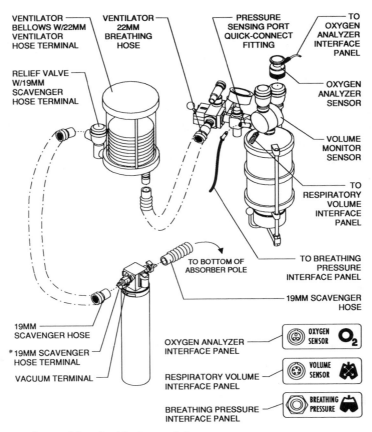

VENTILATOR BELLOWS W/22MM VENTILATOR HOSE TERMINAL

VENTILATOR 22MM BREATHING HOSE

PRESSURE SENSING PORT QUICK-CONNECT FITTING

TO OXYGEN ANALYZER INTERFACE PANEL

OXYGEN ANALYZER SENSOR

RELIEF VALVE W/19MM SCAVENGER HOSE TERMINAL

VOLUME MONITOR SENSOR

TO RESPIRATORY VOLUME INTERFACE PANEL

TO BOTTOM OF ABSORBER POLE

TO BREATHING PRESSURE INTERFACE PANEL

19MM SCAVENGER HOSE

19MM SCAVENGER HOSE

19MM SCAVENGER HOSE TERMINAL

VACUUM TERMINAL

OXYGEN ANALYZER INTERFACE PANEL

RESPIRATORY VOLUME INTERFACE PANEL

BREATHING PRESSURE INTERFACE PANEL

OXYGEN SENSOR O₂

VOLUME SENSOR

BREATHING PRESSURE

Scavenger System: Assembly of a Narkomed 4.

Scintillation:

Flash of light exhibited by certain materials (scintillators) when struck by radiation. Light production is proportional to the original radiation. Radioactive samples can be quantified by mixing them with a scintillation solution and counting the light flashes in a scintillation counter.

Scintillation Counter:

See Photomultiplier.

Scopolamine; L-Hyoscine:

Antimuscarinic agent similar to atropine and obtained from the belladonna plant. It is a competitive antagonist of acetylcholine at receptor sites in smooth muscle, cardiac muscle, and exocrine glands. Scopolamine produces mydriasis and paralysis of ocular accommodation. It inhibits secretions of the respiratory tract, including the mouth, nose, pharynx, and bronchi, and is therefore frequently used as a premedicant for anesthesia (in conjunction with a narcotic). Scopolamine causes drowsiness at low doses because it penetrates the blood-brain barrier into the central nervous system much more readily than atropine. In the

528

past, however, it was often used alone in higher doses for sedation, a technique known as "twilight sleep," during which the patient would be somnolent and responsive, but would have no memory of the procedure. Delirium, an adverse side effect caused by scopolamine, may be reversed by physostigmine (Antilirium). *See* Atropine; Physostigmine; Premedication.

SCR:

See Silicon controlled rectifier.

SCRAM:

A type of anesthesia mask. SCRAM stands for selected contour retaining anatomical mask. It is designed for patients who are difficult to fit to a mask. *See* Face mask.

Screen Oxygenator (Mayo Gibbon Pump Oxygenator):

Type of pump oxygenator used for exchange of gases during cardiopulmonary bypass. Gas exchange takes place as the patient's blood flows down a fine-mesh screen that is contained in a high-O_2 atmosphere. *See* Cardiopulmonary bypass.

SD:

See Standard deviation.

SEA:

See Society for Education in Anesthesia.

Secobarbital (Seconal):

Short-acting sedative-hypnotic agent. *See* Barbiturate.

Second:

Standard international unit of time determined by the duration of a specific number of periods of radiation emitted by a cesium 133 atom decaying between two known states. It was formerly defined as 1/86,400 of the mean solar day.

Second Gas Effect:

Phenomenon seen with inhalation anesthesia, particularly during induction, when a high concentration of a primary gas (usually a blood soluble agent) is given in conjunction with a second gas (anesthetic vapor). The rapid uptake of the primary gas accelerates the rate of rise of alveolar concentration of the second gas; i.e., the constituents of the alveolar gas that do not leave the alveoli and enter the blood as rapidly as the primary gas form a larger percentage of the remaining alveolar gas volume. The second gas effect is best illustrated by the administration of 75% N_2O/1% halothane/24% O_2. Because N_2O crosses the alveolar membrane much more rapidly than halothane, the gas remaining in the alveoli has a higher concentration of halothane. If the second gas is also highly soluble, the second gas effect is negligible; however, a rapid transfer of both agents to the blood creates an increase in inspired volume. Gas is drawn down the trachea to replace alveolar gas, which has crossed into the lung. *See* Concentration effect.

Secondary Emission:

Liberation of electrons from a material that has been struck by a high-velocity electron. Secondary electrons can be accelerated by an electromagnetic field and go on to strike another metal surface, causing further secondary emission, thereby leading to an electron avalanche or cascade. *See* Photomultiplier.

Secondary Fibrinolysis:

See Primary fibrinolysis.

Secondary Lobule (Respiratory Lobule):

Anatomic unit of the lung surrounded by connective tissue septa and consisting of a small cluster of terminal bronchioles together with the respiratory tissue it supplies. *See* Conducting airways.

Secondary Winding:

See Transformer.

Sedation:

Drowsy state of consciousness that allows an individual to respond to commands appropriately. The patient may fall asleep spontaneously unless stimulated. *See* Conscious sedation.

Sedimentation:

Tendency of free particles in a liquid to clump together under the influence of gravity or centrifugal force.

Seebeck Effect:

See Thermocouple.

Segmental Atelectasis:

See Atelectasis.

Segmental Block(s):

Imprecise term usually used to mean an epidural block of levels T10–L1. It is imprecise because "segmental block" has also been used to mean either a unilateral or bilateral paravertebral block of one or more levels of the sympathetic chain.

Segmental Wall Motion Abnormalities (SWMA):

Using the ability of the transesophageal echocardiograph to demonstrate real time-cardiac wall motion. Normal patterns of wall motion have been determined. When a segment of the cardiac wall moves abnormally, it is believed to be a sensitive indicator of myocardial ischemia. *See* Transesophageal echocardiography.

Seizure:

State of excessive, uncontrolled overactivity affecting part or all of the central nervous system. *See* Epilepsy.

Seldinger Technique:

Method of placing a catheter (of the same size as the bore of the needle) into a vessel via a puncture needle and stylet (guidewire). The Seldinger technique was originally designed for arterial catheterization with injection of contrast medium. This method has since been used to insert an endotracheal tube following placement of the guidewire through the cricothyroid membrane and upward into the mouth. The wire is then used to guide the tube for proper placement. A variation of the Seldinger guidewire, the J-wire, has a curved tip that is able to bypass a partial obstruction in a vessel.

Selectivity:

Ability of a device, such as an electric circuit, to discriminate among specific frequencies.

Self-Inflating Bag:

See Breathing bag.

Self-Propagating Flame:

Combustion process by which fuel is mixed with air at a rapid rate so a flame travels from the point of ignition. The flame continues to burn after the original point of ignition has cooled. *See* Cool flame.

Self-Taming of Succinylcholine:

Technique of administering succinylcholine to attenuate muscle fasciculation. A small dose is administered (one-fifth to one-tenth the total dose), and the patient is observed for fasciculation before the remainder is given. Controversy exists as to whether total fasciculation is decreased with this technique.

Self-Test Capability (Self-Calibration; Calibration Signal):

Built-in feature of many sophisticated electronic monitors whereby the monitor is able to generate a signal internally (cal signal) that acts precisely like the signal it is meant to acquire, display, or record. The unit can therefore be checked without being attached to a patient.

Sellick Maneuver:

Procedure used to block regurgitation of stomach contents into the esophagus during a rapid sequence intubation technique. It involves pressing on the cricoid cartilage of the trachea to compress the esophagus. *See* Rapid sequence induction.

SEM:

See Standard error of the mean.

Semiautomated Record Keeping:

Constantly evolving technique of automating chart keeping during anesthesia. In its simplest form, it directly couples, through appropriate electronics, the signals put out by the various monitors and records them in human readable form on a chart. The major obstacle to overcome is appropriate artifact rejection. *See* Anesthetic record.

Semiconductor:

Material that resists the flow of an electric current more than a conductor but less than an insulator. Unlike most materials, semiconductors also have a negative temperature coefficient of resistance, i.e., as the temperature rises, the relative resistance of the material decreases. The rare elements germanium and selenium are examples of a semiconductor. Semiconductors are important in solid-state electronics. In certain semiconductors, there is an absence of an electron (a "hole") in the orbit of an atom. This hole functions as a positive charge carrier. Because some semiconductors have a relative overabundance of holes (p-type material) and others have a relative overabundance of electrons (n-type material), differences of potential can be set up by layering wafers of these materials. The interface of the two materials, the pn junction, functions as a rectifier of alternating current as electrons flow only across the junction when the polarity is in the same direction as the junction (e.g., negative source attached to n-material).

Semipermeable Membrane:

Membrane that allows certain particles and solvents to pass through but excludes other particles and solvents. *See* Osmotic pressure.

Sensitivity:

Criterion for evaluating diagnostic tests. It is the number of true positives (TP) detected by the test TP + the number of false-negatives (FN) missed by the test × 100 to give a percentage (TP/TP + FN × 100). *See* Specificity; Validity.

Sensitization:

See Habituation.

Sensor:

Device used to detect changes in physically measurable parameters, such as temperature, pulse, and air flow.

Septic Shock:

See Shock.

Septicemia:

Condition caused by the persistent presence of pathogenic microorganisms and their toxins in the blood. Regional anesthesia is contraindicated in the presence of septicemia, as any bleeding at the injection site would be contaminated by the offending microbes and would therefore be an immediate threat to the nerve trunks in the area.

Sequential Multiple Analyzer (SMA 1260; SMA 660):

See Automated analysis instrument.

SER (Sensory Evoked Response):

See Evoked potential.

Series Circuit:

Type of electrical connection in which the same current flows in all elements of the circuit providing a single path; the voltage drop, however, is different across each element depending on its individual resistance. *See* Parallel circuit.

Serotonin (5-Hydroxytryptamine, 5-HT):

Vasoactive substance distributed throughout the central nervous system in nerve endings, hypothalamus, and enterochromaffin cells of the gastrointestinal tract. High concentrations of serotonin are found in the platelets. Excessive amounts of serotonin may be secreted by carcinoid tumor cells. *See* Carcinoid syndrome.

Serpasil:

See Reserpine.

Serum, Blood:

Clear fluid part of the blood plasma with fibrinogen removed.

Serum Osmotic Pressure:

See Osmotic pressure.

Servomechanism:

Device that automatically corrects the performance of a system by a feedback mechanism.

Sevoflurane:

Inhalational anesthetic that is considered nonirritating, is pleasant-smelling, and provides rapid induction and awakening because of its low blood solubility. Its chemical formula is $C_4H_3F_7O$.

Shake Test:

See Foam test.

Shape Factor "A":

Element of the regression equation used to determine the magnitude of the hypoxic ventilatory response (HVR); "A" serves as an index of HVR hypoxia. *See* Hypoxic ventilatory response.

Sheriff of Nottingham Syndrome:

See Intracerebral steal syndrome.

Shift Register:

Discrete circuit for storing digital data. A typical shift register has 1024 locations, each capable of storing one word (usually a byte of 8 bits). In the recirculate mode, the shift register can provide a "freeze" (unchanging) trace of a particular few seconds of an electrocardiogram (ECG). (The pattern stored is constantly fed back to the electron beam.) In the unit mode, a continuous real-time ECG can be displayed. With two shift registers, a continuous ECG can be compared on the screen with a desired portion of a previous ECG. *See* Figure.

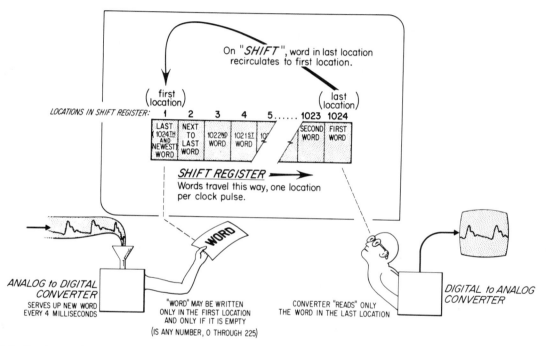

Shift Register: Shift register operating in the recirculate mode, in which the word in the 1024 slot is recycled to the number 1 slot and the word sequence is reread. Only if there is no word in the first slot (the shift register is in the write and recirculate mode) can the analog-to-digital converter add a new word to the first slot.

Shock:

Condition in which there is a decrease in the function of vital organs due to inadequate blood supply or vascular perfusion. Although it may be the result of many causes, this decreased blood supply ultimately leads to tissue hypoxia, metabolic acidosis, and cellular death. Shock may be classified on the basis of primary cause or the type of functional disturbance produced. Types of shock include hypovolemic, cardiogenic, septic, vasogenic, and neurogenic. Hypovolemic shock is characterized by fluid loss of either blood, plasma, or extracellular fluid, e.g., due to hemorrhage, burns, diarrhea, or dehydration. The body attempts to compensate for this loss by shifting fluid from the intracellular space to the extracellular and intravascular spaces. This shift is mediated by increased sympathetic activity causing a heightened vasomotor tone. The body also attempts to compensate hormonally by releasing aldosterone, which leads to the retention of sodium. These responses are attenuated by administration of a general anesthetic. *Cardiogenic shock* is characterized by an inadequate cardiac output, although a normal blood volume exists. It is most commonly seen after myocardial infarction, although other causes exist such as dysrhythmia, acute valvular failure, or cardiac tamponade. *Septic shock* appears to be due to pathogenic microorganisms or circulating bacterial endotoxins and exotoxins. Although blood volume is usually normal, O_2 is not efficiently utilized by the cells. *Vasogenic shock* occurs when vasodilatation causes the normal blood volume to be inadequate for supplying the vessels. It may follow an anaphylactic reaction, which releases excessive histamine into the blood and produces a strong antigen-antibody reaction. *Neurogenic shock* is associated with syncopal episodes during which the functions of the sympathetic autonomic system are altered and vasodilation results. All types of shock may be involved concurrently. The key element in any type of shock appears to be the loss of effectiveness of the normal mechanisms that control the intravascular space. The clinical signs are instability of pulse, blood pressure, and cardiac function and increasing metabolic acidosis. Treatment of shock involves restoration of adequate circulatory volume, adequate pumping action of the heart (with inotropic drugs or digitalis), and adequate peripheral resistance. In addition, metabolic acidosis must be reversed (by appropriate drug administration), organ function (particularly urine output) must be maintained, and sepsis must be treated with appropriate antibiotics. *See* Table.

Shock: Clinical signs and symptoms of early and late shock (not all may be present at all times).

Parameters	Early	Late
Acid Base	Respiratory Alkalosis	Metabolic and respiratory acidosis
Blood Pressure	+(−) ↓	↓↓↓↓
Cardiac Output	↑↑	↓↓ to ↓↓↓↓
Central venous pressure	+(−) ↑	↓↓ to ↑↑
Mental status	↓	↓↓↓↓
Pulmonary artery pressure	+(−) ↑	↑↑
Pulse	+(−)↑	↑↑↑↑ and weak
Renal	+(−) ↓	↓ to ↓↓↓↓
Respirations	↑↑	↑↑↑
Serum K$^+$	↓	↑
Skin	None specific	None specific

Shock Therapy:

See Electroconvulsive therapy.

Shock Wave:

See Explosion.

Short Circuit:

Electronic connection of low resistance between two points in a circuit in which the resistance is usually higher.

Short-Term Memory:

Logical construct used to describe a part of human memory function. The information must be kept alive by active attention or rehearsal, or it fades out within about 20 seconds. The capacity of short-term memory is restricted, considered to be at best five to nine items. It appears to be specifically associated with awareness. *See* Long-term memory.

Shrader Fitting:

Type of quick disconnect joint in gas lines that allows hoses to be quickly attached and detached from a central gas outlet. Various shapes and diameters are used to prevent cross-connection between gases. *See* Quick connector.

Shunt:

Blood that enters the arterial system without undergoing gas exchange in the lungs. Sources of this blood include bronchial artery blood (collected by the pulmonary veins after perfusion of the bronchi and depletion of O_2) and coronary venous blood (which drains directly into the left ventricle via the thebesian veins). The combination of thebesian and bronchial flow is called *physiologic shunt* or *venous admixture* and measures 1–2% of the cardiac output of the healthy individual. Anatomic shunt refers to a transfer of mixed venous blood from right to left without passing a ventilated area in the lung (cardiac septal defect or patent ductus arteriosus). Atelectatic shunt refers to mixed venous blood that returns to the left side of the heart after passing closed (atelectatic) alveoli and therefore does not come into contact with respiratory gas. Physiologic shunt and ventilation/perfusion abnormalities contribute to the alveolar-arterial O_2 difference. *See* Figure. *See* Alveolar-arterial oxygen difference.

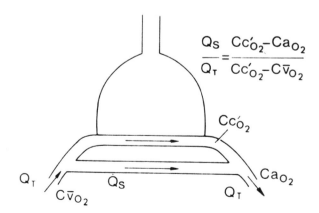

$$\frac{Q_S}{Q_T} = \frac{Cc'_{O_2} - Ca_{O_2}}{Cc'_{O_2} - C\bar{v}_{O_2}}$$

Shunt: Measurements of shunt flow with the shunt equation; QT = total blood flow, Qs = amount of shunted blood/time, Cc'_{O_2} = amount of O_2 in pulmonary capillary blood, $C\bar{v}_{O_2}$ = amount of O_2 in venous blood, Ca_{O_2} = amount of O_2 in arterial blood.

Shunt Equation:

Estimates the amount of physiologic shunt flow in the lungs. *See* Shunt.

SI:

See International system of units.

SIADH:

See Inappropriate antidiuretic hormone (ADH) secretion syndrome.

Sialagogue:

See Antisialagogue.

Sickle Cell Disease:

Congenital condition caused by the production of abnormal hemoglobin S, which is a minor variant of normal hemoglobin. Unfortunately, the minor variation causes the hemoglobin molecule to change configuration in zones of low partial pressure of oxygen. This condition in turn bends, or sickles red blood cells and makes them susceptible to aggregation microthrombi. *Sickle cell trait* occurs in individuals who have only one parent with sickle cell disease. These individuals are still at risk during anesthesia when tourniquets are used on limbs and in any conditions where they face low oxygen tension.

Sickness Impact Profile:

Process to assess the impact of illness. It evaluates such areas as mobility, social interaction, communication, and emotional behavior.

Sick Sinus Syndrome:

Term loosely applied to multiple types of sinus node depression characterized by prolonged sinus pauses, sinus arrest, marked sinus bradycardia, or sinoatrial block.

Side Effect:

Consequence (possibly adverse) of drug administration or a procedure that differs from the desired result.

Side Stream Sampling:

See Mainstream sampling.

Siggaard-Andersen Alignment Nomogram:

Mathematic device for interrelating base excess, total CO_2, and HCO_3 when pH and PCO_2 are known in an arterial sample. *See* Figure. *See* Nomogram.

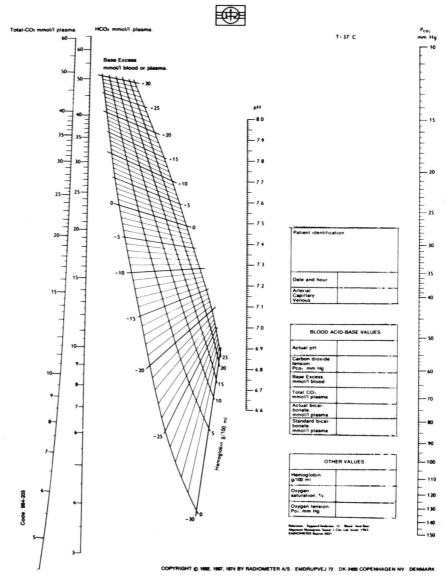

Siggaard-Andersen Alignment Nomogram.

Sigh:

Deep, audible, semivoluntary breath usually in response to a strong emotion. Alternately, in the control of respiration, a sigh is a deliberate, stepwise change in inspiratory volume of two to three times the normal tidal volume repeated on a fairly vigorous basis each hour. The purpose of the sigh is to open terminal airways that have a tendency to collapse during stereotypic ventilation (when respiration delivers exactly the same tidal volume at exactly the same flow rate and flow pattern, breath after breath). *See* Mechanical ventilation.

Sight Glass:

Vertical glass tube attached to a chamber of liquid so the height of the liquid in the chamber is duplicated in the glass tube. It allows the volume of liquid in the chamber to be determined without actually looking into the large chamber. The sight glass was used on early anesthetic vaporizers.

Sign:

Objective evidence perceptible to an examiner and indicative of disease. Signs are, to some extent, measurable and quantifiable. *See* Symptom.

Signal Averaging:

Technique for extracting a signal from random background noise thereby improving the signal-to-noise ratio. Random noise cancels itself out when averaged over an increasing number of trials, whereas a steady strength signal is unaffected by the number of trials averaged. This signal-averaging technique is used in electroencephalogram (EEG) analysis to identify an evoked potential "lost" in the regular EEG activity. The stimulus for the evoked potential is presented repeatedly, and gradually the evoked potential emerges from the background noise. *See* Figure. *See* Evoked potential.

Signal:

Variable parameter used to convey information.

Signal-to-Noise Ratio:

Ratio of the strength of the desired information (signal) in a communication to that of unwanted random sounds (noise). The purpose of most signal-processing equipment is to enhance the signal-to-noise ratio. For example, while using a stethoscope to listen to blood pressure sounds (signal), sounds generated by body movement and the environment (noise) are also heard. *See* Signal averaging.

Significance Level:

Maximum probability of arriving at a type I or type II error when evaluating observations. In practice, a level of significance of 0.05 or 0.01 is common. At 0.05 or 5% level of significance, one is 95% certain of reaching the correct interpretation; at 0.01, or 1%, level of significance, one is 99% certain. *See* Type I error; Type II error.

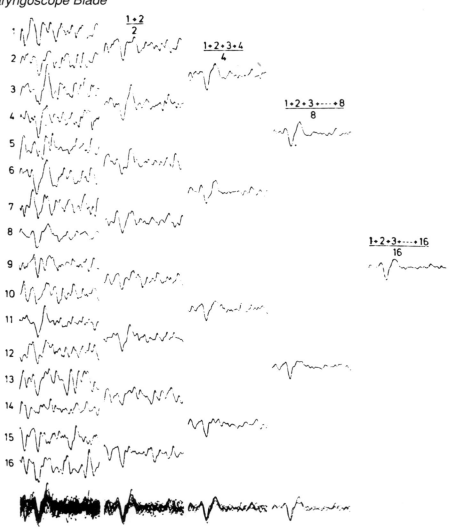

Signal Averaging: Improvement of signal-to-noise ratio by signal averaging. The noise is progressively reduced left to right with the repetition of the signal.

Siker Mirror Laryngoscope Blade:

Modification of the curved laryngoscope blade that incorporates a mirror to allow vision around an obstruction. *See* Laryngoscope.

Silent Gene:

See Dibucaine number.

Silent Zone of Lung:

Area of the lung comprising the small peripheral airways. In healthy individuals this zone contributes only 20% of total peripheral resistance and therefore remains "silent" until significantly diseased.

Silicon-Controlled Rectifier (SCR):

Semiconductor device that permits current flow in one direction when an appropriate signal is applied to one of its electrodes (gate). SCRs are used in many devices as precision switches.

Silicone:

Polymeric organic compound containing silicon. Silicones are heat-resistant, have a high dielectric strength, and are highly water-resistant.

SIMV:

See Synchronized intermittent mandatory ventilation.

Single-Breath Test:

Test to measure the inequality of lung ventilation. A patient takes a single breath of 100% O_2 and then exhales slowly and evenly into an N_2 meter, which rapidly measures the concentration of expired N_2. The expiratory volume is recorded simultaneously. After the first 750 ml are expired (assuming this volume clears the deadspace), the N_2 concentration is measured throughout the next 500 ml. Nitrogen concentration does not increase by more than 1.5% (the alveolar plateau) in healthy individuals. In patients with pulmonary disorders such as emphysema, bronchiectasis, or cancer, the N_2 concentration rises more rapidly. In these patients, there is an uneven dilution of lung N_2 by inhaled O_2. In addition, poorly ventilated regions of the lung, i.e., damaged by disease, receive little or no O_2 from a single breath and empty toward the end of expiration. The single-breath test can be modified to determine closing volume and anatomic deadspace. *See* Figure. *See* Closing capacity; Infrared analyzer; Multibreath test.

Sinister Pattern of Fetal Heart Rate:

See Fetal heart rate terminology.

Sinoatrial Node (SA Node):

Normal pacemaker or determinant of the pulse rate in the heart. From the SA node a wave of depolarization spreads across the atria to the atrioventricular (AV) node. The normal pacemaker action of the SA node depends on the fact that it is the fastest cardiac tissue to depolarize spontaneously. The vagus nerve acts to decrease this spontaneous discharge; higher body temperature increases this rate, and lower temperature decreases it. The rate of discharge is also depressed by digitalis and is increased by sympathetic stimulation or circulating catecholamines. *See* Heart, conduction system of.

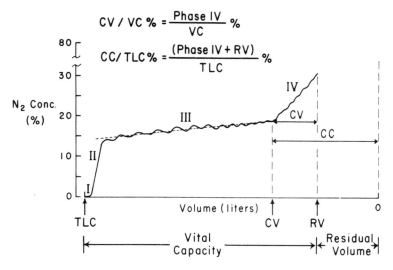

$$CV / VC \% = \frac{Phase\ IV}{VC} \%$$

$$CC / TLC \% = \frac{(Phase\ IV + RV)}{TLC} \%$$

Single Breath Test: Example of single-breath nitrogen curve. Phase I represents dead-space gas, phase II a mixture of dead-space gas and alveolar gas, phase III alveolar gas, and phase IV gas from upper-lung-zone alveoli. Closing volume (CV) is lung volume above residual volume (RV) at which airway closure occurs in dependent lung zones. Closing capacity (CC) = CV + RV. TLC is total lung capacity, and VC vital capacity.

SI Unit:

Standard international unit (from the French Système International d'Unites) that is the agreed on system of measurement or quantification for all scientific and most technical needs. SI units are based on the meter-kilogram-second system (MK) and replace the centimeter-gram-second system (CGS). *See* Table. *See* International system of units.

SI Unit: Prefixes Used with SI Units.

Name of Factor	Prefix	Symbol	Name of Factor	Prefix	Symbol
10	deca-	da	10^{-1}	deci-	d
10^2	hecto-	h	10^{-2}	centi-	c
10^3	kilo-	k	10^{-3}	milli-	m
10^6	mega-	M	10^{-6}	micro-	μ
10^9	giga-	G	10^{-9}	nano-	n
10^{12}	tera-	T	10^{-12}	pico-	p
			10^{-15}	femto-	f
			10^{-18}	atto-	a

Skin Potential Response:

Means of evaluating regional anesthesia block along with such things as temporary regional sympathectomy. The skin potential response is determined by measuring with a sensitive voltmeter, the difference in potential of two points on the skin before and after sympathectomy. *See* Causalgia; Sympathetic nerve block.

Skin Preparation:

Procedure for reducing the bacterial count on the skin by applying an iodine solution or alcohol prior to puncture or incision. This technique does not sterilize the skin. The effectiveness of the reduction of the bacterial count depends not so much on the individual agent but on the vigor and length of time of its application. Although the method has been used for nearly 100 years, the parameters of skin preparation are still controversial.

Slander:

Verbal statement that defames or misrepresents another person. *See* Defamation.

SLEC:

See Spontaneous lower esophageal contractions.

Sleep:

Normal physiologic state associated with relaxation, reduced environmental awareness, mild hypotension, mild bradycardia, and a definite reduction of metabolic state. Different levels of sleep can be distinguished by the ease with which the subject is awakened and by specific changes in the electroencephalogram. Sleep appears to be a required bodily function without which severe and progressive mental disability occurs. *See* REM.

Sleeve:

Form of adaptor used to alter the external diameter of a system component.

Slow Twitch Muscle:

See Type I muscle fiber.

SNDO:

See Standard of diseases and operations.

Snow, John:

English physician credited with being the first specialist in anesthesia. His administration of chloroform to Queen Victoria for childbirth in 1853 was a key element in counteracting the fundamentalist arguments, biblically based, that women must bring forth children in pain. He died in 1858 at the age of 45.

SOAP:

See Society for Obstetric Anesthesia and Perinatology.

Society for Education in Anesthesia (SEA):

Founded in 1984, the Society is made up of anesthesiologists interested in issues related to education in anesthesia. It is accredited by the Accreditation Council of Continuing Medical Education to sponsor continuing medical education or symposia for physicians. The headquarters of the Society is Richmond, Virginia.

Society for Obstetric Anesthesia and Perinatology (SOAP):

Organization founded in 1969, its membership at the beginning of the decade of the 1990s was more than 660 members. The objective of the organization is to provide a forum for discussion for anesthesia-related problems unique to the peripartum period. The address of the organization usually resides with the president of the organization.

Society of Academic Anesthesia Chairmen (SAAC):

Organization for those chairmen of anesthesia whose departments run residency programs approved by the American Accreditation Council for Graduate Medical Education (ACGME) in a university hospital as part of a medical school. Currently, there are approximately 110 members of SAAC, and anyone meeting the qualifications for membership in both SAAC and AAPD may apply for *joint* membership. SAAC is headquartered in Park Ridge, Illinois. *See* Association of Anesthesiology Program Directors (AAPD).

Society of Ambulatory Anesthesia (SAMBA™):

Society chartered in 1985 for anesthesiologists (voting members) and interested other individuals (nonvoting members) to advance the subspecialty of ambulatory anesthesia. SAMBA began the decade of the 1990s with a current membership of 1600 to 1700. The purpose of the Society is to provide education and directions in matters pertaining to ambulatory anesthesia. The Society is headquartered in Park Ridge, Illinois.

Soda Lime:

Widely used absorbent to remove CO_2 from anesthesia rebreathing systems. Soda lime consists of small amounts of sodium hydroxide and potassium hydroxide mixed with a large amount of calcium hydroxide. Inert silica and an indicator dye are also added. Because the mixture of sodium and calcium hydroxide was protected by a patent, competitors used other metal hydroxides (e.g., barium hydroxide) in manufacturing absorbents. This situation led to production of Baralyme, a major competitor of soda lime. Baralyme (barium hydroxide lime) is a mixture of 20% barium hydroxide octahydrate and 80% calcium hydroxide. It may also contain some potassium hydroxide and an indicator dye. Price and handling characteristics usually determine choice of absorbent. *See* Indicator dye.

Soda Lime Canister:

See Carbon dioxide absorption canister.

Sodium (Na):

Alkaline metallic element with atomic number 11 and atomic weight 23. It provides the principal cation of extracellular body fluids. The normal range of serum Na is 135–145 mEq/L.

Since Na has a valence (charge) of 1, the osmotic pressure of serum Na has the same value (i.e., 135–145 mOsm/L of water). The total body content of exchangeable Na in a normal 70-kg man is 2700–3800 mEq. A large proportion of Na (at least 2000 mEq) is extracellular. Intracellular Na is in the range of 10 mEq/L of intracellular water. Excess Na can be easily excreted in the urine (in a normal urine volume), whereas Na balance can be maintained (during Na deprivation) by intake of as little as 10–15 mEq/day. Aldosterone, a mineralocorticoid secreted by the adrenal cortex, helps to regulate Na metabolism in the body. In addition, antidiuretic hormone (ADH) controls the Na concentration of extracellular fluids. *See* Table. *See* Action potential.

Sodium: Factors affecting sodium levels.

Elevated Serum Na	Decreased Serum Na
Dehydration	Diuresis
Primary Aldosteronism	Dilutional
Diabetes Insipidus	Cirrhosis
	Inappropriate ADH syndrome
	Na-losing nephropathy
	Addison disease

Sodium Channel:

Passageway, or pore, in a nerve membrane that allows rapid influx of sodium (Na) ions (necessary for depolarization). In the resting state this "gate" remains nearly closed to Na ion diffusion. When the gate opens, the permeability of the Na channel increases approximately 5000-fold. *See* Ionic channel; Potassium channel.

Sodium Nitroprusside (Nipride):

Rapid-acting, short-term vasodilator administered by intravenous (IV) infusion. (A freshly prepared solution must be used.) Nitroprusside is used to produce deliberate hypotension for surgical procedures and to relieve hypertensive crisis. Nitroprusside dilates both arteriolar and venous smooth muscles. The drug is sensitive to light, and precautions must therefore be taken to ensure that the IV tubing and bottle are covered. Although cyanide is an intermediate breakdown product of nitroprusside, cyanide toxicity is rare. Toxic effects of nitroprusside are related to excessive vasodilation and hypotension. Symptoms include nausea, vomiting, palpitation, and headache. *See* Nitroglycerine.

Software:

Written programs, values, information bits, data, and equations that direct functioning of the computer electromechanics (hardware).

Solenoid:

Electromagnetic switch that usually consists of a coil of wire with a length greater than its diameter. A metal rod slides on the track inside the coil and extends beyond the end of the coil. When current flows through the coil, a magnetic field is created that attracts the rod. The rod moves into the coil; or if the rod is a permanent magnet and polarities are arranged properly, it can be made to extend outside of the coil. The rod contains a contact for making and breaking a circuit.

Solid State:

See Semiconductor.

Solubility:

Relative ability of a given substance (gas, liquid, or solid) to dissolve when mixed with another substance. Solubility is dependent on temperature, pressure, and polarity.

Solute:

Substance dissolved in a solvent.

Solution:

Homogeneous mixture of a solute (liquid, gas, or solid) with a solvent (usually liquid but may be gas or solid).

Solvent:

Substance that dissolves another substance and forms a homogeneous solution.

Somatic Pain:

Type of pain felt in body structures that are expected to experience environmental insult (e.g., the skin). Pain is perceived by specific nerve structures called nociceptors, which are divided into high threshold mechanoreceptors (HTMs) and polymodal nociceptors (PMNs). The former respond only to intense mechanical stimulation, whereas the latter respond to intense thermomechanical and a variety of chemical insults. *See* Nerve conduction; Nociceptor; Visceral pain.

Somatosensory Evoked Potential:

Evoked potential caused by electrical stimulation of a sensory nerve in an extremity. *See* Evoked potential.

Somatostatin:

Hormone found not only in the hypothalamus but also in the D cells of the pancreatic islets and the gastrointestinal mucosa. It has a profound inhibitory effect on growth hormone, as well as other hormones, such as thyroid-stimulating hormone insulin and glucagon.

Sound:

Audible vibrations transmitted through fluids and solids and measured in decibels. Under most ordinary circumstances, sound is transmitted to the human ear by means of vibrations of the air in the range of 20–20,000 Hz/second. *Infrasound* comprises the vibrations below the frequency range of the waves usually perceived as sound (<16 Hz). The speed of sound varies depending on the density of the material through which it is moving, temperature, pressure, and altitude. Sound cannot travel through a vacuum. *Ultrasound* comprises the vibrations above the audible frequency of 20,000 Hz/second and may extend to 10 or 12 mHz. Ultrasonography is used as a valuable diagnostic technique for the detection of abnormalities in various body organs and the evaluation of fetal development. *See* Ultrasound.

SP:

See Substance P.

Space Blanket:

Lightweight nylon sheet with one reflective surface that traps a high percentage of body heat. Because it is lightweight, the space blanket does not interfere with the patient's movement, and it is an effective passive technique for raising body temperature.

Spark:

Visible evidence of an electric current between two electrodes separated by an air gap. Sparks are generated when the potential difference between the electrodes is increased enough that the charged particles present are accelerated to the point at which they strike neutrally charged gas molecules, thereby dislodging electrons. These gas molecules themselves become charged and move in an electric field. The process becomes self-propagating depending on the magnitude of the potential difference, the length of time it is maintained, and the molecular composition of the gas mixture. The potential difference that is just adequate to cause a minimum spark discharge is called the breakdown voltage. The spark discharge is an economic source of ignition, as a large amount of energy is focused in a small volume of gas, heating that portion of the gas rapidly before heat dissipation into the surrounding gas can drop the temperature.

Spark Gap:

Arrangement of electrodes between which a disruptive discharge occurs when a voltage is applied that exceeds a specific predetermined value. A spark gap generator is a type of electrosurgical unit, useful for coagulation, that uses a spark gap to generate radiofrequency waves. *See* Cauterization; Coagulation current.

Sparkover:

See Flashover.

Specific Gravity:

Ratio of the density of a solution at a specific temperature to the density of water at that same temperature.

Specific Heat Capacity:

Heat needed to raise the temperature of the unit mass of a substance by 1°. In SI units, this measurement is in joules per kilogram/kelvin °. Each substance has a specific heat capacity.

Specificity:

Criterion for evaluating diagnostic tests. It is the number of true-negatives (TN) detected by the test   TN + the number of false-positives (FP) detected × 100 to give a percentage: TN/(TN + FP) × 100. *See* Sensitivity.

Spectral Edge Frequency:

See Leading edge analysis.

Spectrometer:

Instrument used to identify the frequency of the components of light emitted by a source. An unknown substance can be heated until it begins to emit light by incandescence. The specific substance can then be identified because each substance emits its own light wavelength. Alternately, a light of known frequency can be passed through an unknown liquid or gas, and the absorption of part of that known spectrum can be used to analyze and determine the unknown substance. Spectrometers are commonly used in the laboratory to detect and quantify the hemoglobin molecule by its absorption of a particular frequency of light.

Spectrophotometer:

Instrument for measuring the relative intensity of various light rays in the spectrum. This measurement aids in identifying unknown substances.

Sphygmomanometer:

Instrument used to determine arterial blood pressure.

Spina Bifida:

Congenital anomaly in which the bony encasement of the spinal cord is not complete. The cord and meninges may or may not protrude through the defect.

Spinal Anesthesia (Subdural Block, Subarachnoid Block):

Form of regional anesthesia in which a local anesthetic solution is deposited into the cerebrospinal fluid in the area of the lumbar vertebrae. The interspace of choice for needle placement is L4–L5. Spinal anesthesia may be used for most surgical procedures done below the level of the diaphragm but may be inadequate for extensive bowel surgery, as it does not block parasympathetic cranial outflow to the intestines. Spinal anesthesia can produce adequate sensory and motor blockade. Even when the blockade is inadequate, the sympathetic trunks may be completely blocked, causing vasodilation and hypotension. *See* Epidural anesthesia; Epidural patch; Hyperbaric solution; Nerve fiber, anatomy and physiology of; Total spinal, accidental.

Spinal Headache:

Known complication of spinal anesthesia ascribed to leakage of cerebrospinal fluid through the hole made in the dura by the spinal needle. (Larger needles and young individuals have a higher incidence.) Conservative treatment includes bed rest, increased fluid intake, and analgesics. Severely affected patients may require an epidural blood patch. *See* Epidural patch; Spinal anesthesia.

Spinal Needle:

Needle usually measuring 20–25 gauge × 3.5 inches used to deposit a regional anesthetic under the dura or to withdraw cerebrospinal fluid by lumbar puncture. The bevel-ended and diamond-point needles are examples of spinal needles. *See* Figure. *See* Epidural needle; Hustead epidural needle.

Spinal Segment:

Portion of the spinal cord that contains a dorsal and ventral nerve root. The segment's name refers to the surrounding vertebra. There are a total of 31 segments in the human (C1–C8, T1–T12, L1–L5, S1–S5, and Co1).

Spinal Shock:

Condition that follows injury or partial transection of the spinal cord. It is characterized by flaccid paralysis and loss of visceral and somatic sensations below the level of the lesion or transection. Tendon and abdominal reflexes are absent as is the plantar response. Bladder and bowel functions are not under voluntary control. A zone of enhanced sensation may be evident above the level of the lesion. The clinical presentation of spinal shock (areflexia) persists from a few days to several weeks when there is a slow return of reflex activity.

Spirometer:

Device used to measure the quantity of air taken into and exhaled from the lungs. With the early mechanical spirometers, the patient's nose was clamped closed, and he or she breathed through a mouthpiece into a bell inverted in a cylinder of water. Movement of the bell was recorded as the air volume inside the cylinder rose and fell with respiration. This apparatus was accurate, but it was also cumbersome and bulky. It has since been replaced by other less accurate mechanical or electric means of determining respiratory volumes. *See* Anemometer, hot wire.

Spironolactone (Aldactone):

Diuretic agent used with other diuretics to reverse hypokalemia and antagonize the effects of aldosterone. Aldosterone acts to conserve sodium and enhances potassium excretion, whereas spironolactone favors sodium excretion and potassium retention. To prevent hyperkalemia, potassium supplements should not be administered in conjunction with spironolactone.

Splanchnic:

Term that pertains to the viscera. Splanchnic circulation comprises the blood flow to the gastrointestinal tract, pancreas, liver, and spleen. Various anesthetic agents (cyclopropane, methoxyflurane, halothane, and isoflurane) reduce this circulation.

549

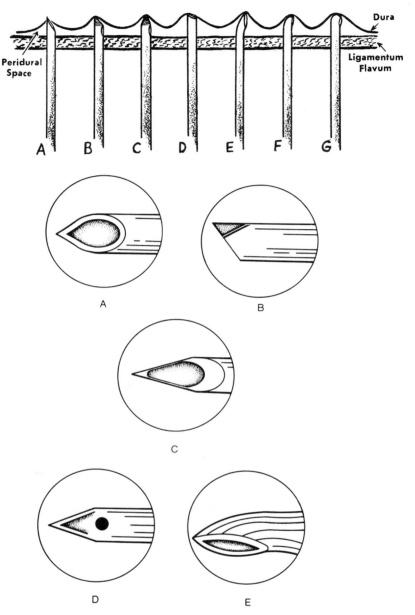

Spinal Needle: Spinal and Epidural Needles: (A) Standard spinal needle with a sharp point that readily punctures the dura. (B) Needle with a solid end and a side opening. (C) Needle with a rounded solid point and a side opening close to its distal end. The Lutz needle has this type of point. (D) Needle with a short, blunt beveled point with rounded edges such as is found on the standard Crawford peridural needles. (E) Needle with a modified huber point as is present on the various Tuohy or Hustead needles. (F) Needle with a directional huber point bent at an acute angle such as is present on the Wagner needle. (G) Needle with an extremely blunt, rounded point and an opening near its end such as is found on the Cheng needle.

Sponge Cuff (Foam Cuff, Kamen-Wilkinson Cuff):

Unusual type of endotracheal tube cuff of large diameter, large residual volume, and large surface area. Pressure against the tracheal wall is determined by the amount of expansion of the foam within the cuff sheath. In order to insert, the cuff must be *deflated,* shrinking the foam to conform to the wall of the tube. *See* Endotracheal tube.

Spontaneous Lower Esophageal Contractions (SLEC):

Physiologic phenomenon in which the lower third of the esophagus made of smooth muscle, demonstrates spontaneous contractions, the magnitude of which decrease with deepening anesthesia. A basis for monitoring depth of anesthesia which is currently considered controversial. In any event, it is not affected by muscle relaxation.

Spontaneous Respiration:

See Ventilation, spontaneous.

Squeeze CO_2:

Measurement of respiratory CO_2 while gentle pressure is exerted on the patient's chest or abdomen in order to force a complete exhalation in those cases where CO_2 production is difficult to evaluate owing to small airway obstruction.

Squint:

See Strabismus.

Stages and Planes of Anesthesia:

System, codified by Guedel, of evaluating a patient's response to anesthesia. This system relates specifically to unpremedicated patients during ether anesthesia. It is no longer clinically applicable because most patients are premedicated, and ether is no longer used. Guedel believed that depth of anesthesia progressed in recognizable increments from consciousness to death by generalized depression. Each increment is identified by changes in the eyes, respiration, muscle tone, response to incision, and pharyngeal and laryngeal reflexes. Stage I (amnesia and analgesia) lasts from onset of anesthesia to loss of consciousness. The pupils are small, the patient's response to pain is altered, muscle tone is normal, and pharyngeal reflexes are unaffected. Stage II (delirium or excitement) lasts from the loss of consciousness to the beginning of rhythmic breathing. The pupils are large, and the eyelid reflex is depressed, muscles are tense, and breathing may be irregular. The patient may cough, struggle, swallow, or vomit. Pharyngeal and laryngeal reflexes are depressed toward the end of this stage. Stage III (surgical anesthesia) is composed of four planes and lasts from the onset of regular breathing to respiratory arrest. Plane 1 includes the time from the onset of rhythmic respiration and absent lid reflex to the cessation of eye movement. During plane 1, the eyes may oscillate or may be eccentrically fixed, and pupillary size changes from dilated to constricted. The vomiting reflex is lost, as is lacrimation. Plane 2 includes the time from absence of eye movement to the beginning of respiratory muscle (intercostal) paralysis. The pupils begin to dilate and become centrally fixed, and muscle tone is decreased. Plane 3 includes the time from the beginning to the completion of respiratory paralysis. Tidal volume is decreased as respiration is accomplished only by the diaphragm. Toward the end of plane 3, the pupils are nonreactive to light. Plane 4 includes the time from complete intercostal paralysis to diaphragmatic paralysis and therefore to cessation of spontaneous respiration. Pupils are dilated and nonreactive. Stage IV (overdosage, apnea) lasts from the onset of diaphragmatic paralysis to cardiac arrest. Most reflexes are absent. Prompt measures must be taken to lighten this inadvertent stage of anesthesia. *See* Figure.

	Respiration Inter-Costal	Diaph-ragm	Ocular Move-ments	Pupils no Pre-med.	Eye Reflexes	Pharynx Larynx Reflexes	Lacri-mation	Muscle Tone	Resp. Response Incision
Stage I			Voluntary Control	◎			Normal	Normal	
Stage II				◎	lid tone	swallow retch vomit		Tense Struggle	
Stage III Plane 1				◎					
Plane 2				◎	corneal pupillary light reflex	glottis			
Plane 3				◎					
Plane 4				◯		carinal			
Stage IV				◯					

Stages and Planes of Anesthesia: The signs and reflex reactions of the stages of anesthesia. The convergency lines indicate progressive loss of the reflex activity as anesthetic depth increases.

Stainless Steel:

Alloy of iron, carbon and chromium that resists corrosion because of a surface coating of chromium oxide that forms on exposure to the atmosphere. This coating is insoluble, self-healing, and nonporous. *See* Steel.

Standard Deviation (SD):

Measure of the dispersion of a series of numbers around their arithmetic mean. It is the square root of the sum of the squared deviation (variance) of each value from the arithmetic mean. (It may also be derived by dividing by one less than the number of squares in the sum of squares rather than taking the arithmetic mean.) A large SD indicates a wide dispersion about the mean, whereas a small SD indicates a distribution close to the mean. For a normal distribution, 68.2770% of all observations lie 1 SD from the arithmetic mean, 95.4570% lie 2 SD from the arithmetic mean, and 99.7370% lie 3 SD from the arithmetic mean. *See* Normal distribution.

Standard Error of the Mean (SEM):

Measurement of data dispersion calculated as the standard deviation (SD) of the sample observations divided by the square root of the number of observations. Large SEMs imply there is a good chance that the mean of the sample is not close to the real mean. The SEM approaches the SD as the number of samples increases.

Standard of Diseases and Operations (SNDO):

Six-digit system for coding diagnoses and surgical procedures formulated by the American Medical Association. *See* ICD.

Standard Temperature and Pressure (STP):

Formal set of conditions to standardize determinants of the physical characteristics of liquids and gases. The conditions correspond to a standard temperature of 0°C (273.15°K) and a standard pressure of 1 atmosphere (approximately 760 mm Hg).

Stat:

Abbreviation for the Latin word *statim*. It is used to indicate that something must be done immediately and without delay. My lunch break is a stat, yours is routine.

State-Trait Anxiety Inventory:

Test consisting of two separate self-reporting scales, each of 20 statements. The respondents indicate to what degree each statement is applicable to themselves. The test attempts to measure both current and general state of anxieties of a test subject.

Static:

Random, unwanted noise present in electric circuits. *See* Signal-to-noise ratio.

Static Flame:

Combustion process in which fuel is combined with O_2 at such a slow rate that the position of the visible flame does not move. A burning candle is an example of a static flame. Even though plenty of wax is available, it melts and burns at such a slow pace that the flame does not consume the entire candle at once. Static flames can ignite explosive gas mixtures such as ether/O_2 when brought into contact with them. *See* Cool flame.

Statistics:

Branch of mathematics that deals with collecting, organizing, analyzing, summarizing, and presenting numeric data.

Status Epilepticus:

Rapid succession of seizures, during which the patient does not regain uninterrupted consciousness or respond to external stimuli. *See* Epilepsy.

Staverman Reflection Coefficient:

Mathematic term expressing the permeability of a membrane to a particular substance. A value of 1 indicates impermeability, and 0 indicates total permeability. This coefficient becomes important when dealing with effects of an oncotic pressure gradient.

Steal Syndrome:

See Intracerebral steal syndrome.

Steel:

Alloy that contains iron and up to 1.7% carbon. Low-carbon steels are malleable, whereas high-carbon steels are brittle. The high-carbon steels are used for tools and high-strength materials even though they are difficult to machine. *See* Stainless steel.

Steinert Disease:

See Myotonia atrophica.

Stelazine:

See Phenothiazine.

Stellate Ganglion:

Star-shaped cluster of nerve cell bodies on the sympathetic trunk formed by fusion of the inferior cervical and first thoracic sympathetic ganglia. It is located on the transverse process of the seventh cervical vertebra and the neck of the first rib. The postganglionic fibers of the stellate ganglion supply blood vessels, sweat glands, salivary glands, retroorbital fat, and heart, and provide pilomotor fibers to the skin of the head, arm, hand, and upper chest. *See* Autonomic nervous system.

Stellate Ganglion Block:

Anesthetic block used to diagnose and treat sympathetic dystrophies of the upper limb and peripheral vascular disease. The landmark for locating the stellate ganglion is the enlarged tubercle of the sixth cervical vertebra (Chassaignac tubercle). Stellate ganglion block dilates the blood vessels of the upper limb and therefore may be performed to aid in some pain relief procedures. The block disrupts the sympathetic nerve supply to the head, upper extremities, and thorax. A successful block is demonstrated on the anesthetized side by Horner syndrome or Horner triad, stuffy nostril, absence of sweating, blushing of the skin, increased lacrimation, and increased temperature of the face and arm. *See* Autonomic nervous system; Horner syndrome.

Stephen-Slater Valve:

See Nonrebreathing valve.

Stereotypic Ventilation:

See Sigh.

Sterilization:

Total destruction and elimination of microorganisms, e.g., bacteria, virus, fungi. Sterilization may be accomplished by different methods, e.g., moist or dry heat, liquid chemical, gas, or gamma radiation depending on the objects to be sterilized. Moist heat in the form of autoclaving is the most dependable method of destroying pathogens. The moisture increases cellular permeability and the heat (>100°C) coagulates protein. Autoclaving, however, may corrode some equipment, deteriorate plastic and rubber, and not penetrate oils, grease, or powder. Dry heat (160°C for 1 hour) may be useful for powder, oil, grease, and glass syringes. Liquid chemical (cold) sterilization is useful for heat-sensitive equipment; however, it is questionable whether a liquid agent can completely sterilize. The gas ethylene oxide (ETO) is used to sterilize anesthetic and respiratory therapy equipment, which is heat- or moisture-sensitive. ETO must be allowed to diffuse out of material such as rubber, however, before tissue contact because it is a strong irritant. Gamma radiation is bactericidal and viricidal. Heat-sensitive objects may be sterilized by this technique. The radioisotope cobalt 60 is commonly used in this method. The items to be sterilized may be prepackaged and remain sterile indefinitely (so long as the package is sealed). Gamma radiation, however, does produce changes in plastics such as polyvinylchloride (PVC). Irradiated PVC articles must not be resterilized with ethylene oxide lest tissue-toxic ethylene chlorohydrin be released. *See* Ethylene oxide sterilization.

Steroid:

See Corticosteroid.

Stethoscope:

Device, invented by Laennec, used during auscultation of sounds in the body. The original stethoscope consisted of a simple wooden tube. The current standard is binaural with the earpieces connected by appropriate tubing to a chest piece that should include both a diaphragm and bell regulated by a valve. The diaphragm is used for high-frequency vibrations, whereas the bell is used for low-pitched sounds and murmurs. The earpieces must fit the ear canal snugly, and the tubing should be as short as possible for efficiency, long enough for comfort, and double-walled to lessen sound distortion. The monaural, or single-ear, stethoscope is used extensively in anesthesia to listen to heart and breath sounds while leaving the other ear free for monitoring alarms. A Ploss valve is used to connect the chest stethoscope and blood pressure stethoscope, automatically switching from one to the other as the cuff is inflated and deflated. *See* Automatic blood pressure device (Dinamap^{TM}).

STI:

See Systolic time intervals.

Stimulus Oxygen Tension (PsO₂):

The partial pressure of oxygen that stimulates hypoxic pulmonary vasoconstriction in the lung. In humans, normal intact lungs have a PsO_2 of 55 mm Hg.

Stoichiometric Mixture:

Chemical mixture in which fuel molecules react completely with O_2 molecules (complete combustion) until no unreacted molecules remain.

Stopcock:

Rotary valve used to redirect or stop flow.

Storage:

Retention of data for later retrieval.

Storage Capacity:

Maximum amount of data or information a memory device is able to retain at one time. *See* Shift register.

Stored Blood:

See Blood storage.

Stovaine:

Obsolete local anesthetic agent synthesized in 1905 (one year before procaine). It was abandoned because it was much more irritating than procaine.

STP:

See Standard temperature and pressure.

Strabismus (Squint):

Abnormality of the coordinating mechanisms of the eye such that the visual axes are misaligned so visual images presented to each eye are not kept on corresponding retinal points. It can be treated surgically with careful muscle shortening.

Strain Gauge:

Instrument for measuring distortions in an object caused by tension, compression, or twisting. This distortion produces a change in the instrument's electronic resistance, capacitance, or inductance that can be quantified to determine the original pressure producing the distortion. (A strain gauge may also be called an extensometer.) *See* Transducer.

Stray Capacitance:

Collection of electric charges of opposing polarity on the two sides of an insulator. It occurs randomly owing to the physical arrangement of components in an electric circuit. Most stray capacitance is undesirable, as it both dissipates energy and produces unwanted feedback of signals throughout an electric circuit. Stray capacitance can be avoided by heavily insulating conductors and by proper routing of electric conduction. *See* Capacitance, electronic.

Stray Inductance:

Casual, unplanned creation of an electromagnetic field around a coiled conductor. Stray inductance can cause unwanted signal transfer and energy loss, as in stray capacitance. *See* Inductance.

Street Ready:

State of patient fitness in which the individual has stable vital signs. Is oriented as to time, place, and person and can be discharged from an outpatient anesthesia facility with an escort.

Streptomycin:

Antibiotic of the aminoglycoside class. Introduced in 1944, it was used against tuberculosis and certain gram-negative microorganisms. Resistance to streptomycin developed rapidly, however, thereby limiting its clinical usefulness for the long-term treatment of bacterial disease. In addition, streptomycin is ototoxic and nephrotoxic. Currently, the use of this agent is limited to unusual infections such as tularemia, bubonic plague, and bacterial endocarditis. Other members of the aminoglycoside class are neomycin, kanamycin, gentamicin, tobramycin, and amikacin; and all produce similar adverse side effects. *See* Aminoglycoside; Antibiotic.

Stress Patterns of Fetal Heart:

See Fetal Heart Rate (FHR) Terminology.

Stridor:

Marked, high-pitched, harsh respiratory sound usually heard during inspiration and caused by acute laryngeal obstruction.

Stroke Volume:

End-diastolic volume of the left ventricle minus the end-systolic volume.

Student *t*-Test:

Statistical measurement that compares two means in an attempt to determine the amount of departure from the standard error of these means. The student *t*-test was developed in 1908 by the statistician Gosset, who published under the pseudonym "Student." The *t*-test is useful for small samples that do not approximate a normal distribution. *See* Standard error of the mean.

Stump Pressure:

Invasive procedure used to measure internal carotid artery stump pressure (ICASP) in the surgically exposed carotid artery. The resulting value provides a relative indication of the adequacy of the collateral circulation to the brain. Stump pressure is normally measured by inserting a small needle immediately proximal to a clamp that occludes the internal carotid artery. The needle is attached to a transducer that directly records pressure. This pressure reading is believed to represent the cerebral perfusion pressure delivered to the cerebral hemisphere on the same side as the clamped vessel. Blood flow is supplied by the internal carotid on the other side and by the vertebral arteries via the circle of Willis. It was believed that a stump pressure of 50 mm Hg or more was a sign of adequate cerebral circulation (collateral flow). It has been shown, however, that this relation is not consistently true. During surgical repair of internal carotid artery occlusion, stump pressures aid in deciding whether or not to shunt a large-bore cannula around the surgical incision site, a technique known as internal carotid shunt.

Stylet:

Wire inserted into the lumen of a tube or catheter to stiffen it in order to facilitate its proper placement. The stylet may also be used to remove foreign material from a catheter, tube, or needle. It may remain inside a needle or catheter to maintain patency.

Stylus:

(1) Heated pointer used to draw tracings on heat-sensitive paper (ECG). (2) Pen-like light source that modifies the display on a computer terminal when it touches the screen.

Subarachnoid Screw (Intracranial Pressure Bolt; Subarachnoid Bolt):

Device for measuring or monitoring intracranial pressure (ICP). A hollow bolt is threaded into a hole in the skull and then through a small dural opening onto the brain surface. The bolt is then attached to a transducer to directly measure pressure. This technique has one advantage over the ventriculostomy catheter in that the screw is easy to insert and does not penetrate brain tissue; it cannot be used, however, to withdraw or sample cerebrospinal fluid. Clinical indications for ICP monitoring include head injuries, hypoxic brain damage, subarachnoid hemorrhage, metabolic coma, stroke, and hydrocephalus. *See* Intracranial pressure measurement; Ventriculostomy catheter.

Subclavian Perivascular Block:

Technique for local anesthetic blocking of the brachial plexus. *See* Brachial plexus block.

Subcutaneous Emphysema:

Air or other gas trapped in the layers of the skin causing an edematous appearance in various body regions. It is most likely to occur because of misplaced insufflating catheters during laparoscopy.

Subcutaneous Pump:

See Subdermal pump.

Subdermal Pump (Subcutaneous Pump):

Complex device implanted under the skin that contains a drug reservoir plus catheter access to either the intravascular space or a body compartment, a pumping mechanism, and an electronic controller. It is used both clinically and experimentally to tonically provide drugs to the body at a controlled rate. For example, intravenous insulin may be administered by the pump based on detection of blood glucose levels. Pain management drugs can be given in the epidural space at a steady rate. Antibiotics can be released continuously. Also referred to as a subcutaneous pump.

Subdural Anesthesia:

See Spinal anesthesia.

Subdural, Subdural Injection:

Interchangeable with intrathecal injection. *See* Intrathecal injection.

Sublimation:

Direct conversion of a solid to a vapor or vice versa with no intervening liquid phase. Dry Ice (solid CO_2) is an example of this physical phenomenon.

Sublimaze:

See Fentanyl.

Subroutine:

See Routine.

Substance P (SP):

An 11-amino acid peptide that plays a role in the transmission of pain. Substance P acts as a sensory neurotransmitter in the dorsal horn. Peripherally, substance P is released from cutaneous nerve endings when pain stimulation is intense, causing vasodilatation and release of histamine from mast cells. *See* Capsaicin.

Substantia Gelatinosa:

See Gate theory of pain.

Succinic Acid:

Breakdown product of succinylmonocholine, one of the final products in the degradation of succinylcholine (succinyldicholine).

Succinylcholine Hypersensitivity:

Phenomenon seen in skeletal muscle that has sustained damage, causing the muscle to be in a catabolic state. It results from direct trauma to the muscle, denervation, burn injury, or simply prolonged forced rest. The hypersensitivity to succinylcholine appears to start after 24 hours from the injury or trauma and has been reported to last up to a year. In those individuals with catabolizing muscle, the administration of succinylcholine causes a huge outpouring of potassium through the muscle membrane into the circulation. Potassium concentration in the serum can increase two to three times the normal level. The effect on the heart is catastrophic: intractable fibrillation often leading to death.

Succinylcholine, Succinyldicholine, Suxamethonium (Anectine):

Depolarizing neuromuscular blocking agent. Its onset of activity is rapid, and its duration of action is short owing to the rapid enzymatic inactivation by plasma pseudocholinesterase. Succinylcholine may be administered both as a single intravenous dose or as a continuous infusion for prolonged procedures to obtain skeletal muscle relaxation. Adverse side effects consist mostly of an extension of the pharmacologic actions of the drug and include bradycardia, increased salivation, and profound or prolonged muscle relaxation, leading eventually to respiratory depression and apnea. Some individuals are sensitive to succinylcholine by virtue of a genetically determined enzyme, atypical plasma cholinesterase. They exhibit prolonged apnea due to a low level of normal cholinesterase. Predisposition may be determined by the "dibucaine number." Other individuals possess an abnormal fluoride-resistant enzyme, or a "silent gene." Patients with a familial history of malignant hyperthermia should be tested for this disorder prior to use of succinylcholine. In addition, because this neuromuscular blocker tends to increase intraocular pressure, it is contraindicated in patients with penetrating eye injuries or acute glaucoma. Lastly, succinylcholine causes a spike-like rise in serum potassium, which pours out of recently damaged or denervated muscle (burns, cord transection). This response can occur within as little as one day after injury and can last up to a year. *See* Dibucaine number; Malignant hyperthermia; Neuromuscular blocking agent; Phase I block; Phase II block.

Succinylcholine Twitch Augmentation:

Effect seen after succinylcholine administration when a single stimulus causes a greater than maximal contraction in a muscle group, innovated by a stimulated nerve. This phenomenon is decreased or abolished by pretreatment with curare.

Succinylmonocholine:

Primary breakdown product of enzymatic hydrolysis (via pseudocholinesterase) of succinylcholine. It is a weak depolarizing agent and is subsequently hydrolyzed to succinic acid and choline by pseudocholinesterase and a liver enzyme. *See* Acetylcholinesterase.

Sudden Infant Death Syndrome (SIDS):

Perplexing, devastating disease that results in infant death, with a peak incidence between 1 month and 1 year. Certain groups of infants (e.g., premature babies, infants who have had bronchopulmonary dysplasia, or those who have had "infant apnea syndrome") are at increased risk. The infant apnea syndrome is the new name for the old self-explanatory "near-miss sudden infant death syndrome." Some of these infants appear to have a decreased response to elevation of arterial CO_2. Although premature infants who are later anesthetized have an increase in postoperative apnea (need apnea monitors) to the postconceptual age of 50 weeks, there is no evidence that general anesthesia triggers SIDS or infant apnea syndrome. There is some connection between families of children who die of SIDS and malignant hyperthermia. *See* Malignant hyperthermia.

Sudomotor Pathway:

Pathway by which sweat glands are innervated.

Sufentanil:

See Fentanyl.

Suggestibility:

See Hypnosis.

Summation:

Combined pharmacologic effect in which the total effect of two or more drugs equals the sum of their individual actions. *See* Antagonism; Synergism.

Sunstroke:

See Heatstroke.

Superconductivity:

Physical phenomenon occurring in many metals and alloys during which there is virtually complete disappearance of electrical resistance when the metals are cooled to temperatures approaching absolute zero. Electrical equipment operating at or near absolute zero can perform an enormous amount of work and yet remain small.

Supercooling (Profound Hypothermia):

See Hypothermia.

Superheating:

Careful heating of a liquid under specific pressure conditions so it remains a liquid beyond its normal boiling point.

Superoxide (O_2^-):

Anion produced by vascular endothelial cells when exposed to soluble or particulate stimuli. Believed to be an agent for cellular damage.

Supersaturated Vapor:

Phenomenon seen when a vapor remains vaporous under a pressure that exceeds the normal amount needed for condensation to a liquid.

Supine Hypotensive Syndrome:

See Aortocaval syndrome.

Supraclavicular Block:

Approach to the local anesthetic injection of the brachial plexus, it uses a small amount of solution but requires elicitation of a paresthesia for proper placement of a local anesthetic solution. There is significant incidence of pneumothorax as a negative sequela. *See* Axillary nerve block.

Supramaximal Stimulation:

See Neuromuscular blockade, assessment of.

Supraspinous Ligament:

See Lumbar puncture.

Surface-Active Agent:

Substance used to reduce surface tension between two liquids or a liquid and solid. Surface-active agents are classified into three categories: emulsifier, wetting agent, and detergent. An emulsifier stabilizes a mixture of two or more liquids that would otherwise be immiscible. Wetting agents are added to water to facilitate penetration into or flow over another surface by reducing the surface tension of water. Detergents concentrate at oil-water interfaces, thereby emulsifying oil. The terms detergent, wetting agent, and emulsifier are often used interchangeably. *See* Surface tension.

Surface Tension:

Physical phenomenon occurring at the interface of two liquids or of a liquid and a gas. The interior molecules of the liquid are attracted by other molecules equally in all directions. At the surface, molecules are attracted toward the interior of the liquid. This uneven pull deforms the surface of the liquid, which acts as if it is covered by an elastic membrane. Surface tension is measured in newtons per meter. *See* Surface-active agent.

Surfactant:

Phospholipid (lecithin and sphingomyelin) produced by type II (septal) alveolar cells. Surfactant helps prevent the collapse of alveoli by decreasing surface tension in the lungs. It forms a thin coating over the alveoli, so they are not pulled in on themselves following expiration. Inadequate amounts of surfactant at birth result in hyaline membrane disease (infant respiratory distress syndrome). Synthetic surfactants (Exosurf) can be administered down the trachea to treat this condition. *See* Infant respiratory distress syndrome.

Surital:

See Thiamylal.

Suxamethonium:

British term for succinylcholine. *See* Succinylcholine.

SVR:

See Systemic vascular resistance.

Swan-Ganz Catheter (Pulmonary Artery Catheter):

Device used for hemodynamic monitoring, usually in cardiac patients. The catheter, introduced into the venous system through the subclavian, femoral, or internal jugular vein, is then advanced to the level of the superior vena cava, then to the right ventricle, and ultimately into the pulmonary artery. The tip of the catheter is flow-directed by an inflatable balloon. The catheter is left in place for continuous monitoring of pulmonary arterial pressure (PAP), cardiac output (CO), and, indirectly, mean left atrial pressure. The Swan-Ganz catheter is available in sizes 5- and 7-French (Fr) for adults (smaller sizes are available for children). The 5-Fr catheter has one pressure lumen at its tip to record PAP, whereas the 7-Fr has two pressure lumens: one at the tip for measuring PAP and one more distally located for measuring central venous pressure (CVP). The catheters come with or without a thermistor that measures cardiac output (CO) by the thermal dilution technique. Newer catheters may also have a pacing port for temporary pacemaker deployment. *See* Figures, Table. *See* Cardiac output.

Swan-Ganz Catheter: Normal Swan-Ganz catheter values.

	PRESSURE IN MMHG
Right Atrium	
Mean	−1 to +7
Right Ventricle	
Systolic	15-25
End Diastolic	0-8
Pulmonary Artery	
Systolic	15-25
Diastolic	8-15
Mean	10-20
Pulmonary Wedge	
Mean	6-12

Sweating:

See Diaphoresis.

SWMA:

See Segmental wall motion abnormalities.

Sympathetic Dystrophy:

See Causalgia.

Sympathetic Nerve Block:

Class of regional anesthetic injections that interrupt transmission in sympathetic fibers and produce vasodilation, increased blood flow, and a rise in skin temperature. Because sympathetic fibers are blocked by a low concentration of local anesthetic, sympathetic block can often be accomplished without affecting sensory or motor nerve fibers. Examples are blocks of the paravertebral lumbar, celiac, and stellate ganglia. These regional blocks may be performed for diagnostic, therapeutic, or prognostic reasons during the first stage of labor and are indicated for use in patients with causalgia, peripheral vascular disease, vasospasm, and abdominal pain due to acute or chronic pancreatitis or pancreatic carcinoma. *See* Autonomic nervous system; Causalgia; Celiac plexus block; Paravertebral lumbar sympathetic block.

Sympathetic Nervous System:

See Autonomic nervous system.

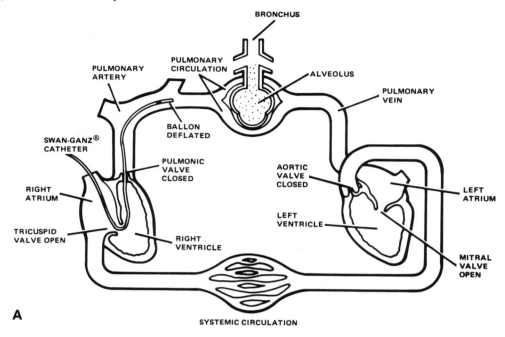

A

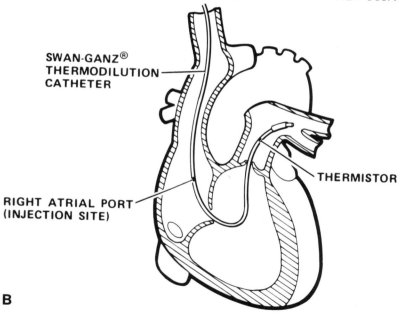

B

Swan-Ganz Catheter: (A) Insertion. (B) Inserted in periphery advancing through pulmonary artery. (C) Catheter placed during surgery. (D) Pressure changes as the catheter moves through the right heart.

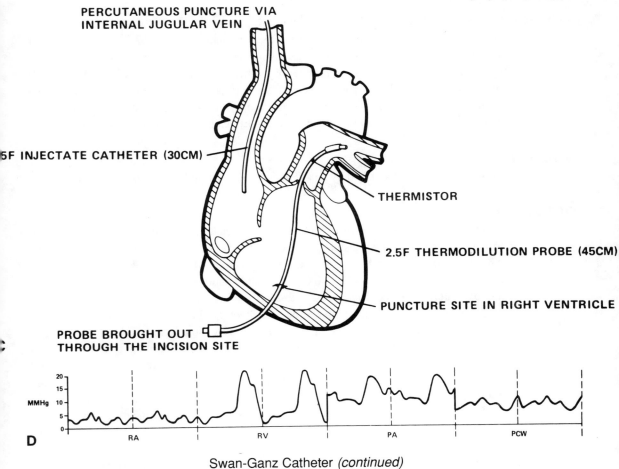

PERCUTANEOUS PUNCTURE VIA
INTERNAL JUGULAR VEIN

5F INJECTATE CATHETER (30CM)

THERMISTOR

2.5F THERMODILUTION PROBE (45CM)

PUNCTURE SITE IN RIGHT VENTRICLE

PROBE BROUGHT OUT
THROUGH THE INCISION SITE

D

MMHg

RA   RV   PA   PCW

Swan-Ganz Catheter *(continued)*

Sympathetic Tone; Parasympathetic Tone:

Basal rates of the activity of the sympathetic and parasympathetic systems, the two components of the autonomic nervous system. Under circumstances that increase or decrease the degree of stimulation of either segment, this tone can be enhanced or decreased. Diethyl ether and cyclopropane were two general anesthetics that maintain or increase sympathetic tone. In addition, the basal level of activity of the sympathetic nervous system is partially regulated by the secretion of epinephrine and norepinephrine. *See* Sympathomimetic drug.

Sympatholytic Agent:

Drug that blocks or reverses the actions of the sympathetic nervous system or sympathomimetic (adrenergic) agents. Phentolamine (Regitine), for example, blocks alpha receptors, thereby counteracting vasoconstriction. *See* Receptor/receptor site.

565

Sympathomimetic Drug (Adrenergic Drug):

Agent that mimics the pharmacologic effects of adrenergic nerve or adrenal medulla stimulation. Some sympathomimetic drugs interact directly with adrenergic receptors (e.g., epinephrine, norepinephrine, isoproterenol). Other agents act indirectly by stimulating the release of norepinephrine from nerve endings (e.g, amphetamine, ephedrine). Sympathomimetic drugs produce mainly vasoconstriction, with some vasodilation, and they generally increase heart rate and blood pressure. *See* Epinephrine; Norepinephrine.

Symptom:

Subjective sensation reported by a patient and not observable by an examiner. *See* Sign.

Synapse:

Junction between two neurons. Impulses are conducted or transmitted from one nerve cell to another at the synapse. Neurons proximal to the synapse are known as presynaptic, whereas those distal to the synapse are postsynaptic. At the synapse there is no direct physical contact between the pre- and postsynaptic neurons; they are separated by a gap of approximately 200–300 angstroms. Axons of the presynaptic neurons release chemical mediators (neurotransmitters) that either block or facilitate impulse transmission. The action of the neurotransmitter is rapidly terminated by either reuptake by the presynaptic membrane or degradation by enzymes in the gap. In the central nervous system two classes of synapses exist; excitatory and inhibitory. Excitatory synapse transmitters (e.g., acetylcholine) cause depolarization in the postsynaptic membrane and thus facilitate impulse transmission, whereas inhibitory synapse transmitters (e.g., gamma-aminobutyric acid, or GABA) hyperpolarize the postsynaptic membrane and thus block neurotransmission. *See* Neuromuscular blockade, assessment of.

Synchronization Mode (Synch Mode; Cardioversion Synchronization):

Electrical modality found on defibrillators used for cardioversion. When activated, the patient's electrocardiogram (ECG) is constantly monitored and the pulse discharge is synchronized with the ECG to avoid the peak of the T wave. Synchronization is done to prevent inadvertent ventricular fibrillation. *See* Cardioversion.

Synchronized Cardioversion:

Treatment for ventricular tachycardia. It requires a defibrillator that can detect the QRS and fires approximately 10 ms after the peak of the R wave, In this way the shock avoids the T wave, which is the electrically vulnerable period when external stimulation may cause further fibrillation.

Synchronized Intermittent Mandatory Ventilation (SIMV):

Similar to intermittent mandatory ventilation (IMV), this type of mechanical ventilation allows the patient to breathe at his or her own rate between mechanical breaths. The mandatory breath of the IMV mode is synchronized to begin at fixed time intervals or at a fixed spontaneous breath count. The efficacy of this technique over routine IMB has been questioned. *See* Assisted mechanical ventilation; Ventilator.

Syncurine:

See Decamethonium.

Syndrome:

Group of signs and symptoms that consistently appear together to characterize a specific disease entity or abnormality.

Synergism:

Combined action of two or more drugs in which the total effect produced is more than the sum of their individual effects. For example, if antibiotic A kills 10,000 bacteria/hour and antibiotic B kills 15,000 bacteria/hour, synergism exists if the concurrent administration of A and B kills more than 25,000 bacteria/hour. *See* Potentiation; Summation.

Syngeneic Transplantation:

See Transplantation.

Syringe:

Cylinder with a plunger and a narrow opening at one end to accept the hub of a needle. A syringe may be plastic or glass and is used for injection, withdrawal, or irrigation. The injecting syringe has been used in medicine for about 120 years.

Syrosingopine (Singoserp):

Closely related to reserpine, this drug is used as an antihypertensive agent.

System, Real-Time:

See Real-time analysis.

Systemic Vascular Resistance (SVR):

Measured as the mean arterial pressure (MAP) minus the right atrial pressure (RAP) divided by coronary output.

Systems Analysis:

Study of any activity, procedure, or technique that improves the flow of information and increases the rapidity of the operation.

Systolic Pressure:

Peak pressure reached in the large arteries due to contraction of the ventricle.

Systolic Time Intervals (STI):

Breakdown of left ventricular systole into time segments. These measurements are a noninvasive method to evaluate myocardial ventricular function. The time intervals are defined as follows: (1) Pre-ejection period (PEP) is the time from the onset of electrical activity in the ventricle (Q wave) until the beginning ejection of blood. (2) Isovolumic contraction time (ICT) is the time between the start of the ventricular pressure rise to the start of ejection. (3) Left ventricular ejection time (LVET) comprises the period from the beginning to the end of ejection. The entire period, from the onset of the Q wave through the end of ejection, is called electromechanical systole (EMS). PEP appears to be an indication of myocardial contractility. The weaker the heart, the longer it takes the ventricle to develop enough pressure to open the aortic valve and begin ejection. PEP encompasses the first derivative of left ventricular pressure measurement (dP/dt), which is a continuous record of the slope of the left ventricular pressure curve and is by itself an index of left heart function. When the contraction is strong, pressure rises quickly, the slope becomes steep, and the dP/dt is short. Indirect measurement of STI requires three simultaneous recordings: electrocardiogram, heart sounds, and peripheral pulse wave.

T

Tachycardia:
Abnormally fast heart rate.

Tachyphylaxis:
Form of drug tolerance that develops acutely with only a few doses of a pharmacologic agent. Observed in both long- and short-acting intravenous anesthetics, the reasons for it remain unknown.

Tachypnea:
Abnormally rapid breathing rate.

Talwin:
See Narcotic; Pentazocine.

Tank Ventilator:
See Iron lung.

TAPSE:
See Tricuspid annular plane systolic excursion.

TEA:
See Tetraethylammonium.

Technetium 99 (^{99}Tc):
Radioactive element (gamma-ray emitter) that may be tagged onto another molecule that has an affinity for a particular body site. When injected intravenously, the ^{99}Tc travels to the target organ e.g., heart, thyroid, liver) and outlines it to a gamma-ray detector placed over the organ. It has been used to outline tumors and differential blood flow patterns, as well as to label albumin to locate the attachment of the placenta. *See* Cold spot imaging.

Technetium 99 (^{99m}Tc) Pyrophosphate (Hot Spot Imaging):
Radioactive compound which when injected intravenously, preferentially concentrates at sites of myocardial infarction. *See* Thallium 201.

TEE:
See Transesophageal echocardiography.

Teflurane:

Fluorinated hydrocarbon that has physiochemical properties (except flammability) similar to those of cyclopropane. After limited clinical trials, interest in its use as a general anesthetic ceased owing to a high incidence of cardiac arrhythmias.

Tegretol:

See Carbamazepine; Trigeminal neuralgia.

Telemetry:

Remote recording or evaluation of information. It usually involves an acquisition system at the measurement site that sends data by automatic sensors to a central location. The most typical application in medicine is the electrocardiographic (ECG) portable telemetry unit, which converts the ECG signal into a radio signal and broadcasts it to a receiver at a remote location. The patient can wear this unit, and free movement is possible without physical attachment to an ECG machine.

Temperature:

Amount or degree of "hotness" or "coldness." Temperature is a measure of the mean kinetic energy of random molecular motions. The temperature of an object determines the direction of heat flow when it is brought into contact with another substance, as heat flows from regions of higher to lower temperatures. Temperature can also be considered the relative amount of vibration of the individual atoms of a substance. As the temperature drops, the vibration decreases. Theoretically, all motion ceases at absolute zero. The concept that relative molecular vibrations account for temperature differentials explains the phenomenon of evaporative cooling. The faster atoms escape into the vapor phase, decreasing the average vibration of the remaining atoms. *See* Celsius scale; Hypothermia.

Temperature Blanket (Heating or Cooling Blanket):

Device for heating or cooling the body by means of surface application of hot or cold temperatures. A typical temperature blanket is composed of two layers of rubberized material that contain coils for the passage of water or a mixture of alcohol and water. Hoses lead from the blanket back to the heating and cooling machine, which usually has both manual and automatic modes of operation. In the manual mode, the device either heats or cools the fluid running through the blanket, cycling on and off depending on a preset temperature. In the automatic mode, a probe placed on or in a patient is used to sense body temperature and cycles the device as required. *See* Figure.

Temperature Coefficient of Resistance:

Specific physical property of a material that is the amount of electrical resistance change per unit temperature change. In general, most materials have a positive coefficient or resistance; as they become hotter, their resistance increases. Semiconductors, however, have a negative coefficient of resistance; their resistance decreases as they become hotter.

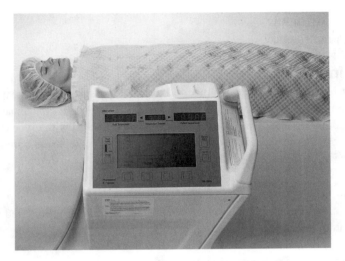

Temperature Blanket: Heating and cooling blanket along with its appropriate hypo/hyperthermia system.

Temporal Disintegration:

See Cannabis.

Tenckhoff Catheter:

Particular type of indwelling peritoneal catheter used for peritoneal dialysis.

Tengesic:

See Buprenorphine.

TENS:

See Transcutaneous electrical nerve stimulation.

Tensile Strength:

Greatest force a material can withstand before it is physically disrupted.

Tensilon:

See Edrophonium.

Tension:

Condition of being taut, strained, stretched, or under pressure.

Tension of a Gas:

See Partial pressure.

Tension Pneumothorax:

See Pneumothorax.

Tension Time Index (TTI):

Means for evaluating cardiac function. It is the measurement of the area under the systolic portion of the aortic pressure curve and is calculated as the mean systolic pressure × duration of systole. This index correlates relatively well with myocardial O_2 consumption. The correlation becomes poorer during exercise, epinephrine administration, or sympathetic activation. *See* Systolic time intervals.

Teratogenesis:

Formation of a defect-anatomic, biochemical, or behavioral-initiated in utero and detected at birth or later.

Tetanic Contraction (Tetanization):

State in which muscle stimulation occurs so frequently that successive contractions fuse together and cannot be distinguished from one another. Critical frequency is the lowest frequency of stimulation at which tetanization occurs. *See* Neuromuscular blockade, assessment of.

Tetanic Stimulation:

See Neuromuscular blockade, assessment of.

Tetanus (Lockjaw):

Acute infectious disease characterized by tonic muscular spasms of the jaws and neck. It is caused by the toxin of *Clostridium tetani,* an anaerobic bacillus. Tetanus has a high mortality rate characterized by autonomic nervous system instability when untreated. Severe tetanus is one of the few conditions that may be treated primarily by an anesthesiologist because of his or her expertise in the areas of muscle relaxants and ventilatory care.

Tetracaine Hydrochloride (Amethocaine; Pontocaine):

Local anesthetic of the ester series. It can be injected or applied topically. Tetracaine is a highly potent drug (10 times more toxic and active than procaine after intravenous injection) that has a long duration of action. It has a slow onset of action when administered as a caudal anesthetic, but its effects are long-lasting. It is commonly used as a spinal anesthetic and as a topical anesthetic for the eyes, pharynx, and tracheobronchial tree. It is rapidly absorbed through mucous membranes and therefore its use should be limited to small areas. There is a great potential for systemic toxicity. *See* EMLA; Local anesthetic.

Tetracyclines:

Class of broad-spectrum antibiotics that has been used clinically since the late 1940s. The closely related tetracycline derivatives include tetracycline (Tetracyn), chlortetracycline (Aureomycin), oxytetracycline (Terramycin), and doxycycline (Vibramycin). Absorption of tetracyclines is incomplete in the gastrointestinal tract and is impaired by milk and milk products, antacids containing aluminum, and oral iron preparations. Administration of tetracyclines is not recommended for pregnant patients or children under 8 years of age because the drug is specifically stored in the growing bones and teeth, resulting in brown discoloration of teeth as they become calcified. *See* Table. *See* Antibiotic.

Tetracyclines.

Generic Name (Trade Name)	Spectrum of Activity	Comments
Tetracycline (Tetracyn) PO IM IV	Broad spectrum including G^- and G^+ microbes, Mycoplasma, Treponema, Borrelia, Leptospira, Rickettsia, Chlamydia and some protozoa, including amebas.	Tetracycline is bacteriostatic except in high concentrations. Its oral absorption is impaired by calcium, oral iron preparations, magnesium and antacids containing aluminum. All of the tetracyclines are stored in the body in growing bones and teeth, thus should not be given to pregnant women or children under 8 yrs of age. Side effects include hypersensitivity reactions, GI disturbances, photosensitivity and superinfections that can lead to staphylococcal enterocolitis. Hepatotoxicity can occur with larger doses, as can nephrotoxicity.
Chlortetracycline (Aureomycin)	Similar to Tetracycline.	Similar to Tetracycline.
Oxytetracycline (Terramycin) PO IM	Similar to Tetracycline. It is used in the treatment of amebiasis.	Oxytetracycline shows a high incidence of GI disturbances.
Demeclocycline (Declomycin) PO	Similar to Tetracycline.	Demeclocycline shows a high incidence of photosensitivity reactions. It has a longer half-life than Tetracycline and is more potent.
Methacycline (Rondomycin) PO	Similar to Tetracycline.	Methacycline has a longer half-life.
Doxycycline (Vibramycin) PO IV	Similar to Tetracycline.	Doxycycline is the best absorbed of the Tetracyclines. It has greater potency, as well as a longer half-life and duration of action. It does not accumulate in the blood in conditions of renal failure and has less impact on intestinal flora than the other Tetracyclines.
Minocycline (Minocin) PO IV	Similar to Tetracycline.	Minocycline has greater potency and a longer half-life than Tetracycline. It can cause vestibular toxicity. It appears to be metabolized almost completely in vivo.

Note: Tetracyclines are rarely used intravenously or topically.

Tetraethylammonium (TEA):

Ganglionic blocking agent currently of no clinical interest.

Tetrahydrocannabinol:

See Cannabis.

Tetralogy of Fallot:

Group of congenital cardiac defects including ventricular septal defect, pulmonary artery stenosis, right ventricular hypertrophy, and overriding aorta. These anomalies are all associated with obstruction of pulmonary outflow to some degree; if severe, the infant may be markedly cyanotic at birth. Most children with this disorder, however, appear cyanotic by 6 months of age. *See* Eisenmenger syndrome.

Tetrodotoxin (TTX):

Marine toxin derived from the Japanese puffer fish, investigated as a possible local anesthetic as it is a highly selective blocker of sodium channels on the exterior of cell membranes. TTX and its derivatives are currently considered too toxic for clinical use.

Thalamus:

Large oval structure located within the diencephalon on either side of the third ventricle. It serves as a relay center for sensory impulses that reach the cerebral cortex from the spinal cord, brainstem, cerebellum, and parts of the cerebrum. The thalamus also aids in the perception of some types of sensation, e.g., pain and temperature. *See* Limbic system.

Thalassemia:

See Anemia.

Thallium 201 (^{201}Tl) imaging:

Nuclear scanning procedure to detect exercise-induced decreased coronary perfusion. The radioisotope ^{201}Tl is injected intravenously at the time of maximum treadmill exercise. Areas of ischemia or scarring of the myocardium appear as defects in the scintigram of the myocardium. After a rest of 4 hours, another image is made of the myocardium. Previous areas of poor perfusion appear normal, whereas infarcted areas still appear poorly perfused at rest. *See* Technetium 99 pyrophosphate.

Thallium 201 (Cold Spot Imaging):

Radiotracer technique used for determining the extent of recent myocardial infarction. It is particularly sensitive during the first 24 hours after the event. It is not as specific as technetium 99 pyrophosphate. *See* Technetium 99 pyrophosphate.

Tham:

See Tromethamine.

Thebaine:

Natural alkaloid found with morphine and codeine in the poppy plant. It has no current clinical use.

Therapeutic Index (Therapeutic Ratio):

Ratio of LD_{50} to ED_{50} in animal experiments. The safety of the drug increases as the ratio increases. In clinical situations, however, the therapeutic ratio is the ratio of the TD_{50} (toxic dose 50%) to the ED_{50}. The estimated TD_{50} is used because a precise determination is both hazardous and unethical and therefore experimentally impossible. *See* ED_{50}; LD_{50}.

Therapeutic Nerve Block:

Injection of a local anesthetic around a nerve in order to treat disease or alleviate pain. An example of a therapeutic nerve block is injection of a local anesthetic into the chest wall to relieve the pain from fractured ribs. *See* Sympathetic nerve block.

Therapeutic Range:

Plasma concentration of a drug with which a satisfactory pharmacologic response (minimal or absent toxicity) is achieved.

Thermistor:

Semiconductor that has a large negative coefficient of resistance. As it is warmed, more current flows through it. A thermistor can be used for temperature measurement or as a controlling unit in electronic circuits. *See* Swan-Ganz catheter; Temperature coefficient of resistance.

Thermocouple (Thermal Junction):

Junction of two dissimilar metals across which an electrical potential is produced when the metals are kept at different temperatures. The potential difference is proportional to the temperature difference, and thermocouples can therefore be used to quantify this difference. If a voltage is applied across the junction of two metals, heat is discharged or absorbed (Peltier effect). Reversing the direction of the voltage reverses this effect. The *See*beck effect is an electromotive force produced when two junctions of dissimilar metals are at varying temperatures in the same circuit. A thermopile is a number of junctions connected together to increase the sensitivity of the thermocouple.

Thermodilution Cardiac Output:

Technique for determining cardiac output. A solution colder than the blood is injected through the proximal port of a multilumen intracardiac catheter (Swan Ganz catheter), and the temperature difference is detected at the distal end of the catheter. The shape of the plotted change in blood temperature is then correlated with cardiac output by computer. *See* Swan-Ganz catheter.

Thermometer, Clinical:

Instrument used to determine body temperature. It operates by the expansion of a mercury column along a scale. It is calibrated between 94° and 108°F or between 35° and 42°C.

Thermopile:

See Thermocouple.

Thermoregulatory Threshold:

Temperature at which centrally mediated, peripheral vasoconstriction occurs as the central temperature drops. This threshold is markedly lowered during anesthesia. The thermoregulatory vasoconstriction that starts to occur at the thermoregulatory threshold is characterized by a threshold value and variable intensity.

Thiamylal (Surital):

Ultrashort-acting barbiturate with pharmacologic properties similar to those of thiopental. *See* Barbiturate; Thiopental sodium.

Thiazides:

Group of diuretic agents useful for controlling hypertension and edema. These agents are to be used with caution in the diabetic patient. In addition, they tend to increase uric acid levels and induce hypokalemia. Serum potassium levels should be monitored closely, and potassium supplementation may be necessary.

Thiethylperazine (Torecan):

Phenothiazine derivative currently useful as an antiemetic agent. *See* Phenothiazine.

Thiopental Sodium (Pentothal):

Oxybarbiturate used primarily as an intravenous anesthetic agent. Currently considered the standard induction agent to which other agents are compared, its action on the brain is enhanced because it is highly lipid-soluble and readily crosses the blood-brain barrier. Thiopental depresses both brain metabolism and O_2 consumption, and it appears to protect the brain against some anoxic insult. Its central nervous system action is thought to terminate mainly by redistribution out of the brain rather than by metabolism. *See* Barbiturate.

Thioxanthene:

Group of antipsychotic drugs similar to the phenothiazine derivatives. Chlorprothixene (Taractan) and thiothixene (Navane) are examples of thioxanthene derivatives. *See* Antipsychotic agent.

Third Party Carriers:

Legal entities such as insurance companies and health maintenance organizations that assume responsibility for medical expense payment to physicians and hospitals.

Third Space:

Body fluid volume that is not intracellular fluid (first space) or extracellular fluid (second space) but, rather, is sequestered to some degree so it cannot easily interact with either. Significant third space fluid is seen with massive ascites, crush injuries, and burns. It is also present in the peritoneum, bowel wall, and lumen of the gastrointestinal tract during abdominal surgery. Third space volume is variable, depending on the extent and duration of surgery or trauma. Significant third space volume causes difficulty in the fluid and electrolyte management of patients. As this fluid is within the body, it ultimately must be mobilized and returned to the circulation so it can be suitably redistributed or excreted. In acute situations, however, because it is not available to the circulation, the fluid may have to be replaced by immediate additions to the circulation.

Thomsen Disease:

See Myotonia congenita.

Thoracic Bioimpedance:

Technique employing four electrodes placed on the neck and chest. One pair places an alternating current into the thorax, and this current is detected by the second pair of electrodes. The resistance to the injected current depends on the fluid characteristics of the thorax. It is possible to calculate stroke volume of the heart using this technique. *See* Figure. *See* Continuous wave doppler ultrasonography.

Thoroughfare Channel:

See Microcirculation.

Thorpe Tube:

See Flowmeter.

Threshold:

Point at which a stimulus just begins to elicit a response. For example, a nerve membrane threshold is the state of membrane polarization just prior to depolarization.

Threshold Block:

See Wedensky effect.

Thrombocytopenia:

Condition in which there is a decrease in the number of platelets. Thrombocytopenia can be the result of decreased production (due to cytotoxic chemotherapeutic agents), increased destruction (disseminated intravascular coagulation), defective maturation (vitamin B_{12} or folate deficiency; myeloproliferative disorders; Wiskott-Aldrich syndrome), altered distribution (massive splenomegaly), or antibody-mediated thrombocytopenia (autoantibodies; alloantibodies). *See* Platelet.

577

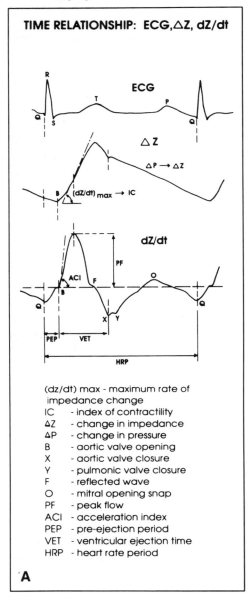

TIME RELATIONSHIP: ECG,△Z, dZ/dt

ECG

△Z

△P → △Z

B (dZ/dt) max → IC

dZ/dt

PF

ACI F

B

O

Q Q

X Y

PEP VET

HRP

(dz/dt) max - maximum rate of
   impedance change
IC   - index of contractility
△Z   - change in impedance
△P   - change in pressure
B   - aortic valve opening
X   - aortic valve closure
Y   - pulmonic valve closure
F   - reflected wave
O   - mitral opening snap
PF   - peak flow
ACI   - acceleration index
PEP   - pre-ejection period
VET   - ventricular ejection time
HRP   - heart rate period

A

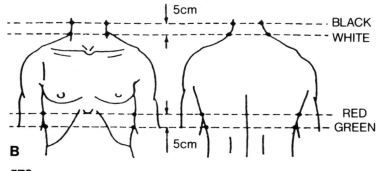

5cm

BLACK
WHITE

RED
GREEN

5cm

B

Thoracic Bioimpedance: (A)
Elements of the measurement
of thoracic bioimpedance. (B)
Placement of bioimpedance
electrodes.

Thromboelastograph:

Device and technique for recognizing and managing coagulopathies. It traces clot strength verses time in a sample of blood. Its use and efficacy is controversial.

Thrombophlebitis:

Inflammation of the wall of a vein associated with the formation of a thrombus. In the practice of anesthesia, thrombophlebitis is most commonly seen in veins that have been used for infusing drugs with irritating qualities, (e.g., thiopental and diazepam). Thrombophlebitis may also be due to blood stasis in the veins of the lower extremities when the patient has been immobile for an extended period.

Thromboxane:

Placental prostaglandin that appears to decrease uteroplacental blood flow and to increase uterine activity, platelet aggregation, and vasoconstriction. *See* Eicosanoids.

Thyroid Cartilage:

Large, prominent cartilage that forms most of the anterior and lateral walls of the larynx. It is attached above to the hyoid bone by the thyrohyoid membrane. Below, it articulates with the cricoid cartilage, but this is variable. The anterior junction between the thyroid and cricoid is formed by the cricothyroid ligament. The thyroid cartilage is open and incomplete posteriorly. *See* Cricoid cartilage; Larynx.

Thyroid Steal:

Obsolete anesthesia induction technique for patients with hyperthyroidism. Tribromoethanol (Avertin) was rectally administered to allow the patient to be quietly "stolen" away to the operating room, thereby preventing anxiety which would trigger catecholamine release and thyroid storm. *See* Thyroid storm; Tribromoethanol.

Thyroid Storm:

Complication of hyperthyroid disease characterized by a sudden massive increase in metabolism, leading to increased O_2 demand, hyperpyrexia, and life-threatening arrhythmias. Treatment includes correction of fluid and electrolyte imbalance and administration of propranolol and other beta-blockers and possibly a short-acting barbiturate (thiopental sodium). *See* Beta blocker; Thyroid steal.

Tibial Nerve Palsy:

Iatrogenic injury seen in patients who have been poorly or carelessly positioned on the operating table. The tibial nerve may be compressed against the head of the fibula by stirrups.

Tic Douloureux:

See Trigeminal neuralgia.

Tidal Volume (TV):

Amount of air that moves into and out of the lungs during each respiratory cycle. *See* Lung volumes and capacities.

Tight Brain:

Condition that results from intracranial hypertension. Usually manifested by bulging of the dura and brain material as a craniotomy flap is removed. Diuretics and hyperventilation may in part relieve this condition. *See* Mannitol.

Time Constant:

Time necessary for a physical characteristic to increase by approximately 63% of its full value or to decrease by 37% of its initial value. In respiratory physiology, the time constant is the time required for a 63% washin (washout) of a new gas from the lungs.

Time Tension Index:

See Tension time index.

Time Units:

See Relative value guide.

Time-Weighted Average (TWA) Gas Sampling:

Method used to determine an average level of trace anesthetic contamination. Ambient atmospheric gas is continuously pumped into an inert bag at a constant low flow rate. The average contamination is determined by analyzing the trace anesthetic concentration in the bag. *See* Grab sample.

Timing Principle:

Technique for rapid induction of anesthesia that uses a single bolus of a nondepolarizing muscle relaxant, which is then followed by administration of an induction agent that is timed to the onset of clinical weakness. *See* Priming principle.

Timolol:

Nonselective beta-blocker with little or no intrinsic sympathomimetic activity and no membrane-stabilizing activity. It is five to ten times as potent as propranolol.

Tissue Solubility:

Quantity of a drug or anesthetic in a tissue at an equilibrium point. The term is often used interchangeably with blood-tissue solubility coefficient.

TIVA:

See Total intravenous anesthesia.

T_{max}:

Time when maximum plasma levels of an administered drug are seen. T_{max} is a composite of rate of absorption and rate of elimination.

To-and-Fro Carbon Dioxide Absorption:

Anesthesia system (obsolete) for the rebreathing of expired gas during which nearly all the CO_2 is absorbed. The absorption canister is placed close to the anesthesia mask or endotracheal tube. CO_2 absorption produces a large amount of heat, which does not dissipate well owing to the limited space between the canister and the patient. This heat may elevate the patient's temperature. Other disadvantages of the to-and-fro system include the possibility of absorber dust entering the patient's respiratory tract and the system's inadequacy for use in head and neck surgery due to the proximity of the surgical field. Advantages of the system include its low resistance and its simplicity. *See* Figure.

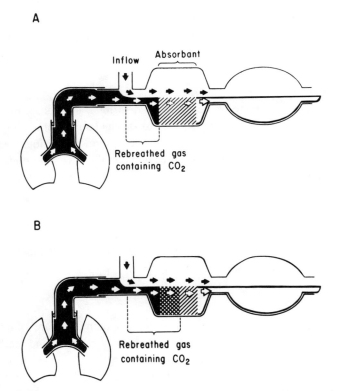

To-and-Fro Carbon Dioxide Absorption: Illustration of the to-and-fro absorber system before (A) and after (B) partial exhaustion of the absorbant. The rebreathed gas containing CO_2 increases as the absorbant becomes exhausted. However, even with fresh absorbant, rebreathing of expired gas (albeit without CO_2) must occur at low inflow rates. Such rebreathing will lower the inspired anesthetic concentration.

Tobramycin (Nebcin):

Antibiotic of the aminoglycoside series useful for treating infections caused by gram-negative organisms. It is closely related to gentamicin, is nephrotoxic and ototoxic, and may enhance neuromuscular blockade. *See* Aminoglycoside; Antibiotic.

Tocodynamometer:

Device for measuring uterine activity that is applied to the maternal abdomen. This force is detected by a variable-resistance strain gauge or similar device, and the resultant pressure is converted into an electrical signal. It is a qualitative rather than a quantitative device.

Tocolytic:

Any of various drugs ranging from β-adrenergic agents such as ritodrine to ethanol to magnesium sulfate and specific prostaglandins, which are administered to inhibit premature labor. Currently, ritodrine is the only β-adrenergic agent approved by the Food and Drug Administration for this purpose.

Tolazoline Hydrochloride (Priscoline):

Weak α-blocking agent with a direct relaxant effect on vascular smooth muscles. It is a cardiac stimulant and produces tachycardia.

Tolbutamide (Orinase):

Oral sulfonylurea hypoglycemic agent used to treat adult-onset diabetes of the insulin-independent type in patients uncontrolled by diet and unable or unwilling to take insulin. Its use is now controversial, as it may have long-term deleterious cardiovascular effects. Tolbutamide may produce an intolerance to alcoholic beverages and various gastrointestinal complaints (less appetite, cramps, nausea, diarrhea). Its use is contraindicated in patients with hepatic or renal insufficiency.

Tolerance:

Need for increasing amounts of a drug to produce the same therapeutic effect as previously possible with lower doses. *See* Tachyphylaxis.

Tomography:

Radiologic technique for forming a roentgenographic picture of one plane or section through a body part. It involves moving both the x-ray tube and the film simultaneously, with the theoretic pivot being at the level of the section desired. This method blurs all other structures above and below the section while leaving the plane of interest in focus. *See* Computerized axial tomography.

Tomomania:

Morbid and unnatural desire to be operated on or, alternately, the tendency for a surgeon to perform an unnecessary operation for a minor ailment.

Tonic Block (Tonic Inhibition):

See Ionic channel.

Tonometer:

Device used to measure pressure or tension. Tonometers may be used to bring a blood specimen into equilibrium with a known concentration of gas. It is usually done in a vibrating or rotating spherical glass cylinder. The resultant sample of blood can then be used to calibrate or check the accuracy of an instrument. Mechanical tonometers are also used to determine intraocular pressure.

Tooth:

Hard, hydroxyapetite projections located in the maxillary and mandibular alveolar ridges of the oral cavity. Teeth are necessary for mastication and proper speech. Enamel, a hard inorganic substance, covers the dentin of the tooth crown. Teeth can be damaged by instrumentation for anesthesia. Claims of tooth injury are one of the leading causes of malpractice actions against anesthetists and anesthesiologists. *See* Figure.

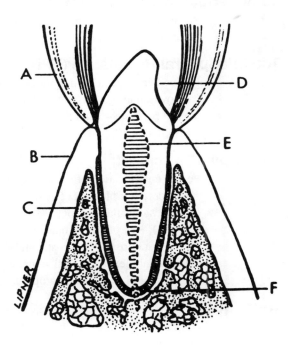

Tooth: Tooth about to be extracted showing the anatomic relationship with the bony structures of the alveolus. (A) Forceps; (B) gingiva; (C) alveolar process; (D) tooth crown; (E) root canal; and (F) root apex.

Topical Anesthesia:

Application of an anesthetic agent directly on the surface to produce numbness or loss of sensation. A local anesthetic spray is used to anesthetize the hypopharynx prior to intubation. Uncontrolled absorption of a systemically active drug is a rare complication of topical anesthetic application. *See* EMLA.

Torecan:

See Thiethylperazine.

Torquemeter:

See Dynamometer.

Torr:

Unit of measurement for pressure equal to 1/760 normal atmospheric pressure. One torr is equal to the pressure needed to support a column of mercury 1 mm high at 0°C and standard gravity on earth (1 torr = 1 mm Hg). On other planets torr would be defined differently.

Tort:

Wrong done by one individual to another individual that may be litigated in a civil action.

Total Intravenous Anesthesia (TIVA):

Growing genre in anesthesia in which the entire anesthetic is delivered by intravenous injection. It includes intravenous analgesics of the opioid class, intravenous induction agents, and muscle relaxants.

Total Peripheral Nutrition (TPN):

Technique for totally replacing nutritional needs without use of the alimentary tract. *See* Amigen.

Total Peripheral Resistance (TPR):

Derived value representing the resistance to flow in the cardiovascular system. In a normal cardiovascular system, arteriolar tone accounts for 60% of the TPR. Clinically, TPR = mean arterial pressure – central venous pressure (CVP) cardiac output (CO) × 80 (TPR = MAP – CVP/CO × 80).

Total Spinal, Accidental:

Feared complication of a spinal anesthetic in which all or nearly all nerve trunks from the spinal cord are blocked. The direct effects can include massive peripheral blood pooling (due to sympathetic blockade), loss of circulating catecholamines (denervation of the adrenals), loss of the sympathetic nerves affecting cardiac rate (sympathetic blockade of T3–T5), and loss of intercostal and diaphragm motion (block of thoracic motor nerves and the cervical plexus). A total spinal can present as respiratory and circulatory collapse. The patient should survive if appropriate cardiopulmonary resuscitation is performed.

Tourniquet:

Device that provides circumferential pressure around a limb to prevent bleeding to or from a distal area. The tourniquet is used during the procedure of exsanguinating a limb (starting at the distal end, progressively wrapping a constrictive band further and further up the limb until the tourniquet site is reached). The current operating room tourniquet is a stiff rubber bladder inflated by O_2 or N_2 to a pressure considerably above arterial blood pressure so the transmission of pressure through muscle mass blocks even the deep vessels. Tourniquets are dangerous if left on too long (>1–2 hour) because nerve trunk compression impedes nerve blood supply and, depending on time and degree, can lead to permanent destruction.

Muscles, bones, ligaments, and tendons tolerate hypoxia better than large nerves. Upon release of the tourniquet, a phenomenon known as *reactive hyperemia* (the opening and filling of all the vascular beds in the limb), which results in tissue swelling, is frequently seen. Patients with sickle cell disease or sickle cell trait, whose limbs may not be totally exsanguinated before application of the tourniquet, pose a functional problem. Any red blood cells (RBCs) remaining in the limb may sickle with RBC clumping. These acidotic RBC masses return to the central circulation when the tourniquet is released and can cause severe cardiac arrhythmias.

Tourniquet Cycling:

Technique of alternate deflation and reinflation of the tourniquet used as part of intravenous regional anesthesia at the end of the procedure, attempting to enhance safety by retarding the peak blood level of the administered local anesthetic.

Toxemia of Pregnancy:

See Eclampsia.

Toxicity:

Quality of being able to cause damage.

Toxiferine:

Derivative of curare and a potent neuromuscular blocking agent not used in clinical practice. It may have been an active ingredient in the original South American arrow poisons.

TPN:

See Total peripheral nutrition.

TPR:

See Total peripheral resistance.

Trace Anesthetic:

Level of anesthetic gas too low to produce overt effects. However, these levels are implicated in the decreased performance in operating room (OR) and dental personnel and the observed increase in stillbirths, spontaneous abortions, and congenital defects of offspring in these individuals as well. The National Institute for Occupational Safety and Health (NIOSH) has proposed a standard for trace anesthetics in ORs of less than 25 parts per million (ppm) for N_2O, 0.5 ppm for halogenated agents, and 2 ppm for halogenated agents when used with O_2 alone. *See* Air sampling.

Trace Freeze Capability (Freeze Trace):

See Oscilloscope; Shift register.

Tracheal Insufflation of Oxygen (TRIO):

Technique for tracheal insufflation of oxygen delivered within 1 cm of the carina. It is a technique used for continuous flow ventilation. It is claimed that it provides adequate arterial O_2 concentrations and adequate removal of CO_2. *See* Apneic oxygenation; Continuous flow anesthesia machine.

Tracheoesophageal Fistula with Esophageal Atresia:

Combination of two serious congenital anomalies that usually occur together (although each may occur alone). There is a discontinuation of the esophagus (a blind proximal pouch) and an opening from near the carina to the lower esophageal segment. In the normal fetus the tracheobronchial tree separates from the primitive foregut during the third to sixth week of life in utero. Interference with the vascular supply of the esophagus during this time apparently results in atresia of the esophagus, whereas failure of complete separation results in a fistula between the trachea and esophagus. The neonate exhibits excessive salivation and nasal secretions. Coughing and cyanosis are evident when these secretions enter the trachea. In addition, hydrochloric acid from the gastric contents may enter the lungs causing a chemical pneumonia, the most severe complication of this disorder. A 30% incidence of other abnormalities, particularly imperforate anus, other gastrointestinal atresias, and heart disease, occur in infants with tracheoesophageal fistula and esophageal atresia. Treatment begins at birth with the correction of fluid and electrolyte imbalances and respiratory and acid-base abnormalities, followed by surgical repair of the fistula. The presence of aspiration or chemical pneumonia renders surgery hazardous or impossible. *See* Figure.

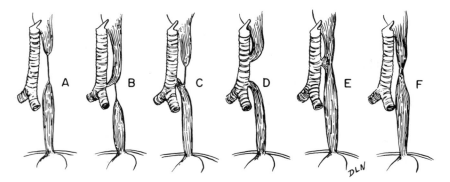

Tracheoesophageal Fistula: Types of congenital esophageal anomalies. (A) Esophageal atresia; (B) esophageal atresia with a proximal segment communicating with the trachea; (C) esophageal atresia with a distal segment communicating with the trachea (approximately 90% of the anomaly occurs with this configuration); (D) esophageal atresia with both segments communicating with the trachea; (E) esophagus has no atresia, but a fistula does exist through the trachea; and (F) esophageal stenosis but no communication with the trachea.

Tracheostomy:

Exterior opening into the trachea created therapeutically to bypass an obstructed airway. Under controlled circumstances, the opening is usually made below the level of the first tracheal ring. For emergencies it is recommended that the opening be created in the membrane between the thyroid and cricoid cartilages in the neck (a surgical procedure known as cricothyrotomy). *See* Larynx.

Tracheotomy:

Incision in the trachea.

Tracking:

Ability of a device to precisely reflect changes in the parameter it is monitoring. For example, an electrocardiography machine may not track rapid atrial fibrillations (the changes are made too quickly and are of such low magnitude that they are ignored by the device).

Traction Reflex:

Phenomenon of hypotension following traction on intraabdominal structures such as the gallbladder, appendix, uterus, or stomach. It appears to be mediated by the autonomic nervous system.

Trademark (Trade Name):

Name or symbol identifying a product that is registered by the government and legally restricted to use by its owner. For example, Fluothane is the trademark for halothane produced by Ayerst Laboratories. No other firm may call its halothane "Fluothane."

Trail Making Test:

Psychometric indicator considered sensitive for detecting brain dysfunction. It provides a measure of visual conceptual abilities and visual motor tracking. *See* Controlled oral word association test.

Train-of-Four:

See Figures. *See* Neuromuscular blockade, assessment of.

Tranexamic Acid:

Antifibrinolytic drug with possible use in controlling postoperative bleeding.

Tranquilizer:

Pharmacologic agent used to promote peace of mind or a more placid outlook on life. The mechanism of action remains obscure. Tranquilizers may be classified as major (antipsychotic) or minor (antianxiety) agents. *See* Antipsychotic agents; Anxiety; Benzodiazepine; Phenothiazine.

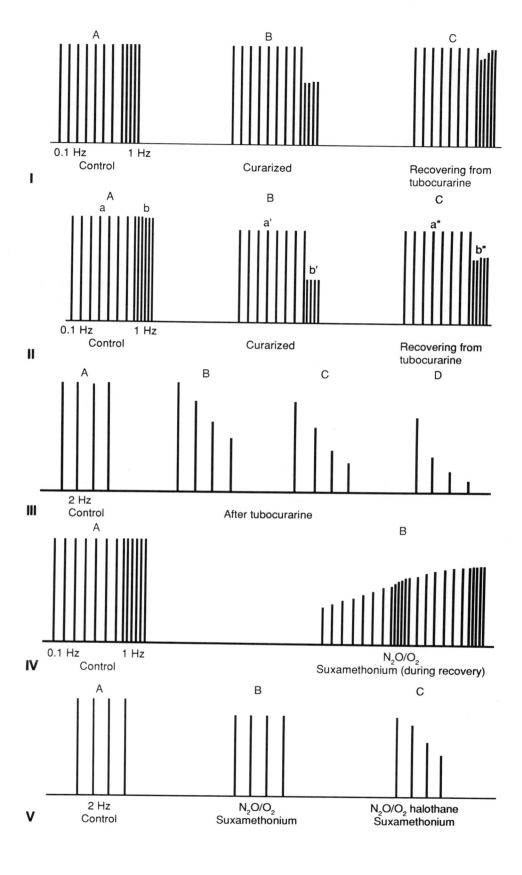

Transcranial Electro Stimulation:

Technique for analgesia using electrodes placed on the scalp to deliver pulses of electrical current. The technique has had mixed results.

Transcutaneous Electrical Nerve Stimulation (TENS):

Technique used to control pain in which the skin associated with an injured area or its nerve supply is stimulated by an electric current of various frequencies, waveforms, current densities, or pulse widths. This treatment has been shown to be beneficial to 15–50% of patients. It is considered an empiric form of therapy and is believed to have low complication rate. It is relatively inexpensive and enables the patient to be in control of his or her own therapy. The basis for the use of TENS is the gate theory of pain, which hypothesizes that the transmission of pain impulses can be interrupted and the perception of pain altered by appropriate stimulation of sites other than the site of origin of the pain. *See* Gate theory of pain.

Transcutaneous Monitoring:

Noninvasive technique in which a sensor, containing a heating element and an O_2 or CO_2 electrode; is attached to the skin surface. The heating element is precisely controlled to warm the skin surface under the sensor, thereby dilating blood vessels and causing gas to diffuse through the skin and underlying tissue. This gas is measured by the electrode. Under the best circumstances (good peripheral circulation, no hypothermia, normal hematocrit, normal systolic pressure, and PaO_2 in the range of 60–100 mm Hg), there is good correlation between the transcutaneous PO_2 measurement and the PaO_2 measurement. Transcutaneous measurement of PCO_2 has a poor correlation to $PaCO_2$. *See* Noninvasive monitor.

Train-of-Four: (I) Diagrammatic illustration of the effect of a small dose of tubocurarine on the twitch height obtained at two frequencies of ulnar nerve stimulation, 0.1 Hz (c.p.s.) and 1.0 Hz. (A) Control muscle twitch before tubocurarine is administered shows no difference in twitch heights at the two rates of stimulation used. (B) During curarization there may be initially no difference in the twitch height at the slower rate of stimulation from that obtained in the control period but a change to the faster frequency results in a sharp decline in twitch height. (C) As recovery progresses the ratio of the twitch height of the faster to the slower frequency gradually approaches unity. (II) Here the twitch heights at the lower rate of stimulation have been depressed. Note ratio b'/a' is less than ratio b"/a" and ratio b"/a" is less than ratio b/a. (III) Diagrammatic illustration of the effect of a small dose of tubocurarine on the isometric muscle twitch response to a train-of-four stimuli at 2 Hz. A shows the control response; B,C and D represent various degrees of curarization. (IV) Diagrammatic illustration of the effect of a small dose of suxamethonium (nitrous oxide/oxygen anaesthesia). When the evoked muscle twitches reappear after complete ablation change from shower to faster frequency does not change the slope of the recovery curve (A) control; (B) during recovery from suxamethonium block. (V) Diagrammatic illustration of the effect of the administration of suxamethonium on the muscle twitch response to the train-of-four stimuli at 2 Hz.

Transducer:

Device that converts a nonelectrical parameter such as light, pressure, or sound into an electrical signal. *See* Figures.

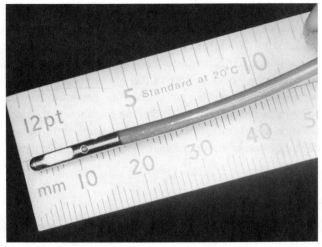

A

Applied physiological pressure

Extracorporeal transducer

Atomospheric pressure, [barometric pressure] communicated to the *back* of the transducer diaphragm. Vent is via fine lumen in the cable carrying wires to monitor.

Applied physiological pressure

Atmospheric vent tube
Transducer

B   Microtransducer catheter

Transducer: (A) Illustration of a microtransducer catheter and (B) its construction.

Transesophageal Echocardiography (TEE):

Technique of echocardiography in which an ultrasonic probe is placed in the esophagus and positioned behind the heart, such that ultrasonic echoes can be bounced off the various moving structures within the myocardium. A rapidly evolving monitoring technique which may become a new "gold standard" for monitoring cardiac performance.

Transfilling:

Hazardous practice of refilling gas cylinders from other cylinders. The danger involves rapid recompression of any gas that may remain in the emptied cylinder, causing a dramatic increase in temperature and resulting in an explosion. All modern anesthesia systems contain check valves that prevent crossfilling (a type of transfilling) between small cylinders that are otherwise connected. *See* Adiabatic.

Transformer:

Electrical device for changing voltage in an alternating current (AC) circuit. The input side (primary coil) and the output side (secondary coil) are coupled by the magnetic fields produced when current flows through a coil of wire. The voltage change is proportional to the number of turns in the coils. A primary with 10 turns and a secondary with 100 turns charge 20 to 200 volts. For both sides, however, the product of voltage × current remains the same. Some losses occur because of the inefficiency of magnetic transfer, so the current × the voltage of the secondary side is slightly less.

Transfusion Filter:

Particulate filter added to transfusion lines to prevent small debris from entering the circulation. The standard in-line filter has a pore size of 170 μm, whereas add-on types can filter particles as small as 20 μm; the latter, however, tend to slow transfusion rates.

Transfusion Reaction:

See Blood types.

Transfusion Therapy:

Direct introduction of fluids into the circulation to restore the volume and functional elements of the blood. Transfusion therapy is divided into three categories: (1) restoration of circulatory volume to maintain adequate cardiac output; (2) restoration of O_2-carrying capacity; and (3) restoration of clotting factors. Volume replacement can consist of crystalloid or colloid solutions. Crystalloids (e.g., lactated Ringer's solution and 0.9% sodium chloride solution) are clear fluids containing dissolved inorganic salts that diffuse easily across semipermeable membranes. Ringer's solution is considered a balanced salt solution because its inorganic salts are present in ratios similar to the normal ratios of those found within the body. Colloids (e.g., albumin, plasma protein precipitate, dextrans, and hetastarch) contain large molecules that are not freely diffusible across semipermeable membranes. Crystalloids distribute themselves out of the circulating volume within a short period and attain a distribution ratio between extracellular fluid and intravascular fluid of approximately 2:1 or 3:1. In contrast, colloids remain in the circulation until metabolic degradation or further hemorrhage occurs. Therefore the practical consideration in volume expansion of the circulation is that crystalloids must be given in a volume two to three times that required to return the circulating volume to normal, whereas colloids may be given on a 1:1 replacement basis. The O_2-carrying capacity is restored with packed red blood cells (RBCs). (Currently, artificial solutions are being studied as substitutes for RBCs.) The functioning RBC increases the O_2-carrying capacity of the blood vastly more than simple

O$_2$ dissolved in serum. If volume is replaced, the otherwise normal individual can withstand an acute loss of at least 20% of the circulating RBC mass before significant compromise is evident. Restoration of clotting factors is possible by administering platelet concentrates, fresh whole blood, or fresh frozen plasma. Usually clotting factors are in such abundance in normal blood that serious bleeding or dilution by massive transfusion must take place before clotting factors drop to such low concentrations as to cause a loss of clotting ability. *See* Table. *See* Albumin; Blood storage; Dextran; Hetastarch; Oxygen carrying capacity; Third space.

Transfusion Therapy: Parenteral infusion solutions.

Solutions	Electrolyte Content (mEq/L)								Glucose (g/L)
	Na$^+$	K$^+$	Ca^{2+}	Mg^{2+}	NH$_4^+$	Cl$^-$	HCO$_3^-$ milliequiv	PO$_4^{2-}$	
Glucose (5%) in water									50
Glucose (10%) in water									100
Isotonic saline (0.9%)	155					155			
Sodium chloride (5%)	855					855			
Ringer solution	147	4	4			155			
Ringer lactate (Hartmann)	130	4	3			109	28		
Dorrow solution (KNL)	121	35				103	53		
Potassium chloride									
0.2% in 5% dextrose		27				27			50
0.3% in 5% dextrose		40				40			50
Modified duodenal solution with 10% dextrose	80	36	5	3		64	60		100
Gastric solution with 10% dextrose	63	17			70	150			100
Ammonium chloride (0.9%)					170	170			
Sodium lactate (1/6 molar)	167						167		
Sodium bicarbonate (1/6 molar)	167						167		
Examples of "maintenance solutions":									
Pediatric electrolyte "No 48" with 5% dextrose	25	20		3		22	23	3	50
Maintenance electrolyte "No 75" with 5% dextrose	40	35				40	20	15	50
Levulose and dextrose with electrolyte (Butler II) .	58	25		6		51	25	13	100
Dextrose (5%) in 0.2% saline	34					34			50
Dextrose (10%) in 0.45% saline	77					77			100

Transillumination:

Technique of passing a bright light through body tissues to allow visualization of subcutaneous structures. Transillumination has been used for many years for viewing air-fluid levels in the sinuses and has more recently been used to identify blood vessels lying deep underneath the skin in the limbs of infants and young children in order to expedite percutaneous puncture.

Transmembrane Signaling:

Various techniques by which cell surface receptors respond to translate information into cellular responses when contacted by neurotransmitters, hormones, growth factors, and similar signals.

Transmission:

Movement, or transfer, of an impulse, disease, genetic trait(s), or signal from one location or individual to another.

Transmural Pressure:

Pressure difference between the inside and outside of a vessel. *See* Laplace law.

Transplantation:

Transfer or grafting of tissue from one location to another. Organ transplantation involves removing a donor organ and transferring it to a recipient. Inherent in the procedure is removal of the diseased organ from the recipient and the ensurance of an adequate vascular connection to the donor organ. Transplantation may involve genetically dissimilar tissue from the same species (allogeneic) or genetically identical tissue (autologous or syngeneic). A xenograft or heterograft is a graft of tissue involving individuals of different species.

Transport:

Movement of biochemical substances across cell membranes. Passive transport occurs in response to concentration gradients. Active transport occurs when a substance is aided (energy is used) for passage through a membrane, at times in the face of a reverse concentration gradient. For example, the "sodium pump" of the nerve cell membrane actively moves sodium from inside to outside the cell membrane in direct opposition to a charge gradient that favors sodium remaining on the inside of the cell.

Transtracheal Anesthesia:

Injection of local anesthetic into the lumen of the trachea via the cricothyroid membrane to produce a cough that effectively spreads the anesthetic. This technique provides excellent topical anesthesia of the larynx and trachea; however, it may initiate bronchospasm.

Transurethral Resection of Prostate (TURP):

Surgical procedure, performed through a cystoscope, for the treatment of benign prostatic hypertrophy. The adenomatous tissue of the prostate is removed up to the false capsule with an electrosurgery loop under direct vision. (The entire prostate is not removed.) TURP poses unique anesthetic problems in that continuous irrigation to keep the surgical field clear is necessary. This irrigating fluid enters the circulation via the many blood vessels opened and then sealed by the electrosurgery loop, and it may cause acute circulatory overload. There is therefore a strict time limit of 1 hour for the entire surgical procedure. Another complication is the possibility of bladder perforation, causing air and fluid to enter the abdominal cavity. This situation causes a great deal of pain (often referred to the shoulder) in the patient who has received a spinal anesthetic. In the patient who has received a general anesthetic for the procedure, bladder perforation is difficult to detect, and significant abdominal distention may occur before the problem is recognized. *See* Referred pain.

Trend Analysis:

Technique for evaluating accumulated data in an effort to determine whether a patient is improving or is remaining stable. A single observation of a patient's condition may not be sufficient for accurate evaluation.

Trendelenburg Position:

Position used during surgery that elevates the pelvis, providing easier access to the urinary bladder, rectum, and vagina. Developed during the late 1800s by Friedrich Trendelenburg, the position is characterized by having the patient head tilted at a 30 to 45 degree angle downward. It has also been used as a treatment for shock. *See* Patient positioning.

Triamterene (Dyrenium):

Oral diuretic agent usually used in combination with the thiazide diuretics. It causes mild sodium excretion and mild potassium retention.

Triazolam:

Benzodiazepine derivative with a short plasma half-life. *See* Benzodiazepine.

Tribromoethanol (Avertin):

Rectally administered general anesthetic used clinically during the 1920s. Drug dose is calculated according to the patient's weight and is given by enema. Respiratory depression occurs in approximate proportion to the dose. Tribromoethanol is reported to aggravate liver and renal disease. It is not used at the present time.

Trichloroethanol:

See Chloral hydrate.

Trichloroethylene (Trilene; Trimar):

Nonflammable, colorless (coloring is sometimes added to distinguish it from chloroform), liquid general anesthetic that is extremely potent owing to its very high gas/oil solubility coefficient. It has a low vapor pressure and is unstable. It decomposes into phosgene and hydrochloric acid when exposed to light or heat and therefore should not be used in systems containing soda lime absorbers. Impure trichloroethylene has been associated with cranial nerve palsies, particularly affecting the fifth cranial nerve. It is currently used around the world to produce analgesia in obstetrics and dentistry.

Trichlorofluoromethane:

See Freon.

Tricuspid Annular Plane Systolic Excursion (TAPSE):

Cardiac performance index determined by transthoracic two-dimensional echocardiography of the right ventricle.

Tricyclic Antidepressant:

Drug used to treat depression. Examples of tricyclic antidepressants are imipramine (Tofranil), amitriptyline (Amitril, Elavil), doxepin (Adapin, Sinequan), desipramine (Norpramin), nortriptyline (Aventyl, Pamelor), and protriptyline (Vivactil). These drugs can cause cardiovascular abnormalities such as tachycardia, some arrhythmias, prolongation of conduction time, and α-blockade. They can also add to the central sedation effect of central nervous system depressants. Severe arrhythmias can result from the combination of halothane, pancuronium, and the tricyclics. *See* Table.

Trieger Dot Test:

Pencil and paper exercise for patients recovering from anesthesia to determine the completeness of that recovery. It primarily checks fine motor coordination and perception. *See* Street ready.

Trifluoperazine Hydrochloride (Stelazine):

Tranquilizer of the phenothiazine group. *See* Phenothiazine.

Trifluoroethyl Vinyl Ether:

See Fluroxene.

Trigeminal Nerve:

Fifth cranial nerve. *See* Cranial nerves.

Trigeminal Nerve Blockade:

See Gasserian ganglion blockade.

Trigeminal Neuralgia (Tic Douloureux):

Painful disturbance (usually without organic cause) in the function of the fifth cranial nerve. It can occur in any of the three divisions of the nerve and is frequently described as the worst possible human pain. Carbamazepine (Tegretol) is used to treat this condition, but frequent adverse reactions limit its usefulness. The only definitive treatment is surgical deafferentation of the affected nerve root. This technique may be implemented as a last resort in a patient disabled by pain due to the permanent sensory loss and, depending on the root involved, the motor complications it produces. *See* Carbamazepine.

Trigger Circuit:

Specific electric circuit that has no output until its input waveform exceeds a specific parameter. When this point occurs, the trigger "fires" a constant output. This circuit is often used to initiate an oscilloscope sweep when the QRS complex is detected across the screen.

Tricyclic Antidepressant.

Generic Name (Trade Name)	Structure	Comments
A. Tricyclic Antidepressants		The tricyclic antidepressants have an onset of action of 1-3 wks and their side effects include atropine-like effects due to their anticholinergic action, orthostatic hypotension, sedation, tachycardia, arrhythmias, and prolongation of AV conduction time. They also may block the antihypertensive action of guanethidine.
Amitriptyline HCl (Elavil)	$CHCH_2CH_2N(CH_3)_2$	Amitryptyline has significant sedative properties while having lower incidence of atropine-like effects than other tricyclics.
Nortriptyline HCl (Aventyl)	$CHCH_2CH_2NHCH_3$	Nortriptyline demonstrates moderate sedation while still possessing some sedative properties.
Doxepin HCl (Adapin)	$CHCH_2CH_2N(CH_3)_2$	Doxepin has a moderate sedative effect and is used as both an antianxiety and antidepressant agent.
Protriptyline HCl (Vivactil)	$CH_2CH_2CH_2NHCH_3$	Protriptyline lacks sedative and tranquilizing properties. It has a more rapid onset of action than the other tricyclics and is particularly suited for withdrawn, lethargic, and depressed patients. There are more cardiovascular effects than with the other tricyclics.

Trimipramine HCL (Surmontil)

Trimipramine is used for the treatment of mild depression.

Imipramine HCl (Tofranil)

Imipramine is less sedative than amitryptiline and doxepin. It is used for the treatment of bed-wetting in children.

Desipramine HCl (Norpramin)

Desipramine has sedative properties like nortriptyline.

B. MAO Inhibitors

1. Hydrazine MAO Inhibitors

   Isocarboxazid (Marplan)
   Phenelzine (Nardil)

The hydrazine MAO inhibitors have a slow onset of action (2–4 wks) and may cause hepatotoxicity. The non-hydrazine MAO inhibitors have a direct amphetamine-like stimulant action, a faster onset of action than the hydrazine.

2. Non-Hydrazine MAO Inhibitors

   Tranylcypromine (Parnate)

MAO inhibitors may or may not cause hepatotoxicity. MAO inhibitors as a class can cause excessive central stimulation, orthostatic hypotension, insomnia, constipation, and paradoxical behavior. They are contraindicated in patients taking meperidine as cardiovascular collapse can occur. Severe hypertension reactions can occur when cheese or other tyramine-containing foods are ingested during tranylcypromine therapy.

597

Trigger Point:

See Myofascial pain syndrome.

Triggered Ventilation:

Mode of operation of a ventilator in which the initial negative pressure generated in the air passageways at the start of patient inhalation activates ventilator function. The sensitivity of the ventilator is usually adjustable.

Trilene:

See Dichloroacetylene; Trichloroethylene.

Trimar:

See Trichloroethylene.

Trimethaphan (Arfonad):

Ultra short-acting, nondepolarizing ganglionic blocking agent that is administered intravenously to produce deliberate, controlled hypotension during some surgical procedures. It is not as easily controlled as nitroprusside, which has replaced it. In addition, trimethaphan may cause respiratory depression and tachycardia.

TRIO:

See Tracheal insufflation of oxygen.

Triple Point of Water:

Point on a pressure-temperature plot where the lines representing the solid, liquid, and vapor phases of water intersect.

Tris:

See Tromethamine.

Trocar:

See Cannula.

Tromethamine (Tham, Tris):

Synthetic buffer solution useful as an alternative drug to sodium bicarbonate for treatment of metabolic acidosis. Its use is advocated when an acute sodium load is inappropriate. Tromethamine, also known as TRIS [tris(hydroxymethyl)aminomethane], is contraindicated during pregnancy or for patients with uremic or chronic respiratory acidosis. It is also available in powder form (THAM-E).

True Capillary:

See Microcirculation.

t-Test:

See Student *t*-test.

TTI:

See Tension time index.

TTX:

See Tetrodotoxin.

Tubocurarine Chloride; *d*-Tubocurarine (Tubarine):

Class leader of the nondepolarizing neuromuscular blocking drugs. Tubocurarine is the active ingredient in curare. Introduced into the clinical practice of anesthesia during the 1940s, it rapidly became popular as an adjunct to anesthesia for the production of muscle flaccidity. The diaphragm is thought to be partially resistant to curare, a characteristic called the respiratory sparing effect of the drug. The drug appears to cause some ganglionic blockade and histamine release. It can therefore produce profound hypotension. Moderate hypothermia diminishes the effect of curare (and other nondepolarizing muscle relaxants), whereas profound hypothermia greatly intensifies it. Equipment for artificial ventilation must be available whenever the drug is used. *See* Neuromuscular blockade, assessment of.

Tuohy Needle:

Large-bore (12- to 19-gauge) needle with a curved tip used in epidural blocks. *See* Epidural needle.

Turbulent Flow:

Type of disorderly fluid flow through a vessel or container in which all the molecules tend to move at approximately the same velocity. Turbulence increases when fluid flow velocity increases. *See* Laminar flow; Reynolds number.

Turnover Time:

A parameter of operating room utilization defined as the time interval between the exit of one patient and the placing of another patient on the room table. *See* Operating room utilization.

TURP:

See Transurethral resection of prostate.

TURP Syndrome:

Any of one or more of the following complications of TURP surgery caused primarily by bladder perforation or intravascular extravasation of irrigating fluid; e.g., pulmonary edema, water intoxication, ammonia and glycine toxicities, hypovolemia, hypervolemia, and coagulopathies. *See* Transurethral resection of prostate.

TV:

See Tidal volume.

TWA:

See Time-weighted average.

Tween 20; Tween 80:

Nonionic chemical agents of low molecular weight that markedly decrease surface tension.

Twilight Sleep:

See Scopolamine.

Twitch Response:

See Neuromuscular blockade, assessment of.

Two-Tailed Test:

Evaluation of a hypothesis that is concerned with values above and below the mean. This evaluation is in contrast to the one-tailed test, which is concerned with values either above or below the mean. Both one- and two-tailed tests are valid only for large samples.

Tympanic Membrane Temperature:

Monitoring technique for temperature in which a small thermocouple is placed in the ear near the tympanic membrane. The temperature of the tympanic membrane is thought to be closely associated with the temperature of the brain. Difficulties associated with the technique involve possible puncture of the membrane and excessive ear wax, which can preclude proper measurement.

Type and Crossmatch:

See Blood types.

Type and Screen:

With this type of blood bank procedure, the potential recipient's blood has been typed as ABO and RH antigens and has been screened against a panel of reagent red blood cells for common antibodies. This procedure is more liberal than the "type and crossmatch" because it frees up bank blood for other patients, as specific units are not held back for specific patients. It is believed statistically that a significant blood transfusion reaction after type and screen with no further compatibility workup is approximately 1 in 10,000. See Blood storage; Blood types.

Type I Error:

Type of error that occurs when one rejects a null hypothesis, although it is true. See Null hypothesis.

Type II Error:

Type of error that occurs when one accepts a null hypothesis, although it is false. *See* Null hypothesis.

Type I Muscle Fiber:

Name for a class of muscle fibers that are structurally capable of continuous and prolonged activity. Also called slow-twitch muscle fibers. Their energy supply comes from oxidative metabolism in mitochondria. *See* Type II muscle fiber.

Type II Muscle Fiber:

Subclass of muscle fibers that appear to be adapted for rapid contraction or high intensity effort. They are also called rapid-twitch fibers. They derive their energy from anaerobic glycolysis.

U

UCR:
See Usual, customary, and reasonable charges.

UL:
See Underwriters Laboratories.

Ultrasonic Fetal Heart Rate Determination:
See Fetal monitor.

Ultrasonic Flowmeter:
See Blood flow, methods for measuring.

Ultrasonic Nebulizer:
See Nebulizer.

Ultrasonography:
Technique of projecting ultrasound waves (i.e., sound energy far beyond the 20 kHz limit of human hearing) in order to probe various depths in the body. Most ultrasonic devices operate at a frequency of greater than 1,000,000 Hz. *See* Ultrasonography, diagnostic.

Ultrasonography, Diagnostic:
Noninvasive method to evaluate tissue density differences associated with certain disorders. Diagnostic ultrasonography is valuable for assessing the size and location of cysts, effusions, and tumors. It can also be used to evaluate fetal development. Its efficacy is based on the patterns of sound reflection caused by different layers of tissue. *See* Sound; TEE.

Ultrasound:
Sounds with a frequency above the human hearing range. *See* Doppler effect; Ultrasonography.

Underwriters Laboratories (UL):
Organization that investigates products for safety at the expense of the requesting manufacturers. Departments of UL include Burglary Protection, Casualty and Chemical Hazard, Electrical, Fire Protection, HAC&R (Heating, Air Conditioning, and Refrigeration), and

Marine. The UL, organized by William Merrill, was called the Underwriter's Electrical Bureau and was incorporated in 1901. Its headquarters are in Northbrook, Illinois.

Unitary Hypothesis of Anesthesia:

Theory stating that the mechanism of action at the molecular level is the same for all inhalation anesthetics.

Unitary Theory of Narcosis:

Concept that all anesthetics cause anesthesia by the same mechanism.

Universal Precautions:

Series of steps to prevent contact between health care practitioners and body fluids from a potentially infectious patient. It includes gowns, gloves and eye shields as necessary. *See* AIDS.

Universal Vaporizer:

See Vaporizer.

Universal Vaporizer Output Calculation (Measured Flow Vaporizer Calculation):

Technique for determining the anesthetic concentration in a fresh gas supply to which the output of a measured flow vaporizer has been added. The computation requires knowing the amount of O_2 flowing to the vaporizer, the vapor pressure of the liquid anesthetic at the temperature of the vaporizer, and the total of all other flows.

Uptake:

Process by which a drug is combined with the blood. The drug may be administered by an intravenous, intramuscular, oral, or inhalational route. Uptake is primarily concerned, however, with the speed of transfer of gaseous anesthetics from the alveolar gas into the alveolar capillary blood.

Urecholine:

See Bethanechol chloride.

Uremia:

Condition caused by the presence of waste products in the blood that are normally excreted in the urine. Signs and symptoms include lethargy, weight loss, vomiting, anemia, pruritus, and an unpleasant taste in the mouth. Uremia is seen during the end-stages of kidney disease or with urinary obstruction.

Urethan:

See Ethyl carbamate.

Urinary Output:

The volume of liquid excreted by the kidneys, usually assumed to be 1 cc/kg/hour or 1700 cc/day in a 70-kg man. Minimum obligatory loss is approximately 500 cc. *See* Methoxyflurane.

Urticaria (Hives):

Allergic manifestation marked by raised, itchy, patchy areas on the skin. It is due to contact with a specific etiologic agent (food, drug, insect, or environmental factor).

Use-Dependent Block:

See Ionic channel.

Usual, Customary, and Reasonable Charges (UCR):

Reimbursement technique used by third-party carriers where reimbursement for physician services is based on individual physician and regional profiles. These averaged payments to physicians are based on geographic and specialty areas. Under conventional schemes of reimbursement, a physician charging more than UCR fees is permitted under certain circumstances to recover from the patient the difference between the payment from the third-party carrier and the fee charged. *See* Relative value guide; Third-party carriers.

Uterine Contractility:

Rhythmic movements of uterine smooth muscle that become more pronounced and more frequent as labor progresses. Uterine contractions may be initiated by any of the smooth muscle cells comprising its musculature. No true pacemaker for the uterus exists. When cells of the uterus contract in a tetanic manner, a contracture occurs, which is a rare condition usually resulting from hyperstimulation of the uterus or from excessive administration of oxytocin. It leads to profound loss of mechanical efficiency and reduction in uterine blood flow. The halogenated anesthetics are potent depressants of uterine activity, whereas routine doses of morphine and meperidine produce no change in contractility. Nitrous oxide, depending on dose, appears to have either no effect or a depressant effect. In general, uterine contractility is independent of direct innervation, but contractions may decrease or stop when efferent impulses to the uterus are blocked early in labor. During the active phase of labor these same doses have little or no effect on uterine contractility. *See* Montevideo unit; Oxytocin.

Uterosacral Block:

See Paracervical block.

V

Vacuum Tube Circuitry:

See Circuit, solid state.

Validity:

Ability of a test used for screening to demonstrate which of a class of individuals have a particular characteristic and which do not. The two components of validity are sensitivity and specificity. *See* Sensitivity; Specificity.

Valium:

Trade name for diazepam. *See* Benzodiazepine.

Valmid:

See Ethinamate.

Valsalva Maneuver:

Forced expiration against an obstruction such as a closed glottis. The physiologic consequences of the Valsalva maneuver are dramatic. Initially, stimulation of the vagus nerve causes bradycardia, and the increased pressure in the chest prevents cardiac filling, followed by a decrease in stroke volume and cardiac output. Tachycardia and elevated blood pressure due to peripheral constriction can occur as well. The momentary venous stasis may lead to dramatic increases in intracranial pressure, which is deleterious, especially to postoperative neurosurgery patients.

Valve:

Device that regulates flow of liquids or gases in a pipe or duct system.

Valvular Heart Disease:

Condition affecting (singly or together) the aortic, mitral, pulmonic, and tricuspid valves of the heart. Valvular heart disease is commonly due to: (1) stenosis, in which the valve becomes less pliable resulting in blood flow obstruction, or (2) regurgitation (i.e., the valve is incapable of closing completely and therefore backflow occurs). Both conditions can occur simultaneously and not to the same extent in any particular valve.

Vapor:

Substance in gaseous form at a temperature below its critical temperature. A vapor can be liquefied by pressure changes without lowering the temperature.

Vapor Pressure:

Pressure constant exerted by a vapor, at a given temperature, that is in equilibrium with its solid or liquid form. The vapor pressure of a volatile anesthetic agent must be known to determine the inspired concentration of the agent via a bubble-through vaporizer. At room temperature (20°C) the vapor pressure of halothane is 242 mm Hg. When a substance is at its boiling point, its vapor pressure equals the atmospheric pressure. *See* Figure. *See* Boiling point; Partial pressure.

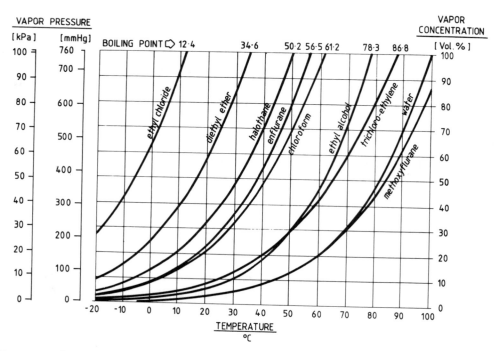

Vapor Pressure: The curve for isoflurane has not been included since it is virtually the same as that for halothane.

Vapor, Saturated:

Equilibrium point between a liquid and its vapor. Additional liquid can be vaporized only if the temperature is raised.

Vaporizer:

Device that converts liquid into vapor. A vaporizer is a necessary component of anesthesia machines that it converts volatile liquids into anesthetic vapors. A vaporizer can be specific for one agent (precision) or used for any liquid anesthetic agent (universal, measured flow).

Its temperature may be automatically (variable bypass), manually (controlled by anesthetist), or passively compensated. A vaporizer may be located outside the breathing system (out-of-circle) on the back bar in series with the flow columns or inside the breathing system (in-circle) in series with the CO_2 absorber. It can bubble gas through a volume of liquid, move gas over the surface of the liquid or a wick, or use a combination of the two techniques. With a variable bypass vaporizer, only a portion of the gas flow to the vaporizer contacts the anesthetic agent. Vaporizers without a variable bypass allow all the gas to contact the anesthetic agent, picking up an unknown amount of anesthetic vapor (determined by temperature, gas flow, and agent partial pressure). *See* Boyle bottle; Copper kettle; Draw-over vaporizer; EMO inhaler; Flagg can; Goldman vaporizer; Vaporizer, draw-over; flow-over; bubble-through.

Vaporizer Capability:

Maximal concentration of anesthetic vapor that can be delivered by a vaporizer. In practice, out-of-system or in-system vaporizers used in a nonrebreathing circuit must have a high capability because no additional anesthetic is added to the gas to be inhaled by the patient.

Vaporizer Circuit Control Valve (VCCV):

Device used on anesthesia machines containing a built-in vaporizer and requiring a measured O_2 flow (copper kettle, Vernitrol). The VCCV directs O_2 through the vaporizer to the machine outlet.

Vaporizer Concentration:

See Vaporizer output.

Vaporizer, Draw-Over, Flow-Over, Bubble-Through:

Types of vaporizers that bring fresh gas (the atmosphere or from an anesthesia machine) into contact with the surface of a volatile liquid anesthetic. The draw-over vaporizer obtains its fresh gas supply from the negative pressure created when the patient inhales, thereby drawing or pulling gas over the surface of the anesthetic. A flow-over vaporizer obtains its fresh gas supply from the positive pressure caused by its in-series attachment to a continuous flow anesthesia machine. The terms *draw-over* and *flow-over* are often used interchangeably. In the bubble-through type of vaporizer, the fresh gas flow is placed under the liquid surface. Therefore equilibration between the liquid and gas is more rapid owing to the creation of many bubble/liquid interfaces. *See* Flagg can; Vaporizer.

Vaporizer, Fluomatic:

Agent-specific vaporizer for halothane (Fluothane). It is a variable bypass, flow-over with wick, out-of-system, temperature-compensating vaporizer previously manufactured by Foregger Company, a former division of Puritan-Bennett. A similar vaporizer, the Fluotec Mark II (or Mark III), is manufactured by Cyprane Limited. *See* Agent specific filling device.

Vaporizer, In-Circle:

See Vaporizer.

Vaporizer, Ohio No. 8:

Flow-over, variable bypass vaporizer that contains a wick but has no temperature compensation. It is used inside the circle system. The quantity of vapor put out by the unit must be controlled by monitoring the clinical signs.

Vaporizer, Out-of-Circle:

See Vaporizer.

Vaporizer Output:

Concentration of anesthetic vapor at the outlet of a vaporizer. Vaporizer output usually refers to an in-circle vaporizer, in which gas entering the vaporizer already contains a significant percentage of anesthetic vapor. Vaporizer concentration, which refers specifically to vaporizers out of the breathing circuit, is the concentration of vapor delivered by the vaporizer when the fresh gas (having no vapor) passes through it. Therefore vaporizer output is equal to vaporizer concentration in an out-of-circuit system. *See* Pumping effect, pressure effect.

Vaporizer, Precision (Agent-Specific Vaporizer):

See Vaporizer, fluomatic.

Vaporizers, "Tec" Series:

Precision vaporizers named according to the specific agent they are designed to vaporize, i.e., Fluotec, Pentec, Ethrec. They are out-of-system, flow-over with wick, variable bypass, and temperature-compensating vaporizers. Three model series have been manufactured thus far: Mark I, II, and III.

Vaporizers, "Vapor" Series:

Group of out-of-circuit, variable bypass, flow-over with wick, precision vaporizers. The "Vapors" are distributed by North American Drager. They are unique in their manual method of temperature compensation. The anesthetist can adjust the concentration of the vaporizer and thereby increase the gas flow as the vaporizing chamber is cooled.

Vaporizer Temperature Compensation:

Appropriate adjustments or modifications needed to counterbalance the heat lost during vaporization of an anesthetic liquid. A constant vapor pressure, with a concomitant constant temperature, is necessary to preserve a stable vapor output. The temperature can be maintained by passive or active compensation. For passive compensation, a good thermal conductor such as copper is used in the body of a vaporizer to aid in maintaining a stable temperature. These copper vaporizers can be mounted to the copper top of an anesthesia machine to efficiently transfer heat. For active compensation, a mechanism such as a variable bypass is used to change the amount of gas exposed to the liquid (useful in out-of-system vaporizers). Only a portion of fresh gas is exposed to the anesthetic liquid; this portion is increased either by a bimetallic spring-operated valve or by a manual control as the temperature of the liquid decreases during vaporization. For active compensation, the vaporizer can also be heated by means of a waterbath or heating coil.

Vaporizer, Universal:

See Vaporizer.

Variable:

Value that is subject to change. For example, in the Henderson-Hasselbalch equation for determining pH, the pKa is a constant, whereas the concentration of bicarbonate is the variable, i.e., it can fluctuate over a wide range and must be directly sampled.

Variable, Dependent:

Unit of information or datum that changes in relation to another value.

Variable, Independent (Experimental Variable):

Unit of information that is directly manipulated and controlled by an investigator.

Variable Patterns of Fetal Heart Rate:

See Fetal heart rate (FHR) terminology.

Variance:

Square root of the standard deviation. It is a measure of the dispersion of values in a normal distribution. *See* Standard deviation.

Vascular Ring:

Type of aortic arch malformation in which the trachea and the esophagus are compressed within a ring-like vascular (aortic) anomaly. The most common vascular ring is caused by a double aortic arch.

Vasoconstriction:

Narrowing of the lumen of a blood vessel. Vasoconstriction may be precipitated by an increased sympathetic nervous system tone, serotonin release by platelets, local metabolic factors (elevated PCO_2, decreased pH), and circulating hormones (epinephrine and norepinephrine). *See* Autonomic nervous system; Epinephrine; Norepinephrine; Receptor/ receptor site.

Vasodilation:

Widening of the lumen of a blood vessel. Vasodilation can be produced by central sympathetic blockade (spinal, epidural), peripheral sympathetic blockade (with ganglionic blocking agents), or direct action on the vessels by drugs (halothane, nitroprusside). The total effect is to decrease peripheral resistance, decrease blood pressure, and store blood in the peripheral capacitance vessels, thereby causing a decrease in blood return to the heart and a decrease in stroke volume.

Vasomotor Center:

Large, diffuse area located in the medulla oblongata, that controls the extent of dilatation of the arterial resistance vessels and the venous capacitance vessels by regulating sympathetic tone.

Vasopressins:

See Antidiuretic hormone; Diabetes insipidus.

Vasospasm:

Constriction of a blood vessel (caused by smooth muscle contraction), thereby reducing its diameter and blood flow. Vasospasm appears to be the endpoint of an intrinsic mechanism for regulating local tissue blood flow. (An extrinsic mechanism also exists that is mediated by the sympathetic nervous system.) Vasospasm can occur in both cerebral and cardiac arteries and is apparently precipitated by only a slight insult or no insult at all. In these circumstances, vasospasm can initiate or worsen infarcts.

Vasoxyl:

See Methoxamine.

VCCV:

See Vaporizer circuit control valve.

VCRII:

See Vital capacity rapid inhalation induction.

Vecuronium:

Steroidal quaternary ammonium nondepolarizing muscle relaxant that has several attributes, including short duration of action and lack of cumulative effect.

Venipuncture:

Introduction of a cannula or needle into a vein, usually by piercing rather than incising the skin. A venipuncture unit composed of a Teflon cannula over a stainless steel needle is typical. The needle penetrates the skin and vein wall, and blood flow back through the needle (flashback) indicates that the vein has been punctured. The cannula is pushed over the needle and threaded into the vein. The needle is then withdrawn, and the cannula end is attached to a fluid line. Other types of venipuncture units include a "through the needle" cannula and a "butterfly." The butterfly is composed of a short stainless steel needle with plastic wings and is applicable to short-term use.

Venous Air Embolus:

See Air embolus; Embolism.

Venous Pressure:

Blood pressure measured in the veins. The peripheral venous pressure is variable and depends on the central venous pressure. *See* Central venous pressure.

Venous Return:

Amount of blood returning to the right atrium from the venous circulation.

Ventilated Lung Volume:

Lung area in communication with air passageways. Its gas composition can therefore be altered by ventilation.

Ventilation and Perfusion, Regional Differences in:

Variations in the amount of ventilation per unit volume received by different segments of the normal lung. When a patient is upright, ventilation to the base of each lung is enhanced; in the supine position, ventilation to the posterior segments is improved. An analysis of diseased lung ventilation has led to the two-compartment analysis in which the lung is considered to have two types of alveoli: fast-ventilated or slow-ventilated. Perfusion studies indicate that the dependent lung is perfused better than the nondependent lung; moreover, perfusion differences are much more pronounced than ventilation differences. Both are caused by gravitational and hydrostatic effects. *See* Pulmonary perfusion, zones of; Ventilation/perfusion abnormality.

Ventilation, Assisted:

Introduction of positive pressure to the upper airways after normal, patient-initiated inspiration has begun. By this technique, flow is increased and tidal volumes are enhanced when the patient has depressed respiration but is still breathing spontaneously. *See* Ventilation, controlled.

Ventilation, Controlled:

Type of respiration that requires neither patient cooperation nor initiation. The patient's tidal volume, respiratory rate, and flow characteristics are determined by the anesthetist and are usually machine settings on a ventilator. Patient acquiescence is usually secured by anesthesia, muscle relaxants, or both. *See* Ventilation, assisted.

Ventilation/Perfusion Abnormality (V/Q Ratio; Ventilation/Perfusion Ratio):

Imbalance in the alveolar ventilation/pulmonary capillary blood flow (V/Q) that occurs either when an excessive amount of blood flows through an alveolus for the volume of alveolar gas that can diffuse into it (decreased V/Q ratio) or when excessive alveolar gas is available for an inadequate blood flow (increased V/Q ratio). The concept is most easily understood at its extremes. When an alveolus or an area of the lung receives no ventilation, all the blood that flows through it is returned to the circulation on the left side without being oxygenated. This condition is known as shunt. At the other extreme, if an alveolus is ventilated but totally unperfused, the condition known as deadspace exists. In a healthy 70-kg man, the normal alveolar ventilation at rest is approximately 4 L/minute and the total perfusion is approximately 5 L/minute. Therefore the V/Q ratio is approximately 4:5, or 0.8. In the ideal lung this ratio would be similar for each individual alveolus. It is a fact, however, that ventilation per cross-sectional area of the lung increases slowly from the top to the bottom in the upright lung, whereas blood flow increases much more rapidly due to gravitational effects. The V/Q ratio ranges from 3.0 at the apex of the lung (which shows an overabundance of ventilation) to a minimum of 0.63 at the base of the lung (which shows a relative overabundance of perfusion or blood flow). During exercise blood flow is more evenly distributed. V/Q differences are not as marked in the supine individual; the anterior lung assumes the characteristics of the apical lung of the upright patient. The difference in PaO_2 from the apex (130 mm Hg) to the base of the lung (90 mm Hg) in the upright lung is 40 mm Hg. Those alveoli that are relatively overventilated cannot aid underventilated alveoli by overloading the blood with O_2 because of the O_2 dissociation curve of hemoglobin. Even at a PO_2 of approximately 90 mm Hg, hemoglobin is nearly 100% saturated. Additional O_2 taken in by the blood going past overventilated alveoli (in which the PO_2 is 140–150 mm Hg) can be dissolved only into the serum, as the hemoglobin is already saturated. The situation with CO_2 is similar but less critical because the dissociation curve of CO_2 and blood is nearly linear in the physiologic range. Therefore alveoli that are relatively overventilated can remove a proportionately higher quantity of CO_2 (almost enough to compensate for the relatively underventilated areas at the base of the lung, which cannot remove as much CO_2). In diseased states in which the V/Q ratio for the overall lung changes drastically, both O_2 delivery and CO_2 removal are greatly affected. An increase in arterial CO_2, however, triggers the compensatory mechanism of hyperventilation. This increase in ventilation is effective in decreasing arterial CO_2 but not in delivering O_2 because of the differences in the O_2 and CO_2 transport noted above. *See* Dead space; Shunt.

Ventilation, Spontaneous:

Natural rate and depth of breathing set by physiologic requirements and performance of an individual.

Ventilator:

Device to assist or control the respiration of a patient. Ventilators can be electrically driven or powered by a compressed gas supply. There are two basic types of ventilators: pressure-limited and volume-limited. In the pressure limited device, gas is delivered to the patient by increasing pressure until some arbitrary pressure limit is reached, at which point the patient is allowed to passively exhale. In volume-limited ventilators, pressure is built up during inspiration until the selected volume of gas has been pushed out of the machine. When this volume is reached, the machine recycles and expiration is allowed to take place. Essentially all of the modern sophisticated ventilators are volume-limited. Volume-limited machines are considered superior to pressure-limited machines in every parameter except compensating for leaks. An older type of ventilator is the flow-generator or flow-limited machine. The machine was set by flow rate in liters per minute for a variable period of inspiratory time. Some intraoperative, pneumatically driven anesthesia machine-mounted units still use this system. *See* Figure. *See* Compression volume.

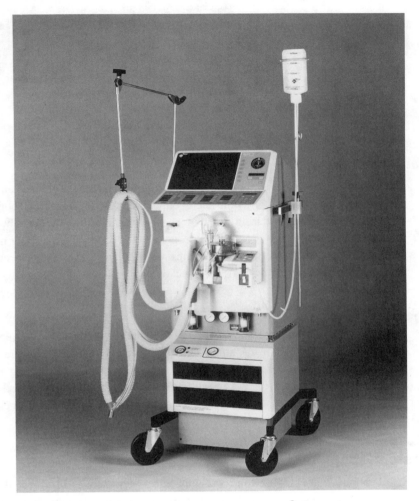

Ventilator: An electrically driven sophisticated ventilator (Bear® 5) with multiple alarms.

Ventimask:

Face mask that delivers precise quantities of O_2 (24%, 28%, 35%, 40%) metered via a Venturi tube. *See* Paradoxical oxygen death; Venturi effect.

Ventricular Fibrillation:

Nonrhythmic, irregular, uncoordinated contraction of segments of the ventricular walls. *See* Figure.

613

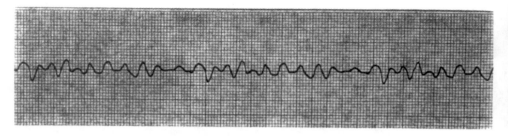

Ventricular Fibrillation.

Ventricular Septal Defect:

Most commonly, a congenital cardiac anomaly in which there is a persistent communica-tion between the right and left ventricle in either the muscular or fibrous portions. Correc-tive surgery performed during infancy or childhood offers the patient an excellent prognosis. Ventricular septal defects may occur as the only abnormality or may be associ-ated with other malformations. Sometimes ventricular septal defects occur because of myocardial infarct damage. *See* Atrial septal defect.

Ventriculography:

Radiographic examination of the ventricles of the brain with the aid of an injection of air or dye as a contrast medium. (A small amount of cerebrospinal fluid is removed and is replaced by the contrast medium.) If air is used as a medium for filling the ventricles, general anesthesia employing N_2O would be hazardous for a variable period following the ventriculography because it diffuses into the air in the ventricles faster than N_2 diffuses out, causing swelling, brain injury, and possibly death. *See* Nitrous oxide.

Ventriculostomy Catheter:

Small cannula that is inserted into the skull (via a burr hole) and is directed through brain tissue into the ventricles of the brain. It is used to measure cerebrospinal fluid pressure, to withdraw fluid for sampling, and to reduce pressure (e.g., in hydrocephalus).

Venturi Effect:

Physical phenomenon describing fluid flow in a tube that has a constriction. Upstream of the constriction, pressure is elevated. Downstream, a partial vacuum and turbulence can be created near the walls of the tube. This effect is useful to dilute O_2 with air in the Ventimask. In addition, the Venturi effect is evident in the mixture of gasoline and air in a carburetor. *See* Ventimask.

Venturi Tube:

See Bernoulli law; Ventimask.

Vernitrol:

Bubble-through, out-of-system, multiagent vaporizer manufactured by Ohio Medical Products. Its mode of operation is similar to that of the copper kettle vaporizer. Passive temperature compensation is accomplished by the mass of metal surrounding the vaporizing chamber. *See* Copper kettle; Vaporizer.

Veronal:

A trade name for barbital. *See* Barbiturate.

Vessel-Rich Group (VRG), Vessel-Poor Group (VPG):

Major subgroups of a circulatory model based on the percentage of cardiac output received. The VRG includes highly perfused organs such as brain, heart, kidney, liver, and endocrine glands. The VRG comprises only 9% of the body mass but receives 75% of the cardiac output. The other divisions of the model are the muscle group, which comprises 50–55% of the body mass but receives only 18% of the cardiac output; the VPG (bones, ligaments, and cartilage), which comprises 22% of the body mass but receives only 1.5% of the cardiac output; and the fat group, which comprises 19% of the body mass but receives approximately 5% of the cardiac output.

Vestibular Folds:

See Laryngospasm.

Vinamar:

See Ethyl vinyl ether.

Vinethene:

See Vinyl ether.

Vinethene Anesthetic Mixture (VAM):

General anesthetic (no longer available in the United States) composed of 75% diethyl ether and 25% vinyl ether. It has a rapid onset of action due to the vinyl ether and low toxicity (compared to vinyl ether alone) due to diethyl ether. *See* Vinyl ether.

Vinyl Ether (Divinyl Ether):

Highly volatile ether preparation that had been used as an induction agent in open-drop applications and for short-term general anesthesia. It can cause liver damage depending on the dose and the duration of administration. Vinyl ether is flammable, explosive, and, because of its high volatility, can cause freezing of tissues if dripped on the face. Vinethene is a trade name for an inhalation anesthetic agent composed of 96% vinyl ether and 4% absolute alcohol. The alcohol renders the product less likely to produce ice formation on the face mask.

Viscera:

Organs within the body cavities (especially in the abdomen). *See* Splanchnic.

Visceral Pain:

Type of pain felt from internal organs and structures not usually exposed to the environment. The pain is usually described as diffuse, and it can be intense and difficult to localize. Internal organs have little painful response to burning, clamping and cutting. Pathologic stimuli, such as stretching, dilatation, inflammation, or ischemia, however, do trigger a pain response. This response is believed not to come from specific pain receptors such as are responsible for pain perception in somatic pain. *See* Somatic pain.

Viscosity:

Resistance to the flow of fluid caused by cohesion of the molecules within the fluid. The unit of absolute viscosity in the CGS system is the poise (P) in which $1 \text{ P} = 1 \text{ dyne sec/cm}^2$. The viscosity of water at 20°C is 1 cP (centipoise). The viscosity of whole blood is 2.7 cP. A viscosimeter is the apparatus used to measure viscosity. *See* Reynolds number.

Vistaril:

See Hydroxyzine.

Visual Analogue Pain Score:

See Visual Analogue Scale.

Visual Analogue Scale:

Type of psychological test used to assess subjective phenomena. Most familiar to anesthesiologists is the Visual Analogue Pain Score. It consists of a 10-cm line, one end of which is labeled by a statement that the symptom or attitude does not exist; at the other end it is labeled with the statement that the symptom or attitude could not possibly be any stronger. The patient is asked to make a vertical line at the point on the horizontal line that represents his or her scoring of the emotion, symptom, or attitude. The vertical line is then measured along the horizontal axis. When used to measure pain, the test appears to be consistent.

Vital Capacity:

Maximal expiratory volume following maximal inspiration. *See* Lung volumes and capacities.

Vital Capacity Rapid Inhalation Induction (VCRII):

Technique for rapid induction with a volatile anesthetic agent. It requires the patient to maximally breath a high concentration of agent at maximum inspiration and expiration until loss of consciousness. Usually unsatisfactory because of coughing and gagging, the technique may become more acceptable with the newer insoluble volatile agents.

Vitalograph:

Device for measuring vital capacity and forced expiratory volume per second (FEV_1). The patient exhales forcefully into a tube connected to the device, producing expansion of a bellows, which drives a pen to mark on a calibrated chart. The chart is moved by an appropriate system during the patient's exhalation so that an x-y plot is obtained.

VMA (4-hydroxy-3-methoxymandelic acid):

Principal metabolite (found in urine) of norepinephrine and epinephrine. Abnormally high levels of VMA may be found in the urine of patients with the adrenal medulla tumor pheochromocytoma, the cells of which can secrete excessive amounts of epinephrine and norepinephrine. *See* Pheochromocytoma.

V_{max}:

See Force-velocity relations.

Vocal Cords:

See Larynx.

Void Space:

Intergranular space in a CO_2 absorber. The void space of fresh soda lime absorbent is approximately 47% of the gross volume. Therefore, a CO_2 canister of 1000 ml has 470 ml of void space. As the fresh soda lime is progressively converted to carbonate by the absorption of CO_2, the void space is filled with water (a byproduct of the hydroxide-carbonate reaction). *See* Carbon dioxide absorption.

Volatile Acid:

Acid in solution, the concentration of which depends on the concentration of one of its components in the gas in contact with the solution. For practical purposes, the only volatile acid of clinical importance is carbonic acid (H_2CO_3), and its concentration depends on the amount of CO_2 in equilibrium with the blood. This parameter, in turn depends on the ability of the lungs to dispose of the CO_2 produced by metabolism.

Volatile Anesthetics:

Any and all of the drugs used to induce general anesthesia that are administered by spontaneous or controlled ventilation. The practice of anesthesia dates from the time diethyl ether anesthetic was administered by spontaneous ventilation to a patient in Boston in 1846. Diethyl ether was the first inhalational anesthetic. Ether acted as the mainstay of the practice of general anesthesia for more than 100 years in the United States. Because of its wide margin of safety, if it were not for its extreme flammability it would still be used today. The standard of inhalational anesthetics as of this writting, is the drug Forane (enflurane) with the agents Sevoflurane and Desflurane on the immediate horizon. *See* Table. *See* Continuous flow anesthesia machine; Pharmacokinetics; Total intravenous anesthesia.

Volt:

Unit of electrical potential difference and electromotive force necessary to produce 1 ampere of current through a resistance of 1 ohm.

Voltage:

Potential energy difference between two points in a circuit expressed in volts.

Volatile Anesthetics: Some volatile anesthetics (agents) and common gases or vapors which have been used in anesthesia.

Substance, formula and molecular mass	Density Gas (sat. vapour) g/L (25°C)	Density Liquid g/ml (RT)	Specific volume* L/g (Vapour) (RTP)	Boiling point °C 1 bar	Vapour pressure kPa (abs) at 20°C	Heat of Vaporisation kJ/g
1 Water H_2O, 18.0	0.60 *Bp*	1.00 *4°C*	1.40	100	2.33	2.45 *RT*
2 Ethyl alcohol $CH_3 \cdot CH_2OH$, 46.1	1.64 *Bp*	0.79	0.53	78.3	5.85	0.92 *RT*
3 Diethyl ether $C_2H_5 \cdot O \cdot C_2H_5$, 74.1	3.03	0.71	0.33	34.6	58.8	0.37 *Bp*
4 Divinyl ether $(CH_2:CH)_2$ O, 70.1	2.86	0.77	0.34	28.3	73.2	0.37 *Bp*
5 Ethyl chloride $CH_3 \cdot CH_2$ Cl, 64.5	2.22 *Bp*	0.92	0.37	12.3	134	0.38 *RT*
6 Chloroform $CHCl_3$, 119	4.89	1.50	0.20	61.2	21.3	0.28 *RT*
7 Trichloroethylene $CHCl: CCl_2$, 131	5.38	1.46	0.18	87	8.6	0.24 *Bp*
8 Halothane $CF_3 \cdot CHClBr$, 197	8.05	1.86	0.11	50.2	32.2	0.15 *Bp*
9 Methoxyflurane $CH_3 \cdot O \cdot CCl_2 \cdot CHF_2$, 165	6.75	1.42	0.15	105	3.06	0.21
10 Enflurane $CHF_2 \cdot O \cdot CF_2CHClF$, 185	7.56	1.52	0.13	56.5	23.0	0.16
11 Isoflurane $CHF_2 \cdot O \cdot CHClCF_3$, 185	7.56	1.50	—	48.5	32	0.15
12 Ethylene $CH_2: CH_2$, 28.1	1.16 *25°C*	0.34	0.851	−104	58.2	0.48 *Bp*
13 Carbon dioxide CO_2, 44	1.85 *RT*	0.77 *RT*	0.543	−78	57	0.15 *RT*
14 Nitrous oxide N_2O, 44	1.85 *RT*	0.79 *RT*	0.543	−88.6	52	0.37 *RT*
15 Cyclopropane $CH_2 \cdot CH_2 \cdot CH_2$, 42.1	1.76 *RT*	0.68 *Bp*	0.571	−33	7.5	0.47 *RT*
16 Oxygen O_2, 32	1.33 *RT*	1.14 *Bp*	0.751	−183	—	0.21 *Bp*
17 Nitrogen N_2, 28	1.17 *15°C*	0.81 *Bp*	0.858	−196	—	0.20 *Bp*
18 Air 29	1.2 *RT*	0.52 *Bp*	0.830	−194	—	0.21
19 Hydrogen H_2, 2.02	0.09 *ST*	0.07 *Bp*	11.9	−253	—	0.45 *Bp*
20 Helium He, 4	0.16 *RT*	0.12 *Bp*	6.01	−269	—	0.025 *Bp*
21 Xenon Xe, 131	5.29 *25°C*	1.75	0.183	−108	—	0.096 *Bp*

Abbreviations: RT = Room temperature: in general, 20°C. BT = Body temperature: circa 37°C. RTP = Value of quantity at 20°C and a pressure of 1 bar. STP = Quantity at 0°C and a pressure of 1 bar. Bp = Boiling point at atmospheric pressure of 1 bar.

*Theoretical specific volume assuming that gases and vapors at 20°C and 1 bar obey ideal gas laws.

Voltage Drop:

Voltage difference measured across the input and output of a device or circuit element. A device offering high resistance to current flow has a high voltage drop measured across its input and output side. *See* Ohm law.

Voltmeter:

Device that measures voltage. Voltmeters can be either analog or digital instruments and can display information via dials, number displays, or cathode-ray tube displays.

Volume Expansion:

Technique of increasing the circulating volume by administering fluid. The fluid can either be a "crystalloid" solution (e.g., lactated Ringer's solution or normal saline) or a "colloid" solution (e.g., albumin solutions). *See* Colloid solutions; Crystalloid solutions; Transfusion therapy.

Volume-Limited Ventilator:

See Ventilator.

Volume of Distribution:

Theoretic volume of body fluid into which a drug would have to be diluted to arrive at a measured plasma concentration.

Volumes Percent:

Concentration of a specific gas in a mixture of gases in terms of its percentage of the total volume.

Vomiting:

See Esophageal reflux.

Von Willebrand Disease:

Familial (autosomal dominant) hemorrhagic disorder that classically has three constituents: prolonged bleeding time, reduced factor VIII levels, and altered in vitro platelet function. *See* Platelet.

VPG:

See Vessel-poor group.

VRG:

See Vessel-rich group.

W

Wagner Needle:

See Epidural needle.

Warburg Apparatus:

Laboratory device that provides controlled conditions necessary for precise manometric determination of O_2 consumption by tissue. The pressure drop caused by O_2 uptake when CO_2 is absorbed is measured in a sealed chamber.

Warranty:

Promise that goods or services meet an agreed upon standard. In medicolegal terms, a prudent health practitioner does not warrant or guarantee results but only that the standard of care for his or her level of skill will not be violated.

Washout:

Continuous process by which a given constituent of a mixture is removed. Lung or alveolar washout of an inhalation anesthetic refers to gradual removal of the anesthetic by continued respiration after administration of the anesthetic ceases. Washout rate of an inhalation anesthetic is determined by the initial concentration in the lungs, respiratory rate and volume, and "resupply" of the lung from anesthetic previously dissolved in the blood. This resupply from the blood continues for a relatively long period, as fat can store a significant amount of halogenated hydrocarbon anesthetics. These gases are gradually released back into the circulation.

Waste Gas System:

See Scavenger system.

Water Balance:

Sum total of water ingressing and egressing from the body during a designated time period (usually calculated for 24 hours). In the normal adult, water leaves the body through a number of routes, including kidneys, respiratory tract, skin, and, to a lesser extent, gastrointestinal tract. The average water loss through the kidneys is approximately 1.5 L/day, whereas the loss through the skin and the respiratory tract is approximately 1 L/day. The loss of water via the respiratory tract increases with an increase in respiratory rate. Water loss through the skin increases (1) in a hot, dry environment, (2) when the patient's body temperature rises, or (3) when the skin is injured, e.g., by burns or large abrasions. Kidney water loss varies with the solute load and with the level of antidiuretic hormone. When the solute load increases (e.g., as in the case of diabetes mellitus when excess glucose is excreted in the urine), the kidney is obligated to excrete sufficient urine to carry the solutes into the bladder. Replacement of water loss is normally accomplished in two major ways: by ingestion (fluid and food) (the average water content of food is between 60% and 97%) or by body metabolism. (The metabolism of approximately 100 calories releases approximately 14 ml of water.) Water balance is best measured by accurate daily weights (1 L water weighs 1 kg or 2.2 lb). *See* Table. *See* Insensate loss; Urinary output.

Water Balance: Routine water exchange in the adult patient.

	Average Daily Volume (ml)	Maximal Daily Volume (ml)
Water gain		
Ingestion		
Fluids	1500–2000	1500/hr
Solids	500–600	1500/hr
Body metabolism	250	1000
Water losses		
Insensible		
Skin	700	1500
Lung	200	
Sensible		
Urine	1000–1200	2000+/hr
Intestinal	200	8000
Sweat	0	2000+/hr

Water Depression Flowmeter:

See Bernoulli law.

Waterston Shunt:

Surgical procedure in which the ascending aorta is anastomosed side-to-side with the right pulmonary artery. This palliative procedure is performed to increase pulmonary blood flow by shunting blood from the systemic circulation to the pulmonary circulation. The Waterston shunt operation is performed on smaller infants than Blalock-Taussig shunt patients. *See* Blalock-Taussig shunt.

Watt:

Standard international unit of power equal to the dissipation of 1 joule of energy per second. It also equals 1 amp × 1 V and is equivalent to 1/746 hp.

Wave:

Curve of an alternating quantity plotted against time. A wave can also be a continuous or transient disturbance that travels through a medium because of the elastic or inertial factors of the medium. When the disturbance is eliminated, the motion ceases.

Waveform:

Shape of a curve generated by plotting the instantaneous values of a variable against time, (e.g., amplitude versus frequency).

Waveguide:

Hollow metal conducting tube used to direct an ultra-high-frequency electromagnetic wave. The wave reflects off the internal surfaces of the guide.

Wavelength:

Distance between two points of corresponding phase on two consecutive wave cycles, represented by the Greek letter lambda (λ). The relation between wavelength, wave velocity, and wave frequency can be stated as λ = velocity/frequency.

Weaning:

Process by which a patient is gradually allowed to resume spontaneous ventilation after controlled mechanical ventilation. Many protocols for weaning exist. The length of the weaning period depends on the chronicity of the respiratory failure, length of time mechanical ventilation is needed, age of the patient, and presence of other body system failures. *See* Table. *See* Intermittent mandatory ventilation; Mandatory minute volume; Mechanical ventilation.

Weaning: Criteria for weaning from controlled ventilation; several schemes exist	
A. Adequate ventilation	
$PaCO_2$	<50 mm Hg
Tidal volume	5 ml/kg
Respiration	<30/mm
Vital capacity	>0.12 ml/kg
Inspire force	>25 ml H_2O
B. Adequate oxygenating	
PaO_2 (100% O_2)	>300 mm Hg
PaO_2 (40% O_2)	>100 mm Hg
PAO_2–PaO_2	<350 torr
Pulmonary shunt	<25%

Wechsler Memory Scale-Revised:

Psychomotor test that measures memory function for adults and adolescents. A series of subtests measure facets of attention and memory, including logical memory, figurative memory, and similar cerebral functions.

Wedensky Effect (Threshold Block):

Fleeting phenomenon seen precisely at the time when the minimum anesthetic concentration (C_m) for local anesthetic is reached at a particular nerve fiber. Repeated stimulation of the nerve distal to the local anesthetic block appears to cause summation of the impulses at the site of the block so that every second or third impulse is conducted through the blocked area. What apparently occurs is that the first and second impulses facilitate passage of the third impulse. The Wedensky effect multiplies the frequency of the train of impulses by one-half, one-third, or one-fourth. As the anesthetic concentration around the nerve rises above C_m, the block becomes increasingly more profound and total block ensues. The Wedensky effect is most frequently seen clinically during recovery from a block because the gradients of local anesthetic concentration change much more slowly. *See* Minimum anesthetic concentration.

Wedensky Inhibition (Wedensky Fade):

Characteristic fade or decrease in muscle movement seen at both slow and fast rates of nerve stimulation during partial paralysis with a nondepolarizing relaxant such as curare. This fade, seen with either repeated single twitches or a "train-of-four," is characteristic of a nondepolarizing agent and may be useful for distinguishing a nondepolarizing from a depolarizing agent. However, this issue is not clear because some "fade" can be observed during the early stages of recovery from total paralysis with a depolarizing agent. This effect disappears, however, as the block continues to decrease. *See* Neuromuscular blockade, assessment of.

Wedge Pressure:

See Pulmonary capillary wedge pressure.

Wells, Horace:

See Morton, William T. G.

Wet and Dry Bulb Hydrometer:

Instrument used to measure relative humidity. It consists of two adjacent thermometers with the bulb of one surrounded by fibers soaking in water. Evaporation of the water from the fibers cools the wet bulb. The rate of evaporation depends on the relative humidity of the surrounding air. The relative humidity is based on the difference in temperature readings of the two thermometers.

Wetting Agent:

Substance that becomes absorbed, thereby decreasing the surface tension of a fluid. It enables solids and liquids to mix and aids in dispersing a liquid on the surface of a solid. *See* Surface tension.

WFSA:

See World Federation of Societies of Anesthesiologists.

Wheatstone Bridge:

Network of precision resistors arranged in a square pattern and used to determine the resistance of an unknown electrical element.

Whiteout:

Endpoint radiologic finding in the completely opaque lung. It can be caused by multiple and diverse conditions (infection, tumor, atelectasis, or pulmonary edema), or severe adult respiratory distress syndrome. *See* Adult respiratory distress syndrome.

White Tube:

Endotracheal tube used for single-lung ventilation. Basically, a variant of the Carlens tube. *See* Carlens tube.

Wide Dynamic Range Neurons:

One of the two groups of cells in the dorsal horn of the spinal cord that functions in the pathway for noxious stimulation from the periphery. They can be activated by either tactile or noxious stimuli. They have large and complex receptive fields. The second group of cells in the dorsal horn are the nociceptive specific (NS) cells, which have limited receptive fields confined to a portion of a dermatome. *See* Gate theory of pain; Nerve fiber, anatomy and physiology of. *See* Wind-up phenomenon.

Windkessel Effect:

Phenomenon of cardiac function, dependent on the elastic recoil of the aorta, in which part of the systolic pulse pressure rise is absorbed by dilatation of this vessel. The systolic pressure rise is never as high as it would be if the vessel walls were rigid; the recoil provides augmentation of diastolic pressure and helps to continue flow along the system.

Wind-Up Phenomenon:

Phenomena seen in dorsal horn wide dynamic range neurons in which repetitive stimulation appears to yield a protracted discharge of these neurons relayed to more central locations. It appears to explain the fact that in some pain states a constant afferent pain input may result in centrally mediated facilitation of the pain state. *See* Wide dynamic range neurons.

Work:

Magnitude of force × the distance moved, measured in joules. One joule equals the work done when a force of 1 newton moves through a distance of 1 m. *See* Horsepower.

Work of Breathing:

Total energy required to ventilate the lungs. It is defined in terms of the O_2 uptake necessary to perform this work. Work is done when expanding the elastic tissues of the lung and chest wall, when displacing the ribs, and when overcoming the resistance to gas flow down the trachea and airways. In various disease states, any or all of these factors may be affected. In normal circumstances, the work of breathing uses 2–5% of the O_2 consumed/minute. With severe respiratory disease, the work increases three- to fivefold.

World Federation of Societies of Anesthesiologists (WFSA):

International anesthesia society initiated in 1955 with a current membership of 85 societies. The WFSA promotes the specialty of anesthesiology by disseminating scientific information and recommending standards for the training of anesthesiologists on a worldwide basis. WFSA members are from major anesthesia societies. World Congress of Anesthesiologists and regional congresses are sponsored by the WFSA.

Wright Respirometer:

Device for measuring the minute volume and vital capacity. It consists of a gas inlet that directs gas flow to strike a small propeller. This propeller spins in the gas stream and is connected to a direct-reading dial by a gear train. The device tends to overread high flow rates and underread low flow rates.

Wrist Block:

Conduction block done at the wrist to block any or all of the ulnar nerve, the medial nerve and the radial nerve, for purposes of anesthesia of the hand.

Wyamine:

See Mephentermine.

X

Xenon-133:

Gamma ray-emitting isotope that is a gas at normal temperature and pressure. It is used to determine regional perfusion in the lung and brain. The xenon is injected intravenously, and its pattern of distribution is determined based on detection of gamma radiation by external scintillation counters. *See* Optical character reader.

Xerography:

Radiographic technique of imaging body tissues (e.g., breast) on selenium-coated metal plates. Xerography is also a copying process in which light passes through the document to be copied and falls on an electrostatically charged plate. This electrostatic charge is dissipated depending on the intensity of the light. A powder with an electric charge is added to the plate. It adheres to the dark areas where the plate has not been discharged. The powder is then transferred to a charged paper where it is heat-fixed. In this manner areas of light and dark can be transferred from one sheet of paper to another.

X-Ray (Roentgen Ray):

Portion of the electromagnetic spectrum of a short wavelength between ultraviolet and gamma rays. X-rays are able to penetrate most substances.

Xylocaine:

Trade name for lidocaine. *See* Local anesthetic.

Y

Yawning:

Involuntary, deep inspiration done with the mouth open and often accompanied by stretching. Yawning is a poorly understood phenomenon, but it has been postulated that it is an automatic reflex operating to reexpand underventilated alveoli after a period of quiet, rhythmic respirations.

Yohimbine:

α-2 antagonist used to treat impotence and orthostatic hypotension. It blocks the action of clonidine and increases the release of norepinephrine.

Yoke Block:

Device that connects a gas source to the yoke of an anesthesia machine by means of a flexible hose. The yoke block takes the place of a small cylinder valve stem. It usually contains holes for the pin-index safety system.

Yoke, Hanger:

Device that supports a gas cylinder and connects it to an anesthesia machine. It allows gas to be piped into the gas delivery system. The hanger yoke usually contains an orifice (which mates up against the gas port of the cylinder valve), a retaining screw, a check-valve assembly, and the pins of the pin-index safety system, which mate into appropriate holes on the cylinder valve.

Y-Piece:

Tube with two inflow ports and one outflow port used to connect the two sides of the anesthesia circle to the endotracheal tube or mask.

Z

Z-79:

Set of standards formulated by the American National Standards Institute (ANSI) to evaluate anesthesia equipment and materials for the purpose of lowering costs and enhancing patient safety. All pieces of equipment that pass inspection are labeled as "meets Z-79 standards or IT" (implant tested).

Zero End-Expiratory Pressure:

Technique of mechanical respiration in which the alveolar pressure is allowed to drop to atmospheric pressure at the end of expiration. *See* Continuous positive airway pressure; Positive end-expiratory pressure.

Zero Order Process (Zero Order Kinetics):

Drug metabolism which occurs when available drug exceeds the capacity of the metabolizing enzymes. The result is the metabolic breakdown of a constant amount of drug per time unit. *See* First order process.

Z Line:

See Actomyosin.

Credits

The illustrations and tables reprinted in this book appear with the permission of the following:

Action Potential (A): Ganong, W.F. 1989. Review of Medical Physiology, 14th ed. Norwalk, CT: Appleton & Lange.

Action Potential (B): Malamed, S.F. 1990. Handbook of Local Anesthesia, 3rd ed., p. 6. St. Louis, MO: Mosby-Year Book, Inc.

Actomyosin: Ganong, W.F. 1983. Review of Medical Physiology, 11th ed. Norwalk, CT: Appleton & Lange.

Acupuncture: Matsumoto, T. 1974. Acupuncture for Physicians. pp. 42–44. Springfield, IL: Charles C. Thomas, Publisher.

Adenosine Triphosphate: Ganong, W.F. 1977. Review of Medical Physiology, 9th ed. Norwalk, CT: Appleton & Lange.

Agent-Specific Filling Device: Dorsch, J.A. and Dorsch, S.E. 1984. Understanding Anesthesia Equipment—Construction, Care, and Complications, 2nd ed., pp. 122–123. Baltimore, MD: Williams & Wilkins Company.

Airway Obstruction (A, B): Standards and Guidelines for Cardiopulmonary Resuscitation and Emergency Cardiac Care. JAMA June 6, 1986, Vol. 225, No. 21, pp. 2841–3044. Chicago, IL: American Medical Association.

Airway Obstruction (C): Finucane, B.T. and Santora, A.H. 1988. Principles of Airway Management, p. 240. Essential of Medical Education Series. Philadelphia, PA: F.A. Davis Company.

Aldrete Score: Reprinted with permission from UMDNJ-Robert Wood Johnson University Hospital, New Brunswick, NJ and Aldrete, JA and Kroulik, D. Nov-Dec 1970. A Postanesthetic Recovery Score, In: Anesthesia and Analgesia—Current Researchers 49 (6):926. Cleveland, OH: International Anesthesia Research Society.

Alpha Stat Management: Reprinted 1990. Editorial Views: Patient CO_2 Managment during Cardiopulmonary Bypass. Anesthesiology 72:4. Philadelphia, PA: J.B. Lippincott Company.

Alveolar End Capillary Difference: West, J.B. 1974. Respiratory Physiology: the essentials, p. 27. Baltimore, MD: Williams & Wilkins Company.

Alveolus: Weibel, E.R. 1970. Morphometric Estimation of Pulmonary Diffusion Capacity. In: J. Appl. Physiol. 11:57. Amsterdam: Elsevier Biomedical Press B.V.

Anesthesia Chart: Courtesy of Mark H. Stein, M.D., Assistant Professor of Anesthesia, University of Medicine and Denistry of New Jersey, Robert Wood Johnson Medical School, New Brunswick, NJ.

Anesthesia Subspecialties: Dripps, R.D., Eckenhoff, J.E., Vandam, L.D. 1988. Introduction to Anesthesia: The Principles of Safe Practice, 7th ed., p. 316. Philadelphia, PA: W.B. Saunders Company.

Anesthesia System, Open: Dorsch, J.A. and Dorsch, S.E. 1975. Understanding Anesthesia Equipment—Construction, Care, and Complications, p. 154. Baltimore, MD: Williams & Wilkins Company.

Arnold-Chiari Deformity: Pryse-Phillips, W. 1978. Essential Neurology, p. 219. New York: Elsevier Science Publishing Company.

Arterialization of Blood: Kinney, J.M. 1960. Arterialization of Blood. Anesthesiology 21:615. Philadelphia, PA: J.B. Lippincott Company.

Arteriole: Ganong, W.F. 1989. Review of Medical Physiology, 14th ed. Norwalk, CT: Appleton & Lange.

Atelectasis: Kent, T.H., Hart, M.N., Shires, T.K. 1987. Introduction to Human Disease, 2nd ed., p. 225. Norwalk, CT: Appleton & Lange.

Automated Anesthesia Record: Courtesy of North American Draeger, Inc., Telford, PA.

Automated Blood Pressure Device: Courtesy of Critikon, a Johnson & Johnson Company, Tampa, FL.

Autonomic Nervous System (table): Daly, B.J. 1980. Intensive Care Nursing. p. 473. Norwalk, CT: Appleton & Lange.

Autonomic Nervous System (figure): Goth, A. 1988. Medical Pharmacology, 12th ed., p. 88. St. Louis, MO: C.V. Mosby Company.

Ayre T-Piece: Dorsch, J.A. and Dorsch, S.E. 1975. Understanding Anesthesia Equipment—Construction, Care, and Complications, 1st ed., pp. 160–163. Baltimore, MD: Williams & Wilkins Company.

Barbituate: Goth, A. 1981. Medical Pharmacology, 10th ed., p. 304. St. Louis, MO: C.V. Mosby Company.

Binary Code: Freedman, A. 1989. The Computer Glossary, 4th ed., p. 61. Point Pleasant, PA: The Computer Language Company, Inc.

Blalock-Hanlon Procedure: Doty, D.B. 1980. Cardiac Surgery, In: Liechty, R.D., Sopor, T.T. Synopsis of Surgery, 4th ed., p. 332. St. Louis, MO: The C.V. Mosby Company.

Blalock-Taussig Shunt: Doty, D.B. 1980. Cardiac Surgery, In: Liechty, R.D. Synopsis of Surgery, 4th ed., p. 332. St. Louis, MO: C.V. Mosby Company.

Blood-Brain Barrier: Seigel, G. 1981. Basic Neurochemistry, 3rd ed., p. 451. Boston, MA: Little, Brown and Company.

Blood Coagulation (table): Ellison, N. 1988. Blood Coagulation and Coagulopathies. In: ASA Annual Refresher Course Lectures, p. 6. Philadelphia, PA: J.B. Lippincott Company.

Blood Coagulation (figure): Barrer, M.J. and Ellison, N. 1977. Platelet Function. In: Anesthesiology 46: 205. Philadelphia, PA: J.B. Lippincott, Company.

Blood Gas Machine: Courtesy of Radiometer America, Inc., Cleveland, OH. The ABL^{TM}-500 is a registered trademark of Radiometer$^®$ A/S.

Blood Type: Greendyke, R.M. 1980. Introduction to Fundamentals of Blood Banking, 3rd ed., pp. 99, 101. New York: Elsevier Science Publishing Company.

Body Fluid (A): Talbot, N.B. Richie, R.H., Crawford, J.D. 1959. Metabolic Homeostasis, p. 5. Cambridge, MA: Harvard University Press. Copyright 1959 by the Commonwealth Fund.

Body Fluid (B): Gamble, J.L. 1954. Chemical Anatomy, Physiology and Pathology of Extracellur Fluid, 6th ed., p. 5. Cambridge, MA: Harvard University Press.

Bourdon Tube Pressure Gauge: Collins, V.J. 1976. Principles of Anesthesiology, 2nd ed., p. 132. Philadelphia, PA: Lea & Febiger, Publisher. (Mushin, W.W., courtesy of Charles C. Thomas, Publisher and Blackwell Scientific Publications, Ltd.)

Boyle Bottle: Courtesy of the Medishield Corporation Limited, Essex, England.

Brachial Plexus Block (A, C): Cousins, M.J. and Bridenbaugh, P.O. 1988. Clinical Anesthesia and Management of Pain, 2nd ed., pp. 399, 401. Philadelphia, PA: J.B. Lippincott Company.

Brachial Plexus Block (B): Labat, G.L. 1928. Regional Anesthesia, 2nd ed. Philadelphia, PA: W.B. Saunders Company.

Bronchoscope, Flexible (A): Courtesy of Olympus Corporation, Lake Success, NY.

Bronchoscope, Flexible (B): Gatell, J.A., et al. 1990. A New Technique for Replacing an Endobronchial Double-Lumen Tube with an Endotrachial Single-Lumen Tube. In: Anesthesiology 73 (2):341. Philadelphia, PA: J.B. Lippincott Company.

Bronchoscope, Rigid (C): Courtesy of Pilling Company, Fort Washington, PA.

Calomel Electrode: Willard, Merritt, and Dean. 1951. Calomel Cell Electrode. New York: Van Nostrand Reinhold.

Capnography: Dripps, R.D., Eckenhoff, J.E., Vandam, L.D. 1988. Introduction to Anesthesia: The Principles of Safe Practice, 7th ed., p. 73. Philadelphia, PA: W.B. Saunders Company.

Carbon Dioxide Absorption Canister: Courtesy of Gibeck-Dryden Corporation, Indianapolis, IN.

Carbon Dioxide Electrode: Courtesy of Professor O. Siggaard-Andersen and Radiometer$^®$ A/S, Copenhagen NV, Denmark.

Cardiac Catherization: Nadas, A.S. 1957. Pediatric Cardiology, 3rd ed., p. 116. Philadelphia, PA: W.B. Saunders Company.

Cardiac Cycle: Guyton, A.C. 1991. Textbook of Medical Physiology, 8th ed., p. 102. Philadelphia, PA: W.B. Saunders Company.

Cardiac Output: Guyton, A.C. 1973. Circulatory Physiology: Cardiac Output and Its Regulation, 2nd ed., p. 9. Philadelphia, PA: W.B. Saunders Company.

Cardiopulmonary Bypass: Dripps, R.D., Eckenhoff, J.E., Vandam, L.D. 1988. Introduction to Anesthesia: The Principles of Safe Practice, 7th ed., Chpt. 25, p. 341. Philadelphia, PA: W.B. Saunders Company.

Cardiopulmonary Resuscitation: Standards and Guidelines for Cardiopulmonary Resuscitation and Emergency Cardiac Care. In: JAMA June 6, 1986, Vol. 225, No. 21, pp. 2918, 2920. Courtesy of the American Red Cross. Copyright 1986, American Medical Association.

Catecholamines: Forsham, P.H. 1986. Basic and Clinical Endocrinology, 2nd ed., Chpt. 11, p. 328. Norwalk, CT: Appleton & Lange.

Caudal Anesthesia: Cousins, M.J. and Bridenbaugh, P.O. 1988. Clinical Anesthesia and Managment of Pain. In: Neural Blockade Pain Management, 2nd ed., p. 373. Philadelphia, PA: J.B. Lippincott Company.

Central Gas System: Reprinted with permission from NFPA 99–90, Health Care Facilities, Copyright 1990, National Fire Protection Association, Quincy, MA 02269. This reprinted material is not the complete and official position of the NFPA, on the referenced subject which is represented only by the standard in its entirety.

Central Nervous System: Chusid, J.G. 1988. Correlative Neuroanatomy and Functional Neurology, 20th ed., p. 81. Norwalk, CT: Appleton & Lange.

Central Venous Pressure: Kaplan, J.A. 1979. Cardiac Anesthesia, p. 79. Orlando, FL: W.B. Saunders Company.

Cerebral Angiography: Courtesy of the Radiology Department, Unversity of Iowa Hospital, Iowa City, IA.

Cerebral Blood Flow (A): Shapiro, H. 1979. Physiologic and Pharmacologic Regulation of Cerebral Blood Flow. 30th Annual Refresher Course Lectures. In: Anesthesiology 5:167. Philadelphia, PA: J.B. Lippincott Company.

Cerebral Blood Flow (B, C): Lassen, N.A. and Tweed, W.A. 1979. Monographs in Anaesthesiology. In: A Basis and Practice of Neuroanaesthesia, Volume 2, pp. 118–119. Amsterdam: Elsevier Biomedical Press B.V.

Cerebrospinal Fluid: Gilman, S., Newman, S.W. et al. 1987. Manter & Gatz's Essentials of Clinical Neuroanatomy and Neurophysiology, 7th ed., p. 219. Philadelphia, PA: F.A. Davis Company.

Chip: Freedman, A. 1989. The Computer Glossary, 4th ed., p. 106. Point Pleasant, PA: The Computer Language Company, Inc.

Circle of Willis: Gilman, S., Newman, S.W. et al. 1987. Manter & Gatz's Essentials of Clinical Neuroanatomy and Neurophysiology, 7th ed., p. 233. Philadelphia, PA: F.A. Davis Company.

Circle System: Dorsch, J.A. and Dorsch, S.E. 1984. Understanding Anesthesia Equipment—Construction, Care, and Complications, 2nd ed., p. 211. Baltimore, MD: Williams & Wilkins Company.

Closing Capacity: Nunn, J.F. 1977. Applied Respiratory Physiology, 2nd ed., p. 118. Surrey, England: Butterworth Heinemann, Subsidiary Reed International.

Colorimetric (A): Courtesy of FENEM Airway Management Sytems, Hollis, NY.

Colorimetric (B): Jones, B.R. and Dorsey, M.J. September, 1989. Equipment, Monitoring, and Engineering Technology III, Disposable FEF^{TM} End-Tidal CO_2 Detector: Minimal CO_2 Requirements. In: Anesthesiology 71 (3A). Philadelphia, PA: J.B. Lippincott Company.

Coma: Shapiro, H.M. 1977. Neurosurgical Intensive Care. In: Anesthesiology, 47:150. Philadelphia, PA: J.B. Lippincott Company.

Computerized Axial Tomography: Courtesy of the Radiology Department, University of Iowa Hospital, Iowa City, IA.

Conducting Airways: West, J.B. 1974. Respiratory Physiology—The Essentials, pp. 5, 7. Baltimore, MD: Williams & Wilkins Company.

Congestive Heart Failure: Kent, T.H., Hart, M.N., Shires, T.K. 1987. Introduction to Human Disease, 2nd ed., p. 141. Norwalk, CT: Appleton & Lange.

Continuous Flow Anesthesia Machine: Courtesy of North American Draeger, Inc., Telford, PA.

Continuous Positive Airway Pressure: Levin, R. 1976. Pediatric Respiratory Intensive Care Handbook, p. 92. New York: Elsevier Science Publishing Company.

Copper Kettle: Dorsch, J.A. and Dorsch, S.E. 1984. Understanding Anesthesia Equipment—Construction, Care, and Complications, 2nd ed., p. 93. Baltimore, MD: Williams & Wilkins Company. Redrawn courtesy of Foregger Medical, former division of Puritan-Bennett Corporation.

Corticosteroid: Modified from Clark, Brader & Johnson: Goth, A. 1988. Medical Pharmacology, 12th ed., p. 554. St. Louis, MO: C.V. Mosby Company.

Cranial Nerves: Krieg, W. 1957. Brain Mechanisms in Diachrome, 2nd ed., p. 59, as modified by Chusid, J.G. 1979. Correlative Neuroanatomy and Functional Neurology, 17th ed. Norwalk, CT: Appleton & Lange.

Cylinder, Gas: Dorsch, J.A. and Dorsch, S.E. 1984. Understanding Anesthesia Equipment—Construction, Care, and Complications, 2nd ed., p. 4. Baltimore, MD: Williams & Wilkins Company.

Defribrillation: Photo courtesy of Physio-Control Corporation, Richmond, VA.

Dehydration: Dell, R.B. (Winters, R.W.) 1973. The Body Fluids in Pediatrics. p. 142. Boston, MA: Little, Brown and Company.

633

Dermatome: Chusid, J.G. 1979. Correlative Neuroanatomy and Functional Neurology, 17th ed. pp. 205–206. Norwalk, CT: Appleton & Lange.

Diffusion Constant: West, J.B. 1974. Respiratory Physiology: The Essentials, p. 24. Baltimore, MD: Williams & Wilkins Company.

Dispersive Electrode: Courtesy of MDT Corporation, Rochester, NY.

Dissociation Constant: Malamed, S.F. 1990. Handbook of Local Anesthesia, 3rd ed., p. 17 from Cohen, S., Burns, R.C. 1987. Pathways of the Pulp, 4th ed. St. Louis, MO: Mosby-Year Book, Inc.

Doppler Effect: Reitan, J.A. and Barash P.G. Noninvasive Monitoring. In: Saidman, L.J. and Smith, N.T. 1984. Monitoring in Anesthesia, 2nd ed. p. 132. Stoneham, MA: Butterworth-Heinemann Publishers.

Double Burst Stimulation: Miller, R.D. 1990. Anesthesia, 3rd ed., Vol. 2, p. 1223. New York: Churchill-Livingstone.

Double-Lumen Tube: Stark, D.C. 1980. Practical Points in Anesthesiology, 2nd ed., p. 297. New York: Elsevier Science Publishing Company, Inc.

Drug Distribution: Price, H.L. 1960. The Uptake of Thiopental by Body Tissues and its Relation to the Duration of Narcosis. In: Clinical Pharmacology and Therapeutics 1:21, p. 21. St. Louis, MO: Mosby-Year Book, Inc.

Einthoven Triangle: Kuida, H. 1979. Fundamental Principles of Circulatory Physiology, p. 45. New York: Elsevier Science Publishing Company.

Electomagnetic Spectrum: Pitt, V. 1977. The Penguin Dictionary of Physics, p. 424. Aylesbury, England: Lawrence Urdang Associates, Ltd.

EMLA: Covino, B.G and Vassallo, H.G. 1976. Local Anesthetics, p. 93. Orlando, FL: W.B. Saunders Company.

Endotracheal Tube (A–G): From Airway Management Products brochure. January, 1991. Courtesy of Mallinckrodt Medical, Inc., Mallinckrodt Anesthesiology Division. Inc., St. Louis, MO.

Endotracheal Tube (table): Dripps, R.D., Eckenhoff, J.E., Vandam, L.D. 1988. Introduction to Anesthesia: The Principles of Safe Practice, 7th ed., p. 190. Philadelphia, PA: W.B. Saunders Company.

Endotrol Tracheal Tube: From Airway Management Products brochure. January, 1991. Courtesy of Mallinckrodt Medical, Inc., Mallinckrodt Anesthesiology Division. Inc., St. Louis, MO.

Epidural Needle: Cousins, M.J. and Bromage, P.R. 1988. Neural Blockade in Clinical Anesthesia and Management of Pain, 2nd ed., Chpt. 8, p. 322. Philadelphia, PA: J. B. Lippincott Company.

Equivalent System of Measurement: From Fluid and Electrolytes. 1970, p. 12. Courtesy of Abbott Laboratories, Abbott Park, IL.

Evoked Potential: From Evoked Potentials in Clinical Practice brochure. Courtesy of Biomedical Division, Nicolet Instrument Corporation, Madison, WI.

Extracorporeal Membrane Oxygenation: Truog, R.D., et al. 1990. Case Reports: Repair of Congenital Diaphragmatic Hernia during Extracorporeal Membrane Oxygenation. In: Anesthesiology 72 (4):751. Philadelphia, PA: J.B. Lippincott Company.

Face Mask: Courtesy of Ambu, Inc., Linthicum, MD.

Fail-Safe Device: Dripps, R.D., Eckenhoff, J.E., Vandam, L.D. 1988. Introduction to Anesthesia: The Principles of Safe Practice, 7th ed., p. 55. Philadelphia, PA: W.B. Saunders Company.

Fetal Circulation: Brown, T.C.K. and Fisk, G.C. 1979. Anaesthesia for Children, Including Aspects for Intensive Care, p. 8. Oxford, England: Blackwell Scientific Publications, Ltd.

Fetal Heart Rate (FHR) Terminology (A): Adapted from Klein, S.L. and Landers, D.F. 1990. Anesthesiology: Problems in Primary Care, 1st ed., Chpt. 24, p. 254. Los Angeles, CA: Practice Management Information Corporation.

Fetal Heart Rate (FHR) Terminology (B, C): Shnider S.M. and Levenson, G. 1987. Diagnosis and Management of Fetal Asphyxia. In: Anesthesia for Obstetrics, 2nd ed., pp. 480–481. Baltimore, MD: Williams & Wilkins Company.

Fiberoptics: Courtesy of Machida Incorporated, Orangeburg, NY.

Flow Control Valve: Dorsch, J.A. and Dorsch, S.E. 1984. Understanding Anesthesia Equipment—Construction, Care, and Complications, 2nd ed., p. 53. Baltimore, MD: Williams & Wilkins Company.

Flowmeter: Courtesy of North American Draeger, Inc., Telford, PA.

Force Velocity Relations: Shimosato, S. 1973. Effect of Halothane on Altered Contractility of Isolated Heart Muscle Obtained from Cats. Nature 45:4. Copyright 1973. New York: Macmillan Magazines Ltd.

Fourier Analysis: Stockard, J.J. 1975. The Neurophysiology of Anaesthesia. In: A Basis and Practice of Neuroanesthesia, Vol. 2, p. 19. Amsterdam: Elsevier Biomedical Press, B.V.

Gate Theory of Pain: Melzack, R. 1965. Pain Mechanisms: A New Theory. In: Science 150:971–979. Washington, DC.: American Association for the Advancement of Science.

Glasgow Coma Scale: Siegel, J.H. and Stene, J.K. 1987. Anesthesia for Critically Ill Trauma Patient. In: Trauma Emergency Surgery & Critical Care as adapted from Lancet 1:879, p. 846. New York: Churchill-Livingstone.

Hemostasis: Ellison, N. Blood Coagulation and Coagulopathies. 1988. In: ASA Annual Refresher Course Lectures, pp. 6–7 (1988 Annual Meeting, San Francisco, CA.) Philadelphia, PA: J.B. Lippincott Company.

Histamine: Goth, A. 1988. Medical Pharmacology, 12th ed., p. 177. St. Louis, MO: C.V. Mosby Company.

Histogram: Klein, S.L. and Klein, V.L. September, 1979. In: Anesthesiology 51 (3):S3. Philadelphia, PA: J.B. Lippincott Company.

Human Immune Response: Stevenson, G.W., et al. 1990. The Effect of Anesthetic Agents on the Human Immune Response. In: Anesthesiology 72 (3):543–554. Philadelphia, PA: J.B. Lippincott Company.

Hydrocephalus: Courtesy of the Radiology Department, University of Iowa Hospital, Iowa City, IA.

Hypoxia: Siesjo, B.K., et al. 1974. Brain Dysfunction in Metabolic Disorder, p. 72. New York: Raven Press, Ltd.

Hypoxic Pulmonary Vasoconstriction: Marshall, B.E. 1990. ACTA Anaesthesiology Scandanavian Vol. 34, Supplementum 94:38. Copenhagen, Denmark: Munksgaard International Publishers, Ltd.

Hypoxic Ventilatory Response: Sahn, S.A., et al. Variability of Ventilatory Responses to Hypoxia and Hypercapnia. In: Journal of Applied of Physiology: Respiratory, Environment and Exercise Physiology 43 (6):1020. Bethesda, MD: The American Physiological Society.

Hysteresis, Lung: Adapted from Scarpelli, E.M. 1988. Surfactants and the Lining of the Lung, 1st ed., p. 58. Baltimore, MD: The Johns Hopkins University Press.

Intercostal Block: Lichtiger, M. and Moya, F. 1978. Introduction to the Practice of Anesthesia, 2nd ed., p. 200. New York: J.B. Lippincott, Company.

Intracranial Compliance: Shapiro, H.M., Drummond, J.C. 1990. Neurosurgical Anesthesia and Intracranial Hypertension. In: Miller, R.D. Anesthesia Vol. II, 3rd ed., p. 1751. New York: Churchill-Livingstone.

Intracranial Hypertension: Shapiro, H. 1979. Physiologic and Pharmacologic Regulation of Cerebral Blood Flow. In: ASA Annual Refresher Course Lectures 5, p. 167. Philadelphia, PA: J.B. Lippincott Company.

Intracranial Pressure Measurement: Shapiro, H.M., Drummond, J.C. 1990. Neurosurgical Anesthesia and Intracranial Hypertension. In: Miller, R.D. Anesthesia Vol. II, 3rd ed., p. 1737. New York: Churchill-Livingstone.

Intravenous Solution (A): Klein, S.L. and Landers, D.F. 1990. Anesthesiology: Problems in Primry Care, 1st ed., p. 63. Los Angeles, CA: Practice Management Information Corporation.

Intravenous Solution (B): Klein, S.L. and Landers, D.F. 1990. Anesthesiology: Problems in Primary Care, 1st ed., p. 340. Los Angeles, LA: Practice Management Information Corporation.

Jackson-Rees Apparatus: Levin, R. 1980. Pediatric Anesthesia Handbook, 2nd ed., p. 49. New York: Elesevier Science Publishing Company.

Jugular Vein: Otto, C.W. 1990. Central Venous Pressure Monitoring. In: Monitoring in Anesthesia and Critical Care Medicine, 2nd ed., pp. 193, 196–197. New York: Churchill Livingstone.

Kidney: Daly, B.J. 1980. Intensive Care Nursing, p. 258. Norwalk, CT: Appleton & Lange.

Labor: Shnider, S.M and Levinson, G. 1987. Obstetric Physiology and Pharmacology, 2nd ed., p. 42. Baltimore, MD: Williams & Wilkins. Reprinted from Friedman, E.A. 1955. Primigravid Labor. A Graphicostatistic Analysis. Obstet Gynecol: Vol 6, No. 6, p. 569. New York: Elsevier Science Publishing Company.

Laminar Flow: Kuida, H. 1979. Fundamental Principles of Circulatory Physiology, p. 20. New York: Elsevier Science Publishing Company.

Laryngeal Mask Airway: Grebenik, C.R, Ferguson, C., White, A. March, 1990. A New Airway in Pediatric Radiotherapy. In: Anesthesiology 72 (3):475. Philadelphia, PA: J.B. Lippincott, Company.

Laryngoscope Blades: Stone, D.J., Gal, T.J. 1990. Airway Management. In: Miller, R.D. Anesthesia, Vol. 2, p. 1277. New York: Churchill-Livingstone.

Larynx (A): Romanes, J. 1972. The Respiratory System. In: Cunningham's Anatomy, 11th ed., p. 482. Oxford, England: Oxford University Press.

Larynx (B, C): Hollinshead, W.H. 1982. The Head and Neck. In: Anatomy for Surgeons, 3rd ed., Vol. I, pp. 414–415. Philadelphia, PA: J.B. Lippincott Company.

Larynx (D, E): Ellis, H.C., Feldman, S. 1988. The Respiratory Pathway Larynx. In: Anatomy for Anaesthetists. 5th ed., pp. 32, 43. Oxford, England: Blackwell Scientific Publications Ltd.

Liquid Crystal: Introduction to LCD Technology brochure, p. 7. Courtesy of Standish Industries, Lake Mills, WI.

Local Anesthesia (A): Adapted from Klein, S.L. and Landers, D.F 1990. Anesthesiology: Problems in Primary Care, 1st ed, p. 125. Los Angeles, CA: Practice Management Information Corporation.

Local Anesthesia (B): Butterworth, J.F. and Strichartz, G.R. April, 1990. Molecular Mechanisms of Local Anesthetics: A Review. In: Anesthesiology 72 (4):729. Philadelphia, PA: J.B. Lippincott Company.

Lumbar Puncture: Bridenbaugh, P.O. and Greene, N.M. 1988. Neural Blockade, 2nd ed., Chpt. 7, p. 241. Philadelphia, PA: J.B. Lippincott Company.

Lung Volume and Capacities: Comroe, J.H., et al. 1962. The Lung: Clinical Physiology and Pulmonary Function Tests, 2nd ed., p. 8. Chicago: Mosby-Year Book, Inc.

Mandible: Klein, S.L. July, 1980. A Dental Primer for Anesthesiologists. In: Anesthesiology Review VII, No. 7, p. 28. Lawrenceville, NJ: Core Publishing.

Mass Spectrometer: Courtesy of Marquette Gas Analysis Corporation, St. Louis, MO.

Morphine: Thorpe, A.H. 1984. Narcotic Intravenous Anesthetics. In: Anesthesia & Analgesia 63 (1):285. New York: Elsevier Science Publishing Company.

Myelin Sheath: Malamed, Stanley, F. 1990. Handbook of Local Anesthesia, 1st ed., p. 5. St. Louis, MO: Mosby-Year Book, Inc.

Narcotics: Jaffe, J.H. and Martin, W.R. 1985. Opioid Analgesics and Antagonists. In: Goodman and Gilman's The Pharmacological Basis of Therapeutics, 7th ed., p. 505. New York: Macmillan Publishing Company.

637

Nerve Fiber: Barash P.G., Cullen B.F., Stoelting R.K. 1989. Clinical Anesthesia, p. 374. Philadelphia, PA: J.B. Lippincott Company.

Neuromuscular Blockade: Gissen A.J. and Katz, R.L. May, 1969. Twitch Tetanus and Posttetanic Potentiation as Indices of Nerve Muscle Block in Man. In: Anesthesiology 30 (5):486. Philadelphia, PA: J.B. Lippincott Company.

Neuromuscular Junction: Sokoll, M.D. and Gergis, S.D. 1977. Neuromuscular Transmission: anatomy, physiology, and pharmacology. In: Refresher Courses in Anesthesiology 5:180.

Neurotransmitter: Eckert R., Randall D., Augustine G. 1988. Animal Physiology: Mechanisms and Adaptions, 3rd ed., p. 170. New York: W.H. Freeman & Company.

Nitrous Oxide: Muskins, W.W. and Jones, P.L. 1987. Compressed Gases and the Gas Laws. In: Physics for the Anaesthetist, 4th ed., Chpt. 8, p. 178. Oxford, England: Blackwell Scientific Publishers Ltd.

Nociceptor: Shrinivasa N.R., Meyer R.A. and Capbell, J.N. April, 1988. Peripheral Mechanisms of Somatic Pain. In: Anesthesiology 68 (4):572. Philadelphia, PA: J.B. Lippincott Company.

Nomogram: Radford, E.P. 1954. Proper Ventilation during Artificial Respiration. In: New England Journal of Medicine 251:877. Waltham, MA.

Opiate: Bailey P.L., Stanley T.H. 1990. Narcotic Intravenous Anesthetics. In: Miller, R.D. Anesthesia, Vol. 1, 3rd ed., p. 284. New York: Churchill-Livingstone.

Opioid Receptor: Bailey P.L., Stanley T.H. 1990. Narcotic Intravenous Anesthetics. In: Miller, R.D. Anesthesia, Vol. 1, 3rd ed., p. 284. New York: Churchill-Livingstone.

Oscillotonometer: From Instruction Pamphlet of Oscillotonometer[R.] Courtesy of Propper Manufacturing Company, Inc. Long Island City, NY.

Oxidative Phosphorylation: Guyton, A.C. 1976. Textbook of Medical Physiology, 5th ed., p. 911. Philadelphia, PA: W.B. Saunders Company.

Oxygen Analyzer: Lauer, J.M. Gas Phase Oxygen Analysis, pp. 5, 25, 29. Courtesy of Teledyne Analytical Instruments, City of Industry, CA.

Oxygen Electrode: From ABL2 Users' Handbook. Courtesy of Radiometer® A/S, Copenhagen, Denmark.

Pacemaker (table 1): Gevirtz, C. June, 1991. Preanesthetic Assessment, Lesson 77. In: Anesthesiology News, p. 33. West Bedding, CT: McMahon Publishing Company.

Pacemaker (table 2): Roizen, M.F. 1990. Anesthetic Implications of Concurrent Diseases. In: Miller, R.D. Anesthesia, 3rd ed., p. 838. New York: Churchill-Livingstone.

Pacemaker (figure A, B): Edmunds, Jr., L.H., Norwood W.I., and Low D.W. 1990. Atlas of Cardiothoracic Surgery, 1st ed., 1990, pp. 15, 19. Philadelphia, PA: Lea & Febiger, Publisher.

Patent Ductus Arteriosus: Liechty, R.D. 1976. Synopsis of Surgery, 3rd ed., p. 551. St. Louis, MO: C.V. Mosby Company.

Patient Controlled Analgesia: Klein, S.L. and Landers, D.F. 1990. Anesthesiology: Problems in Primary Care, 1st ed., p. 316. Los Angeles: Practice Management Information Corporation.

Patient Positioning (table): Poland, J.L., Hobart, D.J., Payton, O.D. 1981. The Musculoskeletal System. In: Medical Outline Series, 2nd ed., p. 83. New York: Elsevier Science Publishing Company.

Patient Positioning (figure A, B): Stark, D.C. 1980. Practical Points in Anesthesiology, 2nd ed., pp. 37–38. New York: Elsevier Science Publishing Company.

Periodic Table: Abrash H.I. and Hardcastle, K.I. 1981. Chemistry. New York: Macmillan Publishing Company.

Pharmacokinetics: Yasuda, N. et al. October, 1990: Reprinted with permission of the International Anesthesia Research Society from "Pharmacokinetics of Desflurane, Seroflurane, Isoflurane and Halothane in Pigs." In: Anesthesia and Analgesia 71 (4):345. New York: Elsevier Science Publishing Company, Inc.

Pharyngolaryngoscope: Diaz J.H., Guarisco J.L., LeJeune F.E. August, 1990. A Modified Tubular Pharyngolaryngoscope for Difficult Pediatric Laryngoscopy. In: Anesthesiology 73: (2):357. Philadelphia, PA: J.B. Lippincott Company.

pH Electrode: From ABL2 Users' Handbook. Courtesy of Radiometer® A/S, Copenhagen, Denmark.

Pneumothorax: Tarhan, S. and Moffitt, E.A. August, 1973. Principles of Thoracid Anesthesia. In: The Surgical Clinics of North America 53 (4):819. Philadelphia, PA: W.B. Saunders Company.

Prostaglandin: Greenspan, F.S. and Forsham, P.H. 1986. Basic and Clinical Endocrinology, 2nd ed., Chpt. 2, p. 22. Norwalk, CT: Appleton-Century Crofts.

Prosthetic Heart Valves: Doty, D.B., Liechty, R.D. and Soper, R.T. 1980. Cardiac Surgery. In: Synopsis of Surgery, 4th ed., p. 564. St. Louis, MO: C.V. Mosby Company.

Pulmonary Artery Catheter: From A Guide to Hemodynamics Monitoring Using the Swan-Ganz Catheter, Application Note 762. Courtesy of Hewlett-Packard Company, Andover, MA and Edwards Laboratories, Division of American Hospital Supply Corporation.

Pulmonary Perfusion, Zones of: West, J.B. 1990. Respiratory Physiology—The Essentials, 4th ed., p. 41. Baltimore, MD: Williams & Wilkins Company. Reprinted with permission from West, J.B., et al. 1964. Distribution of Blood Flow in Isolated Lung; Relation to Vascular and Alveolar Pressures. In: J. Appl. Physiol. 19:723.

Pulmonary Physiology Symbols: Comroe Jr., J.H. 1962. The Lung: Clinical Physiology and Pulmonary Function Tests, 2nd ed., pp. 330–331. Chicago, IL: Mosby-Year Book, Inc. As modified from: Standardization of Definitions and Symbols in Respiratory Physiology. Federation Proceedings 9:603, 1950.

Pumping Effect, Pressure Effect: Dorsch, J.A. and Dorsch, S.E. 1984. Understanding Anesthesia Equipment—Construction, Care, and Complications, 2nd ed., p. 89. Baltimore, MD: Williams & Wilkins Company. As modified from Hill, D.W. 1968. British Journal of Anaesthesia 40:656.

Receptor/Receptor Sites (table): Modified from Ghoneim, M.N. and Mewaldt, S.P. 1990. Benzodiazepines and Human Memory: A Review. In: Anesthesiology 72 (5):927. Philadelphia, PA: J.B. Lippincott Company.

Receptor/Receptor Sites (figure A, B): Greenspan, F.S. and Forsham, P.H. 1986. Basic and Clinical Endocrinology, 2nd ed., p. 333. Norwalk, CT: Appleton-Century Crofts.

Rendell-Baker Soucek Mask: Courtesy of Ohmeda, A Division of BOC Health Care, Inc., Madison, WI.

Respiratory Centers: Barash, P.G., Cullen, B.F., Stoelting, A.K. 1989. Clinical Anesthesia, 1st ed., Chpt. 32, p. 884. Philadelphia, PA: J.B. Lippincott Company.

Retrobulbar Block: Cousins, J.J. and Bridenbaugh, P.O. 1980. Neural Blockade in Clinical Anesthesia and Management of Pain, 1st ed., Chpt. 17, p. 458. Philadelphia, PA: J.B. Lippincott Company.

Reye Syndrome: Lovejoy, F.H., et al. 1974. Clinical Staging in Reye Syndrome. In: Am. Journal of Diseases of Children, Vol. 128:36. Chicago, IL: American Medical Association. As tabulated by Levin, R.M. 1976. Pediatric Respiratory Intensive Care Handbook.

Sanders Injector: Courtesy of Pilling Company, Fort Washington, PA.

Scavenger System: From the Narkomed 4 Operators Manual, Copyright 1991. Courtesy of North American Draeger, Telford, PA.

Shift Register: Bruner, J.M.R. and Wright, J. 1978. Handbook of Blood Pressure Monitoring, p. 109. Chicago, IL: Mosby-Year Book, Inc.

Shunt: West, J.B. et al. 1974. Respiratory Physiology—The Essentials, p. 56. Baltimore, MD: Williams & Wilkins Company.

Siggard-Andersen Alignment Nomogram: Courtesy of Radiometer® A/S, Copenhagen, Denmark.

Signal Averaging: Cooper, R. 1980. EEG Technology, 3rd ed., p. 193. London: Butterworth-Heinemann.

Single Breath Test: Buist, A.S. August, 1975. Current Concepts—New Tests to Assess Lung Function. In: New England Journal of Medicine 293 (9):438. Waltham, MA.

Spinal Needle: Lund, P.C. 1966. Peridural Analgesia and Anesthesia, p. 147. Springfield, IL: Charles C. Thomas, Publisher.

Spinal Needle: Bridenbaugh, P.O. and Greene, N.M. 1988. Neural Blockade in Clinical Anesthesia and Management of Pain, 2nd ed., Chpt. 7, p. 238. Philadelphia, PA: J.B. Lippincott Company.

Stages and Planes of Anesthesia: Reproduced with permission from Gillespie, N.A. 1943. The Signs of Anaesthesia. Anesthesia and Analgesia 22:275. New York: Elsevier Science Publishing Company.

Swan-Ganz Catheter: From Guide to Hemodynamic Monitoring Using the Swan-Ganz Catheter, Application Note 702., pp. 5,9,19. Courtesy of Hewlett Packard Company, Andover, MA and Edwards Laboratories, Division of American Hospital Supply Corporation.

Temperature Blanket: Courtesy of Thermal Products, Baxter-Pharmaseals, Valencia, CA.

Thoracic Bioimpedance: From Technical Specifications CDDP System. Courtesy of BoMed® Medical Manufacturing, Ltd., Irvine, CA.

To-And-Fro Carbon Dioxide Absorption: Eger, E.I. 1974. Anesthetic Systems: Construction and Function. In: Anesthetic Uptake and Action, Chpt. 13, p. 213. Baltimore, MD: Williams & Wilkins Company.

Tooth: Klein, S.L. July, 1980. A Dental Primer for Anesthesiologists. Anesthesiology Review VII, No. 7, p. 27. Lawrenceville, NJ: Core Publishing.

Tracheoesophageal Fistula: Levin, R. 1980. Pediatric Anesthesia Handbook, 2nd ed., p. 139. New York: Elsevier Science Publishing Company.

Train of Four: Ali H.H., Utting J.E., Gray C. 1970. Stimulus Frequency in the Detection of Neuromuscular Block in Humans. British Journal of Anaesthesia 42:970. London: Professional and Scientific Publishers.

Transducer: From MMI Gaeltec's Cardiovascular Series. Courtesy of Medical Measurements Incorporated, Hackensack, NJ.

Vapor Pressure: Mushin, W.W., Jones, P.L. 1987. Physics for the Anaesthetist, 4nd ed., Chpt. 5, p. 114. Oxford, England: Blackwell Scientific Publications, Ltd.

Ventilator: From The Bear® 5 Ventilator brochure. Courtesy of Bear Medical Systems, Riverside, CA.

Ventricular Fibrillation: Adapted from Klein, S.L., Landers, D.F. 1990. Anesthesiology: Problems in Primary Care, 1st ed., Chpt. 29, p. 301, Los Angeles, CA: Practice Management Information Corporation.

Volatile Anesthetics: Mushin, W.W. and Jones, P.L. 1987. Physics for the Anaesthetist, 4th ed., pp. 597–598. Oxford, England: Blackwell Scientific Publications, Ltd. Adapted from Steward, A., et al. 1973. Brit. J. Anaesth. 45:282–293.

Water Balance: Borrow, M. 1977. Fundamentals of Hemostasis, 2nd ed., p. 10. New York: Elsevier Science Publishing Company.